Perspectives on Stress and Wellness Management in Times of Crisis

Rohit Bansal
Vaish College of Engineering, India

A volume in the Advances in Psychology, Mental Health, and Behavioral Studies (APMHBS) Book Series

IGI Global
PUBLISHER of TIMELY KNOWLEDGE

Published in the United States of America by
IGI Global
Information Science Reference (an imprint of IGI Global)
701 E. Chocolate Avenue
Hershey PA, USA 17033
Tel: 717-533-8845
Fax: 717-533-8661
E-mail: cust@igi-global.com
Web site: http://www.igi-global.com

Library of Congress Cataloging-in-Publication Data

Names: Bansal, Rohit, 1982- editor.
Title: Perspectives on stress and wellness management in times of crisis / edited by Rohit Bansal.
Description: Hershey, PA : Medical Information Science Reference, [2023] | Includes bibliographical references and index. | Summary: "Perspectives on Stress and Wellness Management in Times of Crisis presents the most recent innovations, trends, concerns, practical challenges encountered, and solutions adopted in the fields of stress and wellness management. It provides emerging research on stress and wellness management in times of crisis, innovative stress management strategies, and the role and impact of stress management in emotional mental well being and work performance. Covering topics such as cyber incivility, leadership persistence, and work-life balance, this premier reference source is an excellent resource for psychologists, practitioners, industry researchers, business leaders and managers, human resource managers, counselors, students and educators of higher education, librarians, researchers, and academicians"-- Provided by publisher.
Identifiers: LCCN 2023001113 (print) | LCCN 2023001114 (ebook) | ISBN 9781668485651 (hardcover) | ISBN 9781668485668 (ebook)
Subjects: MESH: Stress, Psychological--prevention & control | Stress, Psychological--complications | Health Promotion--methods | Healthy Lifestyle | Psychological Well-Being
Classification: LCC RC49 (print) | LCC RC49 (ebook) | NLM WM 172.4 | DDC 616.08--dc23/eng/20230306
LC record available at https://lccn.loc.gov/2023001113
LC ebook record available at https://lccn.loc.gov/2023001114

This book is published in the IGI Global book series Advances in Psychology, Mental Health, and Behavioral Studies (APMHBS) (ISSN: 2475-6660; eISSN: 2475-6679)

British Cataloguing in Publication Data
A Cataloguing in Publication record for this book is available from the British Library.

For electronic access to this publication, please contact: eresources@igi-global.com.

Advances in Psychology, Mental Health, and Behavioral Studies (APMHBS) Book Series

Harish C. Chandan
Argosy University, USA
Bryan Christiansen
Southern New Hampshire University, USA

ISSN:2475-6660
EISSN:2475-6679

Mission

The complexity of the human mind has puzzled researchers and physicians for centuries. While widely studied, the brain still remains largely misunderstood.

The **Advances in Psychology, Mental Health, and Behavioral Studies (APMHBS)** book series presents comprehensive research publications focusing on topics relating to the human psyche, cognition, psychiatric care, mental and developmental disorders, as well as human behavior and interaction. Featuring diverse and innovative research, publications within APMHBS are ideally designed for use by mental health professionals, academicians, researchers, and upper-level students.

Coverage

- Personality Disorders
- Psychiatry
- Counseling & Therapy
- Addiction
- Emotional Health
- Socialization
- Anxiety
- Cognition
- Treatment & Care
- Trauma & Stress

IGI Global is currently accepting manuscripts for publication within this series. To submit a proposal for a volume in this series, please contact our Acquisition Editors at Acquisitions@igi-global.com or visit: http://www.igi-global.com/publish/.

The Advances in Psychology, Mental Health, and Behavioral Studies (APMHBS) Book Series (ISSN 2475-6660) is published by IGI Global, 701 E. Chocolate Avenue, Hershey, PA 17033-1240, USA, www.igi-global.com. This series is composed of titles available for purchase individually; each title is edited to be contextually exclusive from any other title within the series. For pricing and ordering information please visit http://www.igi-global.com/book-series/advances-psychology-mental-health-behavioral/110200. Postmaster: Send all address changes to above address.

Titles in this Series

For a list of additional titles in this series, please visit: www.igi-global.com/book-series/advances-psychology-mental-health-behavioral/110200

Enhancing Social Justice, Service Delivery, and Advocacy Through Multicultural Counseling Competencies
Keith B. Wilson (University of Kentucky, USA) Si-Yi Chao (University of Kentucky, USA) and Travis S. Andrews (University of Kentucky, USA)
Information Science Reference • © 2023 • 315pp • H/C (ISBN: 9781668461556) • US $215.00

Perspectives and Considerations on Navigating the Mental Healthcare System
Susan Van Alstyne (Centenary University, USA)
Medical Information Science Reference • © 2023 • 300pp • H/C (ISBN: 9781668450499) • US $305.00

Managing Pandemic Isolation With Literature as Therapy
Antonio Cortijo Ocaña (University of California, Santa Barbara, USA) Vicent Martines (ISIC-IVITRA, University of Alicante, Spain) and Veronica Orazi (Università degli Studi di Torino, Italy)
Information Science Reference • © 2023 • 281pp • H/C (ISBN: 9781668447352) • US $240.00

Latinx Mental Health From Surviving to Thriving
Edward A. Delgado-Romero (University of Georgia, USA)
Medical Information Science Reference • © 2023 • 353pp • H/C (ISBN: 9781668449011) • US $305.00

Handbook of Research on Play Specialism Strategies to Prevent Pediatric Hospitalization Trauma
Giulia Perasso (University of Milano-Bicocca, Italy) and Yagmur Ozturk (University of Trento, Italy)
Medical Information Science Reference • © 2023 • 416pp • H/C (ISBN: 9781668450680) • US $425.00

The Role of Child Life Specialists in Community Settings
Genevieve Lowry (Bank Street College of Education, USA) Lindsey Murphy (Missouri State University, USA) and Cara Smith (Missouri State University, USA)
Information Science Reference • © 2023 • 472pp • H/C (ISBN: 9781668450970) • US $245.00

Counseling Strategies for Children and Families Impacted by Incarceration
Kenya Johns (Geneva College, USA)
Medical Information Science Reference • © 2022 • 365pp • H/C (ISBN: 9781799892090) • US $295.00

The Reproduction and Maintenance of Inequalities in Interpersonal Relationships
Tyler Ross Flockhart (Viterbo University, USA) Abigail Reiter (University of North Carolina at Pembroke, USA) and Matthew R. Hassett (University of North Carolina at Pembroke, USA)
Information Science Reference • © 2022 • 332pp • H/C (ISBN: 9781668441282) • US $215.00

IGI Global
PUBLISHER of TIMELY KNOWLEDGE

701 East Chocolate Avenue, Hershey, PA 17033, USA
Tel: 717-533-8845 x100 • Fax: 717-533-8661
E-Mail: cust@igi-global.com • www.igi-global.com

Table of Contents

Detailed Table of Contents

The chapter seeks to provide new and appropriate insights and answers for academic leaders that help them to experience better conditions in times of crisis and unforeseen situations and provide a suitable response to circumstances. Looking to the future, the emergence of an "allostatic leader" with an adaptive capacity to learn and evolve in a crisis, as well as to deal with future stresses and crises, is considered very important. Therefore, first, the concept of allostatic leadership was discussed. Next, the difference between allostatic leadership and adaptive leadership was explained. Then the development of allostatic leaders in crisis and stressful situations has been discussed. Finally, the best allostatic leadership practices are considered for academic leaders to go through crises and unexpected situations. Although these strategies are described in an academic context and in order to face the crises of the new COVID-19 pandemic, they can be equally applied by professionals in other industries facing their own crises.

Employee stress has been explored extensively. However, there remain a dearth of scholarship on how leadership, specifically authentic leadership, helps to reduce employee stress levels in crises, such as the COVID-19 pandemic, in emerging economies, and to ensure employee wellness and performance using the social exchange theory. Using exploratory qualitative design and thematic analysis, data from 32 interviews with public sector employees in Ghana were analysed. Findings demonstrate that authentic leaders exhibit such characteristics as honesty, accountability, self-regulation, relational transparency, objective analysis of information, and valuing followers' contributions to arrive at decisions. These characteristics relate positively to employee job performance, wellness, and stress management.

Businesses have had financial and economic crises in the past, but none have compared to the COVID-19 pandemic, according to industry leaders. There is always a need for consistency, safety, and compassion in situations like COVID-19. Emotional intelligence has long been considered a crucial leadership skill. Now more than ever it is essential to navigate this crisis and establish a new normal. Consider emotional health as water in a glass that, in normal circumstances, might slowly evaporate and that leaders occasionally need to top off. Change, uncertainty, tension, and anxiety, however, behave like holes in the glass during a crisis, allowing water to pour out all over the place. There needs to be more top-down additions made in order to maintain emotional stability. Leadership plays an essential role in difficult situations to guide individuals or the group down the rocky path that lies ahead. Leaders must develop the traits that will enable them to efficiently manage their emotions and, in turn, assist others in managing theirs.

Impulsive buying (IB), of which mood regulation function is well-documented, is among the methods for coping with psychological strain during the COVID-19 pandemic. However, IB is likely to hinder psychological well-being rather than repairing it in vulnerable periods. This study aims to answer: 1. Do negative psychological states promote IB during the pandemic? 2. Does IB lead negative emotions? 3. What is the role of pre-pandemic purchasing style on the process? 4.Does pandemic -related psychological strain fuel post-impulsive purchase negative emotions? A survey was conducted in Turkey with 405 participants. Results revealed that, regardless of pre-pandemic purchasing style, COVID-19-induced anxiety and loneliness promoted IB, and IB was followed by negative affect including guilt, regret, and shame. Furthermore, COVID-19-related anxiety and loneliness were found to fuel the negative affect induced by IB. The findings provide deeper insights into the dysfunctionality of IB for mood regulation and stress alleviation in a highly-stressful crisis period.

There are a variety of stress management techniques that are used to deal with the stressors of life, both short term as well as long term. In this chapter, a special focus will be given to the science of positive psychology for combating stress and related scenarios. The structure of this chapter will begin with the introduction of stress and its related problems from a psychology point of view. This will be followed with a detailed elaboration of some of the commonly used stress management techniques. After laying the initial foundation, the concept and elements of positive psychology will be detailed. The chapter will then put forth a comprehensive picture of the value in action (VIA) 24 character strengths. With relevant examples backed by recent research in positive psychology, effective strategies and techniques of dealing with stress by utilizing our inner potentials will be highlighted in this chapter.

Global rates of stress and mental health distress have reached all-time highs. Given the scale of the problem, the development and dissemination of stress management strategies ought to be accessible, trainable, and low-cost. Growing evidence indicates that the utilization of compassion-based skills has positive effects on stress reduction, enhanced mental wellbeing, and emotional resilience. In this chapter, the science of compassion will be highlighted and reviewed. This chapter explores the psychological and neurobiological foundations of compassion and how those factors can be trainable motivations and behaviors. The science of compassion demonstrates that people can reduce stress in their lives by engendering the perspective taking, emotion regulation, and relational skills within compassionate behaviors. Given contemporary workplace stressors, the application of compassion to address stress and wellbeing in the workplace is explored.

This study aims to investigate the contribution of voluntary simplicity to psychological resilience during the Covid-19 pandemic. Distinctively, the study investigates (1) how a voluntary simplicity lifestyle (VSL) supports psychological well-being in terms of the valuation of life, mental health, and boredom experienced during the pandemic crisis and (2) whether pandemic-induced psychological states encourage the intention for a future VSL. Data were collected in Turkey through an online survey of 541 participants in the Covid-19 period. Analysis results revealed that not all but certain VSL aspects supported psychological resilience by promoting the valuation of life, mental health, and alleviating boredom during the pandemic. Material independency appeared as the most prominent VSL value contributing to psychological resilience. Findings revealed that a high valuation of life and high mental stress during the pandemic motivates individuals for future simple lives. The present study enhances the current knowledge about voluntary simplicity during highly stressful periods.

Resilience is perceived within the context of perceived risk, fear, and vulnerability. The purpose of the theme chosen is to help contribute and help reduce suffering and to improve overall psychological wellbeing while strengthening resilience within guiding resilience principles of practice. COVID-19 continues to ravage the world and so there is a need for interventions that will help in managing the vulnerabilities that arise. The author hopes to contribute to this important topic and to come up with a

Preface

The COVID-19 pandemic is a global public health crisis of a scale not previously experienced in modern times and had a major effect on our lives. In addition to the vast human loss, the pandemic has destructed economic, social, and psychological well-being worldwide. Public health actions, such as social distancing, are necessary to reduce the spread of COVID-19, but they can make us feel isolated and lonely and can increase stress and anxiety. Social distancing and varying levels of quarantine precautions changed individuals' working, studying, socializing, shopping, traveling, cleaning, eating, praying routines and leisure time activities for a significant period. It has led to a global experience of increased levels of distress and anxiety due to social isolations consequences and other tragedies. Many of us are facing challenges that can be stressful, overwhelming, and cause strong emotions in adults and children. The prolonged exposure to stress arising from the crisis is likely to have insidious long-term health effects including increased risk of physical (e.g., chronic disease risk) and mental (e.g., depression, anxiety disorders and post-traumatic stress disorder) health problems and impaired cognitive function.

Stress-management strategies may be a promising approach. Learning to cope with stress in a healthy way will make you, the people you care about, and those around you become more resilient. Addressing stress and wellness during and after the pandemic requires novel approaches to mental/emotional health support and a fundamentally high standard of care compared to current medication alternatives for anxiety and depression disorders.

Accordingly, the book title, *Perspectives on Stress and Wellness Management in Times of Crisis*, is self-explanatory. The book contains eighteen chapters that attempt to mirror the major areas of research on the topic and thus offer valuable findings to practitioners and readers.

Chapter 1 seeks to provide new and appropriate insights and answers for academic leaders that help them to experience better conditions in times of crisis and unforeseen situations and provide a suitable response to circumstances. Chapter 2 demonstrates that authentic leaders exhibit such characteristics as honesty, accountability, self-regulation, relational transparency, objective analysis of information and valuing followers' contribution to arrive at decisions. These characteristics relate positively to employee job performance, wellness, and stress management. Chapter 3 highlights that academic, ecological, societal, and well-being issues wholly add to the stress development. Further, students' stress levels are quite high, and as the number of days' passes, so does their stress level. Yoga and digression therapy, such as devoting time with loved ones and watching television, are also used by learners as coping tactics. Chapter 4 explores the lived experiences of a middle-aged Caucasian production supervisor who worked in the manufacturing industry within the United States and founds that the stress and trauma she endured primarily stemmed from repetitive, prolonged, and cumulative sexual harassment. Chapter 5 specifies job stress as a mediator between cyber incivility and job satisfaction and argues that to enhance satisfaction and reduce job stress, managers need to build an incivility-free environment, the sender should be cautious with the tone of the messages. Chapter 6 explains the importance of emotional intelligence for the leaders to manage people and business effectively in times of crisis. Chapter 7 investigates how negative psychological states promote IB during the pandemic, does IB lead negative emotions, what is the role of pre-pandemic purchasing style on the process, and does pandemic related psychological strain fuel post-impulsive purchase negative emotions. Chapter 8 focuses on the science of positive psychology for combating stress and related scenarios. Chapter 9 enumerates how pandemics in the modern digital era are a stimulus that engenders anxiety, depression and insomnia affecting the global population. The psychological impact can be reduced through bibliotherapy and reposition bibliotherapy as a means of treating distress, boredom, and isolation. Chapter 10 analyzes the factors and consequences of stress in the professional activity of social workers, as well as the changes in the health area caused by the pandemic crisis context in Portugal. Chapter 11 makes an evaluative study of the way individuals and organizations have tried to approach the issue of work and life balance post-COVID and the emerging challenge for people to balance work and home post-COVID after working from home for over two years. Chapter 12 examines the relationship between work-life balance, roles and outcomes expectations, anasakti, mental health, and life happiness among university professors. Chapter 13 explores the factors that influence the "work-life balance" in "remote work" and suggesting ways to maintain "work-life balance" in remote work. Chapter 14 discovers the techniques to manage stress to ensure work-life balance in today's world. Chapter 15 explores the psychological and neurobiological foundations of compassion and how those factors can be trainable motivations and behaviors. Chapter 16 investigates how a voluntary simplicity lifestyle (VSL) supports psychological well-being in terms of the valuation of life, mental health, and boredom experienced during the pandemic crisis, and whether pandemic-induced psychological states encourage the intention for a future VSL. Chapter 17 provides a conceptual framework to guide psychological resilience knowledge and practice regarding COVID-19. Lastly, Chapter 18 documents and suggests methods to manage worries from future crisis or pandemic.

We highly appreciate everyone involved in the publication of this book.

Rohit Bansal
Vaish College of Engineering, India

Chapter 1
Allostatic Leadership:
The COVID-19 Pandemic and Opportunity for Stress Management in the Universities

Esmaeil Jafari
https://orcid.org/0000-0003-3950-8795
University of Shahid Beheshti, Iran

ABSTRACT

The chapter seeks to provide new and appropriate insights and answers for academic leaders that help them to experience better conditions in times of crisis and unforeseen situations and provide a suitable response to circumstances. Looking to the future, the emergence of an "allostatic leader" with an adaptive capacity to learn and evolve in a crisis, as well as to deal with future stresses and crises, is considered very important. Therefore, first, the concept of allostatic leadership was discussed. Next, the difference between allostatic leadership and adaptive leadership was explained. Then the development of allostatic leaders in crisis and stressful situations has been discussed. Finally, the best allostatic leadership practices are considered for academic leaders to go through crises and unexpected situations. Although these strategies are described in an academic context and in order to face the crises of the new COVID-19 pandemic, they can be equally applied by professionals in other industries facing their own crises.

INTRODUCTION

The outbreak of COVID-19 Disease has caused a great deal of fear, anxiety, and worry among people around the world. This has disrupted all aspects of human life, including education, worldwide (Paudel, 2021). Its rapid spread has led to the closure of educational institutions. The United Nations Organization (2020) report shows that the COVID-19 pandemic has caused the largest disruption to education systems in history. Facing the uncertainty and increasing intensity of the COVID-19 epidemic, with a strategic decision by academic leaders and policymakers, universities and higher education institutions moved towards online learning (Khoshbakht *et al*, 2021). Although senior university officials play an important role in university response to crises, in reality, the role of university leaders in creating a

DOI: 10.4018/978-1-6684-8565-1.ch001

culture of trust, collaboration, and shared leadership before a crisis is significantly greater and affects the ability of universities to resist in times of crisis (Kezar *et al*, 2018). In this way, the decision to focus on online teaching and learning requires new transformative learning for all beneficiaries and serious adaptive work, which is stressful, because, in the attitude, values, and beliefs of some beneficiaries, many academic institutions lack the necessary digital infrastructure, while the transition to providing online courses requires fundamental changes. This condition is clearly visible in Iran and other countries in the world (Mousavi & Jafari, 2019)

This stress can have adaptive (usually beneficial) or maladaptive (often harmful) effects depending on time, duration, the intensity of stressors, and individual differences. The acute psychological and biological effects of stress responses are generally adaptive and beneficial. Activation of psychological processes, such as cognitive appraisal, allows individuals to use past experiences and available resources to respond effectively to a threat or challenge. Simultaneous activation of these systems to respond to stressful factors is necessary to maintain mental and physical health. When these systems are disrupted by repeated, chronic, or traumatic stressors or illness or physical injury, responses may be inadequate, and even those responses that are highly adaptive may fail (McEwen, 2004). It is important to note that these biological and behavioral reactions that respond to crises can lead to some kind of survival or success, but do not respond to a stressful or critical situation that tries to develop itself. In this regard, in response to the stress caused by the COVID-19 crisis, academic leaders may cross organizational boundaries at different levels to exert creative influence during change periods (Kezar & Holcombe, 2017). Looking to the future, the emergence of an "allostatic leader" with an adaptive capacity to learn and evolve in a crisis, as well as to deal with future stresses and crises, is considered very important.

The term allostatic leadership describes leaders who consider, respond, adapt, learn, and change all factors in response to situations and demands to optimize their impact and effectiveness in current and future stressful situations (Yarnell & Grunberg, 2017). According to Heifetz et al. (2009), allostatic leaders use their skills and insight to deal with challenging situations and help other people cope with discomfort when they experience the "imbalance" of challenging situations. The basis of the current process is that Cannon observed that the body's ability to adapt in the face of changes is associated with limitations and concluded that the acute and adaptive response is faced with limitations (Burrows, 2015). This was the beginning of further thinking about stress responses, which helped in the search for an ideal and inclusive type of leader. In this type of leadership, a leader changes after learning from challenges and crises. With flexibility, understanding, and compassion, these leaders can create an environment where learning can be pursued in an online or blended environment without any stress on the part of faculty, staff, and students.

Looking to the future, once the current COVID-19 crisis is over, academic leaders may face a dilemma as they rebuild as they are now somewhat perplexed. In this way, what should be done with these online courses that were provided in emergencies to pass academic semesters? Are they modified and preserved in a transformed reality, or discarded as a used agent? Academic leaders with the adaptive capacity to take advantage of emerging strategic opportunities may redefine organizational responsibilities innovatively and use digital technologies to change or eliminate inefficient practices. Perhaps digital resources produced in response to other crises might be used to help disadvantaged students, those with physical and learning disabilities, or to design vocational courses for non-traditional students returning to education after the crisis subsides.

Considering that a leader has an important and influential role in times of change, leading an academic institution during a crisis is stressful. In addition, not much attention has been paid to the concept of allostatic leadership and it is a new concept in the topics related to leadership; therefore, in this chapter, the concept of allostatic leadership will be discussed first. Next, the difference between allostatic leadership and adaptive leadership will be explained and it will be clear how allostatic leadership differs from adaptive leadership in crisis and stressful situations. Then the development strategies of allostatic leaders in stressful and crises have been discussed and it has been determined that strategies such as understanding and strengthening emotional and social intelligence, management and resilience techniques, and developing the dominant response to a given situation can be used in this field. Finally, allostatic leadership best practices are considered for academic leaders to navigate through a crisis and unexpected situation, which include connecting with the scientific and academic community, distributed, collaborative and networked leadership, and communicating mutuality and clearly. Although these practices and strategies are described in an academic context and in order to face the crises of the new COVID-19 pandemic, they can be equally applied by professionals in other industries facing their own crises. These factors require that leaders who are in leadership positions must prioritize these responsibilities immediately after accepting the position, rather than waiting for a crisis to occur.

ALLOSTATIC LEADERSHIP

In response to the disaster caused by COVID-19, many researchers and academic communities believe that it provides an opportunity to transform a system that faces deep economic and political inequalities and is profoundly environmentally destabilizing. It is not just about adapting to a "new normal" but creating a new system. Although the chaos, uncertainties, and fears of COVID-19 are depressing and daunting, there are opportunities and challenges to develop and present a new way to organize and manage society and its important policies to the public. As Albert Einstein said: "We cannot solve our problems with the same thinking we used when we created them". In this regard, an attempt is made to present a psycho-social approach that is formed in an attempt to identify a type of inclusive leader to highlight the psychological aspects of the leader while taking relevant biological and social factors into account. In this sense, psychological aspects are combined with biological and social factors, which biological factors express what happens within the leader in unexpected situations, and social factors express the influence of leaders on others (Day, 2011). According to this framework, while working, a person experiences pressures, some of which are related to individual characteristics and some to the organizational structure. Lewin's field theory states that each person's behavior is a function of his or her "life space". Lewin's field theory suggests that people's behaviors are a function of the psychological and biological aspects of the person and their physical, psychological, and social environments. In fact, one of the principles of Lewin's field theory is that during the analysis of behavior, the totality of situations should be considered. This psychosocial conceptualization is very important for understanding people in different roles - including the role of leader (Yarnell & Grunberg, 2017).

According to Levin's emphasis on the conditions that make up the living space, it is clear that physical and psychological stressors strongly affect the environment and an individual's biological and psychological factors influence his immediate and long-term responses to stressors and stressful situations. Furthermore, in stressful situations, leaders become more influential, and followers turn to leaders for guidance and direction (Heifetz, 2000). Therefore, considering what is known about stress and stress responses is critical to understanding effective leaders and their behaviors. Considering this context, stress literature is worth attention as a source of information to achieve the research goal of identifying a type of inclusive leader. These stress responses can have different effects under the influence of various factors, and in order to respond to stressful situations, a person may use the experiences and resources related to past crises to help preserve the health of people.

In this direction and in order to face the uncertainty and increasing intensity of the COVID-19 epidemic, with a strategic decision by the leaders and macro-politicians, universities and higher education institutions moved towards online and blended learning (Khoshbakht et al., 2021). In this direction, moving towards online and distance learning requires a collective wisdom with the participation of all stakeholders, which is a manifestation of crisis conditions. This stems from the fact that many institutions did not have the hardware and software equipment to make courses electronic before Covid-19. On the other hand, many stakeholders were confused and resistant to digital tools. However, a quick response by academic leadership was essential to effectively manage the crisis, and it sent a clear message to all beneficiaries that leaders understood the COVID-19 crisis, took it seriously, and were taking steps to address it. In this regard, as Kezar and Holcombe (2017) state, the quick response of some academic institutions to crises is due to the rapid response of some academic institutions to present crisis was facilitated by the existence of authentic systems of shared leadership enabling local decision-making. According to Kazar and Holcombe (2017), organizations that use a shared leadership model benefit from a greater degree of agility, innovation, and collaboration and in the face of crises, they benefit from institutions that rely on an outdated and inflexible hierarchical leadership paradigm. Traditional autocratic leadership models are appropriate when faced with technical problems. When we face complexities and uncertainty during pandemic crises (e.g., COVID-19), these models are inadequate, because they do not address real-time problems and put these institutions at a strategic disadvantage. In this direction, the emergence of the allostatic leader as a type of flexible leadership style with an adaptive capacity to learn and evolve in crisis and unexpected cases can be considered very important.

To better understand the concept of allostatic leadership, McEwen (2005) introduced the terms "allostasis" and "allostatic load" to provide a unified explanation of stress responses that are sometimes beneficial and sometimes detrimental. This can explain the stress responses (i.e., including psychology, biology, and social environments) related to the current chapter, its psycho-social perspective, and search for a way to describe a type of inclusive leader that effectively responds to the challenging and stressful environment. To better understand this type of leadership, a distinction must be made between a situation or condition that is stabilizing to maintain survival (homeostasis) and a situation or condition that is changing to maintain stability (allostasis) (McEwen, 2005). Allostasis involves several biological systems and adaptive processes that are generally adaptive in the short-term and over time and in response to various stressors, repeated responses and adaptations to stressors lead to changes and readjustment of homeostatic dimensions and ranges. This process of reaction, adaptation, and change is the main feature of allostasis (Yarnell & Grunberg, 2017). Allostasis' emphasis on adaptation and change for survival distinguishes it from homeostasis, which involves a return to a baseline after a challenge and an acute response. A factor sometimes referred to as "adaptation", but it involves a short-term change, not a lasting change like allostasis. In general, allostasis refers to change to become stronger and respond more effectively to future challenges. It is different from short-term or acute adaptation, and it is different from homeostasis. In this regard, response, adaptation, and change in response to stressors and experience are central to the concept of allostatic leaders. Allostatic leadership is an optimal strategy for creating ideal leaders, and other types of effective leaders can serve as an umbrella.

Allostatic Leadership and Adaptive Leadership

There are many books and academic journals that discuss different types of leadership such as adaptive, affiliative, authoritative, autocratic, charismatic, facilitative, participative, servant, situational, strategic, transformational, and virtuous (Blanken, 2017; Boyatzis & McKee, 2005; Day & Antonakis, 2012; Raza, 2017; Thornton, 2013). Each of these leadership styles has different competencies and describes different types of effective leaders. However, the growing list of leader types raises questions about the value of disaggregating leader types in different ways and whether, in contrast, there is a way to describe an inclusive type of leader that can serve as an umbrella over different types of leaders. This does not mean that other leadership styles are not valuable; rather, they may be best suited to individual leaders, specific groups of followers, and situations, but still, be summed up under a broader term and description.

Along with this thinking, the higher education system was also accompanied by changes. One of the suggestions for using the COVID-19 crisis as a springboard to address the concept of academic leadership was the term allostatic leadership. However, many researchers considered the allostatic leadership response to be something similar to the adaptive leadership response. Heifetz et al. (2009) state that "adaptive" leaders use their skills and insight to deal with challenging situations. They manage themselves depending on the demands of the environment and help others to cope with discomfort when they experience the "imbalance" of challenging situations. Although adaptive leaders respond effectively to challenging situations, it is not clear that they learn and change from these adaptations and experiences. They may do so, or alternatively, they may return to their previous state (similar to a return to homeostasis).

Although the adaptive leader can effectively respond to a situation or challenge, this type of leader is not well prepared for future challenges. Ideal leaders must adapt, learn and change as a result of their experiences in different situations and environments, changing aspects of themselves to prepare them to respond optimally to future situations. In other words, leaders must become "allostatic leaders" who learn and change to face future challenges. In fact, biological and behavioral responses or adaptations that are focused on performance in acute and challenging situations are faced by adaptive leaders with an appropriate and varied response to specific situations to optimize success and survival. However, it cannot be an effective type of leadership in stressful and unexpected situations; because it does not involve learning, growing or changing with experience. Indeed, when these systems are disrupted by repeated, chronic, or traumatic stress or disease or physical injury, the responses may be inadequate and even those responses that are highly adaptive may be lost (McEwen, 2005). The ideal leader—or "allostatic leader"—responds, adapts, learns, and changes with experience to become even more effective in subsequent situations.

The basis of the present process is that Cannon also observed that the body's ability to adapt in the face of changes is associated with limitations and concluded that the acute and adaptive response is faced with limitations (Burrows, 2015). This was the beginning of further thinking about stress responses, which helped in the search for an ideal and inclusive type of leader. In this type of leadership, a leader learns from challenges and crises and then changes, while in adaptive leadership, the leader may face the challenge of survival after repeated challenges. The ideal leader becomes stronger and better prepared for new challenges after repeated responses, adaptation, learning, and change (Yarnell & Grunberg, 2017).

In this case, there is an opportunity for those academic leaders who are goal-oriented, risk-taking, and long-term and strategic to seek success in the educational environment and gain a competitive advantage (Fernandez and Shaw, 2020). It is time for academic leaders to be brave enough to disrupt long-standing patterns of behavior, challenge institutional opinions and norms and change the existing situation. With flexibility, understanding, and compassion, these leaders can create an environment where the transition to learning in an online and blended environment is followed without any stress from faculty members, staff, and students, and this process is done successfully.

Allostatic Leadership and COVID-19

As an ambiguous and complex threat, COVID-19 represents a crisis challenge that has been responded to in part by higher education leaders using experiences gained during the pandemic (Bouffard, 2020). As universities, in response to the impending crisis, focused on distance learning in Spring 2020, some higher education leaders and policymakers used a toolbox of intellectual stimulation, ideal influence, and inspiration to help faculty, staff, and students, which contributed to the higher education landscape threatened by the Covid-19 pandemic (Fernandez & Shaw, 2020a). Faced with limited resources, these leaders needed to rapidly rebuild systems to maintain academic quality and equity and inspire a growth mindset in all beneficiaries. Therefore, to successfully navigate the COVID-19 pandemic and advance their institutional mission, academic leaders needed to use a set of short-term tactical behaviors and more visionary and creative strategic skills to review and redesign old policies and practices. During the pandemic, these higher education leaders were able to tactically guide faculty in their efforts to create stability, continuity, and adaptability in their courses, which were quickly redesigned for remote delivery, by building a foundation of resilience and flexibility. For some faculty, this required fundamental changes in their attitudes, values, and beliefs (Heifetz & Laurie, 2001), especially for those who have historically been skeptical about online learning.

Using a distributed leadership style and focusing on the long-term vision of universities, strategic allostatic higher education leaders were able to benefit from a greater degree of faculty collaboration, innovation, and creativity to overcome the barriers to educational access, technological expertise, and digital equity that emerged with the rapid transition to distance education. Training, support, and resources were urgently needed for faculty and students suddenly immersed in online teaching and learning as a result of the pandemic. It is a credit to these decisive, collaborative, transformative, and resourceful leaders that usable online courses were made available to students who also showed remarkable flexibility in this course.

Some of the courses that were hastily redesigned for distance learning in the spring of 2020 were mediocre at best and they certainly weren't as good as online courses thoughtfully and intentionally designed and offered by institutions with accredited online programs. However, given the circumstances, and everyone's focus on the health, safety, and well-being of the family, a tactical transition to distance learning was an emergency strategy needed to make it through the end of the semester. In such a situation, the allostatic leader's focus is on building infrastructure across higher education institutions. Were there enough computers? Did all students, faculty, and staff have access to the Internet? For distance education to be effective, allostatic higher education leaders must use their academic collective skills and talents, including in dealing with those who are digital skeptics and resistant to teaching with technology (Harris, 2010). This optimism and vision transfer, accompanied by a kind of assurance, encourages a strategically distributed leadership style, collaboration, and inclusiveness.

Although the term allostatic leader, which originates from the field of social sciences and stress literature, may not be well known in the literature of higher education, it can be used to depict the principles related to the types of effective leadership (Yarnell & Grunberg, 2017). Specifically, these allostatic leaders are willing to change with experience to become more effective in subsequent situations; because they admit that mistakes are inevitable and are ready to fail fast, learn and move forward. These leaders are willing to change course as the crisis evolves (Kerrissey & Edmonson, 2020). While this type of leadership focuses both strategically on the vision and mission of the institution and the health and well-being of the university community, it tries to learn to adapt and make bold decisions and sets of policies and strategies with incomplete information in real time to overcome a challenge for which there was no plan and no time to prepare.

Developing Allostatic Leaders

Despite the long debate about whether leaders are born or made, the current thinking in the leadership field is that leaders can be developed. In the university environment, the development of effective, value-oriented, and results-focused leaders is critical to overcome many challenges that promote and sustain systems of higher education and focus on best delivery and practices. In order to formulate thoughtful policies, effective academic leaders are needed. Wise allocation of resources, addressing existing needs and inequalities, focusing on optimal results, and encouraging people to perform appropriate behaviors are the things that a leader should focus on. General education about strategies, providing best practices (administrative and executive), equity in the allocation of resources, addressing existing needs and inequalities, focusing on optimal results, and encouraging people to perform appropriate behaviors are among the things that a leader should focus on.

Understanding and Strengthening Emotional and Social Intelligence

This section discusses how stress affects emotional and social intelligence and how an allostatic leader can respond in that context. For decades, leaders and managers of many organizations have been advised to leave their emotions at the door when they enter their offices. However, in recent years, empirical research has shown that such advice was incorrect and impractical (Nafukho et al., 2016). There is no strategy to prevent the influence of emotions on the behaviors and actions of employees in the workplace (Druskatet al., 2006). Based on neuroscience research findings, emotions are an integral part of cognitive reasoning without which the brain cannot set priorities and make decisions (Damasio, 1994). In this regard, the ability to understand and express oneself, understand others and relate to them, manage one's own and others' emotions, and use emotions as a source of information is what is generally referred to as emotional intelligence (EI) (Bar-On, 2006). A review of empirical literature shows that EI is a set of skills for effective leadership (Johnson, 2005). Effective leaders manage their own and others' emotions better and use followers' emotional support to achieve organizational goals. As Roy (2015) pointed out, this is because leadership involves constructive and creative influences, relationships, and emotions, all of which are reciprocal between leaders and followers.

The best strategy to achieve this level of awareness is to plan for it, practice potential responses, and then interact/respond when ready. An example of this level of awareness would be regarding difficult communication such as dealing with unprofessional behavior. As Nafukho et al. (2016) state, leaders must equip themselves with EI skills and be effective in responding to unexpected and stressful crises in their workplace, especially in social skills and relationship management. This process may seem difficult every time a leader needs to interact with a follower, but the allostatic leader is able to integrate and automate these steps to reduce the energy, effort, or time required for each interaction. Practice is critical to achieving this level of EI as it allows the leader to anticipate the emotions/feelings/reactions of others and plan and respond accordingly. The allostatic leader tries to understand a different perspective and how context affects not only feelings but also thoughts and behaviors and then matches their answers with what is observed. This ability is part of social intelligence (SI). Like EI, SI is important for a leader (Yarnell, & Grunberg, 2017). The social skills of leaders make them perform better in stressful situations (Halverson et al., 2004).

As mentioned earlier, an allostatic leader is more inclusive than an adaptive leader; therefore, the allostatic leader has the flexibility to learn and change to respond with increased effectiveness to any situation. Given that in times of crisis, most interpersonal interactions are likely to take place under stressful conditions, a leader needs to understand how stress is experienced by people's ability to manage emotions effectively. Therefore, the allostatic leader must understand the Lewinian domain (B, P, and E) and take steps to be better prepared for any situation. Allostatic leaders certainly experience stress, but they develop effective strategies to help minimize the burden of stress and prevent physical, behavioral, or mental collapse.

Stress Management and Resilience Techniques

This section discusses how the allostatic leader can work to reduce personal stress levels to minimize its impact and prevent burnout. Stress reduction requires optimizing the elements of Lewin's equation. In other words, to reduce stress, health-promoting behaviors (B), cognitions and emotions (P), and social environment (E) should be targeted.

According to Yerkes-Dodson Law (inverted U model), there is a special relationship between work pressure and our performance, as our performance depends on our level of stress and anxiety. Peak performance occurs when we experience a moderate amount of stress and when the amount of pressure and stress exceeds a certain limit, our performance decreases (Yarnell, & Grunberg, 2017). Stress management usually refers to reducing high levels of stress that impair performance and health, including physical and mental well-being. The literature addressing adverse psychological outcomes following the 2003 SARS-CoV-1 epidemic found significant emotional distress in 18–57% of employees (Maunder et al, 2006). Examples of factors identified as stress factors include worry for family, fear of contagion, Job stress, and interpersonal isolation. Two years after the SARS-CoV-1 epidemic, employees reported significant levels of burnout, psychological distress, and post-traumatic stress. Also, employees faced burnout, which includes emotional exhaustion, depersonalization, and a diminished sense of personal accomplishment (Callahan et al, 2018).

In the context of the COVID-19 pandemic, employees who have experienced previous crises can deal with traumatic events such as the death of family members, friends, and colleagues. These important events will contribute to the stress caused by the COVID-19 crisis that the academic environment is facing (Heath et al., 2020). A broad strategy that can help regulate or manage stress to bring it within the range of optimal performance is allostatic leadership. Allostatic leaders are most effective when they can generate moderate arousal in themselves and others. This shows that when there is no social support from leaders and peers, more stress and more unfavorable work results occur (Burke et al., 2012). Allostatic leaders seek social support for themselves and create or contribute to an environment in which people feel supported; for example, people who feel well supported to carry out their tasks, contribute their views as a valued member of the team, offer a counterpoint or different perspective, and speak up when the situation calls for it. Managing stress can be difficult and is an ongoing process. Allostatic leaders understand how health-promoting behaviors and cognitions can be used to reduce stress for themselves and others. An allostatic leader uses these techniques to optimize performance and minimize burnout. While a certain amount of stress can be managed, stress is inevitable even in allostatic leadership. Therefore, an allostatic leader must develop dominant responses that are effective in stressful situations and social support provides a clear mechanism for effective responses.

Developing the Dominant Response to a Given Situation

The COVID-19 pandemic reached a global scale in 2020 and required a response from leaders around the world. Although the virus is a pervasive problem, world leaders have varied considerably in their responses, leading to mixed results in terms of virus reduction, public health, and economic stability. One explanation for this inconsistency is that leaders have adopted different approaches to understanding the crisis, which in turn have driven their method of decision-making and communication (Crayne & Medeiros, 2021). It is the act of explaining what styles and actions crisis leaders are likely to take in times of crisis. This action can bring with it different effects that these approaches to COVID-19 have and affect society. Therefore, today there is a need to practice dominant responses to specific situations. In fact, the goal is to identify the most likely responses to a specific crisis and stressful situation, depending on knowledge, skills, and practice, which may be correct or incorrect (Zajonc & Sales, 1966). In this regard, allostatic leaders must be sure to develop "right" and "best practices" as dominant responses, because many of their decisions and actions are made under stress and even when a stressful environment or factor may lack challenges. The reality is that others (followers and observers) watch, judge, and evaluate the leader, and these are all conditions that maximize the performance of dominant responses. The simplest strategy to develop the desired dominant responses is repetitive practice.

To develop as an allostatic leader, it is important to identify specific areas that need improvement and change behavior or thinking gradually; for example, when they tend to become defensive at the time of obvious criticism from followers. The leader can initially not provide a response at all, but instead, take all the information in and take some time to process exactly what is being conveyed. Then, the leader can work out what the first response is likely to be. Once that response is reviewed, make a judgment as to whether that response is necessary for the situation. In addition, it can be evaluated whether responding in that way improves effective interactions with followers or not. Otherwise, the cause of the response must be coordinated (e.g., what the leader could do better or how to change based on feedback and/or the situation) and what alternative response is needed to be effective.

Various studies show that individual factors may also affect how people respond to crises and stressful situations (Delahaij et al., 2010). For example, tenacious people are more effective in stressful situations, because they evaluate such situations differently and evaluate them as less threatening, and believe they can control the situation and even learn from it (Kobasa, 1979). By acting on these control perceptions, tenacious people will have more mastery experience in stressful situations. According to Bandura (1997), mastery experiences create self-efficacy beliefs, which is an important predictor of behavior and performance, because it affects the goals people adopt, the way people try to achieve those goals and the resilience they show in trying to achieve them (Bandura, 1990). Therefore, it can be said that different types of responses can be tried until the person acts better than the defensive state, practices the correct response, and finally tries to have a more effective dominant response in the future.

Allostatic Leadership Practices

The characteristics of an effective academic leader in the face of challenges are not limited to responsibility, reliability, honesty, etc. that have been described before (Fernandez & Shaw, 2020). In a crisis, best practices should be applied to increase the capacity to face future challenges and minimize damage, and adapt, learn, and change with experiences and challenges. This is necessary for crises for this type of leadership.

Connecting with the Scientific and Academic Community

Perhaps there has never been a more important time to focus the leadership debate on the relationship between leaders and beneficiaries. The list of possible reasons for such a change is long. First, to recognize that the world is mired in a leadership crisis (Gandolfi & Stone, 2018). Second, leadership has become increasingly difficult, complex, and multifaceted for organizations of all types globally (Gandolfi & Stone, 2016). Third, the crisis caused by Covid-19 has increased the scope for the emergence of leadership that can focus on the growth, needs, and well-being of people (Ruiz-Palomino et al, 2022). Therefore, at this point and during unexpected crises that create stressful conditions, it is very important for the leadership to communicate, empathize, empower, participate, and accompany the people in general and university beneficiaries. In this regard, an effective leader is potentially very desirable for organizations of any type and industry in the 21st century, especially in a crisis.

It seems that servant leadership, which is one of the basic messages of divine religions and involves followers in different dimensions (e.g., relational, moral, emotional, spiritual), has received more attention today than any other type of leadership. This type of leadership, first of all, seeks to develop followers based on the altruistic and moral orientations of leaders (Greenleaf, 2002). When followers' well-being and growth are prioritized, they in turn are more engaged and effective in their work. Servant leaders see themselves as stewards of organizations (Van Dierendonk, 2011), and unlike performance-oriented leadership approaches that often consider beneficiaries as a profitable factor (Sendjaya, 2015), servant leaders focus on long-term sustainable performance. In this regard, academic leaders put the interests of others above their own (Doraiswamy, 2012).

Servant leadership, which emphasizes empowerment, participation, and collaboration, can be used specially and more effectively in university leadership (Wheeler, 2012), because of the higher applicability of this leadership style in times of crisis (Doraiswamy, 2012). In the face of the new coronavirus pandemic, academic leaders are forced to quickly overcome any common biases they may have and quickly assess the current reality that students, faculty, and staff are experiencing real problems in their daily lives. Therefore, considering that during a crisis, the stress level is high for everyone, university leaders must be able to speed up to create an adaptive environment (Heifetz & Laurie, 2001); therefore, they can balance the stress of others and themselves. In this case, university leaders can best adjust the stress among all beneficiaries and in return, get full support from these them during the crisis.

Leaders at all academic levels must act with calmness, courage, and humility in a crisis to strengthen relationships with people inside and outside the institution (Garcia, 2006). In universities where there might be a culture of mutual mistrust and rift between faculty and administration, now, is the time to put the mistrust aside (Dever & Justice, 2020) and take advantage of this type of true shared governance. Without mutual trust, there is no transformative change. Some academic leaders may even use the crisis as an opportunity to reestablish past relationships and forge new relationships with those who hold opposing views. Communicating with people at all academic levels during a crisis allows a leader to be truly transformative and collaborate meaningfully (Fernandez & Shaw, 2020).

Building relationships and mutual trust in a crisis is not easy and requires academic leaders to be authentic and non-judgmental active listeners, accept advice and criticism, and express their opinions clearly by speaking from the heart and promoting psychological security. (Kezar et al., 2018). In a crisis, leaders may be called upon to resolve interpersonal and task-related conflicts as they arise, whereas they should encourage healthy debate provided it is effective (Robbins & Judge, 2018). Investing in relationships during a crisis strengthens the bond between students, faculty and staff, and the university. An investment that is fully realized after the crisis has passed, because the relationships created in a crisis with meaningful interaction can be long-term and result-oriented when the crisis subsides (Kezar et al., 2018).

Distributed, Collaborative, and Networked Leadership

Considering that academic environments often include different faculties and departments, a leader alone cannot have many successful activities in times of crisis (Dumulescu & Muţiu, 2021). In this regard, the academic leader should be the one who determines the organizational strategy and priorities and at the same time creates and forms a team to provide the basis for the participation of the beneficiaries in the decision-making process through delegating authority and giving responsibility to other people. Indeed, in times of crisis, the academic leader gives the team the autonomy to take responsibility for their own decisions based on the characteristics of their faculty/departments. Such distributed leadership can be more effective in improving the quality and speed of decisions and at the same time increase the feeling of empowerment and motivation of each team (Kezar and Holcombe, 2017). In this case, a university leader can choose team members based on their personality traits and not just the skills and competencies of the members, because regardless of competencies, one's personality traits are very important in times of crisis.

Decisions made by academic leaders jointly and with the cooperation of beneficiaries can help them find solutions that are compatible with the crisis and make local decisions with the benefit of greater organizational agility, innovation, collaboration, and joint support (Fernandez & Shaw, 2020). The collaborative leadership paradigm helps the university to respond to the crisis through distributed leadership and increasing responsibility at every organizational level (Kezar and Holcombe, 2017). In addition, distributed leadership means creating connections between people at all levels of the organization who are facing the challenges of a crisis. Beyond that, teams stay motivated because they have more freedom to solve the problem compared to a university that implements a top-down leadership model. With sufficient resources, these teams are allowed to operate in an atmosphere of trust and participate in problem-solving, innovation, and change. Therefore, the role of leaders in the orientation of the academic environment by finding the most appropriate solutions for empowerment, developing a culture of trust, and orientating towards solutions that lead to effective results is critical (Kezar et al., 2018).

Certainly, network leadership (joint, collaborative, and distributed) is the new requirement of educational environments (Azorín, 2020) and networks are at the forefront of resilience action in the fight against COVID-19 and other crises in the university environment. The Covid-19 crisis has led to the emergence of collaboration networks and academic solidarity, which has caused a fundamental change in the behavior of beneficiaries (from individuality to collective) and has formed a magnificent example of social participation that proves the power of professional capital. A new chapter in educational leadership is currently being written due to COVID-19. A leadership order is changing that is more distributed, collaborative, and networked. Academic leaders have a central role in making a safe, principled, and collective transition so that all beneficiaries see better days.

Communicating Mutuality and Clearly

Leaders must communicate clearly and frequently with all beneficiaries while knowing that merely sending a message to the beneficiaries is not important, but the medium through which the message is sent is also important. Communication media differ in richness and since information and data are important in the current crisis, it is necessary to use more than one communication channel (Robbins & Judge, 2018). In the current and similar crises where leaders are unable to communicate face-to-face, they should consider live-streaming updates or messages of encouragement to beneficiaries. The communication channel chosen by the leadership should also consider the preferences of the beneficiaries, and therefore communication with the staff and students as the main beneficiaries of the university may be done through different channels. Faculty and staff may prefer leadership updates via email, while students, many of whom are born in Generation Z, may prefer to receive their updates through a variety of social media platforms (or text messages), or relatively new communication channels. These types of messaging tools, apps, and social media are useful for communicating with all beneficiaries to create a sense of community, belonging, and trust, and reduce anxiety (Cowen, 2020). Communication in a crisis is a delicate balancing act, because communication and lack of proper messaging may cause worry and anxiety (Field, 2020).

The most important factor in the discussion of a leader's relationship with academic beneficiaries is the component of the leader's integrity and credibility in a crisis. If the leader is not authentic, the delivered message will not be considered valid. Academic leaders must be able to communicate a persuasive and thoughtful shared vision for universities that is realistic and achievable after the crisis is over, and that can inspire faculty, staff, and students. The process of communicating to present a compelling vision of the future requires a dynamic and collaborative process (Ancona et al, 2007). The leader's stated strategic vision must be aligned with organizational goals and consistent with the organizational mission to assure all beneficiaries that they are following the situation and have a strategy to resolve the crisis. Leaders must determine how the organization's strategy and vision will be implemented and share it as more information and the impact of actions become known. Academic leaders' actions should be transparent in crises so that the university community is clear about the direction the university is moving. At such times, leaders must understand the complexities of the Covid-19 pandemic, gather information as it becomes more accessible, and communicate these complexities to all beneficiaries while articulating potentially acceptable solutions. By communicating effectively with all beneficiaries, academic leaders gain the trust of faculty, staff, and students and acquire organizational and academic commitment in pursuing strategic opportunities and alternative and sustainable solutions.

In this regard, it is very important to support the welfare of students and other beneficiaries. This means communicating clearly with beneficiaries about changing conditions and expectations, as well as using positive assumptions when communicating with beneficiaries about their non-participation or willingness to participate (Netolicky, 2020). Paying attention to this requires that leaders support beneficiaries through clear expectations and structures that also consider their needs and feedback.

CONCLUSION

This pandemic has shown us that we are one community, one humanity, and leadership is for all of us. Now is the time to think about what it means to be a leader. We can reach out and support each other as much as we can, even though isolation seems to go against our biology. We can carefully consider where we get our information and how we respond to them. We can all lead by example, by clear communication with one another, and by the clarity of purpose and coherence of action. There is no time more important than now to be kind to ourselves and each other. We are in a time of adaptation and evolution, by necessity. When we come out on the other side, society, work, and education may well be reformed.

Given the importance of connecting with all beneficiaries as individuals and building mutual trust, distributing leadership responsibilities among situationally aware teams, and communicating clearly and regularly, academic leaders can take comfort in the knowledge that they are not expected to be perfect. There is no such thing as a perfect academic leader, but those leaders who have the flexibility and adaptive capacity to learn and evolve as a result of a crisis will be able to respond to future challenges more effectively and with less effort, and they might just make great leaders. In this regard, what should the universities of the world do to prepare for the next pandemic? The universities must form a better understanding of the potential for the emergence of a new leadership strain. Allostatic leadership" is an ideal type of leadership for our academic institutions (Yarnell & Grunberg, 2017), whose basic component is the ability to learn and change. By committing to these important leadership practices and trying to develop themselves, university leaders emerge from crisis to rebuild and thereby help university communities in times of crisis and stress.

REFERENCES

Ancona, D., Malone, T. W., Orlikowski, W. J., & Senge, P. M. (2007). In praise of the incomplete leader. *Harvard Business Review*, *85*(2). PMID:17345683

Antonakis, J. (2012). Transformational and charismatic leadership. *The Nature of Leadership*, 256-288.

Azorín, C. (2020). Beyond COVID-19 supernova. Is another education coming? *Journal of Professional Capital and Community*, *5*(3), 381–390. doi:10.1108/JPCC-05-2020-0019

Bandura, A. (1990). Perceived self-efficacy in the exercise of control over AIDS infection. *Evaluation and Program Planning*, *13*(1), 9–17. doi:10.1016/0149-7189(90)90004-G

Bean-Mellinger, B. (2017). *Six leadership styles*. Academic Press.

Berkman, L. F., & Syme, S. L. (1979). Social network, host resistance, and mortality: A nine-year follow-up of study of Alamed county residents. *American Journal of Epidemiology*, *109*(2), 186–204. doi:10.1093/oxfordjournals.aje.a112674 PMID:425958

Boyatzis, R., Boyatzis, R. E., & McKee, A. (2005). *Resonant leadership: Renewing yourself and connecting with others through mindfulness, hope, and compassion*. Harvard Business Press.

Burke, R. J., Moodie, S., Dolan, S. L., & Fiksenbaum, L. (2012). *Job demands, social support, work satisfaction and psychological well-being among nurses in Spain.* ESADE Business School Research Paper, (233).

Burrows, V. (2015). *The medicalization of stress: Hans Selye and the transformation of the postwar medical marketplace*. City University of New York.

Callahan, K., Christman, G., & Maltby, L. (2018). Battling burnout: Strategies for promoting physician wellness. *Advances in Pediatrics, 65*(1), 1–17. doi:10.1016/j.yapd.2018.03.001 PMID:30053918

Crayne, M. P., & Medeiros, K. E. (2021). Making sense of crisis: Charismatic, ideological, and pragmatic leadership in response to COVID-19. *The American Psychologist, 76*(3), 462–474. doi:10.1037/amp0000715 PMID:32772539

Day, D. V. (2011). Leadership development. The SAGE Handbook of Leadership, 22, 37-50.

Delahaij, R., Gaillard, A. W., & van Dam, K. (2010). Hardiness and the response to stressful situations: Investigating mediating processes. *Personality and Individual Differences, 49*(5), 386–390. doi:10.1016/j.paid.2010.04.002

Dever, C., & Justice, G. (2020). *Coming together in crisis times.* Retrieved from https://www.insidehighered.com/advice/2020/03/27/during-pandemic-crisis-faculty-and-administrators-must-move-beyond-thei
r

Dumulescu, D., & Muţiu, A. I. (2021). Academic leadership in the time of COVID-19—Experiences and perspectives. *Frontiers in Psychology, 12*, 648344. doi:10.3389/fpsyg.2021.648344 PMID:33959076

Fernandez, A., & Shaw, G. (2020). Leadership in higher education in an era of new adaptive challenges. In *INTED2020 Proceedings* (pp. 61-65). IATED. 10.21125/inted.2020.0037

Fernandez, A. A., & Shaw, G. P. (2020). Academic leadership in a time of crisis: The Coronavirus and COVID-19. *The Journal of Leadership Studies, 14*(1), 39–45. doi:10.1002/jls.21684

Field, K. (n.d.). Lessons from campuses that closed after natural disasters. *The Chronicle of Higher Education*.

Gandolfi, F., & Stone, S. (2016). Clarifying leadership: High-impact leaders in a time of leadership crisis. *Revista de Management Comparat International, 17*(3), 212.

Gandolfi, F., & Stone, S. (2018). Leadership, leadership styles, and servant leadership. *Journal of Management Research, 18*(4), 261–269.

Garcia, H. F. (2006). Effective leadership response to crisis. *Strategy and Leadership, 34*(1), 4–10. doi:10.1108/10878570610637849

Greenleaf, R. K. (2002). *Servant leadership: A journey into the nature of legitimate power and greatness*. Paulist Press.

Harris, A. (2010). Distributed leadership: Evidence and implications. *The principles of educational leadership and management*, 55-69.

Heath, C., Sommerfield, A., & von Ungern-Sternberg, B. S. (2020). Resilience strategies to manage psychological distress among healthcare workers during the COVID-19 pandemic: A narrative review. *Anaesthesia*, *75*(10), 1364–1371. doi:10.1111/anae.15180 PMID:32534465

Heifetz, R. A. (2000). *Leadership without easy answers*. Harvard University Press.

Heifetz, R. A., Heifetz, R., Grashow, A., & Linsky, M. (2009). *The practice of adaptive leadership: Tools and tactics for changing your organization and the world*. Harvard Business Press.

Heifetz, R. A., & Laurie, D. L. (2001). The work of leadership. *Harvard Business Review*, *79*(11). PMID:10174450

Kerrissey, M. J., & Edmondson, A. C. (2020). What good leadership looks like during this pandemic. *Harvard Business Review*, *13*(1).

Kezar, A., Fries-Britt, S., Kurban, E., McGuire, D., & Wheaton, M. M. (2018). *Speaking truth and acting with integrity*. American Council on Education. https://www.acenet.edu/Documents/Speaking-Truth-and-Acting-with-Integrity.pdfnoe

Kezar, A. J., & Holcombe, E. M. (2017). *Shared leadership in higher education*. American Council on Education.

Khoshbakht, F., Mohammadi, M., Naseri, R., Mirghafari, F., Safari, M., Roosta, F., & … . (2021). Evaluating the Health-Oriented Attitude of Parents of Elementary School Students towards the Reopening of Schools in the Corona Crisis. *The Journal of Educational Research*, *8*(42), 33–48.

Kobasa, S. C. (1979). Stressful life events, personality, and health: An inquiry into hardiness. *Journal of Personality and Social Psychology*, *37*(1), 1–11. doi:10.1037/0022-3514.37.1.1 PMID:458548

Maunder, R. G., Lancee, W. J., Balderson, K. E., Bennett, J. P., Borgundvaag, B., Evans, S., Fernandes, C., Goldbloom, D., Gupta, M., Hunter, J., McGillis Hall, L., Nagle, L., Pain, C., Peczeniuk, S., Raymond, G., Read, N., Rourke, S., Steinberg, R., Stewart, T., ... Wasylenki, D. A. (2006). Long-term psychological and occupational effects of providing hospital healthcare during SARS outbreak. *Emerging Infectious Diseases*, *12*(12), 1924–1932. doi:10.3201/eid1212.060584 PMID:17326946

Maunder, R. G., Leszcz, M., Savage, D., Adam, M. A., Peladeau, N., Romano, D., Rose, M., & Schulman, R. B. (2008). Applying the lessons of SARS to pandemic influenza. *Canadian Journal of Public Health*, *99*(6), 486–488. doi:10.1007/BF03403782 PMID:19149392

McEwen, B. S. (2004). Protection and damage from acute and chronic stress: Allostasis and allostatic overload and relevance to the pathophysiology of psychiatric disorders. *Annals of the New York Academy of Sciences*, *1032*(1), 1–7. doi:10.1196/annals.1314.001 PMID:15677391

Mousavi, M., & Jafari, F. (2019). Virtual education in the era of corona virus, opportunities and challenges. *The First National Conference of Applied Research in Education Processes*.

Nafukho, F. M., Muyia, M. H., Farnia, F., Kacirek, K., & Lynham, S. A. (2016). Developing emotional intelligence skills among practicing leaders: Reality or Myth? *Performance Improvement Quarterly*, *29*(1), 71–87. doi:10.1002/piq.21215

Netolicky, D. M. (2020). School leadership during a pandemic: Navigating tensions. *Journal of Professional Capital and Community*, *5*(3/4), 391–395. doi:10.1108/JPCC-05-2020-0017

Paudel, P. (2021). Online education: Benefits, challenges and strategies during and after COVID-19 in higher education. *International Journal on Studies in Education*, *3*(2), 70–85. doi:10.46328/ijonse.32

Robbins, S. P., Judge, T. A., & Breward, K. E. (2018). *Essentials of Organizational Behavior Ottawa*. Pearson.

Ruiz-Palomino, P., Yáñez-Araque, B., Jiménez-Estévez, P., & Gutiérrez-Broncano, S. (2022). Can servant leadership prevent hotel employee depression during the COVID-19 pandemic? A mediating and multigroup analysis. *Technological Forecasting and Social Change*, *174*, 121192. doi:10.1016/j.techfore.2021.121192 PMID:34538969

Sendjaya, S. (2015). *Servant leadership research. In Personal and Organizational Excellence through Servant Leadership*. Springer. doi:10.1007/978-3-319-16196-9

UNO. (2020). *Education during COVID-19 and beyond*. UNESCO.

Van Dierendonck, D. (2011). Servant leadership: A review and synthesis. *Journal of Management*, *37*(4), 1228–1261. doi:10.1177/0149206310380462

Wheeler, D. W. (2012). *Servant leadership for higher education: Principles and practices*. John Wiley & Sons.

Yarnell, A. M., & Grunberg, N. E. (2017). Developing "allostatic leaders": a psychobiosocial perspective. In *Leader development deconstructed* (pp. 23–50). Springer. doi:10.1007/978-3-319-64740-1_2

Chapter 2
Managing Stress and Enhancing Employee Wellness and Performance in Times of Crisis:
The Authentic Leader as the "Magic Bullet"

Evans Sokro
https://orcid.org/0000-0002-5692-2886
Central University, Ghana

Theresa Obuobisa-Darko
Ghana Communication Technology University, Ghana

ABSTRACT

Employee stress has been explored extensively. However, there remain a dearth of scholarship on how leadership, specifically authentic leadership, helps to reduce employee stress levels in crises, such as the COVID-19 pandemic, in emerging economies, and to ensure employee wellness and performance using the social exchange theory. Using exploratory qualitative design and thematic analysis, data from 32 interviews with public sector employees in Ghana were analysed. Findings demonstrate that authentic leaders exhibit such characteristics as honesty, accountability, self-regulation, relational transparency, objective analysis of information, and valuing followers' contributions to arrive at decisions. These characteristics relate positively to employee job performance, wellness, and stress management.

INTRODUCTION

The onset of the COVID-19 pandemic, a stressful life situation, has significantly altered human life and resulted in overwhelming uncertainty and new behavioural "norms" such as wearing of face covering, remote working, the way daily activities are carried out, and several changes in work schedules. While some employees have to work full time remotely, others have to combine working remotely and in-person.

DOI: 10.4018/978-1-6684-8565-1.ch002

These changes in work schedules, coupled with the uncertainties surrounding the COVID-19 pandemic have resulted in different psychological conditions like anxiety, depression and stress at the workplace.

Stress, "an unpleasant psychological process that occurs in response to environmental pressures" (Robbins & Judge, 2017, p. 65), can be task-based, role-based, environmental and social. Specifically, it can be as a result of workload, poor supervision, bad bosses and any of these combined, with any diversity issue can lead to stress. While some authors indicate that stress has no negative effect on employee performance (Muis et al., 2021), many scholars opine that stress affect organisations negatively. These negative effects include decline in employee performance (Khan et al., 2022), counterproductive behaviour like extreme anger (De Clercq et al., 2019; Jun et al., 2018), frequent absenteeism (Abdullah & Lee, 2012), and employee wellness (Tsui, 2021; Abdullah & Lee, 2012). Due to these negative effects, the effective management of employee stress has become a strategic activity for managers of organisations. Therefore, there is a call to adopt an appropriate leadership style which will help manage the stress, identify and implement employee wellness programmes to prevent its potential negative effects.

Wellness is a holistic and self-driven process comprising of multi-dimensions of wellbeing, which ultimately promote an optimal, purposeful and improved quality of life (Kumar et al., 2022). Workplace wellness results in environment that supports healthy lifestyles for employees and their families through systems and structures implemented by leaders. Organisations derive several benefits when they ensure employee wellness such as improved employee performance (Ford et al., 2011; Warr & Nielsen, 2018; Wu et al., 2017), stress (Wu et al., 2017; Hoert et al., 2018), employee turnover, improved employee relations and employee health (Hoert et al., 2018). Consequently, leaders have to adopt the appropriate style and implement strategies and programmes to ensure employee wellness to experience all these benefits. The question then is, what leadership style should leaders adopt to ensure employees stress is well managed and enhance employee wellness to increase performance?

Several studies suggest a relationship between leadership and effective management of employee stress and wellness after the pandemic. Leadership is a process not an outcome, where the leader influences other people with the aim of maximising their efforts towards the achievement of goals (Robbins and Judge (2009) by adopting different styles. Leadership styles refer to the relatively stable patterns of behaviour displayed by leaders. There exist different leadership styles and one well recognised and contemporary one is the authentic leadership style. Authentic leadership is a pattern of transparent and ethical leader behaviour that encourages openness in sharing information needed to make decisions while accepting followers' inputs (Avolio et al., 2009). According to Walumbwa et al. (2008), authentic leaders demonstrate four major characteristics: balanced processing, internalised moral perspective, relational transparency, and self-awareness. While the balancing processing characteristic enable the leader analyse data objectively before making decisions, the internalised moral perspective ensures that the authentic leader is guided by internal moral standards which help self-regulate his behaviours (Walumbwa et al., 2008; Beddoes-Jones & Swailes, 2015). Additionally, the relational transparency refers to the authentic leader's characteristic which enables him to present his authentic self, by openly sharing relevant information and feelings appropriate to the situation (Obuobisa-Darko & Domfeh, 2016). Lastly, the self-awareness dimension makes the authentic leader to demonstrate an understanding of one's strengths and weaknesses (Walumbwa et al., 2008).

Leader behaviour is a major determinant of the stress levels of followers (Harms et al., 2017). They assess and identify workplace stressors as well as the first signs of stress in worker. With several stressors at the workplace both leaders and employees are exposed to stress. However, a clear relationship between leadership and stress, with leadership level being inversely related to stress (Sherman et al.,

2012), leaders are able to manage their stress, relate well with their subordinates to better manage that of their followers. Again, employees get stressed when there is an imbalance in work and life (Nam, 2014). Leaders who are self-aware and are able to manage their moods, thus do not suffer from mood swings are in a better position to assist their followers to manage their stress. It is therefore argued that, the adoption of the authentic leadership, a relatively new leadership style and less researched into (Robbins & Judge, 2014), has thus become the "magic bullet" to manage employee stress and improve employee wellness to increase performance post COVID-19 pandemic. It is from this stance that this chapter attempts to answer the question: Which behaviours and strategies of authentic leaders ensure employees' stress management and employee wellness for organisational performance and success post COVID-19 pandemic?

Drawing on the happy-productive worker hypothesis and the social exchange theory, this chapter explains how leaders ensuring employees happiness will cause them to reciprocate by putting in more efforts to perform. The happy-productive worker hypothesis, popularly referred to as the "Holy Grail" of management research, presumes that workers who are happy on the job will become more productive and willing to remain in the organisation than less happy workers (Wright & Cropanzano, 2007). The social exchange theory (SET), a well-known influential theory is used in understanding employee behaviour and clarification of how employees are likely to react in different situation in their work environment. According to the theory, there exists a reciprocal relationship between employees and their leaders. It proposes that all human relations exist on the basis of 'cost-benefit' analysis and a comparison of alternatives based on trust and reciprocity.

Using this to explain the authentic leader, employee stress and performance in crisis period relationship, the argument being made is, the COVID -19 pandemic led to several changes in work schedules and stressful situations which affected employee wellness and their performance negatively. With the authentic leader being self-aware, balancing processing, internalizing moral perspective and relationally transparent, they will relate well with their subordinates and ensure their wellness which will improve their social exchange relationship. These employees, as a result of the improved social exchanges will reciprocate by putting in much effort, to be active in the wellness programmes implemented and this will reduce their stress, improve their wellness and impact positively on their performance.

There are not many studies that adopted the happy-productivity thesis in a crisis like the COVID-19 pandemic. Again, several studies have been carried out using the SET, but not much is known with focus on the authentic leader in crisis like the COVID-19 in developing countries context. Since context matter in research, this research is therefore carried out to make significant contribution to the SET as well as the authentic leadership literature by examining how authentic leaders manage employees in crisis to minimise the negative effect created by the pandemic on employees' stress and its role in ensuring employee wellness and performance in the current emerging economy.

The paper adopts exploratory qualitative research approach by gathering data from public sector employees to determine the relationship between authentic leadership, stress management, employee wellness and performance, post COVID-19 pandemic. The paper proceeds as follows. Following this introduction is the literature review which covers discussion of the happy-productive worker hypothesis and the social exchange theory, authentic leadership, stress and stress management, employee wellness and employee performance. The next section is a description of the methodology used to carry the study, followed by the results, discussion and lastly, conclusion and recommendation.

THEORETICAL FRAMEWORK

The Social Exchange theory (SET) is based on one of the oldest theories of social behaviour, where any interaction between individuals reflects an exchange of resources (Homans, 1958). Therefore, it aims at examining human social behaviours from the perspective of the exchange of resources. Blau (1964), first to use the phrase "theory of social exchange" described it as a kind of social interaction, where the persons involved in these social exchanges believe that they will receive financial or social benefits as a result of the interaction. These social exchanges refer to the "voluntary actions of individuals that are motivated by the returns they are expected to bring and typically do in fact bring from others" (Blau, 1964, p. 91). The theoretical tenets of SET explain that "social behaviour is a series of exchanges" (Chang *et al.*, 2015, p.868) which involve both tangible and intangible resources. These exchanges are based on reciprocity (Chang *et al.*, 2015) which is explained as mutual exchanges that partners perceive as fair (Saglam *et al.*, 2022). Thus, the theory assumes that relationship between individuals are established based on "cost-benefit" analysis and a comparability of alternatives (Nguyen *et al.*, 2016). As a result, individuals compare the potential benefits to costs to incur before performing a behaviour (Blau, 1964; Shin *et al.*, 2017; Tsai and Kang, 2019). It should be noted however that the benefits that one enjoys from the exchange relationship are mostly intangible resources, which result in such benefits such as love, respect, knowledge, information, status, honour and friendship (Cropanzano & Mitchell, 2005; Liao, 2008).

Using the social exchange theory as the theoretical framework for this study, is very significant, in that, the employee who perceives the authentic leader is putting in effort to ensure their wellness and manage their stress will remain committed and engaged and reciprocate by putting in much effort which will reflect in improved performance. The argument therefore is, the adoption of authentic leadership style – a leader who is self-aware, kind, accountable (Yukl, 2010), provides relevant information, involves employees in decision making (Walumbwa, *et al.*, 2008) and very transparent, will help manage employee stress and ensure their wellness and improve performance.

LITERATURE REVIEW

Happy-Productive Worker Hypothesis

The happy-productive worker thesis (HPWT) is considered the Holy Grail of management (Wright & Cropanzano, 2007; Peiró *et al.*, 2021). This is because all things being equal, happy workers are expected to perform better than those who are unhappy or less happy (Wright & Cropanzano, 2007; Cropanzano & Wright, 1999, 2001; Wright et al., 2002; Wright *et al.*, 2007; Zelenski *et al.*, 2008). This explains why proponents of the "happy-productive worker" thesis are convinced that "a happy worker is a good worker" (Hosie & Sevastos (2009). They are good employees because, such employees are sensitive to opportunities, build resources for future performance, more confident and more supportive to colleagues (Zelenski *et al.*, 2008). Contrary to this, less happy and miserable individuals are more pessimistic, sensitive to threats, defensive when with colleagues (Cropanzano & Wright, 2001), display little energy or motivation, and as a result achieve little (Zelenski et al., 2008). Happy employees are therefore sought after by managers. It is therefore prudent that leaders of organisations adopt the appropriate leadership style and characteristics to make employees happy to become sensitive to opportunities and supportive to their colleagues in all circumstances including crisis period, and one of such is the authentic leader.

The argument then is, when authentic leaders remain approachable, encourage openness in sharing information, build trust and accept followers input during discussions, they will be happy and therefore have positive emotions, reduce stress, improve their wellness and this will have a positive impact on their performance. It is therefore hypothesised that authentic leadership will cause employees to be happy and this will have a positive impact on their performance, wellness and stress levels.

AUTHENTIC LEADERSHIP

Different schools of thought on leadership have evolved over time. From the 'Great Man' (1840's) and 'Traits' theories (1930's-1940's) to 'Behavioural' theories (1940's-1950's) to 'Transformational' leadership (1970's) (Bolden, et al. 2003) and in recent past, authentic leadership which was introduced by Bill George, a management expert. Authentic leadership is relatively new and there is less research on it than the other forms of leadership (Robbins & Judge, 2014). With the minimum research that focus on this leadership style (Robbins & Judge, 2014), scholars are yet to agree on one common definition. Authentic leadership according to Walumbwa et al. (2008) refers to "…a pattern of leader behaviour that draws upon and promotes both positive psychological capacities and a positive ethical climate, to foster greater self-awareness, and internalized moral perspective, balanced processing of information, and relational transparency on the part of leaders working with followers, fostering positive self-development". (94).

Beddoes-Jones and Swailes (2015) developed the three-pillar model of authentic leadership which are self-awareness, ethics and self-regulation, Walumbwa et al. (2008) had earlier developed a four-model version which included self-awareness, balanced processing, internalised moral perspective and relational transparency. This paper adopts the four-pillar model developed by Walumbwa, et al. (2008) as this includes the characteristics developed by Beddoes-Jones and Swailes (2015) in addition to other characteristics. It should be noted however that, Walumbwa et al. (2008) initially described authentic leadership as having five distinct but related components, which are self-awareness, relational transparency, internalised regulation, balanced processing of information and positive moral perspective. However, the internal regulation processes and positive moral perspective were combined and named internalised moral perspective which resulted in having the four components. These pillars are briefly explained in the next session.

Self-awareness (SA) refers to 'demonstrating an understanding of how one derives and makes meaning of the world and how that meaning making process impacts the way one views himself or herself over time' (Walumbwa et al, 2008, p.95). From another perspective, Ilies et al. (2005) believe that self-awareness reflects an individual's awareness of one's own personal characteristics, values, motives, feelings, and cognitions, as well as a clear understanding of who one is that is one's personality and how others perceive it. Self-awareness therefore is about an individual being conscious of what one is good at and also acknowledging what one is not good at and therefore, yet to learn. Similarly, Valsania (2012) perceives self-awareness to be an individual's awareness of his/her values, emotions, identity and goals as well as how their actions affect others they relate with. Therefore, self-awareness can reflect an individual's consciousness of his/her values, motives, feelings which reflect in how he makes meaning of the world and the people he relates with. Some values exhibited the authentic leaders include honesty, altruism, kindness, fairness, accountability and optimism (Yukl, 2010).

Balanced processing (BP), the authentic leaders' characteristic which makes them 'objectively analyse all relevant data before coming to a decision' (Walumbwa et al., 2008, p. 95). This characteristic make the authentic leader analyse information received objectively before making decisions (Gardner, et al., 2005) and also cause their followers to seek views from others that challenge their existing positions (Walumbwa et al., 2010). As a result of this characteristic, the authentic leader seeks information from all including his subordinates in making decisions.

Internalised moral perspective refer to an internalised and integrated form of self-regulation (Walumbwa et al., 2008). A self-regulated individual is self-discipline, keeps his ego in check, does not suffer from mood swings, and remains approachable even when facing significant challenges and consistently acts as a role model for others (Beddoes-Jones & Swailes, 2015). This characteristic, not imposed by society, organisation or any group of individuals makes the leader behave in an ethical manner and makes ethical decisions (Walumbwa *et al.*, 2008). Relational transparency refers to presenting one's authentic self (as opposed to a fake or distorted self) to others (Walumbwa *et al*, 2008, p.95). The authentic leader thus develops authentic relations with followers, which lead to building trustful relationship between themselves and their followers (Gardner, *et al.*, 2005; Clapp-Smith, *et al.*, 2009).

STRESS AND STRESS MANAGEMENT

Scholars are yet to agree on the definition of employee stress due to its highly subjective nature (Hall *et al.*, 2012) and therefore there are inconsistencies and differences in the definitions (Bacchus, 2008). While Steigleder et al. (2023) define stress as a process in which a person reacts to internal or external demands while the resources for coping with it seem limited, Kihara and Mugambi (2018) defined it as a psychological and physical reaction to prolonged internal and/or environmental conditions in which individual's adaptive capabilities are over extended (p. 2383). Similar to Kihara and Mugambi's (2018) definition, Robbins and Judge (2017) explained stress as an unpleasant psychological process that occurs in response to environmental pressures (p. 659). In the view of Seaward (2019), stress reflects a form of unpleasant emotional reaction developed by individuals as a result of perceived exposure to threat in or outside work environmental and/or internal conditions, to which such persons lack adequate response. Though there are slight differences, it can be observed that stress reflects a reaction to conditions or situations where an individual employee feels a discrepancy in the demands on the resources, skills and capabilities of the employee which may result in anxiety.

Causes of stress have been classified in different ways. Robbins and Judge (2017) into three main environmental factors, organisational factors and personal factors (Robbins & Judge, 2017). Environmental factors include economic uncertainty, political uncertainty, technological change while organisational factors include task demands, role demands, and interpersonal demands, while personal factors include family problems and economic problems. For Saleem et al (2021), there are two main streams of stress. Job related which refers to how stressful psychosocial aspects of work environments, like role conflict, increased workloads, lack of autonomy, and lack of social support cause job strains and eventually hinders performance. The second, environmental source refers to how the employees' abilities, their physical environment as well as a person-environment 'misfit' affect their level of stress and their performance (Saleem *et al.*, 2021).

Even though contemporary organisations are known to cause employees stress, there has been an increase in the level of employee stress due to the COVID-19 pandemic (Rothan & Byrareddy, 2020; Oruh *et al.*, 2021). This is as a result of crisis-related stressors such as poor work conditions, health risks, job loss, job insecurity, and delayed payment (Hill, 2020; Oruh et al., 2021). Others include one's inability to cope with work demands, lack of engagement or opportunity to express grievances due to fear of being laid off (Seaward, 2019). Another major cause of stress in this post pandemic period is work life imbalance. Working from home, as a result of technological advancement, may result in an imbalance between employees' work and family life which results in stress (Nam, 2014) due to employees' inability to separate work life from home life as they work from home.

Although stress is typically discussed in the negative, it has few positive outcomes. For instance, some employees cite pressure of heavy workload and deadlines as positively challenging them to put in much and also enhance their quality of work and satisfaction derived thereof (Robbins & Judge, 2017). On the contrary several researchers indicate that increased stress leads to reduced productivity (Halkos & Bousinakis, 2010), depletes employees' cognitive and emotional resources (Liao *et al.*, 2022), and job satisfaction (Ajayi, 2018). Due to these adverse effects, employee stress needs to be managed.

EMPLOYEE WELLNESS

Employee wellness is not just a responsibility but also the required investment for an organisation (Dhobale, 2009). Wellness has been defined as "a state of complete physical, mental and social well-being and not merely the absence of disease or infirmity" (World Health Organization Constitution, 2014, p. 1). It refers to the complex and multifaceted nature of physical, mental, and emotional health and well-being of employees and their personal resources (ability, knowledge, motivations) to strive toward well-being; and wellness programmes as a process whereby firms offer wellness services to employees (Solnet *et al.*, 2020, p. 940).

Wellness is often defined as a means and not an end, which is aimed at individual holistic health state including emotional and physical wellbeing (Corbin & Pangrazi, 2001; Varga *et al.*, 2021). Organisations usually put in place wellness programmes to ensure their employees wellbeing. Wellness programmes include the practices and activities which enable employees to adopt healthy behaviours and modify unhealthy lifestyles to achieve a balanced emotional, social, physical spiritual and intellectual health (Zhang et al., 2014). Such activities may include health promotion activities, onsite clinical care, biometric screening, other occupational health service (Zhang, 2018), on-site fitness centres, healthy selections in company cafeterias, health assessments, and employee assistance plans (Kumar et al., 2009).

Due to the benefits of employee wellness to organisations, leaders endeavour to implement such plans to enjoy these benefits as individuals and as organisations. Some of these are improved performance (Ott-Holland et al., 2019; Kumar et al., 2009), engagement (Mattke et al., 2013) employee motivation (Mattke et al., 2013), lower turnover (Berry et al., 2010; Varga et al., 2021), job stress (Abdullah & Lee, 2012; Hoert et al 2018) and good physical health (Kumar et al., 2009).

Scholars and practitioners agree that wellness programmes can only be effective if the organisation is focused on the health and wellness of its employees (Berry et al., 2010) which is a significant role of the leader. The authentic leader who knows and takes ethical decisions, due to his internalised moral perspective characteristic, will choose to implement significant wellness programme which ensure employees' wellness and happiness.

EMPLOYEE PERFORMANCE

Armstrong (2006) defined performance as the "accomplishment, execution, carrying out, and working out of anything ordered or undertaken" (p. 498). In the view of Motowidlo and Kell (2012) it is "the total expected value to organisation of the discrete behavioural episodes that an individual carries out over a standard period of time"(p.92). Similarly, Bandura and Lyons, (2014) indicated that performance reflects employee behaviour which results in such employees doing more above and beyond regular task expectations and freely getting involved in voluntary, helpful behaviour to support organisational goals. Contrary to Motowidlo's (2003) and Motowidlo and Kell's (2012) definition of performance as a behaviour, Viswesvaran and Ones (2000) define performance as "scalable actions, behaviours and outcomes that employees engage in or bring about that are linked with and contribute to organisational goals" (p. 216). Thus, in the view of Viswesvaran and Ones (2000) performance could be described as both a behaviour and an outcome.

Performance is made up of three broad dimensions: Contextual performance, Counterproductive work performance and Task performance (Koopmans, *et al.*, 2011, 2012; Rotundo & Sackett, 2002; Viswesvaran & Ones, 2000). Koopmans, *et al.* (2011) originally presented a fourth dimension of performance known as adaptive performance which refers to an employee's ability to adapt to changes in a work system or work roles (Griffin et al., 2007).

Adaptive performance includes solving problems creatively, dealing with uncertain and unpredictable work situations, learning new tasks, technologies and procedures, and adapting to other individuals, cultures or physical surroundings (Koopmans et al., 2011, p.862). An individual's ability to adapt in performing his task is seen in the ability to cope with, respond to, and/or support changes that affect the execution of task assigned (Griffin et al., 2007). However, Koopmans, et al. (2012) indicated that "adaptive performance does not appear to be a separate dimension, but rather an aspect of contextual performance" (, p.21).

Contextual or extra-role performance refers to behaviours that are not considered in job descriptions (Peiró et al., 2021) and it is defined as "behaviours that support the organizational, social, or psychological environment in which the technical core functions" (Koopmans et al., 2011, p. 861). This confirms Hosie and Nankervis (2016, p.426) definition of contextual performance as a behaviour that involves cooperation and helping others in the organisation and those that ultimately contribute to organisational effectiveness. Contextual performance therefore refers to behaviour that contribute to the organisational effectiveness by providing a good environment in which task performance can occur.

Counterproductive Work Behaviour is defined as behaviour that harms the wellbeing of the organisation or its members (Koopmans et al., 2011; Rotundo & Sackett, 2002). It includes behaviours like absenteeism, off-task behaviours, theft and substance abuse (Koopmans et al., 2011), gossiping about people at their organisations, talking badly about people behind their backs, or spending time on personal issues (Bai, Lin & Wang, 2016). The last dimension of performance is Task Performance which is traditionally the focus of individual performance (Koopmans et al., 2012) and usually included in job description and therefore prescribed (Viswesvaran, 2001; Peiró et al., 2021). It refers to the proficiency (i.e. competency) with which one performs his/her assigned job that is formally recognised as part of their jobs (Borman & Motowidlo, 1993; Koopmans, et al., 2011). It is described as job-specific task proficiency, technical proficiency, or in-role performance (Koopmans et al, (2011). Behaviours that are usually used to describe task performance include work quantity and quality, job skills and job knowledge (Rotundo & Sacket, 2002). Employee task performance can thus be explained as the execution of roles assigned with proficiency (job specific, technical, in-role, behaviour) that contributes to the organisation's success. Even though there are different dimensions of performance, this chapter describes it as a composite variable and explain it as a process that reflects employee behaviour which results in accomplishment of task assigned, which may be expectations to support organisational goals.

With the characteristic of balanced processing (Walumbwa, 2010, 2008), authentic leaders seek and accept suggestions from subordinates when making decisions. Literature confirms that employees whose opinions are sought when decisions are being made, reciprocate by being engaged (Obuobisa-Darko & Domfeh, 2019) which result in an increase in performance (Ohemeng et al., 2020; Anitha, 2014). Again, employees who perceive their leaders to be interested in their wellness, will reciprocate by putting in much effort to achieve set target (Obuobisa-Darko, & Domfeh, 2019; Ilies et al., 2007)). It can therefore be deduced and concluded that, the adoption of authentic leadership style will result in improved wellness and performance.

METHODOLOGY

Study Design, Sampling and Data Collection

This study adopts the exploratory qualitative research approach which helps to understand individual beliefs and values, cultures, experiences, and situations (Creswell & Poth, 2016; Hunter, McCallum, & Howes, 2019; Kalu & Bwalya, 2017). Qualitative research is also useful for exploring complex social phenomena that are difficult to measure with quantitative studies (Kalu & Bwalya, 2017; Yin, 2013). As the method of understanding the unique, dynamic and holistic nature of human beings (Creswell, 2014), this research approach is suitable for discovering how authentic leaders manage stress and ensure wellness of their followers in organisations. The qualitative research also allows flexibility in obtaining rich data from the participants in varied ways. Data were gathered by using semi-structured interviews as it guarantees flexibility in interacting with the study participants. This interview strategy not only allow the researcher to build rapport and interact freely with the interviewees, but also helps the interviewees to provide deep insight as they tell their stories (Patton, 2002).

The participants of the study were employees of the Public sector in Ghana. Potential participants were contacted via emails and phone calls inviting them to participate in the study. The principal aim and objective of the study including other relevant information were clearly explained to them. They were assured that participation in the study was completely voluntary and all information provided were confidential. Participants were asked to respond to an interview guide that has been designed based on the key research question the study seeks to answer. While a total of 46 individuals agreed to participate in the study after the initial contacts, only 32 participated in the study. All participants completed a consent form. Examples of the interview questions include do you see the characteristics of authentic leadership in your leader? Do you think these characteristics have any effect on how stress is managed and how it ensures wellness? Does your leader objectively analyse all relevant data before coming to a decision and accept information from subordinates? Does it influence your performance in any way? Tell me some of the causes of work stress, in your view can stress affect your performance and wellness level? and what strategies help you manage stress?

Majority of the interviews were conducted via telephone whiles a few were conducted in-person during lunch break at a location suggested by the respondents. The interviews lasted between 29 and 45 minutes each and were digitally recorded with the consent of the interviewees.

DATA ANALYSIS

Data was analysed using thematic analysis as this approach is valuable for gaining in-depth insight of the social phenomena of interest (Braun & Clarke, 2006). Thematic analysis is a method used by researchers for identifying, analysing and interpreting patterns of meaning within qualitative data. It is useful for recognising patterns within and across data in relation to participants' lived experience, views and perspectives, behaviour and practices (Clarke, Braun, & Hayfield, 2015). This method uses open coding by breaking down, classifying. examining, comparing, and conceptualising data (Ngulube, 2015; Nowell *et al.*, 2017). Themes were generated to capture relevant information that helped addressed the research question. As suggested by Fusch and Ness (2015), the analysis was stopped at the point of saturation of the data.

RESULTS AND DISCUSSION

This exploratory qualitative study sought to provide insights on the role of authentic leaders in managing employees' stress and ensuring wellness. The findings of the study are based on employees' views, experiences and opinions regarding how their leaders exhibit authentic leadership characteristics and how this influence how stress is managed, their wellness and performance. The thematic categories that emerged from the data analysis regarding employees' perceptions of how authentic leaders manage their stress and ensure their wellbeing and performance are authentic leader characteristics, objective analysis of data, self-regulation and relational transparency, stress management and performance.

Authentic Leader Characteristics

Authentic leaders are deeply aware of their personal values and beliefs, they are self-confident, genuine, reliable and trustworthy. They also focus on building the strengths of followers, broadening their thinking, and creating a positive and engaging organizational setting (Ilies, Morgeson, & Nahrgang, 2005). They are also described as genuine people who are true to themselves and what they believe in. They engender trust and develop genuine connection with others. Because people trust them, they can motivate others to high levels of performance rather than letting the expectations of others guide them, they are prepared to be their own person and go their own way (George *et al.*, 2007). According to George (2004) the five dimensions of authentic leadership include pursuing purpose with passion, practicing solid values, establishing enduring relationships, leading with heart and demonstrating self-discipline. Begley (2001, p. 354) adds that authentic leadership represents "a genuine kind of leadership – a hopeful, open-ended, visionary and creative response to circumstances". The respondents indicated that their leaders largely exhibit the authentic leadership characteristics:

My boss is honest, he treats us fairly in terms of work assignments, performance appraisal, payment of performance bonuses and employee recognition. He is accountable and ensures accountability at the workplace. Each of us is accountable for the outcomes of our assigned duties. (Participant 4)

Yes, he is fair, accountable and optimistic. He is just frankly honest, a trait I appreciate so much and wish every leader exhibits. (Participant 15)

My boss relates very well with his subordinates. He is honest and accountable and fair in dealing with subordinates. (Participants 18)

These characteristics according to the interviewees have impacted their wellness and performance in diverse ways:

Knowing that your leader is authentic promotes quality of life at work, and it makes me emotionally and psychologically sound. It is easy to approach and discuss issues with him or her, both personal and work-related matters that have direct or indirect effects on work performance outcomes. (Participant 3)

It does feel good to know that your leader is aware of the situations around and more when the leader actually shows empathy to your situation. (Participant 6)

Objective Analysis of Data

It is mandatory for authentic leaders to objectively analyze all relevant data before arriving at a decision. Such leaders also welcome followers' views that challenge their decisions, thoughts, and actions (Gardner *et al.*, 2005). They are noted for brainstorming, weighing options and encouraging their followers to suggest innovative ways of finding solutions to organizational challenges. This leadership characteristic has the potential of motivating followers to be strongly committed to carrying out the request of the leader. This demonstrate to followers that their views, opinions and contributions are valued and taking onboard in major decisions which impact their work outcomes. While majority of our interviewees confirm that their leaders objectively analyze data and considers their views in decision making, a very few of them think otherwise:

He practices the open-door policy and allow employees to suggest ways of dealing with difficult work situations as well as receiving input from subordinates regarding work designs and work flexibility arrangements. It makes me feel inclusive and valued as my suggestions are always taking on board in decision making. (Participants 18)

Hmmm, my leader doesn't listen to anyone at the unit. She takes all decisions alone and doesn't welcome the views of the rest of us.... it's like a one man show at the department. Well, sometimes I wonder if she is even mindful of the negative effect of this behavior on teamwork. Nursing is all about teamwork and as my leader doesn't take input from anyone, this will negatively impact work performance, service delivery and client satisfaction. (Participant 5)

Self-Regulation and Relational Transparency

A key aspect of self-regulation is the assessment of current behavior against set goals, whereby discrepancies between current states and end goals prompt the modification of thoughts and actions to enhance the possibility of goal attainment (Yeow & Martin, 2013). Individual behaviors are regulated using different psychological processes including feedback seeking, goal setting and self-monitoring (Guillaume *et al.,* 2014). Similarly, team behaviors are also regulated by team goal orientation, team monitoring and tracking progress towards collective goal attainment (Rapp et al., 2014). Relational transparency on the other hand, reflects the notion that an individual must act in accordance with one's true self (Luthans and Avolio, 2003). It is defined as "valuing and achieving openness and truthfulness in one's close relationships" (Gardner et al., 2005, p. 357). Algera and Lips-Wiersma (2012) maintain that being true to 'self-in-relationship' is one of the essential components of authentic leadership. Establishing enduring relational transparency is consistent with relational orientation and practicing solid values according to Gardner et al. (2011). Even though sharing of information is a key component of authentic leadership, Gardner et al. (2005) argue that leaders are often required to be relatively transparent in expressing their true emotions and feelings to followers. Thus, they are required to regulate and minimize displays of inappropriate or potentially damaging emotions that can have negative effect on followers. The participants of the study agreed that self-regulation and relational transparency are important attributes of effective leaders. They do not only influence how the leader relates with others and manages his/her own emotions, but also affect employees' wellness and ensure trust in management:

Being emotionally balance is important for my wellness. Emotional balance requires that the leader compartmentalise his/her emotions knowing where and how to interact with others, the people he/she is interacting with and the reasons and goal for the interactions. (Participant 12)

Exactly, faking is stressful so if you remain open and transparent, it helps in stress reduction and management. Being who you are in all situations is critical in demonstrating to your subordinates that you can be trusted; this ensures followers trust in leadership. (Participant 16)

Self-awareness of the leader is a reflection of his capacity to self-regulate. Thus, making the leader better at defusing tension and creates the environment for continuous dialogue. (Participant 1)

Empathy and understanding the other person's perspective is essential in reducing misunderstanding and conflict situations. (Participant 8)

One respondent reported that his manager relates well with followers but there is evidence of lack of emotional maturity in his behaviour. This assertion is supported by the response below:

Even though my leader is always approachable, he often experiences mood swings and his responses to issues are not predictable. You are therefore not sure of how he will react in one situation or the other. Of course, negative reactions could result in holding back on information and suggestions regarding work. This could slow down workflow and work processes. (Participant 10).

STRESS MANAGEMENT AND PERFORMANCE

According to the study participants, the sources of work stress include excessive workload, unhealthy work climate, role conflict, autocratic leadership, unfair appraisal, unfair disciplinary procedures and outcomes, inadequate resources, unfavourable work schedules, unplanned activities and meeting unrealistic deadlines. The findings of this study add to the work of Değirmenci et al. (2023) who found that excessive workload, role ambiguity, decrease in the number of customers, time pressure, long working hours, role conflict, low and unsteady income, closing the workplace for a long period and job insecurity are the major antecedents of stress at the workplace. The management of stress can be at the individual or organisational level (Robbins & Judge, 2017). Robbins and Judge (2017) comment further that individual employees are mainly responsible for reducing stress levels by adopting strategies such as time-management techniques, physical exercise, relaxation techniques, and social support networks. Employees can manage their time effectively to reduce stress by maintaining to-do lists, prioritising activities, doing the hard tasks first, and blocking out distraction-free time to accomplish tasks (Robbins & Judge, 2017). Employees' views on the effect of stress on job performance and wellness are expressed below:

Stress impact performance negatively. In recent time, most workers are doing long hours to meet targets, get extra hours of pay to help cater for the family needs or probably using absolute working tools etc. Assuming you know for sure that come what may you will not be dismissed from your job or suffer reduction in income, you can opt to reduce number of hours or sometimes work from home. You would have the peace of mind to perform better and be innovative. (Participant 20).

Effective stress management helps enhance performance, improve relationship with colleagues and superiors. Similarly, the use of technology has positive impact on how work is done. It facilitates fast delivery of tasks. Inadequate stress management strategies on the other hand, have negative effect on social relationship as it does not promote work-life balance. (Participant 10)

For example, the reduction of the work week to 3 days in the office and 2 days' work from home reduced the financial stress associated with daily commuting to work. Use of technology allowed workers to remain productive from anywhere including home. (Participant 8)

In relation to what strategies help respondents manage stress, majority of them reported that they manage stress via relaxation techniques, more sleep, talking to close friends and sometimes saying no to unimportant requests. Certainly, employees can benefit from social support network, through friends, family and colleagues who will be ready to share individuals' problems and offer suggestions to help manage stressful situations. Certain organisational activities and practices cause stress and this calls for leadership actions to facilitate its management. Such activities pertain mostly to task and role demands. Some strategies to manage these include improved employee selection and job placement, training, goal-setting, redesign of jobs, increased organisational communication, employee involvement, employee sabbaticals, and wellness programmes (Robbins & Judge, 2017). In addition, using proactive measures such as early support, providing workers with clear messages, aftercare attention and actively monitoring and protecting their wellbeing and concerns can be effective in managing employee stress (Greenberg et al., 2020). This assertion was confirmed by the interviewees:

Communicating, for example during the recent high rises in food and fuel prices, the leader spoke and empathise with the staff and actually took steps to get some extra financial support for the staff to cushion them during that period. This brought some relief in the area of financial stress. (Participant 8)

Participants also indicated that their organisations also use new technologies, work-life balance, effective communication and workplace diversity to manage stress. Adoption of proactive measures in managing employees' stress and ensuring their wellness including availability of adequate support from the organisation could reassure employees that the organisation cares about them and are interested in their wellbeing. The perception of positive treatment from the leadership of organisation can trigger the norm of reciprocity (Blau, 1964), where employees are obligated to pay back the organisation's favourable treatment with improved performance, organisational commitment, and organisational citizenship behaviours (Ridwan *et al.*, 2020).

IMPLICATIONS

Theoretically, this study contributes to the social exchange theory (Blau, 1964; Chang *et al.*, 2015; Homans, 1958) by providing evidence suggesting that employees often reciprocate favourable treatment from organisational leadership through improved performance, organisational commitment, psychological attachment, and intentions to remain in the organisation. Thus, leaders in organisations that seek to derive the best from their employees and maximise their human capital must adopt the authentic leadership style. Such leaders are "individuals who act in accordance with deep personal values and convictions to build credibility and win the respect and trust of followers by encouraging diverse viewpoints and building networks of collaborative relationships with followers and thereby lead in a manner that followers recognise as authentic" (Avolio et al., 2004, p. 806). They therefore attain high levels of authenticity and as a result know who they are, what they value, believe in and act upon those values and beliefs when interacting with others. In the same vein, it reinforces the claim of the happy-productive worker hypothesis. Thus, happy workers tend to outperform those who are less happy., Ultimately, the behavioural characteristics displayed by authentic leaders can relate positively to conducive organisational climate, satisfying manager-subordinate relationship and employee psychological wellbeing.

Practically, authentic leadership plays a significant role in employee work-related outcomes including stress management and wellness. As echoed by Walumbwa *et al.* (2008), authentic leader behaviour helps to promote positive psychological capacities and a positive ethical climate, which could influence employee performance and wellness. Organisations that desire to attain set goals, become more effective and achieve sustainable competitive advantage must not ignore authentic leadership style of governance at the workplace.

LIMITATIONS AND SUGGESTION FOR FUTURE RESEARCH

This study is not without limitations. Hence, the findings reported should be interpreted in light of the following limitations. First, the study did not focus on the entire public sector but only collected data from some selected institutions including health, education, and statistical service. It is therefore recommended that further studies could be carried out with focus on other public sector organisations to confirm how employees' perception of authentic leadership plays out in managing employees' stress and ensure their wellbeing and performance. Again, a comparative study between public and private sector organisations could be carried out to ascertain if there are differences in the outcome of the study. The study attempted to establish a link between authentic leadership, stress management, employee performance and wellness. Future studies could employ a mixed methods study design to investigate this association as the mixed method study design overcomes the weaknesses inherit in a single method study design.

CONCLUSION

Authentic leadership has been linked with a number of positive work outcomes at the individual level, including performance, creativity, work engagement and job satisfaction (Giallonardo, 2010; Grandey *et al.*, 2005). It has also been cited as one major way for effective stress management in crisis such as the pandemic (Sultana *et al.*, 2020). The findings of this study revealed that the characteristics of authentic leadership such as honesty, accountability and relational transparency are largely evident among the public sector organisations. Authentic leaders, the present study contends are able to analyse all data received objectively before making any decision (Gardner, *et al.*, 2005; Walumbwa et al., 2008). They are also able to analyse information on the causes of stress, be it organisational, environmental, or personal factors and identify the best strategy to adopt to manage it. Therefore, it can be concluded that the adoption of the authentic leadership style will facilitate the management of employees' stress and ensures their wellness.

REFERENCES

Abdullah, D. N. M. A., & Lee, O. Y. (2012). Effects of wellness programs on job satisfaction, stress and absenteeism between two groups of employees (attended and not attended). *Procedia: Social and Behavioral Sciences*, *65*, 479–484. doi:10.1016/j.sbspro.2012.11.152

AjayiS. (2018). Effect of stress on employee performance and job satisfaction: A case study of Nigerian banking industry. *Available at* SSRN 3160620. doi:10.2139/ssrn.3160620

Anitha, J. (2014). Determinants of employee engagement and their impact on employee performance. *International Journal of Productivity and Performance Management*, *63*(3), 308–323. doi:10.1108/IJPPM-01-2013-0008

Armstrong, M. (2006). A handbook of human resource management practice (10th ed.). Kogan Page.

Avolio, B. J., Walumbwa, F. O., & Weber, T. J. (2009). Leadership: Current theories, research, and future directions. *Annual Review of Psychology*, *60*(1), 421–449. doi:10.1146/annurev.psych.60.110707.163621 PMID:18651820

Bacchus, D. N. (2008). Coping with work-related stress: A study of the use of coping resources among professional *Black women. Journal of Ethnic & Cultural Diversity in Social Work*, *17*(1), 60–81. doi:10.1080/15313200801906443

Beddoes-Jones, F., & Swailes, S. (2015). Authentic leadership: Development of a new three pillar model. *Strategic HR Review*, *14*(3), 94–99. doi:10.1108/SHR-04-2015-0032

BerryL.MirabitoA. M.BaunW. B. (2020). What's the hard return on employee wellness programs? SSRN.

Blau, P. M. (1964). *Exchange and power in social life*. John Wiley and Sons.

Bolden, R., Gosling, J., Marturano, A., & Dennison, P. (2003). *A review of leadership theory and Competency frameworks*. Centre for leadership studies, University of Exeter. Retrieved on January 21, 2023 from http//: centers.exeter.ac.uk/cls/documents/mgmt.sandardspdf

Braun, V., & Clarke, V. (2006). Using thematic analysis in psychology. *Qualitative Research in Psychology*, *3*(2), 77–101. doi:10.1191/1478088706qp063oa

Burke, R. J., & Richardsen, A. M. (2014). Corporate wellness programs: An overview. In Corporate wellness programs: Linking employee and organizational health. Edward Elgar Publishing.

Chang, H. H., Tsai, Y. C., Chen, S. H., Huang, G. H., & Tseng, Y. H. (2015). Building long-term partnerships by certificate implementation: A social exchange theory perspective. *Journal of Business and Industrial Marketing*, *30*(7), 867–879. doi:10.1108/JBIM-08-2013-0190

Clarke, V., Braun, V., & Hayfield, N. (2015). Thematic analysis. *Qualitative Psychology: A Practical Guide to Research Methods, 3*, 222-248.

Corbin, C. B., & Pangrazi, R. P. (2001). Toward a uniform definition of wellness: A commentary. *President's council on physical fitness and sports research digest.*

Creswell, J. W. (2014). *Research Design: Qualitative*. Quantitative and Mixed Methods.

Creswell, J. W., & Poth, C. N. (2016). *Qualitative inquiry and research design: Choosing among five approaches*. Sage publications.

Cropanzano, R., & Mitchell, M. S. (2005). Social exchange theory: An interdisciplinary review. *Journal of Management*, *31*(6), 874–900. doi:10.1177/0149206305279602

Cropanzano, R., & Wright, T. A. (1999). A 5-year study of change in the relationship between well-being and job performance. *Consulting Psychology Journal*, *51*(4), 252–265. doi:10.1037/1061-4087.51.4.252

Cropanzano, R., & Wright, T. A. (2001). When a" happy" worker is really a" productive" worker: A review and further refinement of the happy-productive worker thesis. *Consulting Psychology Journal: Practice and Research, 53*(3), 182-199.

De Clercq, D., Haq, I. U., & Azeem, M. U. (2019). Time-related work stress and counterproductive work behavior: Invigorating roles of deviant personality traits. *Personnel Review*, *48*(7), 1756–1781. doi:10.1108/PR-07-2018-0241

Değirmenci, B., Durmaz, Y., Fidanoğlu, A., & Değirmenci, S. (2023). Psychological effects of COVID-19 phobia on industrial consumers: A case study in Turkey. *Journal of Business and Industrial Marketing*, *38*(1), 170–187. doi:10.1108/JBIM-04-2021-0221

Dhobale, R. S. (2009). Stress Management Training: A Boon to Employee Wellness! *The IUP Journal of Soft Skills*, *3*(1), 39–44.

Fisher, C. D. (2010). Happiness at work. *International Journal of Management Reviews*, *12*(4), 384–412. doi:10.1111/j.1468-2370.2009.00270.x

Ford, M. T., Cerasoli, C. P., Higgins, J. A., & Decesare, A. L. (2011). Relationships between psychological, physical, and behavioural health and work performance: A review and meta-analysis. *Work and Stress*, *25*(3), 185–204. doi:10.1080/02678373.2011.609035

Fusch, P. I., & Ness, L. R. (2015). Are we there yet? Data saturation in qualitative research. *Qualitative Report*, *20*(9), 1408. doi:10.46743/2160-3715/2015.2281

Gardner, W. L., Avolio, B. J., Luthans, F., May, D. R., & Walumbwa, F. (2005). "Can you see the real me?" A self-based model of authentic leader and follower development. *The Leadership Quarterly*, *16*(3), 343–372. doi:10.1016/j.leaqua.2005.03.003

Gardner, W. L., Cogliser, C. C., Davis, K. M., & Dickens, M. P. (2011). Authentic leadership: A review of the literature and research agenda. *The Leadership Quarterly*, *22*(6), 1120–1145. doi:10.1016/j.leaqua.2011.09.007

George, B. (2007). *True north: Discover your authentic leadership*. Jossey-Bass.

George, B., Sims, P., McLean, A. N., & Mayer, D. (2007). Discovering your authentic leadership. *Harvard Business Review*, *85*(2), 129. PMID:17345686

Giallonardo, L. M., Wong, C. A., & Iwasiw, C. L. (2010). Authentic leadership of preceptors: Predictor of new graduate nurses' work engagement and job satisfaction. *Journal of Nursing Management*, *18*(8), 993–1003. doi:10.1111/j.1365-2834.2010.01126.x PMID:21073571

Greenberg, N., Docherty, M., Gnanapragasam, S., & Wessely, S. (2020). Managing mental health challenges faced by healthcare workers during covid-19 pandemic. BMJ, 368, 2-4.

Guillaume, Y. R., Van Knippenberg, D., & Brodbeck, F. C. (2014). Nothing succeeds like moderation: A social self-regulation perspective on cultural dissimilarity and performance. *Academy of Management Journal*, *57*(5), 1284–1308. doi:10.5465/amj.2013.0046

Halkos, G., & Bousinakis, D. (2010). The effect of stress and satisfaction on productivity. *International Journal of Productivity and Performance Management*, *59*(5), 415–431. doi:10.1108/17410401011052869

Hall, J. C., Everett, J. E., & Hamilton-Mason, J. (2012). Black women talk about workplace stress and how they cope. *Journal of Black Studies*, *43*(2), 207–226. doi:10.1177/0021934711413272 PMID:22457894

Harms, P. D., Credé, M., Tynan, M., Leon, M., & Jeung, W. (2017). Leadership and stress: A meta-analytic review. *The Leadership Quarterly*, *28*(1), 178–194. doi:10.1016/j.leaqua.2016.10.006

Hill, B. (2020). Coronavirus: Origins, signs, prevention, and management of patients. *British Journal of Nursing (Mark Allen Publishing)*, *29*(7), 399–402. doi:10.12968/bjon.2020.29.7.399 PMID:32279552

Hoert, J., Herd, A. M., & Hambrick, M. (2018). The role of leadership support for health promotion in employee wellness program participation, perceived job stress, and health behaviors. *American Journal of Health Promotion*, *32*(4), 1054–1061. doi:10.1177/0890117116677798 PMID:27920214

Homans, G. C. (1958). Social behavior as exchange. *American Journal of Sociology*, *63*(6), 597–606. doi:10.1086/222355

Hosie, P. J., & Sevastos, P. (2009). Does the "happy-productive worker" thesis apply to managers? *International Journal of Workplace Health Management,* 2(2), 131-160.

Hunter, D., McCallum, J., & Howes, D. (2019). Defining exploratory-descriptive qualitative (EDQ) research and considering its application to healthcare. *Journal of Nursing and Health Care*, *4*(1).

Ilies, R., Morgeson, F. P., & Nahrgang, J. D. (2005). Authentic leadership and eudaemonic well-being: Understanding leader–follower outcomes. *The Leadership Quarterly*, *16*(3), 373–394. doi:10.1016/j.leaqua.2005.03.002

Ilies, R., Nahrgang, J. D., & Morgeson, F. P. (2007). Leader-member exchange and citizenship behaviours: A meta-analysis. *The Journal of Applied Psychology*, *92*(1), 269–277. doi:10.1037/0021-9010.92.1.269 PMID:17227168

Iskamto, D. (2021). Stress and its impact on employee performance. *International Journal of Social and Management Studies*, *2*(3), 142–148.

Jun, W. H., Yang, J., & Lee, E. J. (2018). The mediating effects of social support and a grateful disposition on the relationship between life stress and anger in Korean nursing students. *Asian Nursing Research*, *12*(3), 197–202. doi:10.1016/j.anr.2018.08.002 PMID:30130592

Kalu, F. A., & Bwalya, J. C. (2017). What makes qualitative research good research? An exploratory analysis of critical elements. *International Journal of Social Science Research*, *5*(2), 43–56. doi:10.5296/ijssr.v5i2.10711

Khan, H., Abbas, J., Kumari, K., & Najam, H. (2022). Corporate level politics from managers and employees perspective and its impact on employees' job stress and job performance. *Journal of Economic and Administrative Sciences*.

Kihara, L. N., & Mugambi, H. (2018). Effect of stress management strategies on employees' performance in the public service. *The Strategic Journal of Business & Change Management*, *5*(2), 2382–2405.

Koopmans, L., Bernaards, C., Hildebrandt, V., van Buuren, S., van der Beek, A. J., & de Vet, H. C. (2012). Development of an individual work performance questionnaire. *International Journal of Productivity and Performance Management*, *62*(1), 6–28. doi:10.1108/17410401311285273

Koopmans, L., Bernaards, C. M., Hildebrandt, V. H., Schaufeli, W. B., De Vet, H. C., & Van Der Beek, A. J. (2011). Conceptual frameworks of individual work performance: A systematic review. *Journal of Occupational and Environmental Medicine*, *53*(8), 856–866. doi:10.1097/JOM.0b013e318226a763 PMID:21775896

Kumar, A., De Bruyn, A. J., & Bushney, M. J. (2020). The employee wellness and employee engagement relationship in a parastatal. *Journal of Contemporary Management*, *17*(1), 1–15. doi:10.35683/jcm19094.53

Kumar, S., McCalla, M., & Lybeck, E. (2009). Operational impact of employee wellness programs: A business case study. *International Journal of Productivity and Performance Management*, *58*(6), 581–597. doi:10.1108/17410400910977109

Liao, H., Liang, R., He, H., Huang, Y., & Liu, M. (2022). Work stress, burnout, occupational commitment, and social support among Chinese pediatric nurses: A moderated mediation model. *Journal of Pediatric Nursing*, *67*, e16–e23. doi:10.1016/j.pedn.2022.10.009 PMID:36307294

Liao, L. F. (2008). Knowledge-sharing in R&D departments: A social power and social exchange theory perspective. *International Journal of Human Resource Management*, *19*(10), 1881–1895. doi:10.1080/09585190802324072

Luthans, F., & Avolio, B. J. (2003). Authentic leadership development. *Positive Organizational Scholarship*, *241*(258), 1–26.

Mattke, S., Schnyer, C., & Van Busum, K. R. (2013). A review of the US workplace wellness market. *Rand Health Quarterly*, *2*(4), 7. PMID:28083279

Motowidlo, S., & Kell, H. (2012). Job Performance. In *Handbook of Psychology* (pp. 82–103). Wiley Online Library.

Muis, M., Nai'em, M. F., Arsin, A. A., Darwis, A. M., Thamrin, Y., & Hans, N. A. P. (2021). The effect of multiple role conflicts and work stress on the work performance of female employees. *Gaceta Sanitaria*, *35*, S90–S93. doi:10.1016/j.gaceta.2020.12.025 PMID:33832638

Mullins, L. J. (2007). *Management and organisational behaviour*. Pearson education.

Nam, T. (2014). Technology use and work-life balance. *Applied Research in Quality of Life*, *9*(4), 1017–1040. doi:10.100711482-013-9283-1

Ngulube, P. (2015). Qualitative data analysis and interpretation: systematic search for meaning. *Addressing research challenges: Making headway for developing researchers, 131*, 156.

Nguyen, B., Chang, K., Rowley, C., & Japutra, A. (2016). Organizational citizenship behavior, identification, psychological contract and leadership frames: The example of primary school teachers in Taiwan. *Asia-Pacific Journal of Business Administration*, *8*(3), 260–280. doi:10.1108/APJBA-01-2016-0010

Nowell, L. S., Norris, J. M., White, D. E., & Moules, N. J. (2017). Thematic analysis: Striving to meet the trustworthiness criteria. *International Journal of Qualitative Methods*, *16*(1), 1–13. doi:10.1177/1609406917733847

Obuobisa-Darko, T., & Ameyaw Domfeh, K. (2016). Authentic Leadership and Employee Engagement the Mediating Role of Trust: A Framework for Future Research and Practice. *International Journal of Business and Management*, *4*(9), 312–320.

Obuobisa-Darko, T., & Domfeh, K. A. (2019). Leader behaviour to achieve employee engagement in Ghana: A qualitative study. *International Journal of Public Leadership*, *15*(1), 19–37. doi:10.1108/IJPL-04-2018-0018

Ohemeng, F. L., Obuobisa Darko, T., & Amoako-Asiedu, E. (2020). Employee engagement and task performance in state-owned enterprises in developing countries: The case study of the power sector in Ghana. *Journal of Public Affairs*, *20*(2), e2021. doi:10.1002/pa.2021

Oruh, E. S., Mordi, C., Dibia, C. H., & Ajonbadi, H. A. (2021). Exploring compassionate managerial leadership style in reducing employee stress level during COVID-19 crisis: The case of Nigeria. *Employee Relations: The International Journal*, *43*(6), 1362–1381. doi:10.1108/ER-06-2020-0302

Ott-Holland, C. J., Shepherd, W. J., & Ryan, A. M. (2019). Examining wellness programs over time: Predicting participation and workplace outcomes. *Journal of Occupational Health Psychology*, *24*(1), 163–179. doi:10.1037/ocp0000096 PMID:28872333

Patton, M. Q. (2002). Two decades of developments in qualitative inquiry: A personal, experiential perspective. *Qualitative Social Work: Research and Practice*, *1*(3), 261–283. doi:10.1177/1473325002001003636

Peiró, J. M., Montesa, D., Soriano, A., Kozusznik, M. W., Villajos, E., Magdaleno, J., . . . Ayala, Y. (2021). Revisiting the happy-productive worker thesis from a Eudaimonic perspective: A systematic review. *Sustainability, 13*(6), 3174.

Rapp, T. L., Bachrach, D. G., Rapp, A. A., & Mullins, R. (2014). The role of team goal monitoring in the curvilinear relationship between team efficacy and team performance. *The Journal of Applied Psychology*, *99*(5), 976–987. doi:10.1037/a0036978 PMID:24865579

Ridwan, M., Mulyani, S. R., & Ali, H. (2020). Improving employee performance through perceived organizational support, organizational commitment, and organizational citizenship behavior. *Systematic Reviews in Pharmacy, 11*(12).

Robbins, S. P., & Judge, T. A. (2009). *Organisational behaviour* (13th ed.). Pearson, Prentice Hall.

Robbins, S. P., & Judge, T. A. (2017). *Organizational Behavior* (Global Edition). Pearson.

Rotundo, M., & Sackett, P. R. (2002). The relative importance of task, citizenship, and counterproductive performance to global ratings of job performance: A policy-capturing approach. *The Journal of Applied Psychology*, *87*(1), 66–80. doi:10.1037/0021-9010.87.1.66 PMID:11916217

Saglam, Y. C., Çankaya, S. Y., Golgeci, I., Sezen, B., & Zaim, S. (2022). The role of communication quality, relational commitment, and reciprocity in building supply chain resilience: A social exchange theory perspective. *Transportation Research Part E, Logistics and Transportation Review*, *167*, 102936. doi:10.1016/j.tre.2022.102936

Sahoo, S. R. (2016). Management of Stress at Workplace. *Global Journal of Management and Business Research. Administrative Management*, *16*(6), 1–8.

Saleem, F., Malik, M. I., & Qureshi, S. S. (2021). Work stress hampering employee performance during COVID-19: Is safety culture needed? *Frontiers in Psychology*, *12*, 655839. doi:10.3389/fpsyg.2021.655839 PMID:34512434

Savard, Y. P. (2023). Work-family spillover of daily positive affect onto performance: The moderating role of domain identity salience. *European Review of Applied Psychology*, *73*(2), 100819. doi:10.1016/j.erap.2022.100819

Seaward, B. L. (2019). *Essentials of Managing Stress* (2nd ed.). Jones & Bartlett Learning.

Sherman, G. D., Lee, J. J., Cuddy, A. J., Renshon, J., Oveis, C., Gross, J. J., & Lerner, J. S. (2012). Leadership is associated with lower levels of stress. *Proceedings of the National Academy of Sciences of the United States of America*, *109*(44), 17903–17907. doi:10.1073/pnas.1207042109 PMID:23012416

Shin, J. T., Jeong, M., Oh, H., & Tierney, E. (2017). Exploring determinants of meeting planners' commitment to the business relationships with destination management companies. *Journal of Convention & Event Tourism*, *18*(2), 135–158. doi:10.1080/15470148.2016.1237317

Sinding, K., & Waldstrom, C. (2014). *Organisational Behaviour*. McGraw-Hill Education.

Solnet, D., Subramony, M., Golubovskaya, M., Snyder, H., Gray, W., Liberman, O., & Verma, R. (2020). Employee wellness on the frontline: An interactional psychology perspective. *Journal of Service Management*, *31*(5), 939–952.

Steigleder, J., Buhr, L., Ehm, J. H., Gawrilow, C., & von Suchodoletz, A. (2023). Changes in subjective stress experiences and self-efficacy beliefs of preschool teachers in Germany: A longitudinal study during 12 months of the COVID-19 pandemic. *Teaching and Teacher Education*, *124*, 104015. doi:10.1016/j.tate.2023.104015 PMID:36628186

Sultana, U. S., Tarofder, A. K., Darun, M. R., Haque, A., & Sharief, S. R. (2020). Authentic Leadership effect on Pharmacists Job stress and satisfaction During COVID-19 Pandemic: Malaysian Perspective. *Talent Development & Excellence*, *12*, 1824–1841.

Tsai, J. C. A., & Kang, T. C. (2019). Reciprocal intention in knowledge seeking: Examining social exchange theory in an online professional community. *International Journal of Information Management*, *48*, 161–174. doi:10.1016/j.ijinfomgt.2019.02.008

Tsui, P. L. (2021). Would organizational climate and job stress affect wellness? An empirical study on the hospitality industry in Taiwan during COVID-19. *International Journal of Environmental Research and Public Health*, *18*(19), 10491. doi:10.3390/ijerph181910491 PMID:34639791

Varga, S., Mistry, T. G., Ali, F., & Cobanoglu, C. (2021). Employee perceptions of wellness programs in the hospitality industry. *International Journal of Contemporary Hospitality Management*, *33*(10), 3331–3354. doi:10.1108/IJCHM-12-2020-1417

Viswesvaran, C., & Ones, D. S. (2000). Perspectives on models of job performance. *International Journal of Selection and Assessment*, *8*(4), 216–226. doi:10.1111/1468-2389.00151

Walumba, F. O., Wang, P., Wang, H., Schaubroeck, J., & Avolio, B. J. (2010). Psychological processes linking authentic leadership to follower behaviours. *The Leadership Quarterly*, *21*(5), 901–914. doi:10.1016/j.leaqua.2010.07.015

Walumbwa, F., Avolio, B., Gardner, W., Wensıng, T., & Peterson, S. (2008). Authentic leadership: Development and validation of a theory-based measure. *Journal of Management, 34*(1), 89–126. doi:10.1177/0149206307308913

Warr, P., & Nielsen, K. (2018). *Wellbeing and work performance. In Handbook of well-being*. DEF Publishers.

World Health Organization. (2014). *Constitution*. https://www.who.int/about/who-we-are/constitution

Wright, T. A., Cropanzano, R., & Bonett, D. G. (2007). The moderating role of employee positive well-being on the relation between job satisfaction and job performance. *Journal of Occupational Health, 12*(2), 93–104.

Wright, T. A., Cropanzano, R., Denney, P. J., & Moline, G. L. (2002). When a happy worker is a productive worker: a preliminary examination of three models. *Canadian Journal of Behavioural Science/ Revue canadienne des sciences du comportement, 34*(3), 146-150.

Wu, C. H., Chen, I. S., & Chen, J. C. (2017). A study into the impact of employee wellness and job satisfaction on job performance. *International Journal of Organizational Innovation, 10*(2), 253–269.

Xu, J., & Thomas, H. C. (2011). How can leaders achieve high employee engagement? *Leadership and Organization Development Journal, 32*(4), 399–416. doi:10.1108/01437731111134661

Yeow, J., & Martin, R. (2013). The role of self-regulation in developing leaders: A longitudinal field experiment. *The Leadership Quarterly, 24*(5), 625–637. doi:10.1016/j.leaqua.2013.04.004

Yin, R. K. (2013). Validity and generalization in future case study evaluations. *Evaluation, 19*(3), 321–332. doi:10.1177/1356389013497081

Zelenski, J. M., Murphy, S. A., & Jenkins, D. A. (2008). The happy-productive worker thesis revisited. *Journal of Happiness Studies, 9*(4), 521-537.

Zhang, T. C., Kandampully, J., & Choi, H. Y. (2014). The role of employee wellness programme in the hospitality industry: A review of concepts, research, and practice. *Research in Hospitality Management, 4*(1 & 2), 45–54. doi:10.1080/22243534.2014.11828313

Chapter 3
Managing Stress Among Learners During the Crisis in India:
A Qualitative Approach

Deepanshi Aggarwal
Maharshi Dayanand University, Rohtak, India

Seema Rathee
Maharshi Dayanand University, Rohtak, India

ABSTRACT

The virus outbreak is the utmost recent massive worldwide crisis of health. This novel virus sickness is terrifying and distressing for the whole world. This virus has impacted all the sectors of the economy, and the education sector is no exception. Thus, the primary goal of this chapter is to highpoint the stress levels among learners and to determine the ways out in order to manage stress among learners during the pandemic in order to make learning effective. Information regarding the levels of stress and the coping way out of the stress among learners during pandemic will be gathered from a variety of reliable periodicals, websites, articles, and other e-content. According to the study's findings, academic, ecological, societal, and well-being issues wholly add to the stress development. Further, students' stress levels are quite high, and as the number of days passes, so does their stress level. Yoga and digression therapy, such as devoting time with loved ones and watching television, are also used by learners as coping tactics.

INTRODUCTION

"Instead of rushing unconsciously into your day set aside a few minutes to sit quietly with yourself. Make sure you are calm, centred with your intention for the day. This way you are prepared for a harmonious positive experience"

DOI: 10.4018/978-1-6684-8565-1.ch003

The virus outbreak is the utmost recent massive worldwide crisis of heath and continually expanding virus. In footings of wide-reaching analysis, the contemporary virus has surpassed previous pandemics. This marks the first time that the entire universe has been touched at the same moment severely in a very short period of time. Due to the high mortality rate of COVID-19 and accompanying issues such as fiscal instability, employment uncertainty, anxiety, this novel virus sickness is terrifying and distressing for the whole world. Equally the virus and its comprehensive consequences continue to reveal internationally and in our communal, it is natural for individuals to have a varied array of views, emotions, and responses. We have to recognise that the virus is more than simply a medical concern; it also has a societal, behavioral, and cognitive effect on individuals. Anxiety, sleep issues, fear and other sorts of psychiatric illness are linked to being isolated and wearing masks. Many learners face psychological challenges as a result of the pandemic's expansion, which impacted their grades as well as their whole disposition. Nations all over the world put draconian controls on their residents in an attempt to limit the spread. The government switched its offline educational system to e-learning, closing public gathering locations and imposing travel restrictions. The most distressing component is quarantine. Living under quarantine, commonly referred as lockdown, can also have serious mental consequences for everyone. The effects of quarantine on three elements of mental health are significant: individuality, competency and connectivity. Every problem is being dominated by stress.

Stress, according to Hans Selye, is "the nonspecific response of the body to any demand". Everyone is subjected to stress at a certain point in their lives. "Stress as a scientific concept suffers the problem of being too widely known and too poorly understood," stated Hans Selye, a physicist who popularised the conception of stress. Regardless of being one of the utmost ubiquitous experiences of human, stress is astonishingly challenging to quantify. Stress, in accordance to scientists, "is a force or event that disrupts normal stability, equilibrium, or functioning". In today's world, stress has become an intrinsic element of lifespan, it affects individuals of all ages and is no longer constrained to adults. COVID 19s contribute to higher learner stress. Beyond an uncertainty, the most frequently stated barrier to academic performance is stress. Some sorts of distress can actually be good for our health since they sharpen our thoughts and reflexes and push us to grow and progress. But when stress persists for an extended duration, it can become a burden or even a health concern.

Thus, the primary goal of this paper is to highpoint the stress levels among learners and to determine the way outs in order to manage stress among learners during pandemic in order to make learning effective.

REVIEW OF LITERATURE

Bokde *et al* (2020) in their research study highlights the impact of pandemic and lockdown on the educational institutions as well as on the students. Furthermore, the research suggested some measures to overcome with the impact of this adversity and concluded that some hygiene related factors and socio-economic are required to reshape the education sector. *Jena (2020)* in his research study shows the core effects of Covid on education sector along with the steps taken by higher education authorities for the undisrupted educational services. In addition to this, suggestions are provided to rebuild the educational sector. The results of the study revealed that MHRD have launched many virtual platforms which helps in turn in the smooth educational services. Mahapatra and Sharma (2020) the study uncovers the challenges faced by the students during covid while learning and the policy measures to cope out with those challenges. Tarkar (2020) in her research study explains the influence of pandemic on education sector in a crisp manner along with the suggestive methods to overcome from this pandemic. Tari and Amonkar (2021*)* in their research study discusses the pros and cons of the pandemic on the education sector accompanied by the measures taken by policymakers for the continuous educational services. Further, the study suggests some tips how to recover from this adversity. Rubilar and Oros (2021) in their study they identify the events which teachers/tutors perceived as a threat in online learning due to virus outbreak. Wirkus *et al* (2021) in their research study investigates the coping strategies of stress for learners during pandemic in Poland. By collecting the data from 577 participants from 17 universities the study concluded that the young students having lowest coping skills. Banjanirat (2022) examines the levels of stress and the influence of stress on the learners of Thailand. After collecting the required data from 270 students and applying Multiple Regression tool the study revealed that 45.60 percent learners have high level of stress. Panis (2022) in this study author discusses about the stress management of schoolteachers during pandemic in aborlan north. After collecting the data from 39 permanent teachers the results of the study revealed they all are in high stress. According to a review of the literature, the majority of the studies on stress management in the education sector during pandemics were conducted outside of India, and the studies that were conducted in India were usually focused on assessing the influence of pandemic on education sector, what challenges are faced by learners and teachers both during pandemic, and the level of stress experienced by learners and teachers during pandemic. *The current study attempts to fill a vacuum by highlighting the levels of stress among learners during a pandemic in India, as well as approaches to manage stress among learners during a virus outbreak in India.*

Research Method

The research design of the study is descriptive in nature. A Qualitative approach will be adopted to achieve the aforementioned objectives of the study. To acquire data on the current study, researchers combed through many reports from national and international agencies on the Covid-19 pandemic. Information regarding the levels of stress and the coping way out of the stress among learners during pandemic, will be gathered from a variety of reliable periodicals, websites, articles and various other e-contents etc.

Level of Stress

Despite the fact that stress is a basic human instinct, it was discovered that determining and quantifying stress is challenging because "there has been no description of stress that everyone accepts" and "people have very different beliefs about their concept of stress." They further claim that defining stress without mentioning positive stress, "its bodily repercussions, or the body's inherent fight-or-flight reaction is insufficient. Stress levels can be classified based on the current scenario" (Veena, 2016).

Acute stress

Acute stress is the most common sort of stress that everyone experiences at a certain time during their lives, and it is triggered by recent or anticipated events. It could be good or detrimental. It appears unexpectedly as a consequence of unexpected or upsetting events. It normally goes away by itself or after the stressful incident is over. Acute stress somehow doesn't normally cause serious health problems. For example, students' stress preceding writing tests or exams; experiencing a rollercoaster ride can cause acute stress, but in a delightful way. The excitement of a fun event is a type of positive acute stress. A car collision is a generator of acute negative stress. There is absolutely nothing problematic with enduring acute stress as soon as it does not last too long or happens on a continuous basis. This form of stress is common and easy to recognise. Jena (2020) lists the following as indicators of acute stress:

Ø Stomach pain, including heartburn, diarrhoea, and reflux of acid.
Ø Amplified pressure of blood and rate of heart.
Ø Chest pain or breath shortness.
Ø Headaches, backache, and pain in jaw.

Because acute stress is so frequent and seems to last for such brief period of time, it is usually simple to manage and cure.

Acute Episodic Stress

Acute episodic stress is a recurrent type of stress that occurs repeatedly. People suffering with this stress are frequently overpowered by it and struggle to manage it. This is the type of stress that comes and goes, occasionally in a rhythm. Individuals that experience this stress are virtually constantly in "full panic mode," are frequently irritated and worried, and might be predisposed to persistent upsetting. It is characterized with concern and anguish over things that are happening to you or around you. If you are a "type A" personality, you may be more prone to this. Type A people are gregarious, motivated, meticulously ordered, highly status-conscious, intolerant, nervous, practical, and obsessed with scheduling. Individuals with Type A dispositions are massively high "perfectionists". You may experience a heightened feeling of earnestness and a desire to complete tasks that may turn into overpowering. For instance, instead of studying continuously throughout the time, students have the option of studying the evening before a test. Because it has become a habit, this form of stress is episodic. The symptoms of episodic stress are similar to those of acute stress, although they might be more severe or persistent. According to the American Psychology Association (2020), "some symptoms of long-term episodic stress include: chronic headaches or migraines, hypertension, and heart disease. People who suffer from episodic stress often regard it as a regular part of life and may be unaware of its detrimental effects".

It has been stated that acute episodic stress sufferers may have difficulty obtaining counselling since they are acclimated to experiencing its symptoms and regard them as normal.

Chronic Stress

Chronic acute stress is defined as continuous stress that wears you down. Chronic stress is more likely if there is no end in sight, if there is no way out. It frequently arises in response to situations that appear depressing and out of your control, such as a broken marriage, a toxic job, or poverty. This type of stress has an influence on your health and can result in heart problems, strokes, or even cancer, among other concerns. Chronic stress needs seeking help. Chronic stress treatment can be tough, and it almost always necessitates the support of an expert in order to achieve long-term progress in healing.

Diverse Stressors Among Learners Throughout Pandemic

Everyone, however, processes it differently and possesses their own set of stressors. The authors' recent analysis found the following usual stressors:

Academic

This could be the utmost frequent longstanding stressor for learners. Leaners life has many benefits, but it also has its drawbacks. These compressions can induce unease and episodes of sadness in people who are now experiencing depression or who are predisposed to it. One of the chief types of stress in the learning process of students has been identified as academic stress. It is undeniably among the most critical difficulties that the current leaners are facing during COVID 19. It is also becoming an increasingly stressful issue for both teachers and pupils. Without a doubt, management of stress has been one of the cornerstones for learners' dedication to their academic achievement, pupil associations with class mates, and the more they try or concern, the less they can study efficiently (Albers et al, 2017). When they try to relax, all they can think about is studying. Some people are afflicted by academic stress and are unable to spend time with their families. Even if it appears untroublesome at first, if not remedied, it will have a negative impact on the learner performance.

Class Planning and Credit Loading

Scheduling classes for multiple disciplines might be tough. Trying to sign up for classes at times that are convenient for you and ensuring that you are having all of your mandatory classes are just a few of the numerous factors to consider. For the first time, some students may be designing their own schedules. You might be confused regarding how many credits to acquire, or which class durations are best for your academic success. You may grow irritated with yourself if your schedule is not what you imagined after a few weeks of classes.

Approaches for Dealing with Stress Caused by Class Planning and Credit Loading

If your schedule is becoming burdensome, keep in mind that it is not permanent. Your existing lessons will cease, and you will need to create a completely new schedule in a matter of weeks or months. Take advantage of this prospect to create a timetable that is well well-matched to your needs. Create your schedule adaptable.

Exams and Grades

Another source of stress for learners is academic achievement. You might sense heaviness to achieve grades in your classes for a variety of reasons, including satisfying the outlooks of educators, parents, and even yourself. Better grades satisfy your wish to continue your education and pursue your preferred profession. You may perhaps study constantly but become so stressed about taking an examination that you are incompetent to perform well. Fear of not studying enough is one of the reasons of exam stress. Furthermore, due to the increasing workload and significant difficulties of harmonizing your educations, private duties, work schedule and social life might be hard-hitting. As a result, this is also a source of stress.

Approaches to Overcome from Exams and Grades Stress

Tackling education stress might be difficult because you are continuously fenced by your stresses and by the same token stressed peers. However, you are there to acquire and propagate, not to receive consecutive A's on your report card. Rather of focusing on grades, prioritise your education. If you take your studies seriously, grades will follow. Study as considerable as you can. Concentrate on only one exam at a time. Avoid thinking about your next exam. Consider the subject matter, not the exam. Do not visualize the exam while studying. Study in the same area where you will take the test or do timed practise questions. Whether it's hiring a teacher to assist clarify topics, having someone double-check your work, finding someone to help you study more efficiently can make all the difference.

Health

According to an APA (2020) survey, 63 percent of respondents describe "health-related problems" as a source of stress, following academic stress. Concerns with health, in particular, may be a big stressor for college learners since they believe it affects academic performance. It was also found that over 30 percent of learners' academic performance was hampered by a medical disease tend to range from allergies to bronchitis. Irrespective of whether the root is a unpretentious cold, a psychological health circumstance, or a prolonged sickness, one thing stays constant: being unwell can make it tough to be consistent with your studies. If you are infectious, you ought to escape going to class, which means you will miss out on valuable info from your educator. Even if you are not infectious but are simply tired, you may lack the stamina to concentrate on the instruction, learning, and projects.

Approaches to Sustain the Health as a Learner

If an illness is spreading on your institution or in your community, try to evade interaction with anybody who is susceptible, wash-down your hands regularly, and keep an eye on other preventative measures. Wearing a mask, social alienation, sanitising, not sharing your items, and not having a gathering were all options in the current COVID 19 scenario. Accept that, despite your best efforts, you may become ill on occasion. If you do get sick, take upkeep of yourself by resting as much as possible and taking antibiotics before returning to your usual activities. Maintain a healthy diet. Eat well and eat correctly. Caffeine, for instance, might aggravate the physical symptoms of test stress.

Personal

The exertion of creating societal connectedness is additional source of stress. Afterward you enter college, your connections with friends, family members, and your significant other may alter. Learners usually dearth the time and/or prospect to form interpersonal ties. Academia might be more essential than it has ever been, and dealing with the challenges that come with it may leave you with less energy to give to your dear ones. Feeling separated from your support network, on top of juggling with educational duties, might generate stress in your life.

Approaches to Maintain Rapport in Institution

Make a conscious effort to exclusively associate with the individuals whose company you love. Your time at campus is too short to dedicate it communicating with individuals you don't get along with. Whether you're working on a group assignment online or participating in a class discussion through chat, you have the option to be judicious about who you devote additional energy to. You can establish lifetime friends in college, so focus your time and attention on the connections that are important to you. Enriched direction for new-fangled graduate learners, more leeway in prerequisites, and strengthening the starring role of faculty advisors/councillors are some strategies for reducing stress.

Finances

Traditional schooling has become increasingly expensive in recent times. Whenever coupled with other costs such as accommodation, meals, and literature, leaners may surface fiscal problems. You may be concerned about money even though you qualify for financial help, receive aid from family members, or work during the school year. Learners may face further stress as a consequence of the learner debts they must return after graduation. Debt can be a burden before you finish schooling as it might influence your funds for ages later college as well as during it. Parallel to being bodily and possibly expressively alone, you may also be financially alone. Rent, food, gas, and amusement are all suddenly your financial responsibility. When you are not in class, you may find that you need to work part-time. Even if you take a fellowship, a credit, or a "full ride" to assist you in paying for it wholly, there will still be calls made, queries, documentation, and cut-off date to meet in order for the cash to keep flowing.

Approaches to Overcome Stress from Finances

Positive thinking has been demonstrated in studies to increase physical well-being, reduce emotions of sadness, and reduce levels of distress. Remember the reason you decided to seek a degree in the initially and remind oneself that it may result in better job opportunities after you graduate. Professionals continue to feel that education is an investment worth making in the long run.

Family Life

For voluminous leaners, college is the initial period they have resided far from home or spent any considerable amount of time away from their family. Aside than that, it's a strange setting. The whole thing is different, including the meals, individuals, and alive arrangements. Nevertheless, most learners adjust to their novel surroundings devoid of issue, the first few weeks of college can be difficult. Even if you are ecstatic about the changes, this is true. Keep in mind that even favourable changes can cause tension. In college life, you must strike an equilibrium amid college, private, and additional responsibilities. Academic loads at all stages of learning frequently upsurge and demand additional work. Trying to preserve with that on uppermost of your occupation and personal commitments might complement extra strain to your day — particularly if your family and work commitments are so arduous that you fall behind on your academic work. It can be especially difficult for non-traditional learners to strike that balance. While customary leaners may be concerned about missing another phone call from their parents, non-traditional learners may have children of their own to care for. Instead of education, you may need to devote your energies to fiscally sustaining your family or considerate for ailing parents or kids if you have any.

Approaches to Balance Family and Work Life

These tactics might assist you in establishing boundaries between different aspects of your life so that you can give each one the attention it requires. Remember that being able to adjust to new issues and requests is equally vital. If you believe you won't be able to make required changes to your plans, you may feel more anxious.

Effective Stress-Reduction Techniques

Face the Stressor

The utmost operative way to deal with stress is to address the source of it instantaneously. If your chaotic timetable is producing your anxiety, take a step back and contemplate what you can do. If a traditional university isn't meeting your scheduling demands, ponder joining to a virtual institution that may be a well fit.

Time Administration

One of the most important stress-relieving approaches is proper time management. Time must be utilised wisely, whether for recreation, labor, or study. Learners should be capable to create and adhere to a schedule. Pick a soothing pause amid study and work though if it's only breathing period. Creating a timetable and utilizing while effectively reveals aims and primacies. Learners should continuously strive to prepare in advance and avoid procrastination in order to properly handle stress. Nevertheless, if they are pushing themselves too thin and falling behind, it is at all times best to remain cool and engrossed. As a result, create a "To Do" list or a calendar, preserve track of cut-off date and timetables, and mug up to say "No." in order to reduce stress.

Being Well-Organized

In academic life, organization is critical for dealing with stress. Stress can be greatly decreased by keeping academic notes organized, submitting assignments on time, and staying on top of all deadlines. Always maintain an organized system for taking notes, preserving track of assignments, and further vital materials. Accordingly, individuals be able to create a nice learning atmosphere in which they can concentrate and complete tasks. Furthermore, if they are well ordered, they can provide the peacetime of mind that originates with knowing where everything is, memorizing cut-off date and exam dates, and letting go the mind of some psychological clutter.

Sleep, Workout, and Diet

Stress can be greatly reduced with regular exercise, a balanced diet, and adequate rest. Leaners necessarily be well-rested so that the stress can be relieved, and they may live a stress-free life.

Surround Yourself with Dear Ones

Encircle yourself with individuals with whom you love spending time. If you don't discourse regarding what's upsetting you, presence of dear one makes you feel at comfort can reduce a proportion of stress. A mug of coffee with dear ones is all you requisite to return your stress levels to normal. Anxiety might also worsen if a person is isolated. You immediately feel a lot better after confiding in someone you trust. Aside from the physical benefits of stress management, learners can also get advantage from better-quality affiliations dear ones.

Relax a Bit

Between lectures, assignment, and other obligations, you might find that the mainstream of your days is occupied with strategies, actions, and duties that must be completed. Take a pause if you're feeling overwhelmed by everything you need to do. Plan an evening where you don't need to do anything, just to read a novel or to watch some comedy movies. "Every day may not be good, but every day contains something good. Try to find it."

Seek Expert Help

You might find yourself in need of further assistance than your precious ones can provide, or you may be dealing with circumstances that are too abundant for you to manage. Don't be scared to strive for professional aid. Even if you are an active learner, your institution most certainly has many support tools accessible to assist you.

Findings and Conclusion

People are also exhausted and anxious owing to the confinement during COVID-19. Learner s are suffering academically. All of this contributes to a disturbance in their mental condition. According to the study's findings, academic, ecological, societal, and well-being issues wholly add to the stress development. Further, students' stress levels are quite high, and as the number of days' passes, so does their stress level. Yoga and digression therapy, such as devoting time with loved ones and watching television, are also used by learners as coping tactics. Academic elements are the utmost key stressors, requiring the necessity for precise and concentrated approaches to significantly reduce the load of stress on students. The operative usage of current student welfare services, the creation of more "student-friendly" environments, and regular periodic extra - curricular activities with universal participation can all be effective stress relievers. Further, the majority of studies showed students favoured include management of stress education in the curriculum, thus actions should be taken to integrate it. Students' health is a big concern, so promoting good food and lifestyle practises must be stimulated. Furthermore, instructors, parents, and even learners themselves should be conscious that unrealistic academic attainment expectations can contribute to stress. In conclusion, consistent study habits and appropriate preparation can assist students in avoiding stress and increasing the effectiveness of their learning.

REFERENCES

Albers, B., & Pattuwage, L. (2017). Implementation in education: Findings from a scoping review. Evidence for Learning, 10.

Almojali, A. I., Almalki, S. A., Alothman, A. S., Masuadi, E. M., & Alaqeel, M. K. (2017). The prevalence and association of stress with sleep quality among medical students. *Journal of Epidemiology and Global Health*, *7*(3), 169–174. doi:10.1016/j.jegh.2017.04.005 PMID:28756825

American Psychological Association (APA). (2020, May 30). *Stress in the time of COVID 19*. APA.

Babicka-Wirkus, A., Wirkus, L., Stasiak, K., & Kozłowski, P. (2021). University students' strategies of coping with stress during the coronavirus pandemic: Data from Poland. *PLoS One*, *16*(7), e0255041. doi:10.1371/journal.pone.0255041 PMID:34310649

Banjanirat. (2022). Stress and burnout during crisis. *Journal of Higher Education*, *97*(8), 1603-1609.

Bansal, R. (2017). Challenges and future trends in commerce education in India. *International Journal of Techno-Management Research*, *5*(3), 25–35.

Bansal, R. (2018). Stress management at workplace. *International Journal of Techno-Management Research*, *5*(04), 29–32.

Bansal, R., Gupta, A., Singh, R., & Nassa, V. K. (2021, July). Role and impact of digital technologies in E-learning amidst COVID-19 pandemic. In *2021 Fourth International Conference on Computational Intelligence and Communication Technologies (CCICT)* (pp. 194-202). IEEE. 10.1109/CCICT53244.2021.00046

Bansal, R., Shuklaa, G., & Pruthi, N. (n.d.). *Higher education sector in India: Disruptions by COVID-19 and post covid trends*. Academic Press.

Bayram, N., & Bilgel, N. (2008). The prevalence and socio-demographic correlations of depression, anxiety and stress among a group of university students. *Social Psychiatry and Psychiatric Epidemiology*, *43*(8), 667–672. doi:10.100700127-008-0345-x PMID:18398558

Bokde, V., Kharbikar, H. L., Roy, M. L., Joshi, P., & Ga, A. (2020). Possible impacts of COVID-19 pandemic and lockdown on education sector in India. *Food and Scientific Reports*, *1*(Special Issue), 30–33.

Brooks, S. K., Webster, R. K., Smith, L. E., Woodland, L., Wessely, S., Greenberg, N., & Rubin, G. J. (2020). The psychological impact of quarantine and how to reduce it: Rapid review of the evidence. *Lancet*, *395*(10227), 912–920. doi:10.1016/S0140-6736(20)30460-8 PMID:32112714

Currie, C., Molcho, M., Boyce, W., Holstein, B., Torsheim, T., & Richter, M. (2008). Researching health inequalities in adolescents: The development of the Health Behaviour in School-Aged Children (HBSC) family affluence scale. *Social Science & Medicine*, *66*(6), 1429–1436. doi:10.1016/j.socscimed.2007.11.024 PMID:18179852

Dangi, R. R., & George, M. (2020). Psychological perception of students during COVID-19 outbreak in India. *High Technology Letters*, *26*(6), 142–144.

Eisenberg, D., Gollust, S. E., Golberstein, E., & Hefner, J. L. (2007). Prevalence and correlates of depression, anxiety, and suicidality among university students. *The American Journal of Orthopsychiatry*, *77*(4), 534–542. doi:10.1037/0002-9432.77.4.534 PMID:18194033

Fink, G. (2010). Stress: definition and history. *Stress Science: Neuroendocrinology, 3*(9), 319-328.

Freitas, A. R. R., Napimoga, M., & Donalisio, M. R. (2020). Assessing the severity of COVID-19. *Epidemiologia e Serviços de Saúde: Revista do Sistema Unico de Saúde do Brasil*, *29*, e2020119. PMID:32267300

Hunsley, J., Elliott, K., & Therrien, Z. (2014). The efficacy and effectiveness of psychological treatments for mood, anxiety, and related disorders. *Canadian Psychology*, *55*(3), 161–176. doi:10.1037/a0036933

Jena, P. K. (2020). Impact of Covid-19 on higher education in India. *International Journal of Advanced Education and Research*, *5*(3), 77–81.

Jennings, M. L. (2009). Medical student burnout: Interdisciplinary exploration and analysis. *The Journal of Medical Humanities*, *30*(4), 253–269. doi:10.100710912-009-9093-5 PMID:19865808

Kraag, G., Zeegers, M. P., Kok, G., Hosman, C., & Abu-Saad, H. H. (2006). School programs targeting stress management in children and adolescents: A meta-analysis. *Journal of School Psychology*, *44*(6), 449–472. doi:10.1016/j.jsp.2006.07.001

Lewis, J., & Webster, A. (2021). *Sort your brain out: boost your performance, manage stress and achieve more*. John Wiley & Sons.

Mahapatra, B., & Bhorekar, K. K. (2021). Analyzing the Economic Depression Post-COVID-19 Using Big Data Analytics. In *Emerging Technologies for Battling Covid-19* (pp. 309–325). Springer. doi:10.1007/978-3-030-60039-6_16

Mayordomo-Rodríguez, T., Meléndez-Moral, J. C., Viguer-Segui, P., & Sales-Galán, A. (2015). Coping strategies as predictors of well-being in youth adult. *Social Indicators Research*, *122*(2), 479–489. doi:10.100711205-014-0689-4

Panis, E. (2022). Implementation of School Learning Continuity Plan (SLCP) in Selected Public Secondary Schools of Aborlan North District in the Division of Palawan. *Journal of World Englishes and Educational Practices, 4*(3), 1-13.

Singh, R., & Bansal, R. (2020). Industry 4.0 in India: Challenges & opportunities. *New Paradigm in Business & Education, 160*.

Singh, R., & Bansal, R. (2020). Study of privatisation in Indian higher education: Pros & cons. *New Horizons in Commerce, IT & Social Sciences*, 91.

Tari, S., & Amonkar, G. (2021). Impact of covid on higher education in India. *Educational Resurgence Journal*, *2*(5), 22–27.

Tarkar, P. (2020). Impact of COVID-19 Pandemic on Education System. *International Journal of Advanced Science and Technology*, *29*(9), 3812–3814.

Thompson, A., & Gaudreau, P. (2008). From optimism and pessimism to coping: The mediating role of academic motivation. *International Journal of Stress Management, 15*(3), 269–288. doi:10.1037/a0012941

Vargas Rubilar, N., & Oros, L. B. (2021). Stress and burnout in teachers during times of pandemic. *Frontiers in Psychology, 12*, 756007. doi:10.3389/fpsyg.2021.756007 PMID:34899498

Veena, J. (2016). Short-term exposure to enriched environment rescues chronic stress-induced impaired hippocampal synaptic plasticity, anxiety, and memory deficits. *Journal of Neuroscience Research, 95*(8), 1602–1610. PMID:27862185

Wang, C., Pan, R., Wan, X., Tan, Y., Xu, L., Ho, C. S., & Ho, R. C. (2020). Immediate psychological responses and associated factors during the initial stage of the 2019 coronavirus disease (COVID-19) epidemic among the general population in China. *International Journal of Environmental Research and Public Health, 17*(5), 1729. doi:10.3390/ijerph17051729 PMID:32155789

Yasmin, H., Khalil, S., & Mazhar, R. (2020). COVID 19: Stress management among students and its impact on their effective learning. *International Technology and Education Journal, 4*(2), 65-74.

Chapter 4
Managing Stress and Overcoming Traumatic Workplace Betrayals

Denise Gates
Arkansas State University, USA

ABSTRACT

The purpose of this chapter was to explore the lived experiences of a middle-aged Caucasian production supervisor who worked in the manufacturing industry within the United States. The chapter emphasized the stress and trauma she endured, which primarily stemmed from repetitive, prolonged, and cumulative sexual harassment. It offered the salient themes that emerged as the participant discussed traumatic institutional betrayal as well as the stress that resulted from working in a culture that condoned sexual harassment and ignored pay disparities. Strategies to overcome stress and marginalization were discussed.

INTRODUCTION

Research suggests that happy workers are more productive (Albrecht & Marty, 2020; Luthans, Luthans, Luthans, 2021; Proto, 2016; Wang & Shi, 2022), so it may be beneficial for scholars and practitioners to explore the events that produce stress in the workplace and examine strategies to overcome said stress or trauma (Gates. 2010; Tyler, 2014). If happy workers are more engaged and more productive (Macey & Schneider, 2008; Albrecht & Marty, 2020), then organizations can enjoy greater success if they contribute to less stress in the lives of employees (Macey & Schneider, 2008; Albrecht & Marty, 2020). Therefore, it may be beneficial for scholars and practitioners to look for ways to eliminate bad stress and help employees strive for more balance (Gates, 2010) so organizational members can enjoy better interactions (Gates, 2003; 2008; 2019; 2021). Level of education also seemed to have a significant influence on level of stress with people at lower educational levels (teachers) reporting more stress than people with advanced degrees (Agai–Demjaha, Karadzinska Bislimovska, Mijakoski, 2015). Perhaps employees with advanced degrees are more adept at understanding emotional intelligence and understanding how to manage relationships which might enhance engagement (Wang & Shi, 2022) and reduce workplace

DOI: 10.4018/978-1-6684-8565-1.ch004

stress (Agai–Demjaha, Karadzinska Bislimovska, Mijakoski, 2015). Overall, stress and conflict remain topics that organizations must tackle and determine how to overcome (Luthans, Luthans, & Luthans, 2021) so that employees can enjoy more productivity.

LITERATURE REVIEW

Traumatic betrayals are betrayals that go beyond the typical betrayal. First noticed in parent-child dyads, betrayal trauma can occur in other relationships. This kind of trauma results when one realizes he/she does not have the life/reality he/she thought he/she had (Schmidt, Adams-Clark, & Freyd, 2023; Tyler 2014). An example of workplace betrayal could be a boss or colleague who steals somebody's work/research and takes credit for it in order to advance his/her own career. Another example of a workplace betrayal trauma could be an employee who has worked with a particular company for years, expecting to retire there, losing his/her job to a less qualified person the employee trained such as the employee's best friend. For some people, the sense of betrayal can be so traumatic that it becomes destabilizing (Guy, 2022; Schmidt, Adams-Clark, & Freyd, 2023).

Betrayal trauma can occur at several levels, such as institutional, parental, partner and interpersonal (Guy, 2022). For example, betrayal trauma can manifest in parent-child relationships. Children who expect their parents to protect them and to be loyal to them may feel betrayed when parents neglect or abandon them. A child who has a parent that sides with an abusive family member over the child complaining of abuse may experience betrayal trauma. People who have experienced betrayal trauma often talk about the betrayal over and over because they are traumatized by it. Similarly, individuals can experience workplace betrayal trauma or institutional betrayal trauma.

Institutional Betrayal

Institutional betrayal refers to the harmful response to reports of workplace abuse, ethical violations, or other illicit acts. When conduct deviates from what organizational members expect, individuals may experience shock, stress, anxiety, or even trauma, depending on the severity of the circumstances (Gates, 2009; 2010; Jablin, 2001; Schmidt, Adams-Clark, & Freyd, 2023). A prevalent type of workplace betrayal encompasses unsolicited and unwanted sexual conduct from a trusted organizational member such as a superior. An employee's relationship with his/her supervisor can vastly shape how he/she experiences an organization (Gates, 2009, 2010, 2011, 2019, 2021). Workplace sexual harassment causes negative psychological outcomes and stress (Fitzgerald, 2022). When organizations don't respond well to complaints about sexual harassment, these encounters compromise the quality of workplace climate and the quality of encounters for survivors of abuse (Fritzgerald, 2022; Guy, 2022; Schmidt, Adams-Clark, & Freyd, 2023). Functioning in workplaces where sexual harassment is the norm and complaints of abuse are ignored can be anxiety-producing or traumatic (Schmidt, Adams-Clark, & Freyd, 2023). These events tend to diminish an employee's job satisfaction, according to Schmidt, Adams-Clark, and Freyd (2023). Ultimately, institutional betrayal decreased job satisfaction, organizational commitment, and increased somatic symptoms. It leads to disengagement due to incivility causing job insecurity (Guo, Qui, & Gan, 2022). However, constructive responses to organizational challenges produced more positive outcomes. Supportive responses to complaints of sexual harassment are characterized as institutional courage. This environment embraces transparency and proactive problem-solving (Schmidt, Adams-Clark, & Freyd, 2023).

Institutional betrayal may also encompass an event that severely deviates from what employees consider the norm. When employees realize the reality they thought they had no longer exists, they feel betrayed (Guy, 2022; Tyler, 2014). Some examples of workplace betrayal could include sexual harassment from a trusted superior, stolen resources, learning that all the members of a team make more money than a given employee to provide the same quality of work to an organization. Betrayal could be stealing someone's research or stealing from someone at work. Workplace betrayal can also encompass reporting a wrongdoing and having those complaints ignored. It may also entail feelings of alienation and being subjected to incivility (LaSala, Wilson, Sprunk, 2016) when complaints are filed such as with whistleblowers. Whistleblowers identify and report incompetent, illicit, or unethical practices in the workplace. Sometimes they experience alienation and stress tied to reporting wrongdoing. Some of these whistleblowers encounter retaliation. Ultimately, people who experience and expose wrongdoing or incivility in the workplace may experience heightened stress and anxiety, resulting in greater disengagement due to being abused and/or reporting the violation (Guo, Qin, Gan, 2021).

When workplace violence as well as unethical or illicit conduct are ignored, organizational members suffer on many levels (Schmidt, Adams-Clark, & Freyd, 2023). The offenses are regarded as more egregious if they are not handled well. "When wrongdoings are reported and institutions turn a blind eye, it harms employees" (Tyler, 2014, p. 43). Organizations need systems in place that promote open communication and constructive problem-solving. "When institutions respond poorly to events such as sexual assaults [or sexual harassment], it increases the victims' emotional distress" (Tyler, 2014, p. 43). Severe emotional distress requires employees to exert more psychological resources (or energy) just to function at work. For some, the stress may cause them to be less engaged and less productive because the stress may compel them to question their job security (Guo, Qin, Gan, 2021). "So assault [including other workplace offenses] is toxic, but institutional betrayal is an additional level of harm," (Tyler, 2014, p. 43). Organizations must understand how to identify, assess, and manage institutional betrayal so as to create strategies for healthier and less stressful outcomes.

Assessing Institutional Betrayal

According to Smith and Freyd (2014), an institutional betrayal questionnaire they devised in 2013 is comprised of the following items: 1) Not taking proactive steps to prevent this type of experience 2) Creating an environment in which this type of experience seemed common or like no big deal 3) Creating an environment in which this experience seemed more likely to occur 4) Making it difficult to report the experience 5) Responding inadequately to the experience, if reported 6) Covering up the experience 7) Punishing you in some way for this experience (e.g., loss of privileges or status) 8) Creating an environment in which you felt discriminated against due to your sexual orientation 9) Responding differently to the situation based on your sexual orientation 10) Expressing a biased or negative attitude toward you and/or the situation based on your sexual orientation (Smith & Freyd, 2014, p. 582).

"This measure assesses individuals' experiences of institutional betrayal surrounding traumatic experiences, typically unwanted sexual experiences (see Table 1 for wording of items). The scale assesses a variety of distinct experiences that may co-occur in a powerful synergistic mix, much as benign and malignant sexism occur together. Importantly, the measure does not assess the degree to which individuals felt betrayed by an institution but rather asks whether the types of institutional inactions or actions described in the following sections occurred" (Smith & Freyd, 2014, p. 582)

The instrument seems to examine the quality of the communication climate as well as the quality of the interactions of people experiencing workplace betrayal. The level of stress may be contingent on the approach organizations take when dealing with concerns. When organizations deny or diminish the experiences of organizational members or fail to create a culture or climate conducive to organizational members being helped and/or taken seriously, organizational members may suffer greater stress and more trauma. Those organizations that implement a constructive strategy to dealing with workplace betrayal may find that organizational members are less prone to stress and trauma. "Systemic trauma must be met with systemic solutions, solutions that carry within them the ability to trans-form women's experiences." (Fitzgerald, 2017, p. 487).

Institutional Courage

The ability to constructively tackle messy workplace matters without denying them, changing the subject when tough topics are broached, or diminishing the experiences of the people complaining takes courage. The concept of institutional courage encompasses the process of openly addressing and being transparent about unethical and/or unlawful workplace violations (Schmidt, Adams-Clark, & Freyd, 2023). Institutional courage is promoted. It "appears to attenuate negative outcomes in both the employee workplace and health domains" (Schmidt, Adams-Clark, & Freyd, 2023, p. 25).

How can employees who have experienced workplace betrayals be socialized and supported? These employees can be encouraged to take advantage of the company's employee counseling services. The company can work to rebuild trust with these employees by displaying consistent and honest behavior. Colleagues should consider being transparent so that employees are not surprised by workplace decisions. Employees may want to seek support outside of the workplace and not rely solely on the workplace for emotional support. These employees may seek to align themselves with colleagues and employers that hold themselves to high ethical standards and work with companies that espouse values similar to the employees' own.

Tyler (2014) suggested that Human Resources personnel exhibit active listening skills when employees come to them was concerns. Workplace betrayals can cause trauma in employees, and the toxic people who inflict traumatic experiences on others need to be managed well. "Trauma can also result from institutional betrayal, such as when an employer ignores or minimizes bad things that have happened" (Tyler, 2014, p. 14). Blaming or invalidating responses from an organization can spur greater trauma. A healthy response, one in which a person is supported, can help them heal and maintain a healthy self-esteem. Listening respectfully and allowing silence for survivors of betrayal to share is recommended. Acknowledge feelings. Ask reflective and supportive questions. Lean in and listen. Don't blame the person. Don't deny the offense. Don't ignore the person or change the subject. Help the individual obtain counseling. "When wrongdoings are reported and institutions turn a blind eye, it harms employees" (Tyler, 2014, p. 43). Institutional courage is encouraged (Schmidt, Adams-Clark, & Freyd, 2023). Healthy workplace interactions (Zhang, Gates, Nealy, & Stark, 2009; Gates, 2003; 2008) are especially important because positive emotions enhance performance and influence the capacity for innovation (Proto, 2016), and innovation may lead to greater workplace success (Carballo & Gates, 2011). Future research needs to examine the prevalence of occupational stress as well as institutional betrayal and determine how professionals are managing them.

RESEARCH QUESTIONS

1) How does the participant in this study experience institutional betrayal?
2) How does the participant in this study experience and manage stress?

METHODS

The purpose of this research is to utilize qualitative research methods (Cresswell, 2003) to conduct in-depth interviews, focus groups, and questionnaires to capture the essence of how 127 professionals experienced their respective workplaces. A total of 71 business students from a midwestern university completed a questionnaire in exchange for extra credit. Another 45 professionals participated in in-depth, one-on-one interviews by phone or Zoom that lasted from 22 minutes to an hour and a half. The 45 people who participated in the interviews were selected using the snowball technique. That means that after each interview, participants were encouraged to submit the names of other professionals who could be interviewed. In addition to the interviews, 20 people participated in two focus groups. The professionals who participated in the study were shown an organizational socialization model (Gates, 2009) published in 2009 by the Publishing House of South China University of Technology. They also were given another document that explained the model. Then participants were asked to indicate how closely the model captured the essence of how they experienced organizational socialization. They were invited to comment on each component of the model.

As the study progressed, interviews revealed more in-depth details about the experiences of the professionals. One salient theme that kept emerging was sexual harassment and traumatic workplace betrayals. A total of 76 of the participants were Caucasian, 43 were African American, 5 were Latino/a, 2 Asians, and 1 Greek. The participants were from Indiana, Texas, Utah, Nevada, Ohio, Missouri, Arizona, Illinois, Michigan, Oregon, Tennessee, Florida, New York, Pennsylvania, Maine, Connecticut, Alabama, Georgia, California, Washington, Virginia, Washington, D.C., Maryland, and Arkansas.

Phone and Zoom interviews were conducted with 45 professionals from a wide range of careers ranging from fortune 100 leaders, bankers, mortgage loan officers, factory workers, professors, deans, government workers, military workers, case managers, pastors, construction workers, business consultants, business owners, pharmacists, general managers of a radio station, etc. The professionals were originally asked about their workplace experiences as they related to organizational socialization and career success. However, during many of the interviews participants divulged details about sexual harassment and traumatic workplace betrayals such as those climates that supported sexism, sexual harassment, racism, and other acts of marginalization. These stress-producing events inspired the present study.

The present study will focus specifically on the traumatic institutional betrayal and stress of a Caucasian, female, production supervisor in her 40s, who earns $60,000 annually. While many people reported experiences with sexual harassment, one woman in particular, a female factory worker employed by a predominately male company, had a compelling encounter with institutional betrayal and stress. She grew up in a working-class family. Her father died of injuries he sustained in the military when she was young, and she recalled that her mother worked in a factory during her childhood. Eager to help support her family, this participant entered the workforce as a factory worker not long after she dropped out of high school. For the sake of discussion, this woman will be referred to as Mandy, which is a pseudonym adopted for the purposes of discussing the stressful workplace events as well as the traumatic workplace betrayals she encountered. She adopted innovative strategies for managing these situations. A 40-minute interview with Mandy was recorded with her consent; she also spoke extensively about her workplace experiences after the recording stopped. The tape-recorded interview with Mandy was analyzed numerous times, until no new themes emerged. The salient themes that emerged centered around the stress she experienced in her workplace as a result of institutional betrayals. Her lived experiences clearly could be characterized as traumatic institutional betrayal and workplace stress.

FINDINGS

The present study focused on the lived experiences of a Caucasian American woman from the United States. She's currently a production supervisor with 18 years of experience in management. She works in the manufacturing industry, and she has been a production supervisor at her current company for three years. She's much happier here than in her previous roles. She said she appreciates her job. "This is the only one that I've been happy with," she said, expressing her gratitude for her present employer. She said that earlier in her career when she was in her 20s and 30s, she was severely sexually harassed, trauma which inspired her to rapidly move from job to job. The stress of being sexually harassed caused a constant cycle of job hopping early in her career.

She tended to leave jobs for better pay or benefits when she wasn't compelled to leave due to sexual harassment. She recalled that two employers terminated her on the spot when they learned of her desire to find better employment. 'Once you tell somebody you had a better opportunity, I would say two of them let me go on the spot," she explained. After that, she stopped advertising plans to leave. She just left. Nevertheless, the most prominent or notable experiences that resonated with her today tended to encompass sexual harassment or other forms of traumatic workplace betrayal as well as the stress that stemmed from it.

Institutional Betrayal: Sexual Harassment

A salient theme the emerged from the interview with Mandy was sexual harassment. After analyzing her interview multiple times, the most prevalent theme was institutional betrayal and sexual harassment. When speaking about her stressful workplace experiences, she said, "It was a very poorly managed company. It was stressful. The management didn't really respect employees," she asserted. "The owner's son called me a BITCH to my face," she revealed. Mandy said she didn't report the offense because "there's nobody to report to if it's the owner's son," she stated. Mandy got support from her immediate family. "I told my brother, and my brother came into the shop [to confront the owner's son]. I just left. I resigned on the spot. I left quickly before anybody got in trouble. I grabbed my stuff and quit that day." Leaving jobs due to sexual harassment or some other form of stress became the norm for Mandy until she landed what resembled her dream job, the job she has today.

Mandy relied on family support to alleviate the pressures of working in a stressful environment. Her older brother comforted her by coming to her job and confronting one of her abusers. "He just wanted to let that guy know you can't go around calling women that [bitch], and he [Mandy's brother] wanted to see if the owner's son would call him that. And the guy did not want to," she laughed. The owner's son harassed Mandy when he had her alone, but he was more reticent about interacting with her when her bother was present to defend her honor.

"He harassed me because I was a woman in a male-dominated workplace," Mandy explained. She didn't witness the boss's son treating her male counterparts in this fashion. The hostile work environment caused Mandy to be less engaged, which may have compromised her level of productivity (Guo, Qin, Gan, 2021). Her concern for safety and job security compelled her to resign from that particular job.

The abuse didn't stop there for Mandy. "In my early 20s, I was sexually harassed a lot. I didn't know, I didn't know better. In your early 20s, you just think that's acceptable behavior. In your late 40s, not so much," Mandy said. "If you report those kinds of things, you get harassed until you quit or they find a reason to fire you," she explained. Essentially, women who resisted sexual harassment in her workplace could expect retaliation if they complained. The work environment would become so hostile or unfavorable that the women resigned on their own, which was essentially constructive termination (Luthans, Luthans, & Luthans, 2021; Lowe, 2018). The workplace was so stressful and hostile that women felt they had no choice but to quit.

When asked about the frequency of her encounters with sexual harassment, the blonde-haired Mandy said, "It's been several times. The boss shows you extra attention or makes several comments to you. Or um if you act like you're offended, then the boss is rude to you, and he doesn't allow you to move up as well," Mandy said. She suggested that the boss at her workplace did not permit her to advance at work unless "you let the sexual advances go." Women were expected to ignore the sexual advances and inappropriate touch if they wanted to be regarded as team players.

"I've only worked in manufacturing in [my] county. That is the basis of my experience. I don't know about everywhere else, but I know for sure that it happened more in my early 20s. When you're older, you know how to stand up for yourself a little more," Mandy indicated. Mandy recalled an encounter whereby she was subjected to unwanted touch from her supervisor. "So, I was bending over," she explained, "to fill up my water bottle, so we had like a water cooler, and I was filling up my water bottle, and my boss came behind me and put his foot in between my legs and touched my vagina with his foot." She recalled the emotional encounter as though it were yesterday. She was still furious with her boss for violating her. "At that point I turned around and pushed him and told him to… 'don't ever touch me again.'" She said her boss stated that he was just kidding, but Mandy didn't find the offense humorous. Mandy said she resigned from that factory shortly after her boss touched her inappropriately. She didn't feel safe at work, and the psychological stress was taking a toll on her personally and professionally. "As a single woman with kids, you got to have that next paycheck, so if a place is feeling unsafe or unstable to me, I will move on very quickly," she explained. She didn't want to risk staying in an unsafe place where she might be fired.

When asked what advice she would offer another woman entering her industry, Mandy said, "Keep to yourself, work hard, do everything they ask you to do, and be on time, be there every day." She said she wishes she had known that the details mattered. As a production supervisor today, she tries to set a good example for her team by being on time and showing respect for others. "Respect matters and being on time matters," she said, "If you want to move up the ladder." Mandy, who considers herself a very spiritual person, tries to practice what she preaches.

Institutional Betrayal: Pay Disparities

Sexual harassment was not the only form of institutional betrayal Mandy endured. She spoke candidly about pay disparities. She stated, "Still in 2023, women are grossly underpaid compared to men for the same jobs…We're still treated very differently even though we're doing what most would consider a male job. We don't get the same benefits as most men doing the same jobs. So, I think that's kind of sad in 2023." Mandy believes that sexism causes her to earn less money than her male counterparts. While she appreciates her current job, equal pay would make it more enjoyable.

DISCUSSION

According to the institutional betrayal assessment by Smith and Freyd (2014), the Caucasian production supervisor with 18 years of managerial experience suffered from institutional betrayal and stress. Her male-dominated industry paid her less money for the same work men did, and contending with sexual harassment was a constant occurrence. She didn't always perceive that she could do much to curtail the abuse short of leaving the organization. Consequently, when she was in her 20s and 30s, she jumped from job to job in search of better pay and benefits as well as a more supportive environment. Because she didn't see her organizations, nor her industry, as taking proactive steps to prevent sexual harassment, she took matters into her own hands. She relied on her family for support, even enlisting the help of her older brother when the boss's son called her a bitch. She felt powerless to complain to the boss because she believed the boss would side with his son over her. Perhaps she could have contemplated taking her concerns to the Equal Employment Opportunity Commission, but she elected to find another job, right after her brother confronted her abuser. Leaving may have been a viable option, but it also has consequences. When employees leave organizations, companies have to pay to locate, hire, and train new employees, and turnover can be costly. A more cost-effective approach for organizations may be to create workplace cultures that are conducive to employees being successful. Healthy organizations embrace talent optimization, and they give their employees the tools to win. Moreover, organizations and employees must ensure that they have good organizational fits before moving forward. Plugging employees into the right positions is imperative if organizations expect employees to thrive (Gates, 2009; 2019). Essentially, companies must set themselves up for success by cultivating healthy cultures and inspiring retention by treating employees with respect in addition to taking advantage of other HR functions.

It appeared that sexual harassment was routine in Mandy's industry as she encountered it in multiple companies within the same county. Inappropriate conduct, sexual in nature, occurred again and again, possibly traumatizing Mandy, the participant in this study. When abuse is repetitive, prolonged, and cumulative, trauma results (Courtois, 2019). Women who complained about the abuse feared retaliation. Consequently, Mandy, learned to stand up for herself and to keep a safe distance between herself and her male colleagues as well as supervisors. In lieu of seeking help from her superiors, she relied on her own devices when problems arose. She didn't want to be fired, so she handled matters personally, or she resigned when problems were too stressful to handle alone. The key to her success was effective communication, always being on time for work, doing what was asked of her when those demands were reasonable, and showing respect for others. She said she tried to model this for her subordinates. However, stellar behavior was no match for the sexual harassment that ensued. In her case, excellence was not always a deterrent to sexism nor sexual harassment.

It was difficult to report sexual harassment and stay at a particular company. She recalled that people had to ignore the abuse if they wanted to advance professionally. She experienced cognitive dissonance in that she, from time to time, tolerated sexual harassment even though the behavior conflicted with her personal standards and contradicted what she knew was right. As a single mother with children to feed, she often did what she thought was best for her family even if it meant sacrificing her immediate happiness. The fear of getting fired or constructively terminated was so pervasive that she tried to conform to the norms of her companies as best she could, although this sometimes caused stress. Her choices were to tolerate or to terminate herself. Complaining was not much of an option because she believed it would result in retaliation or ultimately termination. Consequently, she relied on her family for emotional support. Her older brother was a sounding board for her when she needed to talk. She was strategic in her communication at work, so that she could reasonably enjoy the outcomes she wanted.

To the extent that she had to leave organizations, factories, where she encountered sexual harassment, she was essentially punished in that she had to part ways with the company and lose her seniority. She opted not to stay and try to work through a grievance process because she was certain that companies would become so hostile toward her that she'd practically be pushed out of the company anyway. She preferred to leave on her own terms, empowering herself by finding alternate employment. Uprooting herself and finding another job could prove stressful because she didn't want her respective employers, at the time, to know she was looking for another job. She had learned from past experiences that once she announced that she was seeking another job, she would get fired on the spot. To circumvent the internal processes that she didn't believe would end well for her, she simply moved to another factory. Her work was impeccable by reasonable standards. Because people respected her work, finding another job was not difficult. But she wasn't guaranteed to find a job with the same title or pay. The location may not have always been suitable either. Moreover, learning the ropes at a new company and becoming acquainted with a new team presented a level of stress of its own. Ultimately, however, selfcare, family support, and her faith helped her contend with the stress and pressures of being a factory worker in a predominately male industry. Additionally, during more recent times, Mandy has been upbeat, optimistic, and confident, and people with these personality traits tend to experience less occupational stress, according to Deguchi, Iwasaki, Konishi, Ishimoto, Ogawa, Fukuda, Nitta, and Inoue (2016). She may have experienced more workplace stress earlier in her career because with only limited education, some high school, she was still developing the skills to master workplace challenges (Agai–Demjaha, Karadzinska Bislimovska, Mijakoski, 2015). As a more mature woman, she has honed her interpersonal skills and gained greater emotional intelligence

Mandy, without a doubt, endured sexism and sexual harassment. The psychological resources required to overcome the stress and challenges she faced may have diminished her level of engagement as well as the quality of the work she could have produced under better circumstances (Wang & Shi, 2022). Who knows what Mandy could have accomplished had she been able to enjoy less stressful organizations, ones devoid of sexual harassment and sexism. In other words, contending with sexism and sexual harassment takes a toll on a person, and when people can be free from those realities, they may be able to add greater value to the workplace. Mandy felt discriminated against due to her sex. Being a woman in a male-dominated industry required Mandy to be innovative and creative to overcome her circumstances. She found strategies that worked for her, and she enjoys a more pleasant workplace climate today. Her current employer of three years is much more supportive of her. She attributes the improvement to having learned how to locate an employer that is compatible with her needs and lifestyle as well as gaining the emotional intelligence that equipped her to overcome workplace obstacles she didn't know how to master in the past (Wang & Shi, 2022). She learned how to assert herself or stand up for herself, and the newly found confidence may be helping her to ward off offenders seeking to sexually harass her. Having conquered the problem with workplace sexual harassment, her mission now is to tackle the pay disparity which remains a concern.

Perhaps organizations in the manufacturing industry in the county where Mandy resides can consider creating plans and policies that promote less stressful and less traumatic environments. According to Kawakami, N., Tsutsumi, A., Department of Mental Health. Kitasagato University School of Medicine, The University of Tokyo, Department of Public Health, & School of Public Health (2016), stress tests and plans to enhance workplace environments may result in improved health for employees. These efforts might reduce turnover, enhance engagement, and spur greater productivity.

LIMITATIONS

This study relies on self-report data, and the memories of professionals. However, because the participants are regarded as experts on their lived experiences, the rich, thick, descriptions provided in this study can help enable others to determine if the context is compatible with transferability. Some of the encounters of the production supervisor introduced in this study may resonate with other professionals who contend with similar challenges.

CONCLUSION

The purpose of this paper was to explore the lived experiences of a Caucasian production supervisor in her 40s who worked in the manufacturing industry of a large company in the United States. Mandy, the participant in this study, endured stress and trauma that stemmed from repetitive, prolonged, and cumulative sexual harassment. She worked in a male-dominated industry in which she feared being fired if she complained about abuse after being terminated previously for sharing plans to secure better employment. Mandy experienced traumatic institutional betrayal as well as stress as a result of working in a culture that condoned sexual harassment.

The climate may have felt even more misogynistic when Mandy learned that women at her job were paid significantly less than men for the same work. Men got better pay and better benefits in an environment that already permitted them to marginalize women by sexually harassing them. As a woman, Mandy clearly was at a disadvantage. She learned to be more strategic so she could be successful in her workplace. She had creative and innovative strategies that enabled her to survive in her profession. Mandy relied on family support to cope with sexual harassment. She limited her workplace complaints as a strategy to preserve her job. She learned how to assert herself. She discreetly sought alternate employment when occupational stress resulting from sexual harassment became unbearable. Essentially, the paper identified the stress-producing activities during times of emotional crisis in the workplace and indicated what innovative strategies a woman employed to manage the stress.

REFERENCES

Agai–Demjaha, T., Karadzinska Bislimovska, J., & Mijakoski, D. (2015). Level of Work-Related Stress among Teachers in Elementary Schools. *OA Maced J Med Sci., 3*, 484-488. doi:10.3889/oamjms.2015.076

Albrecht, S. L., & Marty, A. (2020). Personality, self-efficacy and job resources and their associations with employee engagement, affective commitment, and turnover intentions. *International Journal of Human Resource Management*, *31*(5), 657–681. doi:10.1080/09585192.2017.1362660

Caraballo, V., & Gates, D. (2011). *Innovation Among Latinos: Exploring Differences Across Genders*. Universidad y Empresa, Universidad del Rosario.

Courtois, C. A. (2019). *Understanding Complex Trauma, Complex Reactions, and Treatment Approaches*. aaets.org.

Cresswell, J. W. (2003). *Research design: Qualitative, quantitative, and mixed methods approach* (2nd ed.). Sage Publications.

Deguchi, Y., Iwasaki, S., Konishi, A., Ishimoto, H., Ogawa, K., Fukuda, Y., Nitta, T., & Inoue, K. (2016). The Usefulness of Assessing and Identifying Workers' Temperaments and Their Effects on Occupational Stress in the Workplace. *PLoS One*, *11*(5), e0156339. doi:10.1371/journal.pone.0156339 PMID:27227771

Fitzgerald, L. (2017). Still the last great open secret: Sexual harassment as systemic trauma. *Journal of Trauma & Dissociation*, *18*(4), 483–489. doi:10.1080/15299732.2017.1309143 PMID:28375711

Freyd, J. J. (1999, June). *Blind to Betrayal: New Perspectives on Memory for Trauma*. Retrieved from https://dynamic.uoregon.edu/jjf/articles/freyd99.pdf

Freyd, J. J. (2021). What is a Betrayal Trauma? What is Betrayal Trauma Theory? *Definition of Betrayal Trauma Theory*. Retrieved from https://dynamic.uoregon.edu/jjf/defineBT.html

Gates, D. (2003). Learning to play the game: An exploratory study of how African American women and men interact with others in organizations. *Electronic Journal of Communication*, *12*(2-3).

Gates, D. (2008). Business communication: identifying strategies employed by Latino/a or Hispanic Americans within superior-subordinate relationships. *Business Research Yearbook*, *15*(2).

Gates, D. (2009). The managerial communication process: Organizational socialization model. In S. Zhang, D. Gates, C. Nealy, & J. Stark (Eds.), *Managerial communication: Theory and application* (pp. 26–58). The Publishing House of South-China University of Technology.

Gates, D. (2010). Polarity management: Balancing stress and tranquility polarities during a recession. *Business Research Yearbook*, *17*(2), 704–711.

Gates, D. (2019). *Superior-subordinate dialogue: Mastering communication with bosses / Examining communication within and across races and genders*. Lambert Publishing House.

Gates, D. (2020). *Next level learning: Mastering Organizational Socialization*. Lambert Publishing House.

Gates, D. (2021). Exploring Superior-Subordinate Communication from the Perspectives of African American and Latino American Subordinates. In R. D. Johnson (Ed.), *Handbook of Research on Multidisciplinary Perspectives on Managerial and Leadership Psychology* (pp. 148–166). IGI Global. doi:10.4018/978-1-7998-3811-1.ch008

Gates, D. (2021). Mastering Diversity and Gaining a Competitive Advantage on University Campuses. In R. D. Johnson (Ed.), *Handbook of Research on Multidisciplinary Perspectives on Managerial and Leadership Psychology* (pp. 558–570). IGI Global. doi:10.4018/978-1-7998-3811-1.ch028

Guo, J., Qiu, Y., & Gan, Y. (2022). Workplace incivility and work engagement: The mediating role of job insecurity and the moderating role of self-perceived employability. *Managerial and Decision Economics*, *43*(1), 192–205. doi:10.1002/mde.3377

Guy, T (2022). *Betrayal Trauma & CPTSD*. CPTSDfoundation.org

Jablin, F. (2001). *Organizational entry, assimilation, and disengagement/exit*. SAGE Publications, Inc. doi:10.4135/9781412986243.n19

Kawakami, N., & Tsutsumi, A. (2016). The stress check program: A new national policy for monitoring and screening psychosocial stress in the workplace in Japan. *Journal of Occupational Health*, *58*(1), 1–6. doi:10.1539/joh.15-0001-ER PMID:26607455

LaSala, K. B., Wilson, V., & Sprunk, E. (2016, May-June). Nursing Academic Administrators' Lived Experiences with Incivility and Bullying From Faculty: Consequences and Outcomes Demanding Action. *Nurse Educator*, *41*(3), 120–124. doi:10.1097/NNE.0000000000000234 PMID:26673315

Lowe, H. (2018). Constructive Termination in Franchise Law. *Franchise Law Journal*, *38*(2), 267–284.

Luthans, B. C., Luthans, K. W., & Luthans, F. (2021). *Organizational Behavior: An Evidence-Based Approach* (14th ed.). Information Age Publishing, Incorporated.

Macey, W. H., & Schneider, B. (2008). The Meaning of Employee Engagement. *Industrial and Organizational Psychology: Perspectives on Science and Practice*, *1*(1), 3–30. doi:10.1111/j.1754-9434.2007.0002.x

Proto, E. (2016). Are happy workers more productive? *IZA World of Labor: Evidence-Based Policy Making*, *315*. Advance online publication. doi:10.15185/izawol.315

Rachman, S. (2010). Betrayal: A psychological analysis. *Behaviour Research and Therapy*, *48*(4), 304–311. doi:10.1016/j.brat.2009.12.002 PMID:20035927

Smidt, A.M., Adams-Clark, A.A., & Freyd, J.J. (2023) Institutional courage buffers against institutional betrayal, protects employee health, and fosters organizational commitment following workplace sexual harassment. *PLoS ONE, 18*(1). doi:.pone.027883 doi:10.1371/journal

Smith, C., & Freyd, J. (2014). Institutional Betrayal. *The American Psychologist*, *69*(6), 575–587. doi:10.1037/a0037564 PMID:25197837

Tyler, K. (2014). Listening Skills. *HRMagazine*, *59*(2), 42–43.

Wang, F., & Shi, W. (2020). The effect of work-leisure conflict on front-line employees' work engagement: A cross-level study from the emotional perspective. *Asia Pacific Journal of Management*, *39*(1), 225–247. doi:10.100710490-020-09722-0

Zhang, S., Gates, D., Nealy, C., & Stark, J. (2009). *Managerial communication: Theory and application*. The Publishing House of South-China University of Technology.

Chapter 5
Cyber Incivility:
An Empirical Study on Job Stress and Job Satisfaction Among Indian IT Professionals

Rajnish Kumar Misra
https://orcid.org/0000-0002-8660-0642
Jaypee Institute of Information Technology, India

Divya Sharma
Lloyd Business School, India

ABSTRACT

Cyber incivility has a detrimental effect on individuals as well as on the organization. In line with the COR theory, the research projected a mediation model in which stress would mediate the association between cyber incivility and job satisfaction. The study focused on IT professionals from the software engineering domain, which includes technical engineers and engineering managers. The outcome specified job stress as a mediator between cyber incivility and job satisfaction. To enhance satisfaction and reduce job stress, managers need to build an incivility-free environment. The sender should be cautious with the tone of the messages. Since an individual on the receiving side generally does not report incivility done by superiors, HR managers should encourage employees to provide feedback to their immediate boss. The implications would help the IT industry in reducing stress and job dissatisfaction and contribute to the limited body of research.

INTRODUCTION

The daily life of IT professional was interrupted and brusquely forced into occupied from home throughout pandemic (Russo *et al.*, 2021). Several software creators were requested to switch their workplace-based settings to new work from home scenario on very short notice which has harmed the well-being of IT Professionals (Ralph, *et al.*, 2020). Although, remote work, *per se,* is not a new term in a software engineer's life. In the late 1990s, researchers started focusing on the opportunities and challenges of work from home scenario and delved into specific practices of software development (Pounder, 1998).

DOI: 10.4018/978-1-6684-8565-1.ch005

In addition, the attributes of asynchronous and remote projects have been premeditated by the "Global Software Engineering Community" (Herbsleb, 2007; Smite *et al.*, 2010). Such research centred on the collaboration of software development groups co-situated in distinctive zones. Nonetheless, the emphasis has been on software teams working together on circulated projects. So far, the studies on work from home scenario have been limited (Russo et al., 2021). The reason for limited research on work from home the scenario is that managers were cynical or unconvinced about remote working due to the concern related to focus, culture, productivity and group cohesiveness (Buffer, 2020). However, the pandemic made numerous individuals to understand that a few feelings of trepidation are groundless (like diminishing productivity) and that they need to face such difficulties until an adequate number of individuals have been immunised, an interaction that might require quite a while. Henceforth, anecdotal proof driving top administrative decisions due to the absence of explicit investigation ought to be enhanced with insightful proof (Mesaglio, 2020).

The Internet has altered the way to connect at workplaces. The speed, ease and efficacy of an electronic system have made it a prevalent way of interaction at the workplace (Kahai & Cooper, 2003). The previous researches state that mailing is the most preferred form of communication as they simplify productivity and coordination (Markus, 1994; O'Sullivan & Flanagin, 2003). Even though email has received numerous rewards for people and associations, utilizing mails to convey message may also be a "double-edged sword".

By focusing on the revolution of "Information Technology" which has changed the "world into a global community", Wriston witnessed, "technology has made us a global community in the literal sense of the term. Mankind now has a completely integrated information marketplace capable of moving ideas to any place on this planet in minutes. Information and ideas will go where they are wanted and stay where they are well treated. It will flee from manipulation or onerous regulation of its value or use, and no government can restrain it for long". The augmented dependency on mail frameworks at the workplace has opened up and given new chances to individuals to take part in bullying or incivility in the work environment. Pearson and Porath (2005, pp. 7) stated that the intricacy of high-tech communications assisted by mails may nourish incivility as individuals "believe that they don't have time to be nice and that impersonal mode of contact does not require courtesies of interaction". Despite the prevalence of mail usage and its possible effect on interpersonal norms of communication, not much investigation has been focused on inspecting online deviant behaviour or incivility at workstations.

There are numerous negative behaviours at workplaces reported in the literature like bullying, aggression, violence, eve-teasing, physical and sexual abuse (Haque et al., 2021). This negative behaviour at the workplace is a growing problem and have gained attention but the focus on incivility is low (Baron & Neuman, 1996; Lim & Cortina, 2005). Incivility is considered to be one of the most common antisocial behaviors in the workplace. Incivility is an extensive phenomenon that can affect the organisation and employee (Giumetti et al., 2016). For instance, incivility impacts the psychological and physical health of an individual and causes lower satisfaction, job withdrawal, intention to quit, increased absenteeism, high turnover, low job performance and stress (Cortina, *et al.*, 2001; Johnson & Indvik, 2001; Porath & Pearson, 2012). It appears that individuals experience negative consequences of bullying and uncivil behaviour (Spadafora *et. al*, 2020). Online rude, impolite, uncivil treatment is widespread (Giumetti et al., 2012). A study conducted among financial employees in Singapore claimed that approximately 90% of the respondents faced cyber incivility (Lim & Teo, 2009). The evidence in the previous study suggests that online incivility at work leads to stress at the end of the working day or even the next morning too (Giumetti *et al.*, 2012).

This study specifically focused on the work from home scenario began at COVID-19 duration. So, here researcher firstly provides the brief of COVID-19. The COVID-19 has troubled the entire world. In December 2019, China reported an eruption of the virus to WHO (World Health Organization) and on January 7th, 2020, the virus was recognized as Coronavirus. The number of corona cases started growing exponentially worldwide. On 23rd January, China declared lockdown in Wuhan with a certain restriction on entry and exit from the state. Soon this lockdown was stretched to other cities and countries. The Aerodromes in different countries like India started the mechanism of screening the people returning from China and positioned those individuals in isolation for testing of Corona (Singhal, 2020). The Indian government took the step of lockdown on March 24th, 2020 to control the community transmission. A significant policy during the COVID-19 pandemic is "social distancing" which necessitates employees to do work from home (Mongey & Weinberg, 2020). Many of the industries followed government advisory and asked employees to do work from home till now. The quantitative study conducted in the year 2020 stated that prolonged work from home scenario is leading to stress because employees were not ready for new normal. The same is being mentioned by the CEO of Microsoft, Satya Nadella in an interview (Singh & Kumar, 2020).

PURPOSE

Apart from a previous investigation, a smaller amount is known about cyber incivility and demands future research and analysis (Akellaa & Lewis, 2019). Consequently, the is to observe the effect of online incivility during the work from home phase on job satisfaction and stress and then to inspect the mediating part of stress in the association between the relationship of cyber incivility and satisfaction with the job (Figure 1). The association between incivility and job dissatisfaction has been reported in the literature (Lim & Teo, 2009). At this point, the researcher framed the research objective:

- To study the mediating effect of stress in the relationship between cyber incivility and job satisfaction.

In this research, the researcher has tried to confirm these findings, with potential mediating processes. In detail, the researcher assumes the association among cyber incivility and dissatisfaction at the job is mediated by job stress. This work from home phase provides a favourable time to study online related phenomenon like cyberbullying or cyber incivility because IT professionals are actively working online from home where the daily life of software engineers was disturbed and brusquely forced into working from home (Russo *et al.*, 2021). This gave a better picture of collecting data and understanding the phenomenon of cyber incivility. Hence, in this study, the researcher discusses the theoretical background, literature review, followed by hypotheses. Further, the study will describe the methodology and result of hypotheses testing. Lastly, the researcher will discuss the implication, limitation, and conclusion of the study.

LITERATURE REVIEW

Theoretical Background

The COR Theory claimed that stress arises from the loss of resources or threats (Hobfoll, 1989). Lack of resources and a high level of demands may reduce a person's resources and this reduction in resource may lead to undesirable outcomes like job stress or job dissatisfaction. The research conducted by Sliter et al, (2010) on face-to-face incivility with COR Theory stated that those who face or experience incivility destroy their mental resources. Thus, Conservation of Resources may also be valuable for considerate the consequence of cyber incivility. Additionally, according to Affective events theory, events like bullying or incivility at workplaces are conjectured to impact employee's attitude towards jobs, which can successively effect job performance. Previous research has supported that incivility has an effect on emotions and consequent vicissitudes in job satisfaction and intention to leave behaviors (Bunk & Magley, 2013; Weiss & Cropanzano, 1996).

Cyber Incivility

Incivility is considered as rude, ruthless, and impolite or disregard for others (Akellaa & Lewis, 2019; Eka & Chambers, 2019). Incivility is a "rude and impolite remark by other individuals and generally measured by asking the individuals to report how frequently they have experienced these types of behaviour" (Cortina et. al, 2001). Historically, these types of behaviour can only occur in person (Giumetti et al., 2012). Nowadays, the usage of technology in organisations among superiors, subordinates, and colleagues has increased. The increase in the usage of "Information and Communication Technologies" (ICT) has endorsed a fresh form of bullying or incivility i.e., cyber incivility at the workplace (Heischman, 2017). Incivility at the workplace can occur both face to face and online. Anderson and Pearson's (1999) defined incivility beyond "physical contexts" (Andersson & Pearson, 1999). It is "communicative behaviour exhibited in computer-mediated interactions that violate workplace norms of mutual respect" (Lim & Teo, 2009). The other previous studies defined it "as discourteous behaviours occurring through information and communication technologies (ICTs) such as email" (Giumetti et al., 2012).

In 2008, Byron differentiated physical and online incivility and said cyber incivility lacks nonverbal, situational cues and contain ambiguous message (Byron, 2008). Because of the ambiguity in the text, the chances of being interpreting the text as uncivil is higher. Then another researcher differentiates and stated that in online incivility, individuals were less worried about acting civilly when they were not actually or physically communicating with each other (Kruger et al., 2005). Online incivility occurs through ICT which includes instant messaging, email, and texts (Andersson & Pearson, 1999). Email is the second most common way of communication among superiors and subordinates (Lim & Teo, 2009). Cyber incivility at the workplace is a recent phenomenon because of the higher usage of emails and text messaging at the workplace (Heischman, 2017) and because of this, the problem can arise from malevolent emails or misconceptions of benevolent messages. The qualitative study conducted by McCarthy (2016) clearly stated that the victims of "cyber incivility" face more severe penalties than "face to face incivility" and a very limited empirical studies examined the effect of cyber incivility.

"I have a different accusation to level at email—it has made us all passive-aggressive. ... It has stifled debate and made office life more stultifying and aggravating than it has ever been." – Kellaway, 2016

Cyber Incivility and Job Satisfaction

The outcome of incivility on satisfaction level has been reported by the preceding researcher (Alola et al., 2021; Laschinger, et al., 2009; Laschinger, et al., 2014; Roy & Mandal, 2021). Cyber incivility at the workplace has also been identified as a cause of job dissatisfaction (Marchiondo et al., 2010; Wright & Hill, 2015). Reio and Ghosh (2009) collected data from 402 workers and claimed the targets of incivility had low job satisfaction and poor physical health. The negative connotation among incivility and satisfaction level in the job has been reported in the literature (Blau & Andersson, 2005). Previous research examined cyber incivility among Singapore employees and claimed that those who were targeted by the superiors had low satisfaction in the job and low commitment towards the organisation (Lim & Teo, 2009). In the ICT context, unclear or ambiguous text can be misunderstood and seems uncivil because the text and email do not convey the non-verbal cues to understand the sender's intent (Byron, 2008). The higher usage of emails and text messaging at the workplace creates a problem from malicious emails or misconceptions of benevolent messages than face-to-face.

Cyber Incivility and Stress

Cyber incivility has been seen as a personal stressor (Chung et al., 2021; Giumetti et al., 2012; Kowalski & Robbins, 2021). Stress is a kind of pressure from the environment which can hinder one's mental and physical health which can affect the individual as well as an organisation (Pandey & Sharma, 2016; Nel, 2019). This has been clearly stated in the literature that whenever an employee experienced cyber incivility, that employee found to report a higher level of stress at work. Cyber incivility has a direct effect on individual's negative emotions namely frustration, anxiety, and confusion (Giumetti et al., 2016). The evidence suggests that online incivility in the work is associated with an advanced level of stress (Giumetti et al., 2016). The field study conducted by Bono (2013) claimed the negative actions as an outcome of incivility i.e., high blood pressure among targets.

Job Stress and Job satisfaction

The literature revealed stress at the job is related to satisfaction in the job (Cooper & Marshall, 1976; Embse et al., 2016; Kowalski & Robbins, 2021; Liu & Ramsey, 2008; Naumann, 1993; Terry et al., 1993; Yang et al., 2021). Job satisfaction is "a reaction that employees have to their work and is firmed by comparing the actual outcomes with the desired one" (Hulin & Judge, 2003). Brief (1998) explained the job-satisfaction model in which both emotions and job situation impact satisfaction. Stress at the job is connected to circumstances in the workplace. Brief (1998) model proposes that incivility is one cause of dissatisfaction and recommends that stress has a vital impact on satisfaction level at the job. The study conducted by Pignata et al. (2014), clearly stated that personnel who established the stress-reduction programs had higher satisfaction in the job. As stated in the literature, cyber incivility has an impact on satisfaction level and stress. In addition, stress has an effect on job satisfaction.

HYPOTHESISED MODEL

Based on the above-mentioned works and research gap, a hypothesised model was developed indicating the hypothesis relationship between job stress, job satisfaction and cyber incivility. Cyber incivility is IV, while job satisfaction is the DV, whereas job stress is shown as the mediator variable. The aim was to observe the mediating effect of online incivility during the work from home scenario and then to inspect the mediating part of stress in the association between the relationship of cyber incivility and satisfaction with the job as indicated in Figure 1.

Figure 1. Hypothesized model
Source: Author

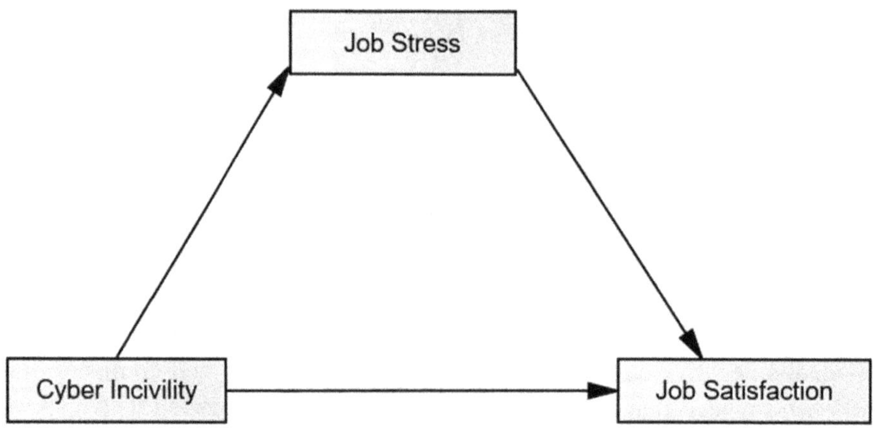

STATEMENT OF HYPOTHESES

The following hypotheses has been framed on the basis of the existing literature:

H1: Cyber incivility has a significant and direct effect on job satisfaction.
H2: Cyber incivility has a significant effect on job stress.
H3: Job Stress mediates the relationship between cyber incivility & job satisfaction.

Given the research gaps, this study is aimed to explore the phenomenon of cyber incivility and explored the effect of cyber incivility on stress and job satisfaction on Indian IT Professionals.

DESIGN

"Data collection is the way of collecting and estimating data on factors of interest, in a built-up way, with the goal that one can answer expressed research questions; test hypotheses framed, and assess results" (De Vaus, 2001). "Primary data refers to the data originated by the researcher for a specific purpose in order to address the research problem whereas secondary data refers to data collected for some other problems apart from the problem at hand" (De Vaus, 2001). In this research, primary data was collected through survey. It explicates the sampling, data and statistical tool used for this study and it gives an account of the philosophical underpinnings that guided the research.

APPROACH

A "cross-sectional quantitative approach" has been conducted by the researcher because in cross sectional study, the researcher measures the exposure and outcome of the participants at the same time. The respondents in cross-sectional study are nominated based on the challenges of IT professionals in terms of negative behaviors during the work from home scenario, "where employees were forced to do work from home and once the respondents have been selected, the researcher follows the study to assess the exposure and the outcomes". For the present study, the researcher chose the purposive sampling design, where, the sample is chosen as per the research question. Therefore, in the present study, the reason behind choosing purposive sampling was that researcher targeted IT Professional where employees were forced to do work from home and the day-to-day life of software engineers was disturbed and forced into remote work from home scenario (Russo et al., 2021). Thus, the researcher chose a sample of Indian IT Professionals.

METHODOLOGY

Participants and Descriptive Statistics

In this study, the questionnaire was distributed to 746 IT Professionals from the software engineering domain, who actively do work from home or follow the formal channel of communication that is ICT (email, text etc.) in India. Fifty six respondents stated that they had not faced any deviant behaviour at the workplace, 64 were dropped from the study because of the incomplete data. So, the final sample consists of 626 IT Professionals from the software engineering domain which include technical engineers and engineering managers, i.e., from positions: entry, mid and senior-level technical and lower, middle and upper management.

The data was received from 634 (85% response rate) engineers from technical and managerial domains. Though, few of the responses were discarded because of the missing data, resulting in 626 useable responses. The sample covers 410 males (65.5%) and 216 females (34.5). The researcher mentioned transgender options in the questionnaire but none of the respondents was transgender. Three hundred fifty-nine (57.3%) participants were lie in the age of 30-39 years, 24.4% (153) of 22-29 years, 14.5% (91) of 40-49 years, and 3.7% (23) of 21 or less. 73.8% (462) respondents have 11-20 years of experience, 16.1% (101) with 21-30 years' experience and 10.1% (63) of 0-10 years. Six levels of position were given to the respondents in which, 63 (10.1%) were in entry-level technical, 356 (56.9%) in mid-level technical, 126 (20.1%) in senior-level technical and 81 (12.9%) in lower-level management.

MEASURING INSTRUMENTS

The three constructs used in the present study are advanced by using measurement scales from previous research. The statements were responded on the "Five-point Likert scale" ("1= Not at all to 5= All the time") for two constructs and ("1- Strongly disagree to 5= Strongly Agree") for one construct. Researcher used the 5-point likert scale because it is likely to be the most common format and here, the respondents gets an option of neutral point which helps them to answer even if they are neither dissatisfied nor satisfied with the statement.

Cyber Incivility

To assess cyber incivility, participants were specified certain potential actions that describe the practice of cyber incivilities such as being sarcastic in emails, belittling remarks, little attention, ignoring, and no answers to queries. Then, contributors read a definition, "The following questions are about being the victim of cyber incivility at work. When the researcher used the word cyber incivility, this means incivility which takes place through e-mail, instant messaging, in a chat room, on a website, or through a text message sent to a cell phone." The researcher assessed this construct with the "cyber incivility scale" industrialised from Lim & Teo (2009) with 14 items. Examples of statements include the supervisor "said something hurtful to you through email", "Used emails to say negative things about you that he/she would not say to you face-to-face", "Made demeaning or derogatory remarks about you through email", "Inserted sarcastic or mean comments between paragraphs in emails", "Put you down or was condescending to you in some way through email", "Sent you emails using a rude and discourteous tone", "Used CAPS to shout at you through email. 8. Not replying to your email at all", "Ignored a request that you made through email", "Replied to your emails but did not answer your queries", "Used emails for time-sensitive messages", "Paid little attention to a statement made by you through email or showed little interest in your opinion", "Not acknowledging that he/she has received your email even when you sent a request receipt function", "Used email for discussions that would require face-to-face dialogue" (pp. 424). An extraordinary reliability of 0.95 was found for this questionnaire. The response rate was on a "5 point Likert scale ranging from 1 to 5 (1= Not at all to 5= All the time"). It is important to measure the reliability, before testing the hypotheses. The most widely used way to test reliability is Cronbach's alpha which establishes the internal reliability of the scale. The range of Cronbach's alpha lies between 0 to 1. The acceptable level is above 0.6 and here the values was 0.991.

Job Stress

The researcher assessed job stress with the "expanded stress scale" established by French et al., (2000) with 3 dimensions i.e., "problem with peer", "problem with supervisor", and "workload" and 18 items. Examples of statements include, "lack of opportunity to talk with other personnel", "lack of opportunity to express negative behavior", "conflict with a supervisor", "lack of support from immediate supervisor", "insufficient time to complete task", "having to work through breaks", "making decisions under pressure" (pp. 171). An extraordinary reliability of 0.76 was found for these dimensions. The question was responded to base on the self-assessment. The Cronbach's value was 0.973.

Job Satisfaction

The researcher assessed job satisfaction with the scale developed from Lim and Teo (2009) with 5 items. Examples of statements include, "I am generally very satisfied with my job", "I am generally satisfied with the kind of work I do in this job", "I seldom think of quitting my job", "Very few people on this job feel that the work is useless or trivial", "Most people on this job are very satisfied with the job". An extraordinary reliability of 0.85 was found for this questionnaire. The responses to the questions based on the self-assessment. The Cronbach's value was 0.971.

Statistical Analysis

The researcher tested a mediation analysis with the help of a bootstrapping method in Structural equation modelling- AMOS, recommended by Preacher and Hayes (2008). Reliability descriptive statistics and structural equation model were conducted for analysis. Bootstrapping technique is a computer-based way of calculating biases, standard errors, and confidence intervals and is proposed by Efron (1979). The entire and indirect outcome of cyber incivility (IV) on job satisfaction (DV) via job stress (mediator) can be smoothly analysed in this method. The researcher tested the hypotheses by simply testing the direct effect of cyber incivility (IV) on job satisfaction (DV) (Figure 2). After that, the researcher entered the mediator variable (job stress) into the model (Figure 3). Further, confidence interval is calculated and if, confidence interval at 95 percent estimated does not include 0, it suggests that indirect effect is statistically significant 5% level.

Procedure and Ethical Consideration

The questionnaire was distributed through email invitation and responses were taken electronically through google forms. Firstly, an informed consent form was completed by the participant to recognize their agreement to join in. The study particularly focuses on the challenges of IT professionals in terms of negative behaviour, where employees were forced to do work from home. Since most of the workforce are interacting online with each other, this phase was ideal for this study as all participants were actively working online from home. The daily life of software engineers was disrupted and brusquely forced into work from home (Russo et al., 2021). This gave a better picture of collecting data and understanding the phenomenon of cyber incivility. The researcher has tested the mediation hypotheses using the "Structural equation model- AMOS".

RESULTS

Instrument Validation

It is important to measure the reliability and validity of the instrument. The researcher verified the reliability as mentioned above. Now, before hypotheses testing, the proposed construct was assessed for validity through confirmatory factor analysis using AMOS. Firstly, the researcher checked the one-dimensionality of the scale by performing an overall measurement model by examining the factor loading of all the item which should be above 0.60 for the established scale (Bagozzi & Yi, 1988). There are several ways of testing the model fit indices. In this study, researcher used RMSEA= .058, CFI= .96, NFI= .90, GFI= .091 and Chisq/df= 1.83. The required level of model fit is achieved. "To establish the convergent validity, items in each factor must have loadings over 0.5, and composite reliabilities (CR) should be over 0.7 and greater than the respective Average Variance Extracted (AVE)". As shown in Table 1, the examination of CR and AVE coefficients of hypothesized constructs confirmed the convergent validity. Further, "to establish discriminant validity, the square root of the AVE should be greater than the inter construct correlation and the diagonal value of the factors should be greater than the particular rows and columns of that variable" (Zammuto, Krakower, 1991; Spreitzer, 1995). Thus, the validity of the instrument is established. The results of CFA support the convergent and discriminant validity.

Table 1. Convergent and discriminant validity of the construct

	CR	AVE	MSV	PS	WL	PP	CI	JST
PS	0.930	0.770	0.011	**0.878**				
WL	0.907	0.714	0.091	0.079	**0.845**			
PP	0.786	0.556	0.091	0.103	0.301	**0.746**		
CI	0.861	0.614	0.059	0.037	-0.062	0.026	**0.783**	
JST	0.757	0.511	0.059	-0.020	0.077	-0.064	0.242	**0.715**

PS, Problem with Supervisor, WL, Workload, PP, Problem with peers, CI, Cyber incivility, JST, Job satisfaction, CR, Composite Reliabilities, AVE, Average Variance Extracted, MSV, Maximum Shared Squared Variance

Hypotheses Testing

The researcher begins testing the hypothesis by simply testing the direct effect of cyber incivility (IV) on job satisfaction (DV) (Figure 2). The output in Table 2 shows the beta coefficient is -0.86 and has a noteworthy impact on job satisfaction (β=-0.86, p= 0.000).

Figure 2. The direct effect of cyber incivility (IV) on job satisfaction (DV)
Source: Author

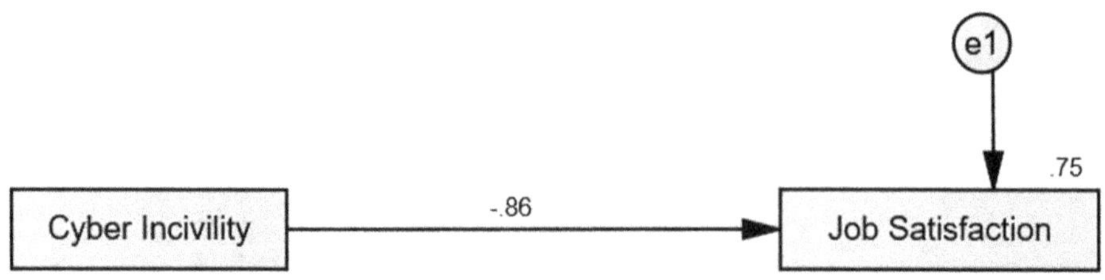

Table 2. The direct effect of cyber incivility on satisfaction level in Job

Est.	S.E.	C.R.	p- value	Result
-.864	.020	-42.950	0.000	Significant

Est, Estimates, S.E, Standard error, P-value, significant

Figure 3. AMOS output showing regression coefficient between variables
Source: Author

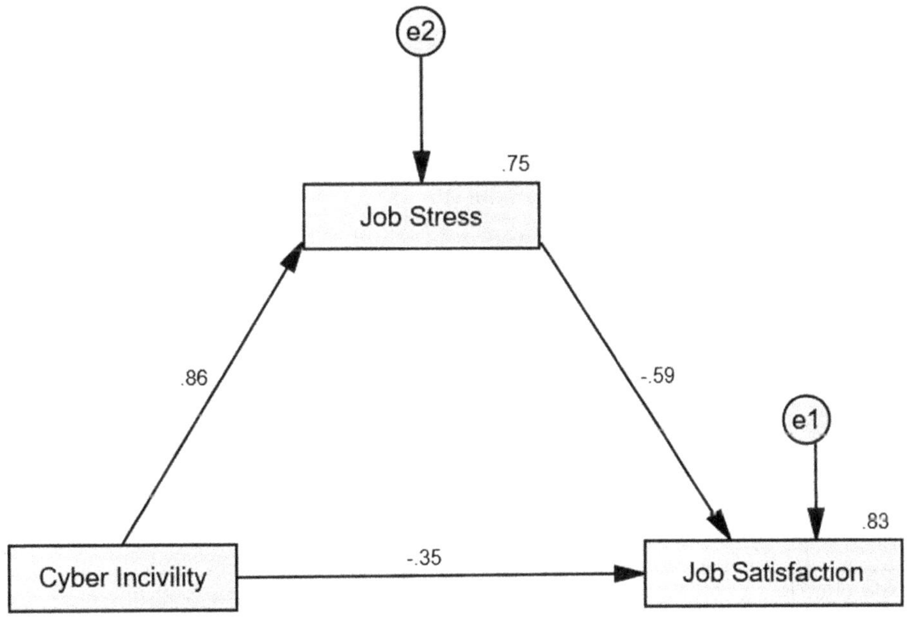

After that, the researcher entered the mediator variable (job stress) into the model (Figure 3). The output in Table 2 shows the beta coefficient is reduced from -0.86 to -0.355 when job stress (mediator) entered into the model and has a noteworthy effect. At this time, conditions of meditation analysis are met. Now the researcher test H2 and H3 to confirm mediation.

Table 3. Hypotheses testing with mediation effects

		Est.	S.E.	C.R.	P-Value	Result
Job Satisfaction	Cyber Incivility	-.355	.032	-10.962	0.001	Significant
Job Stress	Cyber Incivility	.865	.020	43.004	0.000	Significant
Job Satisfaction	Job Stress	-.589	.032	-18.212	0.001	Significant

Est, Estimates, S.E, Standard error, P-value, significant

Table 4. Hypothesis testing for a direct effect of cyber incivility and satisfaction in the job

Est.	S.E.	C.R.	P-Value	Result
-.355	.032	-10.962	0.001	Significant

Est, Estimates, S.E, Standard error, P-value, significant

Table 5. Hypothesis testing for a direct effect of cyber incivility and job stress

Est.	S.E.	C.R.	P-Value	Result
.865	.020	43.004	0.000	Significant

Est, Estimates, S.E, Standard error, P-value, significant

This was observed from the model that the direct effect of Cyber incivility is reduced from -0.86 to -0.35 after job stress (mediator) entered the model (β=-0.35, p= 0.001).

H1: Cyber incivility has a significant and direct effect on job satisfaction.

Result: H1 is accepted.

H2: Cyber incivility has a significant effect on job stress.

Result: H2 is accepted.

H3: Job Stress mediates the relationship between cyber incivility and job satisfaction.

Result: H3 is accepted.

Table 6. Hypothesis testing for the causal effect of job stress on job satisfaction

Est.	S.E.	C.R.	P-Value	Result
-.589	.032	-18.212	0.001	Significant

Est, Estimates, S.E, Standard error, P-value, significant

The form of mediation is known as "partial mediation" as we can see the effect of IV on DV is significant after mediating variables entered the model. Since, the aforesaid steps 1, 2, and 3 have already met the criteria as mentioned in the hypotheses 1, 2, and 3 simultaneously; so to test the step 4 another structural model is to be tested where, the researcher implemented bootstrap method to study the indirect effect in the mediation model. In bootstrapping method, the resampling of the existing data is executed. It is run on AMOS software and set 95% confidence interval (CI). After executing the bootstrapping technique, the generated p values and confidence interval (CI) of the parameters are considered along with the standardized regression weights to understand the model path effects. The confidence interval at 95 percent estimated does not include 0 and it suggests that indirect effect is statistically significant 5% level. Table 2 to 6 shows the results of total, indirect, and direct effect.

DISCUSSION

Taken together, the result of the current study supports the hypotheses. Incivility at the workplace harms individuals in terms of stress. Whereas most of the research focused on face to face incivility, the present research extended the literature by concentrating on cyber incivility, which includes instant or text messages and email. By applying the COR and AET theory, the present study inspected the consequence of cyber incivility. The outcome of the study claimed that those individuals who experienced online incivility tend to report job dissatisfaction through the experience of job stress.

This study has analysed the arbitrating impact of stress on the association between cyber incivility and job satisfaction and the result clearly indicates that job stress is a mediator between online incivility and satisfaction in the job. The finding of the study supported by previous research on the face to face incivility in relation to job satisfaction (Laschinger, et al., 2009) and job stress (Giumetti et al., 2012). This study suggests that personnel's who experience incivility or others who behave badly at work with them may report job stress, which leads to job dissatisfaction. Hence, the aforesaid objective is in line with the past studies and the result of it is supported (Cooper & Marshall, 1976; Embse et al., 2016; Giumetti et al., 2012; Laschinger, et al., 2009; Laschinger, et vbal., 2014; Liu & Ramsey, 2008; Naumann, 1993; Nel, 2019; Marchiondo ct al., 2010; Pandey & Sharma, 2016; Terry et al., 1993).

IMPLICATIONS

The current study revealed the association between cyber incivility and stress and job satisfaction by demonstrating the subjective perception of individuals who experienced incivility behaviour as the channel through which cyber incivility exerts its impact on employees' stress and job satisfaction. As a practical implication, to enhance job satisfaction or reduce job stress, effective managers or leaders need to find ways to improve or reduce incivility at the workplace by making bullying or incivility-free environment. In general, this can lead to higher satisfaction in a job. Further, the finding of this research clarifies that negative behaviour triggers job stress and job satisfaction which has practical relevance, so while communicating, the sender should be very careful with the tone of the messages all the time. The workplaces should create a platform where an employee can easily discuss issues when communicating online. By providing such opportunities to the employees, there will be awareness regarding netiquette and acceptable behaviour. Further, generally, individuals do not report incivility done by superiors, so, human resource managers should encourage feedback on their immediate boss. This would help the organization in identifying the bully at an early stage. Early detection of a perpetrator allows the the HR to counsel the perpetrator appropriately.

The judgement of the study specifies the impact of cyber incivility on the stress and satisfaction among employee. This finding has a possible implication in various fields, including IT Professionals and education. For example, if managers treat their employees poorly through technology like email, they may be more likely to avoid online sync-ups. To evade these matters, administrators should ponder executing online etiquette strategies to provide cognisance about the possible way for miscommunication online. Furthermore, workers should give special consideration to their online correspondences and rearticulate any cases that could be misperceived as being offensive. Technology companies have effectively begun the tools that can assist users to refrain from sending uncivil mails. For instance, the feature of Gmail ''Undo Send' which permits to prevent mails from being sent as long as 30 seconds after user hits send" is beneficial for users. Such an element may permit senders "to review the note before it is sent and drop the message from being sent inside a 30-second time window if the message is seen to be uncivil". This is also an attention-grabbing example that exemplifies "how changes in technology may help individuals refrain from being uncivil online".

Given the considerable undesirable effects brewing up among employees due to deviant behaviour in the Indian arena (D'Cruz & Rayner, 2014), this study may be obliged to investigators, academicians, practitioners, government authorities or policy and lawmakers to comprehend that such issue needs to be recognised and halted by taking instant action. However, the law for the protection against sexual harassment exists in the legislation, but no law in India precisely deals with bullying or incivility in the workplace, even though bullying is ranked on the top amongst all other types of negative behaviours at workplaces (Giorgi, et al., 2016; Wilson, 1991) and in 2003, Gary Namie clearly stated that it is supposed to be "three times more prevalent than sexual harassment" (pp. 2). Thus, there is a need to provide awareness among the Indian masses about the extent of online bullying or incivility phenomenon. So, an organisation should state clear norms regarding appropriate and acceptable email communication which can deliver a powerful message regarding the intolerance for cyber incivility among employees (Grant, 2019).

LIMITATIONS AND RECOMMENDATIONS

Although this investigation makes numeral contributions to the writing, certain limitations should be considered in order to properly infer the findings. The nature of the study is cross-sectional and this bound the researcher to test causal relationship i.e. recursive. So, a future researcher should longitudinally analyse the hypotheses, which will help to reveal how job stress, cyber incivility, and job satisfaction association will change over time. Longitudinal data is needed to confirm and generalise the findings of the present study. The respondents in the current investigation came from the software engineering industry, which may have a unique feature not found in other industries. Thus, there is a need to study the model in other cultures and samples like higher educational professionals or B-school, engineering faculties or some other sectors to generalize the findings. There can be some other variables for the cyber incivility-satisfaction associations, such as sleep disorders, post- traumatic stress disorder, low organisational commitment, intention to leave, and the well-being of employee. The researcher invites future researchers to examine potential relationships. Future studies can also do a comparative study among different cities or states in relation to the prevalence of cyber incivility. In this study, researcher takes all type of ICT but the future researcher should examine all kinds of ICT as there are numbers of ICT, like messages, email, video calls and text. So, future researchers can explore each form of ICT as a separate construct and compare them. Additionally, future studies can compare the workplace that has ICT usage with no ICT usage workplaces which will help to understand which form of incivility is more harmful, i.e., "face to face incivility or cyber incivility".

CONCLUSION

In conclusion, this study contributed and emphasis on the research related to cyber incivility. Since, the use of online communications present at most workstations, their potential glitches remain an issue that grants the consideration of the researcher. Theoretical work on the incivility recommends that such practices can be twisted into different types of aggression. This work could be protracted to an online setting to regulate whether cyber incivility intensifies traditional incivility or physical violence. This study signified an initial phase in investigating the consequence of cyber incivility on stress at job and satisfaction in the job. From the research point of view, this study extends the body of knowledge in terms of the role of cyber incivility and individual consequences.

REFERENCES

Akellaa, D., & Lewis, V. (2019). The Modern Face of Workplace Incivility. *Organization Management Journal*, 1-7. doi:10.1080/15416518.2019.1604202

Alola, U. V., Avcı, T., & Öztüren, A. (2021). The nexus of workplace incivility and emotional exhaustion in hotel industry. *Journal of Public Affairs*, *21*(3), e2236. doi:10.1002/pa.2236

Andersson, L., & Pearson, C. (1999). Tit for tat? The spiralling effect of incivility in the workplace. *Academy of Management Review*, *24*(3), 452–471. doi:10.2307/259136

Bagozzi, R. P., & Yi, Y. (1988). On the evaluation of structural equation models. *Journal of the Academy of Marketing Science*, *16*(1), 74–94. doi:10.1007/BF02723327

Baron, R., & Neuman, J. (1996). Workplace violence and workplace aggression: Evidence on their relative frequency and potential causes. *Aggressive Behavior*, *221*(3), 161–173. doi:10.1002/(SICI)1098-2337(1996)22:3<161::AID-AB1>3.0.CO;2-Q

Blau, G., & Andersson, L. (2005). Testing a measure of instigated incivility. *Journal of Occupational and Organizational Psychology*, *78*(4), 595–614. doi:10.1348/096317905X26822

Bono, J., Glomb, T., Shen, W., Kim, E., & Koch, A. (2013). Building positive resources: Effects of positive events and positive reflection on work stress and health. *Academy of Management Journal*, *56*(6), 1601–1627. doi:10.5465/amj.2011.0272

Brief, A. (1998). *Attitudes in and Around Organizations*. Thousand Oaks ed. CA. *Sage (Atlanta, Ga.)*.

Buffer. (2020). *The 2020 state of remote work*. Retrieved from https://lp.buffer.com/state-of-remote-work-2020

Bunk, J. A., & Magley, V. J. (2013). The role of appraisals and emotions in understanding experiences of workplace incivility. *Journal of Occupational Health Psychology*, *18*(1), 87–105. doi:10.1037/a0030987 PMID:23339748

Byron, K. (2008). Carrying too heavy a load? The communication and miscommunication of emotion by email. *Academy of Management Review*, *33*(2), 309–327. doi:10.5465/amr.2008.31193163

Chung, H., Quan, W., Koo, B., Ariza-Montes, A., Vega-Muñoz, A., Giorgi, G., & Han, H. (2021). A Threat of Customer Incivility and Job Stress to Hotel Employee Retention: Do Supervisor and Co-Worker Supports Reduce Turnover Rates? *International Journal of Environmental Research and Public Health*, *18*(12), 6616. doi:10.3390/ijerph18126616 PMID:34205422

Cooper, C. L., & Marshall, J. (1976). Occupational sources of stress: A review of the literature relating to coronary heart disease and mental ill health. *Journal of Occupational Psychology*, *49*(1), 11–28. doi:10.1111/j.2044-8325.1976.tb00325.x

Cortina, L., Magley, V., Williams, J., & Langhout, R. (2001). Incivility in the workplace: Incidence and impact. *Journal of Occupational Health Psychology*, *6*(1), 64–80. doi:10.1037/1076-8998.6.1.64 PMID:11199258

D'ambra, A. M., & Andrews, D. R. (2014). Incivility, retention and new graduate nurses: An integrated review of the literature. *Journal of Nursing Management*, *22*(6), 735–742. doi:10.1111/jonm.12060 PMID:23927565

D'Cruz, P., & Rayner, C. (2014). The incidence of interpersonal workplace bullying in India"s ITES-BPO sector. *Indian Journal of Labour Economics*, *57*(2), 221–242.

De Vaus, D. (2001). Research design in social research. *Sage (Atlanta, Ga.)*.

Efron, B. (1979). Bootstrap methods. Another look at jackknife. *Annals of Statistics*, *7*(1), 1–26. doi:10.1214/aos/1176344552

Eka, N. G., & Chambers, D. (2019). Incivility in nursing education: A systematic literature review. *Nurse Education in Practice*, *39*, 45–54. doi:10.1016/j.nepr.2019.06.004 PMID:31382114

Embse, V., Sandilos, N., Pendergast, L., & Mankin, A. (2016). Teacher stress, teaching-efficacy, and job satisfaction in response to test-based educational accountability policies. *Learning and Individual Differences*, *50*, 308–317. doi:10.1016/j.lindif.2016.08.001

French, S. E., Lenton, R., Walters, V., & Eyles, J. (2000). An Empirical Evaluation of an Expanded Nursing Stress Scale. *Journal of Nursing Measurement*, *8*(2), 161–178. doi:10.1891/1061-3749.8.2.161 PMID:11227582

Giorgi, G., Perminiene, M., Montani, F., Fiz-Perez, J., Mucci, N., & Arcangeli, G. (2016). Detrimental effects of workplace bullying: Impediment of self-management competence via psychological distress. *Frontiers in Psychology*, *7*. Advance online publication. doi:10.3389/fpsyg.2016.00060 PMID:26913013

Giumetti, G., McKibben, E., Hatfield, A., Schroeder, A., & Kowalski, R. (2012). Cyber incivility @ work: The new age of interpersonal deviance. *Cyberpsychology, Behavior, and Social Networking*, *15*(3), 148–154. doi:10.1089/cyber.2011.0336 PMID:22304404

Giumetti, G., Saunders, L., Brunette, J., Di Francesco, F., & Graham, P. (2016). Linking Cyber Incivility with Job Performance Through Job Satisfaction: The Buffering Role of Positive Affect. *Psi Chi Journal of Psychological Research*, *21*(4), 230–240. doi:10.24839/2164-8204.JN21.4.230

Giumetti, G. W., Hatfield, A. L., Scisco, J. L., Schroeder, A. N., Muth, E. R., & Kowalski, R. M. (2013). What a rude e-mail! Examining the differential effects of incivility versus support on mood, energy, engagement, and performance in an online context. *Journal of Occupational Health Psychology*, *18*(3), 297–309. doi:10.1037/a0032851 PMID:23834445

Grant, A. (2019, Feb 15). *No, you can't ignore email. It's rude.* Retrieved from The New York Times: https://www.nytimes.com/2019/02/15/opinion/sunday/email-etiquette.html

Hair, J., Black, W. C., Babin, B. J., & Anderson, R. E. (2013). *Multivariate Data Analysis*. Pearson Education Limited.

Haque, M. R., Hafiz, R., Azad, A. A., & Adnan, Y. (2021). Crime Detection and Criminal Recognition to Intervene in Interpersonal Violence Using Deep Convolutional Neural Network with Transfer Learning. *International Journal of Ambient Computing and Intelligence*, *12*(4), 14. doi:10.4018/IJACI.20211001.oa1

Heischman, R. (2017). *Face to Face and Cyber Incivility*. Academic Press.

Herbsleb, J. (2007). Global software engineering: The future of sociotechnical coordination. In *Proceedings of the Future of Software Engineering Conference* (pp. 188–198). IEEE.

Hobfoll, S. (1989). Conservation of resources: A new attempt at conceptualizing stress. *The American Psychologist*, *44*(3), 513–524. doi:10.1037/0003-066X.44.3.513 PMID:2648906

Hulin, C., & Judge, T. (2003). Job attitudes. In Handbook of Psychology: Industrial and Organizational Psychology. Wiley. doi:10.1002/0471264385.wei1211

Johnson, P., & Indvik, J. (2001). Rudeness at work: Impulse over restraint. *Public Personnel Management*, *30*(4), 457–465. doi:10.1177/009102600103000403

Kahai, S. S., & Cooper, R. B. (2003). Exploring the core concepts of media richness theory: The impact of cue multiplicity and feedback immediacy in decision quality. *Journal of Management Information Systems*, *20*(1), 263–299. doi:10.1080/07421222.2003.11045754

Kellaway, L. (2016, March 13). *Email: The weapon wielded by the passive aggressive colleague.* Retrieved from Financial Times, https://www.ft.com/content/dee75f5e-e635-11e5-a09b-1f8b0d268c39

Kowalski, R. M., & Robbins, C. E. (2021). *The Meaning, Prevalence, and Outcomes of Cyberbullying in the Workplace. In Handbook of Research on Cyberbullying and Online Harassment in the Workplace*. IGI Global.

Kruger, J., Epley, N., Parker, J., & Ng, Z. (2005). Egocentrism over e-mail: Can we communicate as well as we think? *Journal of Personality and Social Psychology*, *89*(6), 925–936. doi:10.1037/0022-3514.89.6.925 PMID:16393025

Laschinger, H., Cummings, G., Wong, C., & Grau, A. (2014). Resonant leadership and workplace empowerment: The value of positive organizational cultures in reducing workplace incivility. *Nursing Economics*, *32*(1), 5–44. doi:10.1111/j.1365-28 PMID:24689153

Laschinger, H., Leiter, M., Day, A., & Gilin, D. (2009). Workplace empowerment, incivility, and burnout: Impact on staff nurse recruitment and retention outcomes. *Journal of Nursing Management*, *17*(3), 302–311. doi:10.1111/j.1365-2834.2009.00999.x PMID:19426367

Lim, S., & Cortina, L. (2005). Interpersonal mistreatment in the workplace: The interface and impact of general incivility and sexual harassment. *The Journal of Applied Psychology*, *90*(3), 483–496. doi:10.1037/0021-9010.90.3.483 PMID:15910144

Lim, V., & Teo, T. (2009). Mind your E-manners: Impact of cyber incivility on employees' work attitude and behavior. *Information & Management*, *46*(8), 419–425. doi:10.1016/j.im.2009.06.006

Liu, X., & Ramsey, J. (2008). Teachers' job satisfaction: Analyses of the teacher follow up survey in the United States for 2000–2001. *Teaching and Teacher Education*, *24*(5), 1173–1184. doi:10.1016/j.tate.2006.11.010

Marchiondo, K., Marchiondo, L., & Lasiter, S. (2010). Faculty incivility: Effects on program satisfaction of BSN students. *The Journal of Nursing Education*, *49*(11), 608–614. doi:10.3928/01484834-20100524-05 PMID:20509588

Markus, M. L. (1994). Electronic mail as the medium of managerial choice. *Organization Science*, *5*(4), 502–527. doi:10.1287/orsc.5.4.502

McCarthy, K. A. (2016). Is rudeness really that common? An exploratory study of incivility at work. *Journal of Organizational Computing and Electronic Commerce*, *26*(4), 364–374. doi:10.1080/10919392.2016.1228362

Mesaglio, M. (2020, March). *4 actions to be a strong leader during COVID-19 disruption.* Retrieved from https://www.gartner.com/smarterwithgartner/4-actions-to-be-a-good-leader-during-covid-19-disruption/

Mongey, S., & Weinberg, A. (2020). *Characteristics of Workers in Low Work-From-Home and High Personal-Proximity Occupations.* White Paper.

Namie, G. (2003). Workplace bullying: Escalated incivility. *Ivey Business Journal*, *68*(2), 1–6.

Naumann, E. (1993). Antecedents and consequences of satisfaction and commitment among expatriate managers. *Group & Organization Management*, *18*(2), 153–187. doi:10.1177/1059601193182003

Nel, E. (2019). The impact of workplace bullying on flourishing: The moderating role of emotional intelligence. *SA Journal of Industrial Psychology*, *45*(0). Advance online publication. doi:10.4102ajip.v45i0.1603

O'Sullivan, P. B., & Flanagin, A. J. (2003). Reconceptualizing flaming and other problematic messages. *New Media & Society*, *5*, 67–93.

Pandey, S., & Sharma, V. (2016). Understanding Work-Related Stress, Job Conditions, Work Culture and Workaholism Phenomenon as Predictors of HR Crisis: An Empirical Study of the Indian IT Sector. *International Journal of Human Capital and Information Technology Professionals*, *7*(2), 13. doi:10.4018/IJHCITP.2016040105

Pearson, C. M., & Porath, C. L. (2005). On the nature, consequences and remedies of workplace incivility: No time for "nice"? Think again. *The Academy of Management Executive*, *19*(1), 7–18. doi:10.5465/ame.2005.15841946

Pignata, S., Boyd, C., Gillespie, N., Provis, C., & Winefield, A. (2014). Awareness of organizational stress-reduction interventions: The impact on employee wellbeing and attitudes. *Stress and Health, 32*, 231–243. doi:10.1002mi.2597 PMID:25066108

Porath, C., & Pearson, C. (2012). Emotional and behavioral responses to workplace incivility and the impact of hierarchical status. *Journal of Applied Social Psychology, 42*, 326–357. doi:10.1111/j.1559-1816.2012.01020.x

Pounder, C. (1998). Homeworking: No longer an easy option? *Computers & Security, 17*(1), 27–30. doi:10.1016/S0167-4048(97)80246-5

Preacher, K., & Hayes, A. (2008). Asymptotic and resampling strategies for assessing and comparing indirect effects in multiple mediator models. *Behavior Research Methods, 40*(3), 879–891. doi:10.3758/BRM.40.3.879 PMID:18697684

Ralph, P., Baltes, S., Adisaputri, G., Torkar, R., Kovalenko, V., Kalinowski, M., Novielli, N., Yoo, S., Devroey, X., Tan, X., Zhou, M., Turhan, B., Hoda, R., Hata, H., Robles, G., Milani Fard, A., & Alkadhi, R. (2020). Pandemic programming: How COVID-19 affects software developers and how their organizations can help. *Empirical Software Engineering, 25*(6), 4927–4961. doi:10.100710664-020-09875-y PMID:32952438

Reio, T. Jr, & Ghosh, R. J. (2009). Antecedents and outcomes of workplace incivility: Implications for human resource development research and practice. *Human Resource Development Quarterly, 20*(3), 237–264. doi:10.1002/hrdq.20020

Roy, M., & Mandal, A. (2021). A Comparative Study on The Influence Of Job Satisfaction On Deviant Workplace Behavior In Private And Government Educational Institutes. *Psychology and Education Journal, 58*(5), 2850–2862.

Russo, D., Hanel, P. P., Altnickel, S., & Van Berkel, N. (2021). The Daily Life of Software Engineers during the COVID-19 Pandemic. doi:10.1109/ICSE-SEIP52600.2021.00048

Singhal, T. (2020). A Review of Coronavirus Disease-2019 (COVID-19). *Indian Journal of Pediatrics, 87*(4), 281–286. doi:10.100712098-020-03263-6 PMID:32166607

Sliter, M., Jex, S., Wolford, K., & McInnerney, J. (2010). How rude! Emotional labor as a mediator between customer incivility and employee outcomes. *Journal of Occupational Health Psychology, 15*(4), 468–481. doi:10.1037/a0020723 PMID:21058859

Smite, D., Wohlin, C., Gorschek, T., & Feldt, R. (2010). Empirical evidence in global software engineering: A systematic review. *Empirical Software Engineering, 15*(1), 91–118. doi:10.100710664-009-9123-y

Spadafora, N., Frijters, J. C., Molnar, D. S., & Volk, A. A. (2020). Do little annoyances relate to bullying? The links between personality, attitudes towards classroom incivility, and bullying. *The Educational and Developmental Psychologist, 37*(1), 30–38. doi:10.1017/edp.2019.20

Spreitzer, G. M. (1995). Psychological empowerment in the workplace: Dimensions, measurement, and validation. *Academy of Management Journal, 38*(5), 1442–1465. doi:10.2307/256865

Terry, D. J., Nielsen, M., & Perchard, L. (1993). Effects of work stress on psychological well-being and job satisfaction: The stress-buffering role of social support. *Australian Journal of Psychology*, *45*(3), 168–175. doi:10.1080/00049539308259135

Weiss, H. M., & Cropanzano, R. (1996). Affective Events Theory: A theoretical discussion of the structure, causes and consequences of affective experiences at work. In B. M. Staw & L. L. Cummings (Eds.), *Research in organizational behavior: An annual series of analytical essays and critical reviews* (Vol. 18, pp. 1–74). Elsevier Science/ JAI Press.

Wilson, C. B. (1991). US businesses suffer from workplace trauma. *The Personnel Journal*, *70*(7), 47–50.

Wright, M., & Hill, L. (2015). Academic incivility among health sciences faculty. *Adult Learning*, *26*(1), 14–20. doi:10.1177/1045159514558410

Yang, S. Y., Chen, S. C., Lee, L., & Liu, Y. S. (2021). Employee Stress, Job Satisfaction, and Job Performance: A Comparison between High-technology and Traditional Industry in Taiwan. *The Journal of Asian Finance. Economics and Business*, *8*(3), 605–618.

Zammuto, R. F., & Krakower, J. Y. (1991). *Quantitative and qualitative studies of organizational culture*. JAI Press.

Chapter 6
Importance of Emotional Intelligence for the Leaders to Manage People and Business Effectively in Times of Crisis

Abirami K.
Department of Business Management, Erode Arts and Science College (Autonomous), India

Jayasudha S. M.
Department of Business Management, Erode Arts and Science College (Autonomous), India

ABSTRACT

Businesses have had financial and economic crises in the past, but none have compared to the COVID-19 pandemic, according to industry leaders. There is always a need for consistency, safety, and compassion in situations like COVID-19. Emotional intelligence has long been considered a crucial leadership skill. Now more than ever it is essential to navigate this crisis and establish a new normal. Consider emotional health as water in a glass that, in normal circumstances, might slowly evaporate and that leaders occasionally need to top off. Change, uncertainty, tension, and anxiety, however, behave like holes in the glass during a crisis, allowing water to pour out all over the place. There needs to be more top-down additions made in order to maintain emotional stability. Leadership plays an essential role in difficult situations to guide individuals or the group down the rocky path that lies ahead. Leaders must develop the traits that will enable them to efficiently manage their emotions and, in turn, assist others in managing theirs.

INTRODUCTION

Although businesses have had financial and economic crises in the past, none have compared to the Covid-19epidemic, and it has changed world drastically. Coronavirus-related societal and economic problems, as well as other catastrophic occurrences like unfavorable weather patterns brought on by

DOI: 10.4018/978-1-6684-8565-1.ch006

climate change and global warming, particularly in the US and China, make the world a hostile place for enterprises. As a result, in order to compete, business organizations must implement restructuring procedures to address economic issues. The modern business climate presents enterprises with additional challenges, including globalization (Pak et al., 2020). As a result, multinational corporations are being forced to implement change management strategies due to cultural, social, managerial, and economic developments. For this, companies are aligning their workforce with cultural and economical diversity. Employees may not adapt well to the substantial change management procedures that business executives implement to be competitive in the current chaotic and dynamic operating environment (Sageder & Feldbauer-Durstmüller, 2019). Therefore, to effectively manage change amid crises, unique leadership techniques are required. Regarding how leaders handle the change management processes in their commercial organizations, emotional intelligence is a key idea in the literature on change management and leadership (Mansaray, 2019). The literature on the connection between emotional intelligence and leadership in influencing change management during a crisis is examined in the current study. It suggests a mechanism for evaluating how well two leadership philosophies transformational and transactional can ensure effective change management in enterprises during times of crisis (Tang, Yin & Nelson, 2010).

In the past or before Covid-19, majority of managers have learned the value of Emotional Intelligence (EQ) in cultivating followership and enhancing performance. Lack of self-control, empathy, or the capacity to engage with or influence others frequently results in catastrophic leadership failures; recent standout instances include Travis Kalanick of Uber, Adam Neumann of WeWork, and Elizabeth Holmes of Theranos (Mark Nevins, 2020). Steve Jobs may be the exception to the rule that owners cannot generate success without a strong sense of EQ. Steve Job's greatest achievement as a leader may have been managing to construct a firm that could withstand his caustic brilliance (Schwantes, 2020). Emotional intelligence (EI) is significant and won't go away any time soon. It can be understood from the track records of Mayor Bill DeBlasio of New York City, Elon Musk of Tesla, and Mark Zuckerberg of Facebook, each of whom appears to struggle with understanding how to effectively engage crucial stakeholders? Leaving aside famous people, the world has changed dramatically in this turbulent year of 2020, making EI an even more important skill for all leaders and managers in both public and private enterprises (Sanchez-Ruiz et al., 2021).

Even under the best circumstances, maintaining emotional ties with our team by regulating our own emotions can be difficult. It's become significantly more difficult when add the brand-new realities of the post-Covid-19era. The strains of remote work which added additional, perplexing pressure and friction to our lives. "Social distance" is a deeply unnatural state that makes developing and sustaining relationships much more challenging (Goodlet, 2022). The continual coverage in the news of rising infection rates, societal unrest, and failing corporations makes us all feel existentially anxious. Employees now expect and need to be heard and understood more than ever. They yearn to feel cherished and safe. Beyond "the stats," they seek a deeper relationship with their superiors. In a manner effective leadership has always involved high levels of EI. It is important to develop and practice this skill in the post-pandemic era because remote and hybrid work is still prevalent and it might be difficult to engage people and establish trust (Koçak, 2021). Hence the leaders and the mange should be good enough in the emotional intelligence. With this backdrop the present chapter has made an attempt to explain the importance of emotional intelligence for the leaders to manage people and business effectively in times of crisis.

WHAT EXACTLY IS EMOTIONAL INTELLIGENCE?

The foundation of emotional intelligence is self-awareness. It begins with the capacity to recognize the feelings someone is going through at the moment. However, the key is to comprehend how those feelings might influence how a person behaves, responds, and decides or makes decisions based on the impact of the feelings (Chin, Anantharaman & Tong, 2011). The second level of emotional intelligence, according to Gurprriet Singh, managing director, APAC Regional Leader of Leadership & Succession, Russell Reynolds Associates, is social awareness or being aware of how others feel and how those feelings may affect their behaviors or choices (Dash, 2022). EQ is the capacity to regulate and channel emotions, foster better interpersonal connections, maximize positive behavior in challenging circumstances and cultivate the capacity to access positive, self-driving emotions that eventually result in positive outcomes. EQ will assist leaders in providing and receiving useful feedback. In the post-COVID era, EQ will be more crucial than ever as work becomes more flexible, occasionally more remote, and almost certainly more ambiguous (Rodrigues, Ribeiro & Gomes, 2022). Similar to how traditional, "hard" leadership talents are taught and developed, EQ should be developed. Businesses should assist managers and leaders in identifying and understanding their EQ traits, and if these traits do not come naturally, in developing them so that they can lead with empathy.

IMPORTANCE OF EMOTIONAL INTELLIGENCE FOR LEADERS DURING CRISIS TIMES

When dealing with challenging events, emotional intelligence is crucial because an emotionally intelligent leader would react to adversity in a cool, collected manner. Leader who has emotional intelligence is better at controlling their own emotions as well as those of others when under stress or strain. The growing risk of burnout is a serious trend that modern leaders must take into account (Aguilar Yuste, 2021). Since the pandemic is a novel situation, many business executives are ill-prepared to handle the demands this new work era places on their character and as persons. Future leaders will still need the "traditional" leadership abilities, knowledge, and experience that propelled them to the top of their organizations, but if they want to inspire and motivate their teams and foster a culture of trust within them, they'll also need to have a higher level of EQ (Altamirano, & Collazo, 2020). Although EQ is not a new idea and many gifted leaders would have already used it in their capacity, its relevance and utility have grown even more crucial with the arrival of the COVID pandemic. Because of this, Coronavirus has avoided shining a sharp light on areas where leaders need to grow and develop. According to a global study report, 2020Work will be more flexible in the future (Semenets-Orlova, 2021). In the future, three out of four employees would welcome more flexibility and a combination of office-based and remote work, and 75% of them believe businesses must maintain the newfound autonomy and flexibility (Dirani, 2020). However, the way managers lead their teams and executives run their businesses will also need to alter in this new era of flexible work. To fulfill changing employee expectations, there will be more emphasis on leaders building "soft skills" like empathy and trust. As a result, around 77 percent of workers want their leaders to demonstrate greater empathy and a helpful attitude, while more than 50 percent of managers and leaders claim they require assistance in adjusting to and reaching these new standards (Mysirlaki & Paraskeva, 2020). To combat the Covid-19pandemic, the globe is making extraordinary efforts. Leaders are working to keep mission-critical activities moving forward, but, inevitably, companies will eventually have to deal with a black swan event. Effective leaders should always prepare the things that they know to be ready for the things they do not know in a highly volatile situation (Alonazi, 2020).

Nearly all large businesses have business continuity plans, fallback procedures, and desktop protocols in place so they can continue their essential operations. It can be difficult to keep staff engaged and motivated during a crisis, and it has been described as a leadership art. Emotional intelligence is one of a leader's most critical abilities for achieving these objectives. To be ready for the things they do not know, leaders should plan, apply, and work with what they already know (Baesu, 2019). The Covid-19pandemic catastrophe and the subsequent recovery will certainly call for a unique set of abilities. After a few months of the Covid-19pandemic crisis, the business world has a good idea of the talents that will be needed from leaders in the future, even though they do not yet know exactly what those skills will be. Hence, the authors have examined how leaders can prepare for, employ, and profit from the four categories of emotional intelligence identified by Daniel Goleman such as self-awareness, self-management, social awareness, and relationship management. Each of these domains can support a leader in managing stress, emotional reaction, and unexpected effects while dealing with any crisis (Dirani, 2020).

Elements of Emotional Intelligence

The core interpersonal and personal competencies that make up emotional intelligence were defined by psychologist Daniel Goleman, who also explained why EQ is just as crucial to success as IQ with five components as Self-awareness, Self-regulation, Motivation, Empathy, Social skills or relationship management (Jacob Morgan, 2021; ICAEW Insights, 2021). Self-awareness is the ability to recognize and comprehend an individual's emotions, including what an individual is feeling and why, as well as how they affect those around them. It forms the cornerstone of sound judgment and decision-making, enabling people to make the best decisions in all spheres of life. Knowing own virtues or moral compass, as well as own strengths and limitations, is another aspect of self-awareness (Görgens-Ekermans, & Roux, 2021). The next stage after self or emotional awareness is Self-regulation. It skillfully controls those emotions, especially the negative ones. This component always is respectful of others and makes an effort to maintain control. Practice remaining calm if an individual tends to have emotional outbursts by taking a step back and taking a deep breath. Additionally, it's critical to uphold an individual's moral standards and take responsibility for actions (Future Talent Learning, 2021). The third "personal" component, motivation, is about the desire to advance and succeed. It involves holding an individual to high standards and perseveringly pursuing objectives. Thereby individuals can develop their assertiveness skills and be prepared to seize chances as they present themselves. Discovery the fine in any situation, even those that didn't go fine, and being hopeful and flexible are other significant apparatus of motivation. Empathy is a fourth component that made individuals able to put their feet in another person's shoes and consider a problem from their point of view is a crucial interpersonal skill. It's crucial to understand and respond to others' feelings, even if an individual disagrees with them, in addition to being aware of their own (Jacob Morgan, 2021). A crucial component of empathy is communication, so pay close attention to what an individual and others say when people speak or act. One more important part of empathy is relating to multiplicity and completeness. The term "people person" is frequently used to describe someone who has strong social or relationship skills. They are dependable team associates and certain speakers who are uniformly skillful at pay attention to others as they are at talking for themselves. They also make outstanding leaders, inspirational and hopeful others, competently handling transformation and divergence, and giving recognition where recognition is due. As a result, these five components are playing a major role in shaping a person's behavior towards a group as well as individually (Tasha Eurich, 2018). In the times of the Covid-19crisis how these components have been helping the managers to manage themselves and their team has been explained as follows.

Role of EQ Components in Shaping Leaders' Emotional Intelligence to Manage People and Business Better in the Covid-19Crisis

Self-Awareness

Self-awareness is regarded as being crucial because it enables people to more fully grasp their internal feelings, preferences, resources, and intuitions. It also enables them to comprehend the emotions of those around them. Self-awareness is divided into two categories. Internal self-awareness, or how individuals see them, falls under the first category, while outward self-awareness, or how others see someone, falls under the second. Leaders who perceive themselves through the eyes of their followers are more effective. The relationships are better, and the workers are happier with them. To effectively lead, one needs actively engage in both: recognizing oneself and obtaining feedback to understand how others view one. High self-awareness individuals are frequently the ones that maintain balance (Semenets-Orlova, et al., 2021). Typically, leaders believe that as they gain experience, their level of self-awareness will rise, but that is not always the right case. Experience can cause leaders to overestimate their level of self-awareness and might give them a false sense of confidence about their performance. Leaders with much experience may not question their presumptions. A leader is more inclined to exaggerate his strengths and capabilities as his power increases. Schlegel and Mortillaro (2019) mentioned that self-awareness is the component of EI that leaders find least enjoyable or time-consuming. Only when a leader becomes adept at knowing himself can they collaborate with others effectively. A leader will be more creative, confident, and able to make wiser judgments, forge deeper connections, and communicate more effectively when they see themselves clearly when the leaders are less prone to steal, cheat, and lie. Having happier workers will increase his effectiveness. However, only 15% of leaders possess this ability, even though the majority of them believe they are self-aware (Eurich, 2018). It is crucial to understand how our beliefs, motivations, aspirations, actions, and reactions fit into our surroundings and what kind of an impact they have on other people (Rivers, 2020). Goleman (2013), states that knowing one's sentiments put one in control. The majority of the personnel are working from home offices during the Covid-19pandemic. The employees' productivity is not equal. When people are participating in online meetings, their children's noise can frequently be heard, giving the impression that they are not paying attention to the conversation. Small errors that had never happened before began to appear. A leader is upset by all of these. How they handle these circumstances is the question.

Oates, (2021), One should be aware that employees are unable to concentrate on their tasks as they formerly did during a crisis when their health and the welfare of their family are at stake. To prevent the same mistake from happening again, leaders should examine each error individually and, where practical, add extra controls to the process. Leaders should speak assertively with their staff in situations where additional controls are ineffective and errors result from a lack of concentration, outlining the consequences of their error while instilling confidence in them that finding a solution to the issue is a shared objective. It is necessary to consider performance and target settings differently. The goal is to work together as a team and battle for survival. Individual goals should be given less weight than team-based, communal goals with shorter time horizons. In actuality, the total is bigger than the parts.

Businesses that can maintain employee motivation and engagement in the first half of 2020 will benefit from the global economy in the second half of that year (Jeremy Sutton, 2021). The good news is that one can increase self-awareness. A leader should work to increase his self-awareness because it is linked to better happiness, personal and social control, and job and relationship satisfaction. A person's anxiety, tension, and sadness will be lessened the higher their level of self-awareness. There are other ways to increase self-awareness, but we'll focus on the most crucial ones. Analyze our actions and reactions that an individual doesn't like and try to change them by taking an impartial look at ourselves. It's interesting how we interpret our values, interests, and goals. Keep a journal because some of the responses and actions might not be welcomed by others. Keep a journal and record every instance in which someone disagreed with an individual. The journal can also be used for self-analysis. '' It enables individuals to recognize, define, and embrace their feelings and thoughts. It aids in our life as self-discovery of what values us, what is our want, and what functions for us (Caroline Forsey, 2018).

After determining the actions and reactions that require improvement, jot down our objectives, strategies, and top priorities. Making a strategy is helpful when beginning to develop the skills. It is usually beneficial to conduct daily introspection. Even if people have begun to advance their abilities, it will take time. To get a clear image of where people stand in the process, practice self-reflection. Self-awareness is not necessarily increased through introspection. Because most individuals do it poorly, it can occasionally be ineffectual. Clearing the mind of unpleasant thoughts and bad energy is facilitated by engaging in mindfulness practices like meditation (Bergner, 2021). The ability to plan and concentrate on the tasks at hand is much easier once unpleasant emotions have been released. This also promotes effective teamwork. In contrast to daydreaming, ruminating, or getting lost in thought, mindfulness is being aware of both environment and within. The goal of meditation is to train the mind to concentrate on one thing, such as the breath, a mantra, or a feeling, and to let thoughts pass by without clinging to them. Both methods can aid in raising our awareness of our internal state and responses to situations (Showry & Manasa, 2014). They can also aid in recognizing thoughts and emotions and help one avoid becoming sucked into them. Yoga is another activity. Yoga aids in teaching the mind self-control, acceptance, and awareness. Taking psychometric and personality tests can reveal the characteristics, thought processes, and responses of a person. If the person filling out the test is honest, the test can yield positive results (Eurich, 2018). Having dependable friends describe an individual. The best test might be there. Even those who know us well may not see things the same way we do. It is never easy to hear something unpleasant. However, if one views criticism as beneficial, one can immediately begin to advance their abilities. People must speak with a range of people to have a complete picture. Because a self-conscious person is aware of when an opportunity is a good fit for him and how to seize it, high self-awareness is an excellent indicator of life's success. Developing listening skills might help an individual become more self-aware. So learn to listen objectively to what another person needs or wants to say by being open to them. This makes it easier to listen to our internal conversations and thoughts with objectivity (Sutton, Williams & Allinson, 2015).

Self-Control

The ability to regulate and adjust responses to prevent unwanted behaviors, promote favorable ones, and accomplish long-term goals is referred to as self-control. To accomplish common goals like decreasing weight, exercising frequently, eating healthily, not procrastinating, giving up bad habits, or conserving money, self-control is crucial. Maintaining healthy behaviors also requires self-control. Our degrees of self-control influence decisions that could have an impact on our health, such as what we eat for breakfast and how frequently we visit the doctor (Restubog, 2011). Being conscious of our emotional condition is a sign of emotional intelligence. Being emotionally intelligent is being aware of the feelings we experience, being able to name them appropriately, and being able to express them without causing harm. We shouldn't or don't have to experience emotional overload. When the information they try to deliver seems uncomfortable, we typically hide our feelings (Imran et al., 2021). Leaders experience this rather frequently, and because they don't consider the entire scenario, their impression of it remains unchanged. The emotion we are most likely to repress in Covid-19 pandemic conditions is dread. Leaders that are emotionally savvy make an effort to comprehend the source of the anxiety and identify ways to lessen it (Kaur, Kremer & Mullainathan, 2010). Bosma et al., (2019), because suppressed emotions lead to stress, which harms our immune system, interpersonal connections, and mental serenity, we must confront and resolve these feelings. Managers' planning and strategy-making abilities are impacted when they are driven by their emotions. The amygdala region of the brain makes decisions when restraint is lacking. Goleman (2013), the prefrontal cortex, the region of the brain in charge of planning and strategy, can be overloaded by this portion of the brain, which is in charge of responding to threats, whether they are real or imagined. Employees anticipate a strategy from their boss during a crisis, not just reactions (Flook et al., 2013; Cornelius, 2017), the prefrontal cortex's ability to exercise control over the amygdala can be strengthened by mental training. This can assist in making leaders more productive and emotionally balanced.

Every leader has at least one crisis that wasn't handled the way they had hoped. Thinking about issues and training the brain with potential solutions is a beneficial activity. We have recently entered an uncharted environment where there is little predictability and our safety is put to the test. The system in which we operate has been completely upended. Leaders frequently encounter problems for which they lack an answer or a workable solution (Gianpiero Petriglieri, 2020). What transpires when a leader is unable to provide an answer? Leaders don't have to have all the answers. Making the best decisions possible given the information at hand is what they need to do. Using the same facts, a more skilled leader can make decisions that are superior to those made by a less skilled one. Employers should voice their concerns to their leaders, and when required, those leaders should admit the lack of simple solutions. They shouldn't become upset if the staff doesn't perform as well amid a crisis. The leaders can take this chance to demonstrate their abilities, set an example, and lead by doing. In challenging situations, self-control helps individuals to make the right choices (Travis Bradberry, 2016). If there are sporadic outbursts or alterations in employees' conduct, leaders should understand. They should keep in mind that everyone has unique circumstances and be considerate of other people's experiences, particularly in cases where a person's employment status may be in jeopardy.

Leaders should take the time to pamper themselves and find something they enjoy doing every day. They cannot take care of others if they are not healthy. The following are the key methods for enhancing self-control:

- Evade all temptation. Distractions can be used to prevent this. Whatever it takes, people should take to divert their attention from the enticing item.
- Even in circumstances where people have felt the impacts of ego depletion, planning can increase willpower.
- By concentrating on one goal at a time, the behaviors can become habits and can be maintained with little effort.

- Meditation is an excellent way to build self-control so that people may better withstand temptations. This method can also teach individuals to slow their thoughts, which can help an individual to regulate any instinctual behavior that interferes with their ability to manage themselves.
- Self-control can be aided by sleep. Our brain cells' capacity to absorb glucose is greatly reduced when we are fatigued. Without glucose, the brain is completely incapable of controlling impulses. What's worse is that we are more likely to reach for sugary snacks to make up for low blood sugar when we don't get enough sleep. Therefore, having a good night's sleep is one of the best decisions we can make if we are trying to exercise self-control over our eating.

Social Awareness

The ability to understand and sympathize with others from different origins and cultures, to understand social and ethical norms for behavior, and to recognize family, school, and community resources and supports are all examples of social awareness (Caldwell, 2009). Cluj Napoca-based business company informed its staff of the demolition of an asbestos-roofed structure nearby in March 2019. Employee access was restricted until management verified that there was no risk and evaluated the air quality. It took three weeks to assess the air quality and sanitize the area. At this time, the staff members worked from home offices and different sites. The management's concern for their employees' well-being during this time allowed them to resolve the crisis more easily. Employees were aware that the management prioritized their health and allowed them to concentrate on their regular tasks. With the Covid-19pandemic, they are now dealing with a comparable issue from one year prior. Employees have faith that their managers are kind and look for the best solutions (Murray, 2020). Investors constantly put leaders under a lot of strain as they watch the financial damage the Covid-19pandemic is causing. But employees don't want to know how much the infection is costing the business; they want their boss to act in the same ways that they have in the past (D'Auria & De Smet, 2020). People need to believe that the leader is sympathetic to their plight. Making workers feel safe and cared for will aid leaders in focusing the staff on maintaining operations as effectively as feasible. Many workers do better in a physical setting with face-to-face interaction. Their engagement and sense of being adequately equipped to perform their job could be negatively impacted by switching to a home office. These workers must speak with their manager every day while also transferring some aspects of the office culture to remote work. In a crisis, a good leader should act quickly (Glotzbecker, 2022) and must adapt his management techniques and work schedule to the demands of the team and the current circumstances.

The following are the key methods for enhancing self-control:

- Understanding the value of listening: While the majority of leaders believe they listen well, the reality is that they are frequently too preoccupied with planning their next move to pay attention to what others are saying. Before hearing someone out, good listeners avoid making assumptions about what they know or how something works. Leaders may be shocked by what they learn about their team members and company when they begin to listen (Ni, et al., 2022).
- Summarize what was said: The best method to demonstrate that you comprehend what has been said is to state what people heard in their own words and, if necessary, request more information. This helps demonstrate an individual's comprehension of what was stated and lets the other person know that they regard and respect their viewpoint.

- Pay consideration to the tone: To determine how our employees are feeling, pay attention to the tone of their words. This is especially important in virtual meetings because there are no visible indications. The tone of someone's voice can help people to determine how they are feeling and offer a better chance to decide on the best course of action or response. The most effective leaders are sensitive to others' sentiments (Emily Swaim, 2022).
- Leaders should pay attention to body language. Employees occasionally respond positively yet physically show that they don't.
- Keep an eye on the office's pulse: The ability to observe is essential to social awareness. An individual's awareness is based on their surroundings and it might influence how an individual responds to various situations when they pay great attention to what is going on around them.
- Take note of the specifics: The leaders must keep their surroundings in mind and take the time to fully perceive what is in front of them and if they want to connect with their employees. Make frequent visits to the office to check on activity. Understanding employees as people and gauging the team's attitude might be helpful.
- Stop making notes: When leaders are focused on writing in their notebooks, it's simple to overlook anything. In meetings, put down their pen and glance up from their paper (Evelyn Marinoff, 2021).

Relationship Management or Social Skills

Relationship management is a tactic that enables a business to keep up regular connections with its audience. This is one of the most crucial qualities a leader should have amid a crisis. The capacity to motivate others, manage disagreements, promote teamwork, and do all of this while working from home can be quite time-and energy-consuming, but it can also be very rewarding. The leader should serve as the link between individuals; this link can determine whether an organization remains an organization or transforms into a team (Hartmann & Lussier, 2020). Discussions with the team regularly are crucial during the Covid-19epidemic. Leaders should not only discuss daily tasks at these meetings; they should also consider how their staff members are doing. Leaders can communicate by phone, Skype, or online conferencing. Although the Covid-19 pandemic is not going away, the leader's emotional intelligence keeps the team on track. It may be simpler to survive a crisis if there are motivated people around. The role of the leader is to show compassion, provide direction, and get people focused when there is fear (Rebecca Knight, 2020). Finding answers can be aided by keeping team members engaged and keeping them motivated. Leaders should be open and honest with their staff. Forward-thinking solutions can be employed throughout the crisis if the populace is aware of the issues the business is facing and is sure that their opinions count. Implementing a plan or strategy from the team is usually simpler than from the leader (Karimi, Leggat, Bartram & Rada, 2020). Employees go above and beyond to prove that their solution to the problem is a good one. A leader who has emotional intelligence is aware of the need to provide his team with these chances. A leader ought, to be honest. He ought to express to the group his anxieties, issues, and ideas.

All these are possible using collaboration with people. How can collaboration be maintained among people? Communication is important in this situation. This indicates that managers must provide the proper resources to enable teamwork in a digital setting. The advice is to avoid doing this via email because messages may quickly pile up and be lost, plus it's all too easy to forget to reply to a recipient or unintentionally hit "reply all" when it wasn't necessary. It will inevitably cause any workflow to stall (Newman & Ford, 2021). It should be thought of as having several working scenarios with the instruments to implement each of them. It must be made sure that everyone has remote access to the intranet or domain of the organization. Before remote work is assigned, everything must be installed and ready to use. Everyone should have access to the information they require whenever they need it, as this will save them from wasting hours looking for missing or inaccessible documents. To exchange and collaborate on various documents, Google Drive is recommended. Anyone can be given access to any file, whether it's a shared calendar, word document, spreadsheet, or presentation, giving them immediate access to the most recent version of any file (Newman, Ford, & Marshall, 2020).

How may loneliness be avoided while working remotely? Lockdown can be emotionally distressing due to the lack of social interaction. When working from home for extended periods, the loss of social connection at the office, shared lunch breaks, social gatherings, and even the basic "watercooler discussion" can cause feelings of loneliness. Remote workers are feeling more alone in this regard without the typical social gatherings and team-building activities. To give some levity with pet images and life milestones, video lunch clubs and social gatherings are encouraged (Di Blasi et al., 2021). It's a straightforward action to take, but the enthusiastic response from the staff can make one smile. Virtual meetings with the camera on are recommended whenever possible since just seeing a familiar face may make a world of difference. It's simple to set up with options like Zoom, Skype, and Google Hangouts (Gismero-González, 2020). It is advised to use these tools for social occasions as well, for streaming an online workout or hosting a virtual lunch club. It's the ideal approach to maintaining our health while staying in touch with others. It could understand from the previous part that the components of EQ support the individual as well as leaders to mold them into emotionally stable personalities (Khan & Wajidi, 2019).

EMOTIONAL STABILITY

The ability to keep one's emotional equilibrium under challenging conditions is known as emotional stability. It is the antithesis of emotional instability and neuroticism. People with emotional stability can handle minor pressures and strains of daily life without getting emotionally upset, apprehensive, nervous, tense, or angry. Even when under brief emotional strain, they can keep their composure (Hills & Argyle, 2001). They tend to have a very consistent baseline mood, and they typically rapidly return to it after stressful or highly agitated situations. The unstable person, on the other hand, is prone to somewhat wide, frequent, and frequently surprising mood fluctuations that may swing from pole to pole. An emotionally stable person can create a well-rounded and integrated perspective on life's challenges (Baba, 2020). It is possible to build reality-oriented thinking, judgment, and evaluation skills with the aid of this organizing capacity and organized perception. To understand life's facts and the causes and circumstances that lead to unhappy situations in one's life, one develops feelings, perceptions, and attitudes. Such comprehension aids in fostering great ego strength. Several natures and emotions, including pessimism/optimism, anxiety/calmness, aggression/tolerance, dependence/autonomy, emotion/logic, and apathy/empathy, are influenced by this equilibrium (Margetić, 2021).

Role of Emotional Intelligence and Emotional Stability in Managing Crisis Situation

Since Covid-19is an infectious disease, it can pass from one person to another either directly or inadvertently. It is brought on by the recently found novel coronavirus, which was initially detected in Wuhan,

China, in December 2019. The reason for the widespread concern is the dearth of confirmed data and circulating rumors. People are susceptible to crises not just physiologically but also psychologically. Every significant event will have an impact on some people's mental health. According to estimates, up to 80% of people who are touched by a crisis may experience minor distress in the short term, 20–40% will experience a psychological condition in the medium term, and up to 5% may experience a long-term issue. Fortunately, the majority of people impacted will heal naturally without medical help (Greaves and Hunt, 2017). Nobody is certain how the coronavirus will affect the economy in the long run, whether it will decline or continue to spread and affect additional places. Everyone's emotional stability, wit, and intelligence are being put to the test by this upheaval. The most change-resistant individuals prevail, not the strongest or the smartest. Leaders must act with compassion, unheard-of optimism, and adaptability to guide their followers out of this crisis. It might all come down to their usual capacity for self-direction and problem-solving. For some people, the Covid-19outbreak may be stressful. Both adults and children might experience intense emotions due to fear and anxiety about a sickness. People and the community will become stronger as a result of stress management. Those who might react to the stress of the crisis more intensely include, People who are older and those with chronic illnesses are more susceptible to Covid-19, Kids and teenagers, People who are assisting with the reaction to Covid-19, such as medical professionals and other first responders, and those who struggle with substance use issues as well as mental health issues. Thus People who already have a mental health illness should keep taking their medications and pay attention to any new or worsening symptoms. Stress can be managed by taking care of oneself, one's friends, and one's family. The community can become stronger by supporting one another in managing their stress. It can understand that people who are emotionally good and stable can face the crisis wisely as well as sensibly. Hence, all individuals as well as leaders need to develop emotional intelligence skills to combat various crises.

HOW TO DEVELOP EMOTIONAL INTELLIGENCE SKILLS?

If managers and people have skill gaps, they can take steps to improve their emotional intelligence abilities using a variety of methods, such as Journaling, and 360-degree feedback, by practicing active listening skills, Paying Attention to their own and others' Emotions and undergoing online Courses or Training. These are explained as follows:

Journaling

All the leaders, supervisors, and employees should review the day's meetings, tasks, and interactions and be evaluated at the end of the day; thereby they can understand how all these things affect them either positively or negatively. With this, they may identify particular patterns in their behaviors and responses, as well as those of others, by outlining their thoughts. Using this they can comprehend that they excelled where? How are the staff members feeling? Are there particular people or circumstances that irritate managers or people in general, and if so, why? The better, the more introspective they are. For instance, managers or other leaders should be more conscious of their triggers to prevent future outbursts, or they could imitate behaviors that have been shown to increase employee morale.

360-Degree Feedback

In a 360-degree assessment, managers or leaders might ask for input from their staff members or managers, colleagues, and peers in addition to conducting a personal self-evaluation. Through the exercise, they can learn important information about how the followers view the leader's qualities as well as any potential blind spots. According to Jack Zenger, CEO of the leadership development business Zenger Folkman, the 360-degree feedback arrangement will help to improve leaders' self-awareness, which, in turn, can lead to improved workplace effectiveness, reduced stress, and healthier relationships.

Practicing Active Listening Skills

Only 10% of people, according to Psychology Today, listen effectively. Technology, obtrusive background noise, and one's thoughts can all easily divert attention. However, to effectively communicate and lead others, one must have good listening skills. Further, Leaders should engage in active listening to develop their emotional intelligence. Paraphrasing and other non-verbal indicators, such as nodding, should be used to demonstrate the listener's attention to what the speaker is saying. It will be simpler to connect with others and fully comprehend others' views and feelings at work if an individual actively listens to them.

Paying Attention on Own and Others' Emotions

A supervisor or leader must first understand their own emotions to understand those of others. Make a deliberate effort to reflect on their feelings whenever they notice themselves experiencing a particularly powerful emotion, whether it's a happy or bad one. Think for a moment about what is causing them to feel this way and what may have caused such a powerful emotional reaction. This will enable the leaders to better understand their own emotions as well as those of their employees and fellow leaders. They ought to be able to develop a productive team as empathic leaders. All of these are only achievable when the leader listens well.

Online Course or Training

An online leadership course or training may be the best next step for a manager or leader who wants to learn more about emotional intelligence and improve their leadership talents. They can hone their powers, knowledge, and skills as a result. They should take several online courses that are available to working professionals. By doing so, students can interact with a global network of peers who share their interests while also learning new things. Thus, leaders can develop their emotional intelligence to handle various crises. However, there are challenges also being hindrances to developing the emotional intelligence.

CHALLENGES IN DEVELOPING EMOTIONAL INTELLIGENCE

Mental impediments that prevent someone from openly expressing their thoughts and feelings are known as emotional barriers. They have an impact on how someone interprets the actions of others, which in turn has an impact on how someone develops their arguments. As a result, these barriers affect how a person communicates in general. Past personal experiences have a significant impact on perceptions, and they are a major cause of emotional barriers in a variety of communication circumstances. In addition to preventing clear communication, emotional barriers also increase the likelihood of significant confrontations. Additionally, communication obstacles caused by emotions at work significantly reduce productivity, which costs firms a lot of money. When taken into consideration, some of them may result in circumstances that are exceedingly favorable and beneficial, while others quite the reverse. The strongest feelings on the negative end of the emotional spectrum typically block effective communication and result in spectacular failures. Thus it could understand that people's strong motivator is emotion. However, some factors affect individual emotions and make them poor in emotional intelligence. The factors are explained as follows;

Fear

It's believed that fear is the most potent negative emotion in its most basic form. Insecurity and humiliation, two prominent emotional impediments to emotional intelligence, are among its declensions. There are times at work when employees are unable to communicate clearly out of a sense of inferiority or fear of rejection. For instance, at a meeting, staff members might hold back from commenting or offering a suggestion out of fear of coming across as stupid. This may ultimately stop a potentially fantastic concept from coming to fruition and becoming something truly remarkable.

Anger

Anger influences the way the brain substantially interprets things and circumstances, it is a potent adversary of efficient emotion management. A boss or leader would be less logical when they were upset. They become less receptive to other people's viewpoints and less adept at problem-solving as a result. As a result, uncontrolled rage and poor emotion management swiftly affect team cohesion, which affects workplace productivity as a whole. In a professional setting, many teams must collaborate on particular projects. It is essential to go through emotional barriers since a company's success depends on its ability to use emotions effectively.

Feel of Pride

Numerous factors, including pride, might obstruct efficient emotion management and communication. Effective emotion management and communication are severely hampered by stubbornness, the need to always be right or to let one's ego get in the way, as well as the inability to accept when one is mistaken. Teams must collaborate to succeed in today's cutthroat business environment. Teamwork and collaboration are difficult to grow when emotional barriers like pride appear.

Anxiety

This is one of the most prevalent impediments to emotional intelligence development and it shows itself in daily life. The area of the brain necessary for successful emotion control and communication is typically negatively affected. Being nervous clouds our judgment and limits our capacity to act, making anxiety an emotional obstacle to effective communication. As a result, anxiety may hinder professional advancement.

Jealousy

A fundamental barrier to emotional intelligence and good communication is envy or jealousy. They may cause the dissemination of inaccurate information that is emotionally charged. This is a waste of time and other resources, which is bad for the company.

Apathy

Apathy, often known as a lack of employee engagement, is a critical issue for every firm. The ability to take on new initiatives and time efficiency suffers, both of which are essential in the contemporary workplace. Therefore, contemporary businesses should focus on developing better training programs for fostering emotional intelligence and effective communication programs to encourage individual growth, collaboration, and teamwork. These are essential for reducing workplace indifference and inspiring workers in addition to providing major financial advantages.

CONCLUSIONS

The most effective managers value emotional intelligence as a crucial competency for identifying and resolving team member issues. Emotional intelligence is a crucial component of many leadership philosophies because of this. The capacity to comprehend, regulates, and understands others' emotions and views is referred to as emotional intelligence in leadership. According to popular belief, psychologists John Mayer and Peter Salovey coined the phrase in 1990. However, the emergence of leadership responsibilities in the last ten years has increased its appeal. In spite of having burly scientific and communication capability, many leaders lack emotional intelligence. Emotional intelligence becomes an essential component of the skill set as leaders establish the tone of the organization. Lacking emotional intelligence, a leader cannot steer an organization through the turbulent waters of today's complex business climate. Especially after Covid-19, the way individuals and organizations operate has undergone a significant transition as a result of the development of new technology, which is replacing people's employment and pushing companies toward novel approaches and solutions, the outcomes of which are, for the majority of people, still unknown. The transition is already underway, so there is no time to relax. Therefore, both individuals and organizations need to practice emotional intelligence since it increases the likelihood that they will be able to overcome the most frequent obstacles to the future of work.

Technology is a powerful force that is expanding quickly and changing the nature of work. It has the power to develop new and efficient work processes, even though it is being considered as a thread that calls for new talents from all employees. Managers and leaders who have developed emotional intelligence can build skills like empathy that technology often overlooks (Tambe, Cappelli & Yakubovich, 2019) Instead of seeing another person as a being, the goal of empathic talents is to comprehend them. Relationships with new clients, team members, leaders, and other parties might benefit from this in a variety of ways. Building strong relationships seems to be more important for certain organizations than developing technology. Emerging cultural shifts brought on by migration, coupled with the need to widen the economic market, can pose many challenges for businesses and employees. The future of work "musts" includes global emotions, communication, and mutual understanding. Carnevale and Hatak, (2020), told that due to the multicultural nature of the workplace, it is crucial to "understand" other people and their cultures, as well as their language and idioms. Along with the other elements of emotional intelligence, establishing strong social and emotional abilities will contribute to the ability to successfully negotiate on a global scale, which is essential for the success of organizations.

The future of employment depends on people acquiring unique abilities and new skills. Workplaces are stretched to the limit as a result of rapid change, client demands, new regulations, and management structures and styles; they are compelled to revise their job descriptions and look for fresh talent. Employees can learn new abilities to help them deal with forthcoming issues by practicing Emotional Intelligence methods and approaches and growing awareness of it in the workplace (Chakravorty, & Singh, 2020). A more nuanced approach like Emotional Intelligence, will produce extraordinary new talent and drive performance and well-being. A new breed of highly skilled workers will emerge as a result of significant employee turnover and job changes. Employee stress levels are rising annually as a result of high expectations, pressure, and lengthy workweeks. Additionally, stress is one of the main factors in extended absences due to illness, which can lead to a toxic workplace, the loss of customers, and the depreciation of important assets like qualified personnel. Employees will become more confident as a result of learning about emotional intelligence and its principles of self-awareness and self-management, which will enable them to operate more effectively. Understanding their emotions can help them manage expectations more effectively and help those who are going through similar problems. Thereby it can control our impulses and authoritatively express our feelings thanks to emotional intelligence. It has numerous advantages for people who are struggling with stress and burnout (Choi, Mohammad & Kim, 2019). According to Drigas & Papoutsi, (2019), 70% of people are thinking about using new self-help techniques to better their abilities and increase their chances of finding a job in the future. With this in mind, impending difficulties can only be handled using techniques that people can swiftly adapt and apply in the workplace. Thus, by assisting people in growing their adaptability, empathy, social skills, and other aspects of emotional intelligence, positive attitudes will be created, which in turn promote productivity, well-being, and a better working environment during times of crisis (Rezvani & Khosravi, 2019). Additionally, managers and leaders should keep in mind that emotions are strong instruments that, when balanced and utilized effectively, can help shape a brighter future for the organization.

REFERENCES

Aguilar Yuste, M. (2021). Leadership and Emotional Intelligence during a Crisis. Revista de Relaciones Internacionales. *Estrategia y Seguridad*, *16*(2), 47–60.

Alonazi, W. B. (2020). The impact of emotional intelligence on job performance during COVID-19 crisis: A cross-sectional analysis. *Psychology Research and Behavior Management*, *13*, 749–757. doi:10.2147/PRBM.S263656 PMID:33061691

Altamirano, M. A., & Collazo, C. E. R. (2020). Leading with emotional intelligence: How leaders of a diverse-based urban college in New York successfully respond to the COVID-19 crisis of 2020. *Communication is Robust when Nations Come Together: The Importance of Collaboration during a Global Crisis.*

Baba, M. M. (2020). Navigating COVID-19 with emotional intelligence. *The International Journal of Social Psychiatry*, *66*(8), 810–820. doi:10.1177/0020764020934519 PMID:32583710

Baesu, C. (2019). Leadership based on emotional intelligence in modern organizations. *The USV Annals of Economics and Public Administration, 18*(28), 73-78.

Bergner, S. (2021). The role of the European Union in global health: The EU's self-perception (s) within the COVID-19 pandemic. *Health Policy (Amsterdam)*. PMID:34802748

Bosma, A. R., Boot, C. R. L., De Maaker, M., Boeije, H. R., Schoonmade, L. J., Anema, J. R., & Schaafsma, F. G. (2019). Exploring self-control of workers with a chronic condition: A qualitative synthesis. *European Journal of Work and Organizational Psychology, 28*(5), 653–668. doi:10.1080/1359432X.2019.1631801

Bradberry. (2016). *Why The Best Leaders Have Conviction*. https://www.forbes.com/sites/travisbradberry/2016/06/28/why-the-best-leaders-have-conviction/?sh=231474001c8d

Caldwell, C. (2009). Identity, self-awareness, and self-deception: Ethical implications for leaders and organizations. *Journal of Business Ethics, 90*(S3), 393–406. doi:10.100710551-010-0424-2

Carnevale, J. B., & Hatak, I. (2020). Employee adjustment and well-being in the era of COVID-19: Implications for human resource management. *Journal of Business Research, 116*, 183–187. doi:10.1016/j.jbusres.2020.05.037 PMID:32501303

Chakravorty, A., & Singh, P. (2020). Work/family interference and burnout among primary school teachers: The moderating role of emotional intelligence. *Decision (Washington, D.C.), 47*(3), 251–264.

Chin, S. T. S., Anantharaman, R. N., & Tong, D. Y. K. (2011). The roles of emotional intelligence and spiritual intelligence at the workplace. *Journal of Human Resources Management Research, 2011*, 1–9. doi:10.5171/2011.582992

Choi, H. M., Mohammad, A. A., & Kim, W. G. (2019). Understanding hotel frontline employees' emotional intelligence, emotional labor, job stress, coping strategies and burnout. *International Journal of Hospitality Management, 82*, 199–208. doi:10.1016/j.ijhm.2019.05.002

Clark. (2020). *8 Ways to Manage Your Team While Social Distancing*. https://hbr.org/2020/03/8-ways-to-manage-your-team-while-social-distancing

Cornelius, J. (2017). *Five minute meditation used to impact workplace meetings* [Doctoral dissertation]. Pepperdine University.

D'Auria, G., & De Smet, A. (2020). Leadership in a crisis: Responding to the coronavirus outbreak and future challenges. *Psychology (Irvine, Calif.), 22*(2), 273–287.

Dash, S. P. (2022). Post Pandemic: The New Advanced Society. *The New Advanced Society: Artificial Intelligence and Industrial Internet of Things Paradigm,* 1-14.

Di Blasi, M., Gullo, S., Mancinelli, E., Freda, M. F., Esposito, G., Gelo, O. C. G., ... Coco, G. L. (2021). Psychological distress associated with the COVID-19 lockdown: A two-wave network analysis. *Journal of Affective Disorders, 284*, 18–26. doi:10.1016/j.jad.2021.02.016 PMID:33582428

Di Blasi, M., Gullo, S., Mancinelli, E., Freda, M. F., Esposito, G., Gelo, O. C. G., ... Coco, G. L. (2021). Psychological distress associated with the COVID-19 lockdown: A two-wave network analysis. *Journal of Affective Disorders*, *284*, 18–26. doi:10.1016/j.jad.2021.02.016 PMID:33582428

Dirani, K. M., Abadi, M., Alizadeh, A., Barhate, B., Garza, R. C., Gunasekara, N., Ibrahim, G., & Majzun, Z. (2020). Leadership competencies and the essential role of human resource development in times of crisis: A response to Covid-19 pandemic. *Human Resource Development International*, *23*(4), 380–394. doi:10.1080/13678868.2020.1780078

Drigas, A., & Papoutsi, C. (2019). Emotional Intelligence as an Important Asset for HR in Organizations: Leaders and Employees. *International Journal of Advanced Corporate Learning*, *12*(1), 58. doi:10.3991/ijac.v12i1.9637

Eurich. (2018). *What Self-Awareness Really Is (and How to Cultivate It)*. https://hbr.org/2018/01/what-self-awareness-really-is-and-how-to-cultivate-it

Eurich, T. (2018). What self-awareness really is (and how to cultivate it). *Harvard Business Review*, 1–9.

Flook, L., Goldberg, S. B., Pinger, L., Bonus, K., & Davidson, R. J. (2013). Mindfulness for teachers: A pilot study to assess effects on stress, burnout, and teaching efficacy. *Mind, Brain and Education*, *7*(3), 182–195. doi:10.1111/mbe.12026 PMID:24324528

Forsey. (2018). *The True Meaning of Self-Awareness (& How to Tell If You're Actually Self-Aware)*. https://blog.hubspot.com/marketing/self-awareness

Future Talent Learning. (2021). *What are the top 5 characteristics of emotional intelligence in good leadership?* https://www.futuretalentlearning.com/en/future-talent learning-blog/what-are-the-top-5-characteristics-of-emotional-intelligence-in-good-leadership

Gismero-González, E., Bermejo-Toro, L., Cagigal, V., Roldán, A., Martínez-Beltrán, M. J., & Halty, L. (2020). Emotional impact of COVID-19 lockdown among the Spanish population. *Frontiers in Psychology*, *11*, 616978. doi:10.3389/fpsyg.2020.616978 PMID:33391136

Gismero-González, E., Bermejo-Toro, L., Cagigal, V., Roldán, A., Martínez-Beltrán, M. J., & Halty, L. (2020). Emotional impact of COVID-19 lockdown among the Spanish population. *Frontiers in Psychology*, *11*, 616978. doi:10.3389/fpsyg.2020.616978 PMID:33391136

Glotzbecker, M. P. (2022). Crisis Leadership: Lessons Learned From the COVID Pandemic. *Journal of Pediatric Orthopedics*, *42*(Suppl 1), S56–S59. doi:10.1097/BPO.0000000000002068 PMID:35405706

Goleman. (2013). *The Focused Leader - How effective executives direct their own and their organizations' attention*. https://hbr.org/2013/12/the-focused-leader

Goleman, D. (1995). *Emotional Intelligence: Why it can matter more than IQ*. Bloomsbury.

Goodlet, K. J., Raney, E., Buckley, K., Afolabi, T., Davis, L., Fettkether, R. M., Jones, M., Larson, S., & Tennant, S. (2022). Impact of the COVID-19 Pandemic on the Emotional Intelligence of Student Pharmacist Leaders. *American Journal of Pharmaceutical Education*, *86*(1), 8519. doi:10.5688/ajpe8519 PMID:34301541

Görgens-Ekermans, G., & Roux, C. (2021). Revisiting the emotional intelligence and transformational leadership debate:(How) does emotional intelligence matter to effective leadership? *SA Journal of Human Resource Management*, *19*, 1279. doi:10.4102ajhrm.v19i0.1279

Groysberg, B., Abrahams, R. A., & Baden, K. C. (2021). *The pandemic conversations that leaders need to have now.* Harvard Business Working Paper.

Hartmann, N. N., & Lussier, B. (2020). Managing the sales force through the unexpected exogenous COVID-19 crisis. *Industrial Marketing Management*, *88*, 101–111. doi:10.1016/j.indmarman.2020.05.005

Hills, P., & Argyle, M. (2001). Emotional stability as a major dimension of happiness. *Personality and Individual Differences*, *31*(8), 1357–1364. doi:10.1016/S0191-8869(00)00229-4

Hunt, P., & Greaves, I. (2017). *Oxford manual of major incident management*. Oxford University Press. doi:10.1093/med/9780199238088.001.0001

Imran, M. K., Fatima, T., Sarwar, A., & Iqbal, S. M. J. (2021). Will I speak up or remain silent? Workplace ostracism and employee performance based on self-control perspective. *The Journal of Social Psychology*, 1–19. PMID:34498546

Insights, I. C. A. E. W. (2021). *The 5 Elements of Emotional Intelligence*. https://www.icaew.com/insights/student-insights/the-5-elements-of-emotional-intelligence

Karimi, L., Leggat, S. G., Bartram, T., & Rada, J. (2020). The effects of emotional intelligence training on the job performance of Australian aged care workers. *Health Care Management Review*, *45*(1), 41–51. doi:10.1097/HMR.0000000000000200 PMID:29742522

Kaur, S., Kremer, M., & Mullainathan, S. (2010). Self-control and the development of work arrangements. *The American Economic Review*, *100*(2), 624–628. doi:10.1257/aer.100.2.624

Khan, M. R., & Wajidi, A. (2019). Role of leadership and team building in employee motivation at workplace. *GMJACS*, *9*(1), 11–11.

Knight. (2020a). *How to Manage a Hybrid Team*. https://hbr.org/2020/10/how-to-manage-a-hybrid-team

Knight. (2020b). *How to Talk to Your Team When the Future Is Uncertain*. https://hbr.org/2020/04/how-to-talk-to-your-team-when-the-future-is-uncertain

Koçak, O. (2021). Does emotional intelligence increase satisfaction with life during COVID-19? The mediating role of depression. Healthcare, 9(11), 1529.

Mansaray, H. E. (2019). The role of leadership style in organisational change management: A literature review. *Journal of Human Resource Management*, *7*(1), 18–31. doi:10.11648/j.jhrm.20190701.13

Margetić, B., Peraica, T., Stojanović, K., & Ivanec, D. (2021). Predictors of emotional distress during the COVID-19 pandemic; a Croatian study. *Personality and Individual Differences, 175*, 110691. doi:10.1016/j.paid.2021.110691 PMID:33518867

Marinoff. (2021). *How to Have Self-Control and Be the Master of Your Life.* https://www.lifehack.org/844012/self-control

Mesaglio. (2020). *4 Actions to Be a Strong Leader During COVID-19 Disruption.* https://www.gartner.com/smarterwithgartner/4-actions-to-be-a-good-leader-during-covid-19-disruption

Morgan. (2021). *5 Components of Emotional Intelligence.* https://thefutureorganization.com/5-components-of-emotional-intelligence/

Murray, L. K. (2020). *How to lead with emotional intelligence in the time of COVID-19.* Johns Hopkins Bloomberg School of Public Health.

Mysirlaki, S., & Paraskeva, F. (2020). Emotional intelligence and transformational leadership in virtual teams: Lessons from MMOGs. *Leadership and Organization Development Journal, 41*(4), 551–566. doi:10.1108/LODJ-01-2019-0035

Nevins. (2020). *Why A Post-Covid World Demands Greater Emotional Intelligence.* https://www.forbes.com/sites/hillennevins/2020/09/29/why-a-post-covid-world-demands-greater-emotional-intelligence/?sh=3d259d0e6bbd

Newman, S. A., & Ford, R. C. (2021). Five steps to leading your team in the virtual COVID-19 workplace. *Organizational Dynamics, 50*(1), 100802. doi:10.1016/j.orgdyn.2020.100802 PMID:36536689

Newman, S. A., Ford, R. C., & Marshall, G. W. (2020). Virtual team leader communication: Employee perception and organizational reality. *International Journal of Business Communication, 57*(4), 452–473. doi:10.1177/2329488419829895

Ni, Y. L., Kuo, C. C., Wu, C. H., Chang, W. H., & Chen, L. H. (2022). How Can We Cope with Self-Control Demands and Enhance Proactive Vitality Management? The Role of Leisure Crafting and Supervisor Recreational Sports Support. *Journal of Happiness Studies, 23*(8), 3961–3980. doi:10.100710902-022-00572-9

Oates, K. (2021). *Leader Empathy, Emotional Intelligence Behaviors and Years of Federal Employment: Predictability of Employee Well-Being* [Doctoral dissertation]. Capella University.

Pak, A., Adegboye, O. A., Adekunle, A. I., Rahman, K. M., McBryde, E. S., & Eisen, D. P. (2020). Economic consequences of the COVID-19 outbreak: The need for epidemic preparedness. *Frontiers in Public Health, 8*, 241. doi:10.3389/fpubh.2020.00241 PMID:32574307

Petriglieri. (2020). *The Psychology Behind Effective Crisis Leadership.* https://hbr.org/2020/04/the-psychology-behind-effective-crisis-leadership

Restubog, S. L. D., Garcia, P. R. J. M., Toledano, L. S., Amarnani, R. K., Tolentino, L. R., & Tang, R. L. (2011). Yielding to (cyber)-temptation: Exploring the buffering role of self-control in the relationship between organizational justice and cyberloafing behavior in the workplace. *Journal of Research in Personality*, *45*(2), 247–251. doi:10.1016/j.jrp.2011.01.006

Rezvani, A., & Khosravi, P. (2019). Emotional intelligence: The key to mitigating stress and fostering trust among software developers working on information system projects. *International Journal of Information Management*, *48*, 139–150. doi:10.1016/j.ijinfomgt.2019.02.007

Rivers, S. E., Handley-Miner, I. J., Mayer, J. D., & Caruso, D. R. (2020). Emotional Intelligence. In R. J. Sternberg (Ed.), *The Cambridge handbook of intelligence* (pp. 709–735). Cambridge University Press. doi:10.1017/9781108770422.030

Rodrigues, C. B., Ribeiro, J. L., & Gomes, D. (2022). Emotional Intelligence and the Impact of the Covid-19 Pandemic on Pharmaceutical Professionals—An Exploratory Study. In *Organizational Management in Post Pandemic Crisis* (pp. 65–87). Springer International Publishing. doi:10.1007/978-3-030-98052-8_4

Sageder, M., & Feldbauer-Durstmüller, B. (2019). Management control in multinational companies: A systematic literature review. *Review of Managerial Science*, *13*(5), 875–918. doi:10.100711846-018-0276-1

Sanchez-Ruiz, M. J., Tadros, N., Khalaf, T., Ego, V., Eisenbeck, N., Carreno, D. F., & Nassar, E. (2021). Trait emotional intelligence and wellbeing during the pandemic: The mediating role of meaning-centered coping. *Frontiers in Psychology*, *12*, 648401. doi:10.3389/fpsyg.2021.648401 PMID:34054650

Schlegel, K., & Mortillaro, M. (2019). The Geneva Emotional Competence Test (GECo): An ability measure of workplace emotional intelligence. *The Journal of Applied Psychology*, *104*(4), 559–580. doi:10.1037/apl0000365 PMID:30346195

Schwantes. (2020). *Steve Jobs: 'Technology is nothing'—here's what he said it really takes to achieve great success*. https://www.cnbc.com/2019/10/05/apple-ceo-steve-jobs-technology-is-nothing-heres-what-it-takes-to-achieve-great-success.html

Semenets-Orlova, I., Klochko, A., Shkoda, T., Marusina, O., & Tepliuk, M. (2021). Emotional intelligence as the basis for the development of organizational leadership during the covid period (educational institution case). *Studies of Applied Economics*, *39*(5). Advance online publication. doi:10.25115/eea.v39i5.5074

Semenets-Orlova, I., Klochko, A., Shkoda, T., Marusina, O., & Tepliuk, M. (2021). Emotional intelligence as the basis for the development of organizational leadership during the covid period. *Studies of Applied Economics*, *39*(5). Advance online publication. doi:10.25115/eea.v39i5.5074

Sutton. (2021). *Assertiveness in Leadership: 19 Techniques for Managers*. https://positivepsychology.com/assertiveness-in-leadership/

Sutton, A., Williams, H. M., & Allinson, C. W. (2015). A longitudinal, mixed method evaluation of self-awareness training in the workplace. *European Journal of Training and Development*, *39*(7), 610–627. doi:10.1108/EJTD-04-2015-0031

Swaim. (2022). *How to Improve Your Self-Control*. https://www.verywellmind.com/psychology-of-self-control-4177125

Tambe, P., Cappelli, P., & Yakubovich, V. (2019). Artificial intelligence in human resources management: Challenges and a path forward. *California Management Review*, *61*(4), 15–42. doi:10.1177/0008125619867910

Tang, H. W. V., Yin, M. S., & Nelson, D. B. (2010). The relationship between emotional intelligence and leadership practices: A cross-cultural study of academic leaders in Taiwan and the USA. *Journal of Managerial Psychology*, *25*(8), 899–926. doi:10.1108/02683941011089143

Chapter 7
Impulsive Buying as a Response to COVID-19-Related Negative Psychological States

Inci Dursun
https://orcid.org/0000-0002-9856-3914
Gebze Technical University, Turkey

Hediye Yürüyen Kılıç
Gebze Technical University, Turkey

Elif Aralık
Gebze Technical University, Turkey

ABSTRACT

Impulsive buying (IB), of which mood regulation function is well-documented, is among the methods for coping with psychological strain during the COVID-19 pandemic. However, IB is likely to hinder psychological well-being rather than repairing it in vulnerable periods. This study aims to answer: 1. Do negative psychological states promote IB during the pandemic? 2. Does IB lead negative emotions? 3. What is the role of pre-pandemic purchasing style on the process? 4.Does pandemic -related psychological strain fuel post-impulsive purchase negative emotions? A survey was conducted in Turkey with 405 participants. Results revealed that, regardless of pre-pandemic purchasing style, COVID-19-induced anxiety and loneliness promoted IB, and IB was followed by negative affect including guilt, regret, and shame. Furthermore, COVID-19-related anxiety and loneliness were found to fuel the negative affect induced by IB. The findings provide deeper insights into the dysfunctionality of IB for mood regulation and stress alleviation in a highly-stressful crisis period.

INTRODUCTION

Since late 2019, the COVID-19 pandemic has affected the whole world and caused the deaths of 5.9

DOI: 10.4018/978-1-6684-8565-1.ch007

million people (WHO, 2022). Governments have taken various precautions to prevent the further spread of the virus, such as home confinement, quarantine, social distance regulations, reduction of social activities, and closure of entertainment venues. These precautions have brought many negative effects across economic, social, and psychological domains. In particular, the direct and indirect adverse effects of the pandemic on the psychological well-being of individuals have been the subject of many studies. Researchers have described the loss of family members, fear of contagion, social isolation, and loss of income or employment for many people as hindering factors for psychological well-being (Morales-Vives et al., 2020). The pandemic has led to increased instances of anxiety, depression, stress, poor sleep quality, loneliness, and boredom (Droit-Volet, 2020; Mazza et al., 2020; Tutzer, 2021). Conversely, individuals have reported benefiting from different coping strategies to release these negative effects and mental states stemming from the pandemic. Coping strategies for addressing COVID-19 related psychological strain can involve behavioral therapy; drug treatments; self-distraction; seeking emotional support from family members and/or loved ones; and complementary therapies such as yoga, meditation, praying, spirituality, or using humor (Dagli, 2020; Fluharty & Fancourt, 2021; Savitsky et al., 2020). Self-distraction strategies involve "focusing more explicitly on doing things to take one's mind off the stressor" (Carver, 1997, pp. 95) and have been identified as the most common coping mechanisms for responding to psychological strain during the pandemic (Park et al., 2020). Accordingly, individuals have detached themselves from COVID-19 related stress through activities such as watching TV, cleaning or tidying up, spending time on the internet, listening to music, reading books, sleeping, exercising, and shopping (Park et al., 2020; Temiz, 2020; Taylor et al., 2020a, 2020b). Shopping, particularly impulsive shopping, has yet to be comprehensively examined as a self-distraction activity in the COVID-19 era.

Impulsive buying refers to "getting a sudden urge to buy something, without advance intention or plan, and then acting on that impulse without carefully or thoroughly considering whether the purchase is consistent with one's long-range goals, ideals, resolves, and plans" (Baumeister, 2002, pp. 670). The mood regulation function of impulsive buying is well accepted in the literature. Studies have shown that individuals tend to engage in impulsive buying when they feel the urge to escape from daily stresses, as well as to regulate and release the increased stress and anxiety levels during crisis periods such as pandemics and natural disasters (DeSarbo & Edwards, 1996; Elliott, 1994; Faber & O'Guinn, 1992; Sneath et al., 2009). For example, a survey of 2000 Americans revealed that impulsive shopping increased 18% during the COVID-19 pandemic, and 72% of individuals reported that it positively affected their mood (Slickdeals, 2020). Similarly, Dursun et al. (2022) reported that 26.5% of their respondents increased impulsive buying and 33% of them reported an increase in their "shopping for therapy" during this time. These findings are not surprising since impulsive buying provides immediate emotional well-being, happiness (Rook & Fisher, 1995), pleasure, excitement, and relief (Gardner & Rook, 1988). However, post-impulse purchase moods are not uniformly positive (Gardner & Rook, 1988, pp. 128) and may also cause economic and psychological side effects such as regret, guilt, and disappointment (Fenton-O'Creevy et al., 2018; Hausman, 2000; Imam, 2013; Santini et al., 2019). Due to its long-term adverse effects, impulsive buying is often considered an irrational and negative type of purchasing behavior (Hama, 2001). Furthermore, adverse effects can be more destructive in crisis periods like the COVID-19 pandemic because individuals are more psychologically and economically vulnerable. Thus, it is crucial to understand the dynamics and consequences of impulse buying in the COVID-19 era.

Although some recent research has focused on panic buying or stocking up (Ahmed et al., 2020; Gupta et al., 2021; Naeem, 2020), few studies have investigated the psychological correlates of impulsive buying during the pandemic (Chauhan et al., 2021; Wang et al., 2020, 2021; Xiao et al., 2020). Consequently, further research is needed to understand how individuals' negative psychological states during the pandemic influenced their impulsive buying behavior and post-purchase affective reactions. In this context, the current study aims to extend previous research in two ways. First, we aim to demonstrate the impacts of COVID-19 related anxiety, social isolation, and loneliness on individuals' impulsive buying behavior during the pandemic. While doing so, we also consider individuals' pre-pandemic shopping style to understand if impulsive buying reactions to COVID-19 stress are merely an extension of individuals' typical purchasing behavior, or a new phenomenon entirely. Second, to uncover the potential negative side effects of impulse buying during the pandemic, we investigate post-purchase negative affective reactions and explore if pandemic-related psychological strain fuels these reactions.

Impulsive Buying During The COVID-19 Pandemic

Impulsive buying is a well-accepted part of consumer behavior, accounting for 62% of supermarket sales and 80% of all sales in certain product categories (Luo, 2005). While early researchers defined impulsive buying as an "unplanned purchase" (i.e., Kollat & Willett, 1967), later studies used a more complete conceptualization focusing on the roles of impulses. Accordingly, impulsive buying occurs when an individual experiences a sudden, often powerful and persistent urge to buy something immediately, typically with diminished regard for the consequences (Rook, 1987). This type of purchase is carried out instinctively and unintentionally due to a struggle between an individual's cravings and willpower (Shahjehan et al., 2012); thus, it is often followed by an emotional reaction (Piron, 1993).

Numerous studies in the consumer behavior and marketing literature have investigated impulsive buying motivators. In their meta-analytic study, Santini et al. (2019) identified demographic factors including income, gender, and age as determinants of impulsive buying tendencies. In their literature review on impulsive buying, Kalla and Arora (2011) categorized the motivators into two groups: (1) consumer-related/internal factors, including self-discrepancy, hedonic needs, mood states, self-regulatory, resource availability, autistic stimuli, social status, and subjective well-being; and (2) shop related/external motivators such as visual stimulus, shopping format, self-service, store environment, discounts, display, shelf space, ambient factors, social factors, and perceived crowding.

Although it is evident that impulsive buying is an emotion-related behavior, researchers have indicated a need for further studies on its relationship with negative emotions, given current contrary findings (Kalla & Arora, 2011; Xiao et al., 2020). It is even more critical to understand the connection between impulsive buying and negative emotions in highly stressful, traumatic periods such as pandemics. However, there is limited direct empirical evidence regarding how impulsive buying occurred due to psychological strain during the COVID-19 pandemic. In this study, we adapted the stimulus-organism-response (S-O-R) framework (Woodworth, 1929) to explain the impacts of pandemic-related negative psychological states on impulsive buying behavior.

Woodworth (1929) proposed the stimulus-organism-response model (S-O-R) as an expanded form of the classical stimulus-response model theory (Pavlov, 1927). This theory was later modified by Mehrabian and Russell (1974) and in Jacoby (2002). In the S-O-R model, "stimulus" represents the environmental elements, "organism" represents the internal structures and processes that occur between the stimulus and the response, and "response" represents the reactions of individuals (Mehrabian & Russell, 1974). Accordingly, the stimuli affect the organism—that is, the affective and cognitive processes of the individuals—which then elicit behavioral responses. The S-O-R model helps to distinguish between the emotions surrounding and perceptions regarding environmental stimuli and the individual responses of consumers (Chen & Yao, 2018). In the consumer behavior literature, the S-O-R model has been employed in many studies on the relationship between store atmosphere and consumer behavior (Bakırtaş, 2013), online experiences and purchase intention (Huang, 2012), unusual buying behavior (Laato et al., 2020), panic buying behavior (Prentice et al., 2020), online shopping behavior (Peng & Kim, 2014), and co-creation in social media communities (Kamboj et al., 2018). The S-O-R model has also been used to explain impulsive buying behavior (Bharathi & Sudha, 2017; Chang et al., 2011; Chen & Yao, 2018; Liu et al., 2020; Ming et al., 2021).

In the COVID-19 context, "stimulus" may comprise a wide range of pandemic-related factors, including the risk of infection, social isolation, and disruptions to well-preferred daily routines. Moreover, the loss of freedom stemming from restriction on movement to slow the spread of the virus has appeared as a common stimulus across many countries and cultures. The "organism" reflects negative psychological states triggered by these common stimuli in the COVID-19 era. Growing evidence demonstrates that the COVID-19 pandemic has created probably interrelated adverse psychological effects including anxiety (Casagrande et al., 2020; Varma et al., 2021; Wang et al., 2020), insomnia (Bartoszek et al., 2020; Casagrande et al., 2020; Hetkamp et al., 2020; Pieh et al., 2020), boredom (Droit-Volet et al., 2020; Tutzer et al., 2021; Yan et al., 2021), stress (Casagrande et al., 2020; Varma et al., 2021; Wang et al., 2020), loneliness (González-Sanguino et al., 2020; Tutzer et al., 2021), depression (Bartoszek et al., 2020; Varma et al., 2021; Wang et al., 2020), fatigue (Bartoszek et al., 2020; Morgul et al., 2020), and decreased well-being (Arslan et al., 2020; Evanoff et al., 2020; González-Sanguino et al., 2020; Pieh et al., 2020). Among all these factors, the current research focuses on anxiety, isolation, and loneliness as negative psychological states experienced during the pandemic representing the "organism" of the S-O-R framework. Here, anxiety represents an excessive and difficult-to-control concern caused by pandemic-related events. It stems from the individual's perception of threats, along with their inability to determine, predict, or control preferred outcomes in certain situations (Barlow, 1988). Anxiety is considered an adaptive process until it becomes a dysfunctional response with negative consequences of persistence or magnitude (Konstam et al., 2005). A significant number of studies have reported COVID-19 related anxiety among various populations (Casagrande et al., 2020; Evanoff et al., 2020; González-Sanguino et al., 2020; Lin, 2021; Varma et al., 2021; Wang et al., 2020). Mazza et al. (2020) found that young people, women, and individuals with an infected acquaintance, and/or a previous history of stressful events were likely to experience higher anxiety, stress, and depression during the early days of COVID-19. Addressing anxiety is critical since it is often associated with serious physiological consequences, including pain, gastrointestinal distress, and cardiopulmonary symptoms (Shevlin et al., 2020).

Self-isolation refers to the separation of uninfected individuals from individuals with communicable diseases to prevent further contagion (Suppawittaya et al., 2020). During a pandemic, however, the state of self-isolation can cause negative repercussions such as disruption of lifestyle or routine, loss of freedom, decreased social contact, and boredom. Although individuals may experience greater free time while in isolation, they may not be able to use this time as they want thanks to the restrictions created by quarantine precautions, which can lead to boredom and depression (Droit-Volet et al., 2020; Martarelli & Wolff, 2020). Individuals who were in isolation during the pandemic reported psychological symptoms such as insomnia, depression, and suicidal tendencies (Lim et al., 2020). Moreover, Taylor et al. (2021) revealed that self-isolation is negatively associated with resilience and optimism and positively associated with negative emotional states.

Loneliness has been one of the most frequently identified psychological states during the pandemic (González-Sanguino et al., 2020; Hoffart et al., 2020; Tutzer et al., 2021). It is defined as a dark and miserable feeling that poses a risk for isolation from society and can generate morbidities such as depression, anxiety, and chronic stress (Banerjee & Rai, 2020). Loneliness involves subjective feelings (Hwang et al., 2020) and is associated with cognition that worsens over time, along with symptoms such as difficulty waking from sleep, suicidal tendencies, and low mood (Cacioppo et al., 2002; Fässberg et al., 2012; Lee et al., 2019).

Following the S-O-R framework, we propose impulsive buying as a behavioral response to the aforementioned negative psychological states. Previous studies provide evidence of linkages between impulsive buying and loneliness (Peng et al., 2020), anxiety (Wang et al., 2020), and social isolation (Lou et al., 2021). Individuals also appear to engage in impulsive buying in an attempt to alleviate these negative emotional states. As indicated by Gardner and Rook (1988, pp. 128), "whether someone is depressed, frustrated, or bored, impulsive buying appears to be an effective tactic for breaking out of an undesirable mood state." Baumeister (2002) explains this phenomenon through the self-control failure argument. Individuals are likely to undermine or lose their capacity to control their actions when they feel upset or depleted by their efforts to control their emotions under changing circumstances, and consequently they behave impulsively (Baumeister, 2002). In the COVID-19 context, it becomes easier for individuals to lose control of their behavior because the intense psychological stress amplifies the goal of feeling better (Baumeister, 2002). A survey of victims impacted by Hurricane Katrina showed that when people feel depressed because of disaster-induced stress, they are more prone to purchase impulsively to cope with their difficult circumstances and/or regain a sense of normalcy (Sneath et al., 2009). For this reason, we propose that individuals are more likely to make impulsive purchases in the COVID-19 era as a response to anxiety, self-isolation, and loneliness, even they had a different purchasing style in the pre-pandemic period. This supposition led to three hypotheses:

H1. COVID-19 induced anxiety is positively related with impulsive buying

H2. COVID-19 induced self-isolation is positively related with impulsive buying

H3. COVID-19 induced loneliness is positively related with impulsive buying

Besides, we expect that individuals who typically engage in impulsive buying will be more likely to do the same during times of crisis than those who are less prone to this behavior. This is because impulsive buying may be a steady personality trait for some individuals, leading them to behave consistently across different situations (Park & Lennon, 2006). Consistently previous research found that the tendency for impulsive buying bolsters the likelihood of such behavior (Ahmad et al., 2019; Barakat, 2019; Kwon & Ahn, 2021; Özer & Gültekin, 2015; Utama et al., 2021). Thus, we proposed:

H4. Impulsive buying in the pre-pandemic period is positively related with impulsive buying during COVID-19 pandemic

Post-Purchase Negative Affect

Consistent with its hedonic nature and mood alteration role, impulsive buying is typically followed by immediate positive emotions such as pleasure, excitement, relief (Gardner & Rook, 1988), and happiness (Rook & Fisher, 1995). However, the literature suggests that after the initial "rush" of an impulsive purchase, individuals may experience negative emotions such as shame (Fenton-O'Creevy et al., 2018), regret (George & Yaoyuneyong, 2010; Hausman, 2000; Hoch & Loewentein, 1991; Imam, 2013; Parsad et al., 2019; Saleh, 2012; Wood, 1998), and guilt (Costa & Laran, 2003, as cited in Santini et al., 2009; Fenton-O'Creevy et al., 2018). These negative emotions stem from post-purchase cognitive evaluation of the appropriateness of the purchase (e.g., financially or socially) and comparison of the present behavior with alternative options (Lee & Cotte, 2009). Individuals may feel guilt when they realize that the impulsive purchase violated their own internal standards of right and wrong (Hanks & Mattila, 2004). After evaluating whether they needed the product or bought the right option, individuals may find the purchase wasteful, redundant (Wood, 1998), or socially unacceptable (Rook, 1987), leading to negative emotions. Therefore, we proposed:

H5. Impulsive buying during COVID-19 pandemic is positively related with post-purchase negative affect.

Furthermore, we predict that post-impulsive purchase negative affect will be stronger for individuals who experience COVID-19 related negative emotional states more intensely. Since emotional states and moods influence how individuals see the world, people in a positive mood on warm and sunny spring days have higher life satisfaction scores than on rainy and cold spring days, which can in turn influence later evaluations of momentary states of mind (Schwarz & Clore, 1983, 1988). Similarly, in the consumption context, individuals in a positive mood have more positive judgments of satisfaction, while individuals in a negative mood are likely to show opposite judgments (Kim & Mattila, 2010). Similarly, Liljander and Strandvik (1997) illustrated that the effect of negative emotions on post-purchase satisfaction is much stronger than that of positive emotions. In the impulsive buying context, Özer and Gültekin (2015) revealed that when individuals make an impulsive purchase in a negative mood, they are less satisfied with the product than those who do the same in a positive mood. Moreover, Li (2015) specified a happy mood has a positive effect on post-impulsive buying satisfaction, while feelings of guilt decrease post-impulsive buying satisfaction. Finally, in Miao and Mattila's (2013) study, participants who experienced a negative pre-purchase mood reported a much higher level of guilt than those who had a positive pre-purchase mood.

These findings can be explained by the role that emotional states play in "various aspects of information processing including encoding and retrieval of information, different strategies used to process information, evaluations, and judgments, and creative thinking" (Bagozzi et al., 1999, pp. 195). According to the model of mood-congruent information recall, people in negative emotional states are likely to learn more about and address negative aspects of their purchases and tend to recall negatively valanced materials regarding their purchase experience because mood-congruent information is over-represented in their memory (Bower, 1981). Furthermore, negative emotions may indicate that individuals are in a problematic situation, which leads them to engage in analytical and detail-oriented processing strategies (Schwarz, 1990). This systematic processing is more likely to result in negative affect after an impulsive purchase, since such purchases are generally not budgeted for and motivated by factors other than utility or need (Hanks & Mattila, 2014). This is especially true during economically vulnerable periods. Based on the empirical evidence and theoretical explanations, we postulate that negative psychological states in the COVID-19 era will fuel the post-impulsive buying negative affect, predicting that:

H6. COVID-19 induced anxiety is positively related with post-purchase negative affect

H7. COVID-19 induced self-isolation is positively related with post-purchase negative affect

H8. COVID-19 induced loneliness positively related with post-purchase negative affect

Control Variables

In previous studies on impulsive buying, various demographic factors such as gender (Atulkar & Kesari, 2018; Utama et al., 2021), age (Badgaiyan & Verma, 2015; Bashar, 2013), marital status (Yang et al., 2011), income (Bashar, 2013; Li et al., 2021; Lui et al., 2022), and education (Mihić & Kursan,

2010; Rana & Tirthani, 2012) were found to impact individuals' impulsive buying behaviors. Thus, these demographic variables were added to the research model as control variables to limit potential confounding effects and enable a more rigorous test of the hypothesized relations. The research model with hypothesized relationships is presented in Figure 1.

Figure 1. Research model

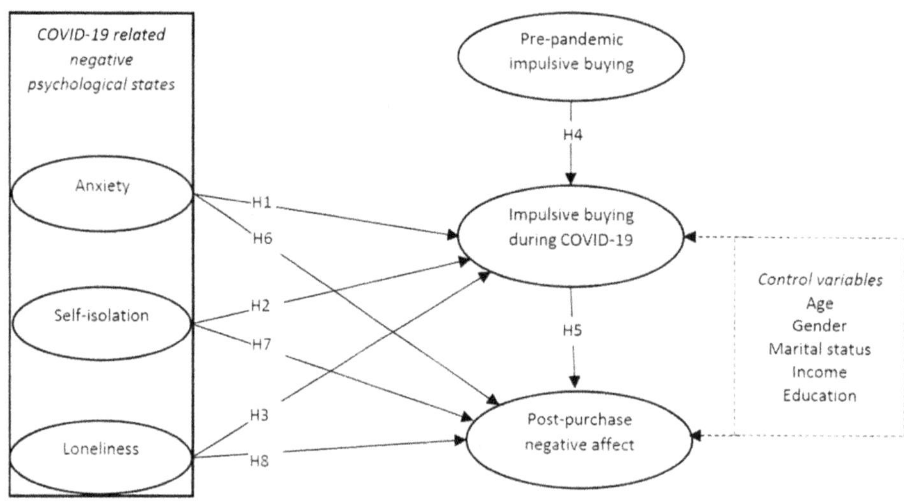

METHOD

Sample and Data Collection Period

Data were collected in Turkey through an online survey using the surveey.com platform. The first COVID-19 case in Turkey was reported on March 11, 2020, with a total of 14.775.634 confirmed cases and 97.666 deaths reported to date (MoH, 2022). To reduce the number of cases and deaths, the Turkish government took preventative measures including closing schools across the country, banning mass gathering events, establishing restrictive measures for public officials (e.g., flexible working arrangements), and imposing additional travel restrictions, curfews, and lockdowns during certain periods (TGA, 2022). Although a controlled normalization stage of the fight against the COVID-19 pandemic began on May 17, 2021 (MoI, 2022), the data for the current study was collected before this process, between January 25 and April 13, 2021. During this period of home confinement precautions and extended national curfews, many sources of entertainment such as cafes, restaurants, event venues, sporting arenas, and game halls were greatly restricted or even closed (İlhan et al., 2021). Thus, the survey period provided an appropriate window of time to assess COVID-19 related psychological stress and its consequences.

Following convenience and snowball sampling procedures, an invitation for the questionnaire was sent through email, social media, and instant messaging applications due to the restricted conditions of the pandemic. A total of 405 valid questionnaires were obtained. Respondents were on average 30,83 years old (standard deviation = 8,91). Of the respondents, approximately 75% were male and 49% were married. In terms of educational attainment, 8% held a primary school education, 27% had graduated from high school, 53% held undergraduate degrees, and 12% held graduate degrees. Finally, 45% of the respondents had a monthly income of more than 5.000₺.

Measures

The survey included six items measuring participants' impulsive buying during the pandemic. The items were adopted from Rook and Fisher (1995) by tailoring the original items to the COVID-19 context. Additionally, participants' pre-pandemic impulsive buying was measured by asking if they often used to purchase impulsively before the pandemic. A nine-item COVID anxiety scale was adopted from Taylor et al. (2020). Loneliness was measured with five items drawn from the UCLA Loneliness Scale by Russell et al. (1978), while isolation was measured with five items adapted from Rubin et al. (2009). Finally, six items were adopted from scales used by Taute and McQuitty (2004) and Valence et al. (1988) to measure post-purchase negative affect. All items were answered on a Likert scale from 1 to 5 with verbal anchors ranging from "strongly disagree" to "strongly agree." with the exception of those eliminated during the validation process, all individual items are displayed in Table 1.

ANALYSES

Scale Validation

Construct validity of the scales was assessed through exploratory factor analysis (EFA) using the principal component analysis and varimax rotation on 31 reflective items measuring research variables. The single item variable "pre-pandemic impulsive buying" was not included in the analysis. The results revealed a five-factor solution which explained 71% of the total variance. After closer examination of the factor loadings, one isolation item and one loneliness item were eliminated from further consideration due to poor loading estimate and cross-loading, respectively. Next, a five-factor solution was suggested by EFA that explained 73% of the total variance. The factor loadings of the individual items to their respective factors were all large (the lowest value was 0.537), providing evidence for the scales' construct validity. The factor loading coefficients are presented in Table 1.

Furthermore, Cronbach's alpha coefficients were all beyond the critical level suggested by Nunnally (1978), providing support for internal consistency (see Table1). After the validation process, the arithmetic mean of the multiple items for each scale was calculated to create composite scales for the research variables. Table 2 displays the descriptive statistics for the composite scales and intercorrelations among variables.

RESULTS

Two linear regression analyses were run to evaluate the hypotheses, holding impulsive buying and post-purchase negative affect as dependent variables, respectively. The first analysis included the control variables, COVID-19 related negative psychological states (i.e., anxiety, isolation, and loneliness), and pre-pandemic impulsive buying as determinants of impulsive buying. As reported in Table 3, the

Table 1. Scale items, factor loadings, and Cronbach's alpha coefficients

Scale	Factor Loadings
Anxiety ***Cronbach's α=0.91***	
I have been worried about catching the virus	0.766
I have been worried that I can't keep my family safe from the virus	0.661
I have been worried that basic hygiene (e.g., handwashing) won't be enough to keep me safe from the virus	0.748
I have been worried that if I touched something in a public space (e.g., handrail, door handle), I would catch the virus	0.819
I have been worried that if someone coughed or sneezed near me, I would catch the virus	0.773
I have been worried that people around me will infect me with the virus	0.809
I have had trouble concentrating because I kept thinking about the virus	0.537
Reminders of the virus have caused me to have physical reactions, such as sweating or a pounding heart	0.539
I have been checking my own body for signs of infection (e.g., taking my temperature)	0.609
Isolation ***Cronbach's α=0.92***	
Because of the COVID-19 pandemic…	
I deliberately canceled meeting my friends/loved ones	0.808
I reduced the amount I go into shops	0.864
I canceled or postponed many social events	0.849
I kept away from crowded places generally	0.794
Loneliness ***Cronbach's α=0.84***	
During the COVID-19 pandemic….	
I found myself waiting for people to call or write	0.554
I felt isolated from others	0.696
I felt as if nobody really understands me	0.840
I felt completely alone	0.849
Impulsive Buying ***Cronbach's α=0.93***	
During the COVID-19 pandemic…	
I often bought things spontaneously	0.779
"Just do it" described the way I bought things	0.824
I often bought things without thinking	0.838
"I saw it, I bought it" described me	0.801
"Buy now, think about it later" described me	0.779
Sometimes I felt like buying things on the spur of the moment	0.777
Post-purchase negative affect ***Cronbach's α=0.95***	
After my impulsive purchases in the COVID-19 period…	
I felt regret and canceled the purchase that I made	0.805
I felt depressed after buying spontaneously	0.855
I felt bad about buying without "checking it out" first	0.866
At times, I have felt somewhat guilty after buying a product because it seemed unreasonable	0.847
There were some things I bought, but I did not show to anybody for fear of being perceived as irrational in my buying behavior	0.800
I had sometimes thought, "if I had to do it all over again, I would…" and felt sorry for something I bought	0.823

Table 2. Descriptive statistics and correlations across individual variables

	Mean (SD.)	1	2	3	4	5	6
1. Anxiety	3.07 (0.97)	1					
2. Isolation	4.17 (0.96)	0.476**	1				
3. Loneliness	2.94 (1.13)	0.481**	0.358**	1			
4. Pre-pandemic impulsive buying	2.29 (1.23)	0.252**	0.015	0.252**	1		
5. Impulsive buying	2.30 (1.05)	0.349**	0.119*	0.359**	0.622**	1	
6. Post-purchase negative affect	2.20 (1.11)	0.389**	0.096	0.368**	0.495**	0.635**	1

** Correlation is significant at the 0.01 level
* Correlation is significant at the 0.05 level

regression model was found to explain 43% of the observed variance in impulsive buying during the pandemic, which is significantly greater than zero (F=29.245; p<0.01).

The results of the first regression analysis showed that after controlling for the impacts of demographic factors, COVID-19-induced anxiety (b=0.154, p<0.01), loneliness (b=0.155, p<0.01), and pre-pandemic impulsive buying (b=0.526, p<0.01) had significant positive effects on impulsive buying. In contrast, isolation was found to have no significant impact. These results supported H1, H3, and H4, while H2 was not supported. According to the standardized beta coefficients, pre-pandemic impulsive buying was the strongest predictor of impulsive buying during the pandemic. A further examination of the results indicated that women were slightly more prone impulsive purchases during the pandemic than their male counterparts (b=0.088, p<0.05). Other control variables appeared to be unrelated to impulse buying.

The second regression model, which included post-purchase negative affect as the dependent variable alongside COVID-19 related negative psychological states (i.e., anxiety, isolation, and loneliness) and impulsive buying as independent variables (while controlling for demographic characteristics), was found to be significant (F=25.652; p<0.01). As reported in Table 3, the overall proportion of observed variance explained in post-purchase negative affect was 40%. As to the effects of individual predictors, impulsive

Table 3. Results of regression analyses

	Dependents Variables					
	Impulsive buying			Post-purchase negative affect		
	Std. B	*t*	*p*	*Std. B*	*t*	*p*
Constant	-	-0.110	0.912	-	0.055	0.956
Control variables						
Age	-0.020	-0.403	0.687	0.044	0.852	0.395
Gender	0.088	20.070	0.039	-0.050	-10.124	0.262
Marital status	0.051	10.029	0.304	0.091	10.761	0.079
Education	-0.010	-0.220	0.826	0.073	10.604	0.110
Income	0.035	0.804	0.422	-0.043	-0.941	0.347
Independent variables						
Anxiety	0.154	20.982	0.003	0.169	30.151	0.002
Isolation	-0.017	-0.352	0.725	-0.097	-10.943	0.053
Loneliness	0.155	30.192	0.002	0.110	20.174	0.030
Pre-pandemic impulsive buying	0.526	110.842	0.000	-	-	-
Impulsive buying	-	-	-	0.517	100.813	0.000
R^2		0.45			0.42	
Adjusted R^2		0.43			0.40	
F		29.245			25.652	
p		0.00			0.00	

buying (b=0.517, p<0.01), anxiety (b=0.169, p<0.01), and loneliness (b=0.110, p<0.05) were found to significantly explain post-purchase negative affect, while isolation had a non-significant effect size. Thus, H5, H6, H8 found support, while H7 had no support. Not surprisingly, impulsive buying during the pandemic appeared as the strongest antecedent of post-purchase negative affect. The results further showed that the control variables had no significant relation to post-purchase negative affect. Empirical findings are visualized in Figure 2.

Figure 2. Empirical findings

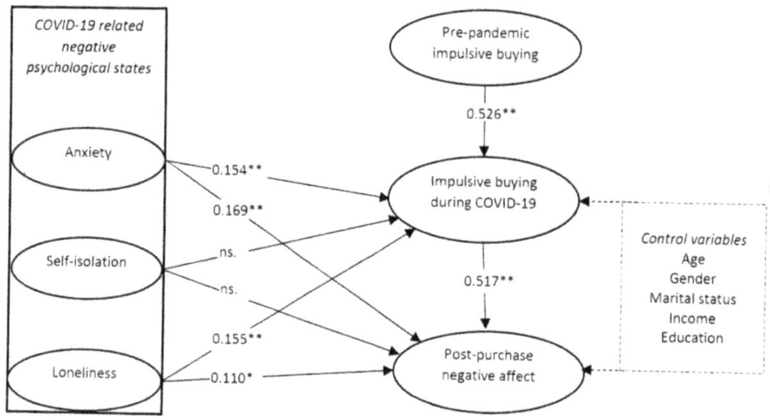

** $p<0.01$; * $p<0.05$; ns $p>0.05$

DISCUSSION

According to the literature that has amassed over the past two years, the precautions taken due to the COVID-19 pandemic have brought severe negative effects on economic, social, and psychological well-being. Individuals who struggle with pandemic-related anxiety, depression, stress, loneliness, and boredom tend to adopt various methods to alleviate the psychological strain. Impulsive buying appears as one of the methods that deserves special attention due to its unintended adverse emotional consequences. Hence, this study aimed to investigate how COVID-19 related anxiety, self-isolation, and loneliness encourage individuals to make impulsive purchases during the pandemic. Meanwhile, pre-pandemic shopping style was also considered to understand whether the impulsive buying response to COVID-19 stress is particularly prevalent in individuals who were already prone to such behaviors in less chaotic times. Finally, we investigated how pandemic-related psychological strain fuels the post-impulsive purchase negative affect to reveal increased emotional distress as a side effect of impulsive buying in the COVID-19 era.

Prior studies noted that impulsive buying is strongly related to the individual tendency for the behavior (Ahmad et al., 2019; Barakat, 2019; Kwon & Ahn, 2021; Özer & Gültekin, 2015; Utama et al., 2021). Consistently, the present study found pre-pandemic impulsive buying to be strongly related to impulsive buying during the pandemic. Moreover, anxiety and loneliness promote impulsive buying even after controlling for the effect of pre-pandemic impulse purchasing behavior. Accordingly, regardless of their previous shopping style or age, gender, marital status, income level, or education, individuals with a higher level of anxiety around COVID-19 are more likely to engage in impulsive buying. Similarly, individuals who feel alienated and isolated from loved ones or their community because of the pandemic are more prone to shop impulsively, even if this behavior does not correspond with their typical purchasing style. It appears that impulse buying is not only an individual trait but also a behavioral response to pandemic-related psychological strain. This response can be attributed to the effort to manage stress and improve mental well-being. Our study contributes to the argument regarding the self-distraction, mood regulation, and stress alleviation roles played by impulsive buying during unpredictable and highly stressful crisis periods (DeSarbo & Edwards, 1996; Elliott, 1994; Faber & O'Guinn, 1992; Sneath et al., 2009) by providing additional empirical evidence from the COVID-19 context.

However, unlike other self-distraction activities or stress coping mechanisms such as yoga, meditation, listening to music, or reading books, impulsive buying has a dark side for individuals. As evidenced in the current study, though impulsive buying may provide fleeting pleasure immediately after purchase, it is later followed by negative affect such as regret, guilt, and shame stemming from cognitive evaluations of purchasing appropriateness. This finding echoes those of several pre-pandemic studies (Fenton-O'Creevy et al., 2018; George & Yaoyuneyong, 2010; Hausman, 2000; Hoch & Loewentein, 1991; Imam, 2013; Parsad et al., 2019; Saleh, 2012; Wood, 1998). Additionally, the present study found that negative post-purchase affective reactions are not only related to the extent of the individual's impulsive buying, but also pandemic induced negative psychological states. Particularly, individuals with a higher level of anxiety and loneliness are more likely to despair after an impulsive purchase, likely because negative emotions yield a negatively biased evaluation of their shopping decision. The results correspond with those of studies demonstrating that individuals feel lower satisfaction (Kim & Mattila, 2010; Liljander & Strandvik, 1997; Özer & Gültekin, 2015) and greater guilt (Li, 2015; Miao & Mattila, 2013) when they make an impulsive purchase while in a negative mood.

It should be noted that the proposed impacts of social isolation on impulse buying and post-purchase negative affect were not confirmed by the data in the present study. This result may be explained by the fact that self-isolation not only increased negative psychological symptoms (Lim et al., 2020) but also limited respondents' shopping opportunities. Moreover, self-isolation provides unexpected free time that can be used for complementary therapies such as yoga, meditation, prayer, and spirituality (Dagli, 2020; Fluharty & Fancourt, 2021; Savitsky et al., 2020), as well as self-distraction activities such as watching TV, cleaning or tidying up, spending time on the internet, listening to music, reading books, sleeping, or exercising (Park et al., 2020; Taylor et al., 2020; Temiz, 2020), instead of impulsive buying.

In sum, COVID-19 generated a wide range of stressors such as the risk of infection of self or loved ones, uncertainty about the length of the pandemic, and changes to well-established daily and social routines, which all caused significant psychological strain. Anxiety and loneliness are among the most common negative states stemming from the pandemic. According to psychological research, individuals benefited from various coping strategies, including impulsive buying, to bolster their mental well-being during this period. The current study revealed that individuals experiencing anxiety and loneliness during the pandemic were likely to engage in impulsive buying regardless of their pre-pandemic buying style. However, linked to anxiety and loneliness, individuals experienced more severe post-purchase guilt, regret, and shame of doing not-budgeted, unnecessary shopping during the pandemic. At this point, it is reasonable to question the functionality of the self-distraction, mood regulation, stress alleviation roles of impulsive buying for individuals, at least in highly stressful crisis periods such as the COVID-19 pandemic. Unlike other stress-coping methods, impulsive buying may create an additional stressor itself. These findings can provide a springboard for further research on dysfunctional consumer behaviors in extraordinary periods, as well for the work of non-governmental organizations, policymakers, counselors, and other professionals who strive to address social needs and alleviate individuals' anxiety and panic (Sun et al., 2021). The findings indicate the importance of informational messages, persuasive campaigns, and public service announcements to reduce dysfunctional behaviors such as impulsive buying and encourage the alternative coping strategies that can reduce psychological strain and enhance resilience during the ongoing COVID-19 pandemic (Dagli, 2020; Polizzi et al., 2020).

LIMITATIONS AND SUGGESTIONS

The contributions of the present study should be interpreted in light of a few important limitations. First, the study was conducted on individuals living in Turkey, so the generalizability of its findings are limited. The negative states experienced by individuals in other countries may vary due to the different pandemic conditions and precautions. Furthermore, this study only investigated three negative psychological states—anxiety, self-isolation, and loneliness—thus, future research should explore other states such as depression, anger, or boredom. Similarly, additional research in this area should also study positive post-purchase emotional reactions. Finally, the present study focused on impulsive buying during the pandemic, when buying opportunities were limited by social distancing mandates and business closures. Thus, "online buying capability" should be incorporated into future research as a moderator factor that is likely to hinder the impulsive buying behavior of older individuals during the pandemic.

REFERENCES

Ahmad, M. B., Ali, H. F., Malik, M. S., Humayun, A. A., & Ahmad, S. (2019). Factors affecting impulsive buying behavior with mediating role of positive mood: An empirical study. *European Online Journal of Natural and Social Sciences*, *8*(1), 17.

Ahmed, R. R., Streimikiene, D., Rolle, J.-A., & Duc, P. A. (2020). The COVID-19 pandemic and the antecedents for the impulse buying behavior of US citizens. *Journal of Competitiveness*, *12*(3), 5–27. doi:10.7441/joc.2020.03.01

Arslan, G., Yıldırım, M., Karataş, Z., Kabasakal, Z., & Kılınç, M. (2020). Meaningful living to promote complete mental health among university students in the context of the COVID-19 pandemic. *International Journal of Mental Health and Addiction*, 1–13. doi:10.100711469-020-00416-8 PMID:33169074

Atulkar, S., & Kesari, B. (2018). Role of consumer traits and situational factors on impulse buying: Does gender matter? *International Journal of Retail & Distribution Management*, *46*(4), 386–405. Advance online publication. doi:10.1108/IJRDM-12-2016-0239

Badgaiyan, A. J., & Verma, A. (2015). Does urge to buy impulsively differ from impulsive buying behaviour? Assessing the impact of situational factors. *Journal of Retailing and Consumer Services*, *22*, 145–157. doi:10.1016/j.jretconser.2014.10.002

Bagozzi, R. P., Gopinath, M., & Nyer, P. U. (1999). The role of emotions in marketing. *Journal of the Academy of Marketing Science*, *27*(2), 184–206. doi:10.1177/0092070399272005

Bakırtaş, H. (2013). SOR paradigması temelinde mağaza atmosferi ve duyguların pazarlamadaki önemi: bir literatür incelemesi. *Karamanoğlu Mehmetbey Üniversitesi Sosyal ve Ekonomik Araştırmalar Dergisi, 2013*(2), 47-55. https://dergipark.org.tr/en/pub/kmusekad/issue/10211/125472

Banerjee, D., & Rai, M. (2020). Social isolation in COVID-19: The impact of loneliness. *The International Journal of Social Psychiatry, 66*(6), 525–527. doi:10.1177/0020764020922269 PMID:32349580

Barakat, M. A. (2019). A proposed model for factors affecting consumers' impulsive buying tendency in shopping malls. *Journal of Marketing Management, 7*(1), 120–134. doi:10.15640/jmm.v7n1a10

Barlow, D. H. (1988). *Anxiety and Its Disorders*. The Guilford Press.

Bartoszek, A., Walkowiak, D., Bartoszek, A., & Kardas, G. (2020). Mental well-being (depression, loneliness, insomnia, daily life fatigue) during COVID-19 related home-confinement—A study from Poland. *International Journal of Environmental Research and Public Health, 17*(20), 7417. doi:10.3390/ijerph17207417 PMID:33053787

Bashar, A., Ahmad, I., & Wasiq, M. (2013). A study of influence of demographic factors on consumer impulse buying behavior. *Journal of Management Research, 13*(3).

Baumeister, R. F. (2002). Yielding to temptation: Self-control failure, impulsive purchasing, and consumer behavior. *The Journal of Consumer Research, 28*(4), 670–676. doi:10.1086/338209

Bharathi, K., & Sudha, S. (2017). Store ambiance influence on consumer impulsive buying behavior towards apparel: SOR model. *Indian Journal of Public Health Research & Development, 8*(4), 4140. doi:10.5958/0976-5506.2017.00329.1

Bower, G. H. (1981). Mood and memory. *The American Psychologist, 36*(2), 129–148. doi:10.1037/0003-066X.36.2.129 PMID:7224324

Cacioppo, J. T., Hawkley, L. C., Berntson, G. G., Ernst, J. M., Gibbs, A. C., Stickgold, R., & Hobson, J. A. (2002). Do lonely days invade the nights? Potential social modulation of sleep efficiency. *Psychological Science, 13*(4), 384–387. doi:10.1111/1467-9280.00469 PMID:12137144

Carver, C. S. (1997). You want to measure coping but your protocol'too long: Consider the brief cope. *International Journal of Behavioral Medicine, 4*(1), 92–100. doi:10.120715327558ijbm0401_6 PMID:16250744

Casagrande, M., Favieri, F., Tambelli, R., & Forte, G. (2020). The enemy who sealed the world: Effects quarantine due to the COVID-19 on sleep quality, anxiety, and psychological distress in the Italian population. *Sleep Medicine, 75*, 12–20. doi:10.1016/j.sleep.2020.05.011 PMID:32853913

Chang, H. J., Eckman, M., & Yan, R. N. (2011). Application of the Stimulus-Organism-Response model to the retail environment: The role of hedonic motivation in impulse buying behavior. *International Review of Retail, Distribution and Consumer Research, 21*(3), 233–249. doi:10.1080/09593969.2011.578798

Chauhan, S., Banerjee, R., & Dagar, V. (2021). Analysis of impulse buying behaviour of consumer during COVID-19: An empirical study. *Millennial Asia*. Advance online publication. doi:10.1177/09763996211041215

Chen, C. C., & Yao, J. Y. (2018). What drives impulse buying behaviors in a mobile auction? The perspective of the Stimulus-Organism-Response model. *Telematics and Informatics, 35*(5), 1249–1262. doi:10.1016/j.tele.2018.02.007

Dagli, R. (2020). Fear and anxiety-coping strategies during COVID-19 pandemic in lockdown. *Journal of International Oral Health: JIOH, 12*(3), 187–188. doi:10.4103/JIOH.JIOH_133_20

DeSarbo, W. S., & Edwards, E. A. (1996). Typologies of compulsive buying behavior: A constrained clusterwise regression approach. *Journal of Consumer Psychology, 5*(3), 231–262. doi:10.120715327663jcp0503_02

Droit-Volet, S., Gil, S., Martinelli, N., Andant, N., Clinchamps, M., Parreira, L., Rouffiac, K., Dambrun, M., Huguet, P., Dubuis, B., Pereira, B., Bouillon, J.-B., & Dutheil, F. (2020). Time and COVID-19 stress in the lockdown situation: Time free,«Dying» of boredom and sadness. *PLoS One, 15*(8), e0236465. doi:10.1371/journal.pone.0236465 PMID:32776990

Dursun, İ., Gökmen Köksal, C., & Tümer Kabadayı, E. (2022). COVID-19 salgını döneminde sürdürülebilir tüketim davranışlarında yaşanan değişim. *Journal of Management and Economics Research, 20*(3), 302–324.

Elliott, R. (1994). Addictive consumption: Function and fragmentation in postmodernity. *Journal of Consumer Policy, 17*(2), 159–179. doi:10.1007/BF01016361

Evanoff, B. A., Strickland, J. R., Dale, A. M., Hayibor, L., Page, E., Duncan, J. G., Kannampallil, T., & Gray, D. L. (2020). Work-related and personal factors associated with mental well-being during the COVID-19 response: Survey of health care and other workers. *Journal of Medical Internet Research, 22*(8), e21366. doi:10.2196/21366 PMID:32763891

Faber, R. J., & O'Guinn, T. C. (1992). A clinical screener for compulsive buying. *The Journal of Consumer Research, 19*(3), 459–469. doi:10.1086/209315

Fässberg, M. M., Orden, K. A. V., Duberstein, P., Erlangsen, A., Lapierre, S., Bodner, E., Canetto, S. S., Leo, D. D., Szanto, K., & Waern, M. (2012). A systematic review of social factors and suicidal behavior in older adulthood. *International Journal of Environmental Research and Public Health, 9*(3), 722–745. doi:10.3390/ijerph9030722 PMID:22690159

Fenton-O'Creevy, M., Dibb, S., & Furnham, A. (2018). Antecedents and consequences of chronic impulsive buying: Can impulsive buying be understood as dysfunctional self-regulation? *Psychology and Marketing, 35*(3), 175–188. doi:10.1002/mar.21078

Fluharty, M., & Fancourt, D. (2021). How have people been coping during the COVID-19 pandemic? Patterns and predictors of coping strategies amongst 26,016 UK adults. *BMC Psychology, 9*(1), 1–12. . doi:10.118640359-021-00603-9 PMID:34266498

Gardner, M. P., & Rook, D. W. (1988). *Effects of impulse purchases on consumers' affective states.* ACR North American Advances.

George, B. P., & Vaoyuneyong, G. (2010). Impulsive buying and cognitive dissonance: A study conducted among the spring break student shoppers. *Young Customers, 11*(4), 291–306. doi:10.1108/17473611011093925

González-Sanguino, C., Ausín, B., Castellanos, M. Á., Saiz, J., López-Gómez, A., Ugidos, C., & Muñoz, M. (2020). Mental health consequences during the initial stage of the 2020 Coronavirus pandemic (COVID-19) in Spain. *Brain, Behavior, and Immunity, 87*, 172–176. doi:10.1016/j.bbi.2020.05.040 PMID:32405150

Gupta, R., Nair, K., & Radhakrishnan, L. (2021). Impact of COVID-19 crisis on stocking and impulse buying behaviour of consumers. *International Journal of Social Economics, 48*(12), 1794–1809. Advance online publication. doi:10.1108/IJSE-03-2021-0163

Hama, Y. (2001). Shopping as a coping behavior for stress. *The Japanese Psychological Research, 43*(4), 218–224. doi:10.1111/1468-5884.00179

Hanks, L., & Mattila, A. S. (2014). The impact of gender and pre-purchase mood on consumer guilt after a travel purchase. *Journal of Travel Research, 53*(5), 625–637. doi:10.1177/0047287513506296

Hausman, A. (2000). A multi-method investigation of consumer motivations in impulse buying behavior. *Journal of Consumer Marketing, 17*(5), 403–426. doi:10.1108/07363760010341045

Hetkamp, M., Schweda, A., Bäuerle, A., Weismüller, B., Kohler, H., Musche, V., Dörrie, N., Schöbel, C., Teufel, M., & Skoda, E. M. (2020). Sleep disturbances, fear, and generalized anxiety during the COVID-19 shut down phase in Germany: Relation to infection rates, deaths, and German stock index DAX. *Sleep Medicine, 75*, 350–353. doi:10.1016/j.sleep.2020.08.033 PMID:32950879

Hoch, S. J., & Loewenstein, G. F. (1991). Time-inconsistent preferences and consumer self-control. *The Journal of Consumer Research, 17*(4), 492–507. doi:10.1086/208573

Hoffart, A., Johnson, S. U., & Ebrahimi, O. V. (2020). Loneliness and social distancing during the COVID-19 pandemic: Risk factors and associations with psychopathology. *Frontiers in Psychiatry, 11*, 1297. doi:10.3389/fpsyt.2020.589127 PMID:33329136

Huang, E. (2012). Online experiences and virtual goods purchase intention. *Internet Research, 22*(3), 252–274. doi:10.1108/10662241211235644

Hwang, T. J., Rabheru, K., Peisah, C., Reichman, W., & Ikeda, M. (2020). Loneliness and social isolation during the COVID-19 pandemic. *International Psychogeriatrics, 32*(10), 1217–1220. doi:10.1017/S1041610220000988 PMID:32450943

İlhan, M. N., Tüzün, H., Kiliç, R., & Yildirim, N. (2021). Nonpharmaceutical interventions in Turkey and worldwide during COVID-19 pandemic. *Turkish Journal of Medical Sciences, 51*(SI-1), 3207–3214. doi:10.3906ag-2106-210 PMID:34590802

Imam, F. (2013). Gender differences in impulsive buying behavior and post purchasing dissonance under incentive conditions. *The Journal of Business Strategy, 7*(1), 23.

Jacoby, J. (2002). Stimulus-organism-response reconsidered: An evolutionary step in modeling (consumer) behavior. *Journal of Consumer Psychology, 12*(1), 51–57. doi:10.1207/S15327663JCP1201_05

Kalla, S. M., & Arora, A. P. (2011). Impulse buying: A literature review. *Global Business Review*, *12*(1), 145–157. doi:10.1177/097215091001200109

Kamboj, S., Sarmah, B., Gupta, S., & Dwivedi, Y. (2018). Examining branding co-creation in brand communities on social media: Applying the paradigm of Stimulus-Organism-Response. *International Journal of Information Management*, *39*, 169–185. doi:10.1016/j.ijinfomgt.2017.12.001

Kim, M. G., & Mattila, A. S. (2010). The impact of mood states and surprise cues on satisfaction. *International Journal of Hospitality Management*, *29*(3), 432–436. doi:10.1016/j.ijhm.2009.10.022

Kollat, D. T., & Willett, R. P. (1967). Customer impulse purchasing behavior. *JMR, Journal of Marketing Research*, *4*(1), 21–31. doi:10.1177/002224376700400102

Konstam, V., Moser, D. K., & De Jong, M. J. (2005). Depression and anxiety in heart failure. *Journal of Cardiac Failure*, *11*(6), 455–463. doi:10.1016/j.cardfail.2005.03.006 PMID:16105637

Kwon, J., & Ahn, J. (2021). The effects of cruise attributes on impulse buying behavior: The mediating role of impulsive buying tendency. *International Journal of Quality and Service Sciences*, *13*(3), 456–470. doi:10.1108/IJQSS-09-2020-0141

Laato, S., Islam, A. N., Farooq, A., & Dhir, A. (2020). Unusual purchasing behavior during the early stages of the COVID-19 pandemic: The stimulus-organism-response approach. *Journal of Retailing and Consumer Services*, *57*, 102224. doi:10.1016/j.jretconser.2020.102224

Lee, E. E., Depp, C., Palmer, B. W., Glorioso, D., Daly, R., Liu, J., Tu, X. M., Kim, H.-C., Tarr, P., Yamada, Y., & Jeste, D. V. (2019). High prevalence and adverse health effects of loneliness in community-dwelling adults across the lifespan: Role of wisdom as a protective factor. *International Psychogeriatrics*, *31*(10), 1447–1462. doi:10.1017/S1041610218002120 PMID:30560747

Lee, S. H., & Cotte, J. (2009). Post-Purchase Consumer Regret: Conceptualization and Development of the PPCR Scale. In A. L. McGill & S. Shavitt (Eds.), *NA - Advances in Consumer Research* (Vol. 36, pp. 456–462). Association for Consumer Research.

Li, B., Hu, M., Chen, X., & Lei, Y. (2021). The Moderating Role of Anticipated Regret and Product Involvement on Online Impulsive Buying Behavior. *Frontiers in Psychology*, *12*, 732459–732459. doi:10.3389/fpsyg.2021.732459 PMID:34975621

Li, Y. (2015). Impact of impulsive buying behavior on postimpulsive buying satisfaction. *Social Behavior and Personality*, *43*(2), 339–351. doi:10.2224bp.2015.43.2.339

Liljander, V., & Strandvik, T. (1997). Emotions in service satisfaction. *International Journal of Service Industry Management*, *8*(2), 148–169. doi:10.1108/09564239710166272

Lim, J., Jeon, S., Shin, H. Y., Kim, M. J., Seong, Y. M., Lee, W. J., ... Park, S. J. (2020). Case of the index patient who caused tertiary transmission of COVID-19 infection in Korea: The application of lopinavir/ritonavir for the treatment of COVID-19 infected pneumonia monitored by quantitative RT-PCR. *Journal of Korean Medical Science*, *35*(6), e79. doi:10.3346/jkms.2020.35.e79 PMID:32056407

Lin, L. (2021). Longitudinal associations of meaning in life and psychosocial adjustment to the COVID-19 outbreak in China. *British Journal of Health Psychology*, *26*(2), 525–534. doi:10.1111/bjhp.12492 PMID:33217144

Liu, B., Song, M., Yang, G., Cheng, S., & Li, M. (2020). RETRACTED: Stimulus organism response model based analysis on consumers' online impulse buying behavior. *International Journal of Electrical Engineering Education*. Advance online publication. doi:10.1177/0020720920940585

Liu, X. S., Shi, Y., Xue, N. I., & Shen, H. (2022). The impact of time pressure on impulsive buying: The moderating role of consumption type. *Tourism Management*, *91*, 104505. doi:10.1016/j.tourman.2022.104505

Luo, H., Chen, J., Li, S., Nie, Y., & Wang, G. (2021). Social exclusion and impulsive buying among Chinese college students: The mediating role of self-esteem and the moderating role of risk preference. *International Journal of Environmental Research and Public Health*, *18*(21), 11027. doi:10.3390/ijerph182111027 PMID:34769547

Martarelli, C. S., & Wolff, W. (2020). Too bored to bother? Boredom as a potential threat to the efficacy of pandemic containment measures. *Humanities and Social Sciences Communications*, *7*(1), 1–5. doi:10.105741599-020-0512-6

Mazza, C., Ricci, E., Biondi, S., Colasanti, M., Ferracuti, S., Napoli, C., & Roma, P. (2020). A nationwide survey of psychological distress among Italian people during the COVID-19 pandemic: Immediate psychological responses and associated factors. *International Journal of Environmental Research and Public Health*, *17*(9), 3165. doi:10.3390/ijerph17093165 PMID:32370116

Mehrabian, A., & Russell, J. A. (1974). *An approach to environmental psychology*. The MIT Press.

Miao, L., & Mattila, A. S. (2013). Impulse buying in restaurant food consumption. *Journal of Foodservice Business Research*, *16*(5), 448–467. doi:10.1080/15378020.2013.850379

Mihić, M., & Kursan, I. (2010). Assessing the situational factors and impulsive buying behavior: Market segmentation approach. *Management*, *15*(2), 47–66. https://hrcak.srce.hr/62289

Ming, J., Jianqiu, Z., Bilal, M., Akram, U., & Fan, M. (2021). How social presence influences impulse buying behavior in live streaming commerce? The role of SOR theory. *International Journal of Web Information Systems*, *17*(4), 300–320. doi:10.1108/IJWIS-02-2021-0012

Ministry of Health Republic of Turkey (MoH-TR). (2022, January 22). *COVID-19 web page*. https://covid19.saglik.gov.tr/

MoI. (2022). *Ministry of Interior (Turkey)*. https://www.icisleri.gov.tr/81-il-valiligine-kademeli-normallesme-tedbirleri-genelgesi-gonderildi

Morales-Vives, F., Dueñas, J. M., Vigil-Colet, A., & Camarero-Figuerola, M. (2020). Psychological variables related to adaptation to the COVID-19 lockdown in Spain. *Frontiers in Psychology*, *11*, 2438. doi:10.3389/fpsyg.2020.565634 PMID:33041929

Morgul, E., Bener, A., Atak, M., Akyel, S., Aktaş, S., Bhugra, D., Ventriglio, A., & Jordan, T. R. (2021). COVID-19 pandemic and psychological fatigue in Turkey. *The International Journal of Social Psychiatry*, *67*(2), 128–135. doi:10.1177/0020764020941889 PMID:32650681

Naeem, M. (2020). Understanding the customer psychology of impulse buying during COVID-19 pandemic: Implications for retailers. *International Journal of Retail & Distribution Management*, *49*(3), 377–393. doi:10.1108/IJRDM-08-2020-0317

Özer, L., & Gultekin, B. (2015). Pre-and post-purchase stage in impulse buying: The role of mood and satisfaction. *Journal of Retailing and Consumer Services*, *22*, 71–76. doi:10.1016/j.jretconser.2014.10.004

Park, C. L., Russell, B. S., Fendrich, M., Finkelstein-Fox, L., Hutchison, M., & Becker, J. (2020). Americans' COVID-19 stress, coping, and adherence to CDC guidelines. *Journal of General Internal Medicine*, *35*(8), 2296–2303. doi:10.100711606-020-05898-9 PMID:32472486

Park, J., & Lennon, S. J. (2006). Psychological and environmental antecedents of impulse buying tendency in the multichannel shopping context. *Journal of Consumer Marketing*, *23*(2), 56–66. doi:10.1108/07363760610654998

Parsad, C., Prashar, S., Vijay, T. S., & Sahay, V. (2019). Role of in-store atmospherics and impulse buying tendency on post-purchase regret. *Journal of Business and Management*, *25*(1).

Pavlov, I. P. (1927). *Conditioned reflexes: An investigation of the physiological activity of the cerebral cortex* (1st ed., G. V. Anrep, Trans.). Oxford University Press.

Peng, C., & Kim, Y. G. (2014). Application of the Stimuli Organism-Response (S-O-R) framework to online shopping behavior. *Journal of Internet Commerce*, *13*(3-4), 159–176. doi:10.1080/15332861.2014.944437

Peng, L., Xia, X., & Su, X. (2020, November). The Effect of Consumer's Loneliness on Impulse Buying in the Internet era: A Model Based on Para-social Interaction. In *2020 2nd International Conference on Economic Management and Model Engineering (ICEMME)* (pp. 843-848). IEEE. 10.1109/ICEMME51517.2020.00173

Pieh, C., O' Rourke, T., Budimir, S., & Probst, T. (2020). Relationship quality and mental health during COVID-19 lockdown. *PLoS One*, *15*(9), e0238906. doi:10.1371/journal.pone.0238906 PMID:32915878

Piron, F. (1993). *A comparison of emotional reactions experienced by planned, unplanned and impulse purchasers*. ACR North American Advances.

Polizzi, C., Lynn, S. J., & Perry, A. (2020). Stress and coping in the time of COVID-19: Pathways to resilience and recovery. *Clinical Neuropsychiatry*, *17*(2), 59. doi:10.36131/CN20200204 PMID:34908968

Prentice, C., Chen, J., & Stantic, B. (2020). Timed intervention in COVID-19 and panic buying. *Journal of Retailing and Consumer Services*, *57*, 102203. doi:10.1016/j.jretconser.2020.102203

Rana, S., & Tirthani, J. (2012). Effect of education, income and gender on impulsive buying among Indian consumer an empirical study of readymade garment customers. *Management*, *1*(12).

Rook, D. W. (1987). The buying impulse. *The Journal of Consumer Research, 14*(2), 189–199. doi:10.1086/209105

Rook, D. W., & Fisher, R. J. (1995). Normative influences on impulsive buying behavior. *The Journal of Consumer Research, 22*(3), 305–313. doi:10.1086/209452

Rubin, G. J., Amlôt, R., Page, L., & Wessely, S. (2009). Public perceptions, anxiety, and behaviour change in relation to the swine flu outbreak: Cross sectional telephone survey. *BMJ (Clinical Research Ed.), 339*(3), b2651. Advance online publication. doi:10.1136/bmj.b2651 PMID:19574308

Russell, D., Peplau, L. A., & Ferguson, M. L. (1978). Developing a measure of loneliness. *Journal of Personality Assessment, 42*(3), 290–294. doi:10.120715327752jpa4203_11 PMID:660402

Saleh, M. A. H. (2012). An investigation of the relationship between unplanned buying and post-purchase regret. *International Journal of Marketing Studies, 4*(4), 106. doi:10.5539/ijms.v4n4p106

Santini, F. D. O., Ladeira, W. J., Vieira, V. A., Araujo, C. F., & Sampaio, C. H. (2019). Antecedents and consequences of impulse buying: A meta-analytic study. *RAUSP Management Journal, 54*(2), 178–204. doi:10.1108/RAUSP-07-2018-0037

Savitsky, B., Findling, Y., Ereli, A., & Hendel, T. (2020). Anxiety and coping strategies among nursing students during the covid-19 pandemic. *Nurse Education in Practice, 46*, 102809. doi:10.1016/j.nepr.2020.102809 PMID:32679465

Schwarz, N. (1990). *Feelings as information: Informational and motivational functions of affective states*. The Guilford Press.

Schwarz, N., & Clore, G. L. (1983). Mood, misattribution, and judgments of well-being: Informative and directive functions of affective states. *Journal of Personality and Social Psychology, 45*(3), 513–523. doi:10.1037/0022-3514.45.3.513

Schwarz, N., & Clore, G. L. (1988). How do I feel about it? Information functions of affective states. *Affect, Cognition and Social Behavior,* 44-62.

Shahjehan, A., Zeb, F., & Saifullah, K. (2012). The effect of personality on impulsive and compulsive buying behaviors. *African Journal of Business Management, 6*(6), 2187–2194. doi:10.5897/AJBM11.2275

Shevlin, M., Nolan, E., Owczarek, M., McBride, O., Murphy, J., Gibson Miller, J., Hartman, T. K., Levita, L., Mason, L., Martinez, A. P., McKay, R., Stocks, T. V. A., Bennett, K. M., Hyland, P., & Bentall, R. P. (2020). COVID-19-related anxiety predicts somatic symptoms in the UK population. *British Journal of Health Psychology, 25*(4), 875–882. doi:10.1111/bjhp.12430 PMID:32458550

Slickdeals. (2022, January 22).) *Slickdeals Survey: Americans Are Spending More During the Coronavirus Pandemic.* https://slickdeals.net/article/news/pandemic-impulse-spending-survey-2020/

Sneath, J. Z., Lacey, R., & Kennett-Hensel, P. A. (2009). Coping with a natural disaster: Losses, emotions, and impulsive and compulsive buying. *Marketing Letters, 20*(1), 45–60. doi:10.100711002-008-9049-y

Sun, X., Su, W., Guo, X., & Tian, Z. (2021). The impact of awe induced by COVID-19 pandemic on green consumption behavior in China. *International Journal of Environmental Research and Public Health*, *18*(2), 543. doi:10.3390/ijerph18020543 PMID:33440719

Suppawittaya, P., Yiemphat, P., & Yasri, P. (2020). Effects of social distancing, self-quarantine and self-isolation during the COVID-19 pandemic on people's well-being and how to cope with it. *International Journal of Science and Healthcare Research*, *5*(2), 12–20.

Taute, H., & McQuitty, S. (2004). Feeling good! Doing good! An exploratory look at the impulsive purchase of the social good. *Journal of Marketing Theory and Practice*, *12*(2), 16–27. doi:10.1080/10696679.2004.11658516

Taylor, S., Landry, C. A., Paluszek, M. M., Fergus, T. A., McKay, D., & Asmundson, G. J. (2020a). COVID stress syndrome: Concept, structure, and correlates. *Depression and Anxiety*, *37*(8), 706–714. doi:10.1002/da.23071 PMID:32627255

Taylor, S., Landry, C. A., Paluszek, M. M., Fergus, T. A., McKay, D., & Asmundson, G. J. (2020b). Development and initial validation of the COVID Stress Scales. *Journal of Anxiety Disorders*, *72*, 102232. doi:10.1016/j.janxdis.2020.102232 PMID:32408047

Taylor, S., Paluszek, M. M., Landry, C. A., Rachor, G. S., & Asmundson, G. J. (2021). Predictors of distress and coping during pandemic-related self-isolation: The relative importance of personality traits and beliefs about personal threat. *Personality and Individual Differences*, *176*, 110779. doi:10.1016/j.paid.2021.110779 PMID:36540361

Temiz, Z. (2020). Nursing students' anxiety levels and coping strategies during the COVID-19 pandemic. *International Archives of Nursing and Health Care*, *6*(4), 150. doi:10.23937/2469-5823/1510150

TGA. (2022, January 22). Türkiye tourism promotion and development agency. *Fight against COVID-19 in Turkey*. https://www.tga.gov.tr/fight-against-covid-19-in-turkey/

Tutzer, F., Frajo-Apor, B., Pardeller, S., Plattner, B., Chernova, A., Haring, C., Holzner, B., Kemmler, G., Marksteiner, J., Miller, C., Schmidt, M., Sperner-Unterweger, B., & Hofer, A. (2021). Psychological distress, loneliness, and boredom among the general population of Tyrol, Austria during the COVID-19 pandemic. *Frontiers in Psychiatry*, *12*, 921. doi:10.3389/fpsyt.2021.691896 PMID:34177672

Utama, A., Sawıtrı, H. S. R., Haryanto, B., & Wahyudı, L. (2021). Impulse buying: The influence of impulse buying tendency, urge to buy and gender on impulse buying of the retail customers. *Journal of Distribution Science*, *19*(7), 101–111. doi:10.15722/jds.19.7.202107.101

Valence, G., d'Astous, A., & Fortier, L. (1988). Compulsive buying: Concept and measurement. *Journal of Consumer Policy*, *11*(4), 419–433. doi:10.1007/BF00411854

Varma, P., Junge, M., Meaklim, H., & Jackson, M. L. (2021). Younger people are more vulnerable to stress, anxiety and depression during COVID-19 pandemic: A global cross-sectional survey. *Progress in Neuro-Psychopharmacology & Biological Psychiatry*, *109*, 110236. doi:10.1016/j.pnpbp.2020.110236 PMID:33373680

Wang, C., Pan, R., Wan, X., Tan, Y., Xu, L., Ho, C. S., & Ho, R. C. (2020). Immediate psychological responses and associated factors during the initial stage of the 2019 coronavirus disease (COVID-19) epidemic among the general population in China. *International Journal of Environmental Research and Public Health, 17*(5), 1729. doi:10.3390/ijerph17051729 PMID:32155789

Wang, S., Liu, Y., Du, Y., & Wang, X. (2021). Effect of the COVID-19 pandemic on consumers' impulse buying: The moderating role of moderate thinking. *International Journal of Environmental Research and Public Health, 18*(21), 1–19. doi:10.3390/ijerph182111116 PMID:34769636

WHO. (2022, January 22). *WHO Coronavirus (COVID-19) Dashboard.* https://covid19.who.int/

Wood, M. (1998). Socio-economic status, delay of gratification, and impulse buying. *Journal of Economic Psychology, 19*(3), 295–320. doi:10.1016/S0167-4870(98)00009-9

Woodworth, R. (1929). *Psychology* (revised edition). Henry Holt.

Xiao, H., Zhang, Z., & Zhang, L. (2020). A diary study of impulsive buying during the COVID-19 pandemic. *Current Psychology (New Brunswick, N.J.)*, 1–13. doi:10.100712144-020-01220-2 PMID:33250615

Yan, L., Gan, Y., Ding, X., Wu, J., & Duan, H. (2021). The relationship between perceived stress and emotional distress during the COVID-19 outbreak: Effects of boredom proneness and coping style. *Journal of Anxiety Disorders, 77*, 102328. doi:10.1016/j.janxdis.2020.102328 PMID:33160275

Yang, D. J., Huang, K. C., & Feng, X. (2011). A study of the factors that affect the impulsive cosmetics buying of female consumers in Kaohsiung. *International Journal of Business and Social Science, 2*(24), 275–282.

KEY TERMS AND DEFINITIONS

Anxiety: An excessive and difficult-to-control concern caused by pandemic-related events.

Impulsive Buying: An unplanned purchasing that occurs because of a sudden, often powerful, and persistent urge to buy something.

Loneliness: A feeling of being disconnected from the world mixed with a sense of emptiness.

Post-Purchase Negative Affect: Negative feelings such as shame, regret, and guilt that arise as a result of individuals find the purchase as redundant and wasteful after evaluating whether they need a product and whether it is the right option.

Self-Distraction Strategies: Strategies that are expressed as focusing one's own mind on doing something to reduce stress.

Self-Isolation: Separation of uninfected individuals from infected individuals to avoid diseases.

Stimulus-Organism-Response (SOR) Model: A commonly used framework for understanding the causes behind individual's behavior, which includes "stimulus" representing the environmental elements, "organism" representing the internal structures and processes that occur between the stimulus and the response, and "response" representing the reactions of individuals. Thank you for your valuable support.

Chapter 8
Positive Psychology:
An Effective Strategy to Combat Stress

Divya Surendran Nair
https://orcid.org/0000-0003-2353-3451
MIT Art, Design, and Technology University, India

ABSTRACT

There are a variety of stress management techniques that are used to deal with the stressors of life, both short term as well as long term. In this chapter, a special focus will be given to the science of positive psychology for combating stress and related scenarios. The structure of this chapter will begin with the introduction of stress and its related problems from a psychology point of view. This will be followed with a detailed elaboration of some of the commonly used stress management techniques. After laying the initial foundation, the concept and elements of positive psychology will be detailed. The chapter will then put forth a comprehensive picture of the value in action (VIA) 24 character strengths. With relevant examples backed by recent research in positive psychology, effective strategies and techniques of dealing with stress by utilizing our inner potentials will be highlighted in this chapter.

INTRODUCTION

Defining Stress

Sita was an efficient and competent employee of her organization. She was associated with her organization for almost a decade and had proved her worth on many occasions. This year the company announced a double promotion with many benefits. Sita was sure she would be considered for this opportunity as she not only fulfilled but also excelled all the benchmarks on which the decision was to be made. However, when the formal announcement of the shortlisted employees was made, Sita was nowhere on the list. Shock would be an understatement for the emotions that Sita went through at that moment. She was extremely frustrated. A constant flow of questions kept on haunting her day and night. Her productivity reduced as she was less focused on her work. She started falling sick very often for no specifically known

DOI: 10.4018/978-1-6684-8565-1.ch008

reason. She started picking up fights and also became over-critical about her decisions. She didn't know what was the reason, but all she could claim was she was stressed!

Pihu was a brilliant student. It was time for the final examinations of her postgraduate course. She was well prepared for the first two papers and was relaxing in her house. A sudden message from her university professor popped up in the inbox of her mobile. This message was a reminder about the sequence of papers. The third paper was supposed to be the first paper tomorrow. This change was already mentioned in the hall tickets given to the students. Pihu panicked as she made the mistake of not going through the hall ticket before. Every student in the group assured the professor that they were aware of this change, and had prepared accordingly. Pihu started sweating and her hands were trembling at a rapid pace. She did not know how to handle this state of affairs. She picked up the notes of the third course as an attempt to face the situation. However, as soon as she glanced at the wall clock, everything seemed to go blank and she collapsed on the floor.

The type of stress that was detailed out by means of Sita and Pihu is quite relatable to most of us. Stress can arise due to any and every reason that can be thought about in this world. Be it a mindless activity, traumatic incident, differences with your boss, conflict with your partner, inability to complete an assignment, or the mere possibility of missing your local train. Stress can be experienced in different ways and the intensity of this experience also varies among individuals. The above mentioned hypothetical examples are a good elaboration of this. Stress can lead to a situation of panic or confusion in some. It can be indicative of a slight or major physical illness in a few individuals with no other specific diagnosis. In a similar way, the coping mechanisms of stress and related aspects are also different. Some might counter the stress in a positive way by empowering themselves, whereas, others might succumb to serious psychological issues. Thus, there is definitely a variety in the way an individual experiences and deals with stress. However, before dwelling into the strategies for dealing with stress, let's begin with the very basic process of understanding the concept of stress in detail.

The word stress originates from "strictus" and "stringere" (Jin, 2012). The meaning of these Latin words can be comprehended as a restricted or limited state that an individual goes through under moments of pressure and challenges (Jin, 2012). In 1950, Hans Selye defined stress as the "nonspecific response of the body to any demand" (Tan & Yip, 2018). Palmer in 1989 defined stress as, "The psychological, physiological and behavioral response by an individual when they perceive a lack of equilibrium between the demands placed upon them and their ability to meet those demands, which, over a period of time, leads to ill-health" (Stainsby & Gandhi, 2018). The world health organization considers stress as any change that leads to a physical, emotional or psychological strain (World Health Organization, 2021).

From all the above mentioned examples, a simplified version for explaining the concept of stress can be stated as follows. Stress is termed as a feeling experienced by an individual that gets triggered through external or internal challenges. These challenges or experiences are said to be stressors. These challenges activate a set of biological and psychological stress responses within the individual that can influence him in a positive or negative way depending on the source and intensity of the stress. One of the crucial elements of this definition is the presence of the word positive in it. This means that stress does not necessarily lead to a negative outcome. Let us understand this with yet another example.

Sameer and Jay are toppers in their college. In the final semester of their course they enroll in an elective subject that has a maximum failure rate. The professor keeps on lecturing the students about the difficulty level of this subject on a daily basis. The professor is sure that most of the students will fail this year in this course no matter what their past records say about their academic achievements. Every interaction of Sameer with this professor is a stressful experience for him. However, to prove the professor wrong, Sameer makes sure to study the subject in depth on a daily basis. He took extra efforts and met experts from the field to get a clarity of the concepts. On the other side, Jay kept on pondering over the professor's statement. Instead of doing something productive, he kept on wondering about the consequences of the predicted failure. When the results were declared, Sameer had topped the university with record marks in the said subject, whereas Jay had failed to clear the paper.

In the above mentioned example, Sameer and Jay went through the same situation. However, the way they dealt with the situation resulted in different outcomes for both of them. Sameer took the stress as a challenge for adding extra efforts to his examination preparation. In this case, the stress was beneficial for Sameer. This type of stress is called eustress. On the contrary, Jay pressurized himself with the burden of unwanted tension that led to a consequence of ultimate failure for him. Thus, stress had a negative impact on Jay. This type of stress is called distress.

STRESSORS

As discussed above, any event can be a potential stressor. However, in general, there are certain prevalences whose intensity is considered to be more stressful in most of the people as compared to others (Monroe & Slavich, 2016). The exposure period also decides the intensity of the stressor and the corresponding response to it. As an illustration, consider this, the stress you experience during your viva when you are unable to answer the questions of the external examiner will vanish the moment your turn is over. However, meeting with an accident that leaves you in a condition where you are not able to move in your entire life will give rise to a stress that is long lasting. Most of the stressors can usually be categorized in one of the following types.

Intense Agonizing Experiences

Here, the stress that a human goes through is extreme and in most of the cases unanticipated. The Russia Ukraine war is an example of such an experience. The trauma, violence, abuse, loss of life and material along with the fear of what will happen next will lead to critical consequences of this type of a stressor. Depression, anxiety and post traumatic disorders have been reported in the victims of this war (Chaaya et al., 2022). Similar experiences that can be categorized under this group can be death of a closed one, sexual abuse, near death experiences, natural calamities etc.

Uncontrollable Experiences

If the predictability of a possible stressful experience is not in our hands, then the impact of the stressor will be very intense and prolonged. For example, a recession in the market can lead to the termination of jobs on an immediate basis without any prior notice. A person who runs his entire family with the support of this job won't be able to handle this shock leading to serious stress-related consequences. However, if he was somewhere or the other able to predict that such a situation might arise in the future and had invested in some solutions that could help him in tackling this scenario, then the stressor won't be able to create an impact on him.

STRESS RESPONSES

The human body is an extremely sophisticated and capable machine. It reacts to a stressor by initiating a stress response. Let us explore a few of the prominent sets of responses initiated by our body when it is subjected to a stressful state.

The Fight or Flight Response

As the name suggests, during a stressful state your body will prepare you to either face the stressor or run away from the stressor in this type of a response. This concept was put forth by Walter B. Cannon (McCarty, 2016). Sympathetic nervous system is active in this type of response. Increased heart rate, blood pressure, respiration related activities are seen as a physiological response under this mechanism (Fight or Flight Response, 2022).

General Adaptation Syndrome

In 1978, Hans Selye put forth the concept of general adaptation syndrome (Selye, 1950). According to Selye, whenever an individual faces a stressful situation, a series of responses is initiated within his body that can be categorized into three phases. The first stage is referred to as the alarm phase. Here, the activation of the sympathetic nervous system takes place. In the resistance phase, the individual will use the fight or flight mechanism for handling the stressful situation. If the individual does not succeed in utilizing the fight or flight response, then the stage of exhaustion comes into picture where the physiological resources diminish (Selye, 1950). To understand this concept in a better way, let's take into consideration a hypothetical situation. Rachel was driving her car in the society premises. Accidently, she lost control of the car and dashed into the nearby vehicles. This led to severe damage to the vehicles that were hit by her car. She started sweating and she could sense her racing heartbeats (alarm stage). The owners of the damaged vehicles demanded money from Rachel that she agreed to pay. However, even after paying the money to the owners she was unable to concentrate on any other work (resistance). Many days have passed by, but Rachel does not feel the confidence to drive any vehicle again. She is experiencing difficulty in sleeping and is often depressed thinking about the past unfortunate incident (exhaustion).

DEALING WITH STRESS THROUGH POPULAR TECHNIQUES

The stressful experiences are not a comfortable zone for any individual to be in. Thus, a variety of strategies are employed for overcoming these stressors and their related experiences. Some of the popular techniques will be explained in the following section.

Biofeedback

This stress management strategy is regarded as one of the most prominent and sorted out techniques for dealing with stress. Since a lot of physiological reactions are involved in the body during a stressful experience, this technique focuses on training the individuals to recognize the onset of their stress and to control it over a period of time. Thus leading to a state of balance. This technique can help people to attain a state of self-awareness and gain mastery to control their physiological responses towards stress in a positive way (Yu et al., 2018). With the help of qualified experts and professional equipment, an array of physiological responses is measured including heart beats, pattern of breathing, activities of brain, muscles etc. (Liza, 2011). The measured aspects are presented in front of the person. This information helps him to understand how a change in his thought process and emotional states can lead to an array of reactions from his body. Training is provided to the person for responding to such changes, for controlling the physiological changes of his system as per his desires.

Relaxation Techniques

These constitute remedial and healing exercises modeled for reducing stress. A variety of strategies come under the umbrella of relaxation techniques. The main focus of most of these techniques is to bring about an overall relaxation of the body by channelizing the thought process in a focused way. One of the most popular relaxation techniques is box breathing (Norelli et al., 2022).

Box Breathing

It is a technique that focuses on controlled breathing activities consisting of four steps. Here, in a systematic way, the individual is asked to go through a series of breathing in, breathing out and holding the breath exercises.

Progressive Muscle Relaxation

Another popular relaxation technique for managing stress and its related consequence is progressive muscle relaxation. This technique is based on the principle that the sympathetic and parasympathetic nervous system cannot be active at the same junction of time. Hence, if there is a state of tension then relaxation cannot take place. Similarly, if there is relaxation then a state of tension won't exist. In the progressive muscle relaxation technique people are involved in a process of creating tension by muscle contraction. This is followed by a subsequent tension releasing activity that ultimately results in relaxation. This constant process repeated over a period of time acts as an immediate stress reliever (Toussaint et al., 2021).

Diaphragmatic Breathing

When an equilibrium is attained between the mind and body a state of relaxation is achieved. This state can be reached through the proper breathing mechanisms which involves the contraction of diaphragm (Consolo et al., 2008). This is one of the best known relaxation techniques for managing stress. Breathing exercises in combination with yoga also is an excellent way of reducing stress and its related consequences (Riley & Park, 2015).

Guided Imagery

In this technique, the power of visualization is used for providing relief from a stressful condition (Bigham et al., 2014). Here, disturbing thoughts and emotions are replaced with positive dimensions of thoughts (Nguyen & Brymer, 2018). As an attempt to create a calm environment, a guided process of instruction is executed for creating a real representation of mental imagery. Imagining oneself to be living in the relaxed environment created through this visualization technique makes this an effective stress reducing strategy.

Cognitive Behavioral Therapy [CBT]

If the source of a problem is known then there are high chances of finding an appropriate solution to it. This is the simple principle of cognitive behavioral therapy. In this strategy, an attempt is made for identifying the various experiences that give rise to a stress response within the participant (Santos-Ruiz et al., 2017). In general, the first step in cognitive behavioral therapy is to make the participant realize that the stress response is an outcome of their own cognitive process. This is followed by a stage of self-monitoring. Finally, the participant is encouraged to make certain modifications in his cognitive process i.e. the way he thinks and perceives the situation for avoiding stress. Let us understand this technique with the help of an example. Shiv has frequent episodes of depression. The therapist motivates Shiv to keep a track of the incidents after which he feels depressed. On analyzing the record diary maintained by Shiv, it was revealed that his office environment was one of the major factors for Shiv's condition. Shiv was never given an opportunity to prove himself and his abilities by his superiors. In the self monitoring phase, the therapist encouraged Shiv to list down the thoughts and emotions he felt whenever his seniors acted unfair to him. Shiv responded by a set of responses like low morale, feeling disgusted, worthless, good for nothing etc. In the last step of this therapy, over a period of time Shiv realized that he can definitely do something to change this stressful situation. He stopped overthinking and was no longer critical about his capabilities. He ignored the demotivating acts of the seniors and started looking out for a new job. Thus, through cognitive behavioral therapy Shiv was successful in managing his stress.

Mindfulness Based Stress Reduction

It is an intervention technique that is carried out in a homogenous or a heterogeneous group over a structured period of few weeks (Grossman et al., 2004). Mindfulness is marked by a gradual and sustained awareness of different activities going on within an individual. This means the individual knows what his current series of thoughts, experiences, feelings etc. are, but is not being critical about the same. In other words, he is paying attention and is highly aware about the meaning of the various sensations he is going through, but is not evaluating or overthinking about it. This technique has been found to be one of the most effective ones for dealing with the different stressors of life (Grossman et al., 2004). In this section, an attempt was made to describe a few of the popular stress management techniques. Now, the focus will shift to the field of positive psychology, which is a promising branch of psychology for dealing with stress.

AN INTRODUCTION TO POSITIVE PSYCHOLOGY

Contemporary psychology is preoccupied with the negative side of life, and interprets the functioning of the person only in terms of a disease model, ignoring almost completely the positive side of life. The widespread wave of depression, negativity and lowered self-esteem among people not only increases the layering of stress and other mental health issues but might also open the doors to serious social, emotional and economic problems. The disease model tries to treat psychological conditions and mental disorders by focusing on the symptoms and diagnosis. Pathology is at the core of the disease model perspective. Here, everything is viewed from the deficit point of view (Terjesen et al., 2004). However, there are various incidents in the history of mankind that show how people overcome life's challenges to emerge victorious. Thus, everything cannot be visualized or perceived from the lens of repairing a defect. Rather, it is equally important to focus on the traits and characteristics that make life better. For instance, trying to treat depression is crucial but getting to know the sources of our inner happiness is also equally important. This perspective is taken into consideration by the domain of positive psychology.

Positive psychology is an applied branch of psychology that focuses on identifying and understanding human strengths and virtues for making life more productive and progressive. It is a scientific approach to study human thoughts, feelings, and behavior, with a focus on strengths instead of weaknesses, building the good in life instead of repairing the bad, and taking the lives of average people up to "great" instead of focusing solely on moving those who are struggling up to "normal" (Peterson, 2008). Most of the times when people are confronted in a situation wherein they have to speak about their strengths and weaknesses, it is easy for most of the lot to focus on their shortcomings rather than their prowess. Positive psychology believes that when an individual is aware about their own strengths it not only enhances a wave of positive emotions among them but also helps in raising their confidence up to the next level. Positive psychology thus aims to initiate a change to cause a re-orientation and turning away from being exclusively busy with repairing the worst things in life, towards developing the best qualities in life. As a science it is based on three pillars. The first is a positive life experience for individuals i.e., exploiting positive emotions. The second pillar is a person's positive physical properties i.e., exploiting positive personality traits, mainly virtues and strengths, but also aptitudes. The third pillar is a positive society i.e., exploiting positive social institutions, those such as democracy, a strong family, and education which promotes positive development (Pluskota, 2014). Positive emotions, wellbeing, strengths, and contentment are some of the major components of this unique branch of psychology.

STRENGTHS - A MAJOR PILLAR OF POSITIVE PSYCHOLOGY

Research is considered a scientific and systematic study. This study is based on facts and validated evidence. This means that every claim needs proof to get acceptance. If this isn't the case, then there are high chances that the said idea will be subjected to heavy criticism. Positive psychology has been criticized on a number of elements. One being, the process of measuring happiness, strengths, contentment, etc. Many researchers also believe these concepts are more suitable in philosophy as compared to psychology (Lazarus, 2003). Martin Seligman, the father of positive psychology however, had a different ideology. He did an extensive study with Christopher Peterson and listed out the famous and well known Values in Action [VIA] classification of strengths and virtues.

So, what exactly do we mean by strengths? Is it a synonym for our talents, or maybe aptitude? Many individuals believe that strength is indeed another word for talent. However, according to experts in positive psychology, these are two different concepts. Let us understand this with a simple example. Rishab is a great dancer. His moves and grace can give a tough competition to professional experts. However, he did not pursue this ability further, nor did he bring this in front of the world through any medium. Dancing in this hypothetical example is what can be referred to as talent. Talents are qualities which are present within us, but they might go unnoticed and unutilized if not channelized properly. However, this isn't the case with strengths. In our day-to-day activities, we use our strengths consciously or subconsciously in a direct or indirect way to handle different situations. For instance, if honesty is Rishab's strength, then no matter what situation, he will always speak the truth. Thus, strengths usually do not fade away as its presence will be marked for sure through the varied experiences that an individual counters. Let us now try and understand the meaning of character strengths and virtues from the positive psychology perspective.

Defining Character Strengths and Virtues

With the help of enormous research-based surveys, Peterson and Seligman identified six elements that were crucial for the development of a good character. These six elements were given the name of virtues. The psychological basis that defines these virtues is referred to as character strengths by these experts. In total, twenty-four character strengths were put forth. Each of these strengths is part of some or the other six virtues. Several inclusion criteria were taken into account before considering a trait as a character strength. Let us now explore some of the main inclusion criteria.

Firstly, strength must be exhibited in a range of dimensions of a person's behavior, and it should be measurable. Secondly, strength should be able to give a sensation of fulfillment of a good life to the individual as well as others. Another inclusion criteria states that every strength should be high on moral values, even if there isn't any obvious benefit attached to it. The next important factor points out strengths to be motivators to others, especially when someone showcases their strengths in person. This means that, whenever a strength is exhibited the onlookers will be intrinsically encouraged to explore their own strengths. Another important criterion for inclusion describes the unidimensional trait of strengths. Here, it is emphasized that strengths do not deteriorate due to the presence of other strengths (Csikszentmihalyi & Csikszentmihalyi, 2006). There are some more inclusion criteria but only some of the prominent ones are mentioned here.

The Six Virtues and Twenty-Four Character Strengths

Wisdom, courage, humanity, justice, temperance and transcendence constitute the six virtues of the value in action (VIA) classification (Niemiec, 2013). The complete list of virtues and their associated character strengths is listed in Table 1. Wisdom virtue deals with cognitive or knowledge prowess. In this virtue, a total of six strengths are included namely, creativity, curiosity, judgment, love of learning, and perspective (Niemiec, 2013). Originality and novelty are the key features of the strength of creativity. Examining and exploring things is a key dimension of curiosity. Making fair decisions, finding evidence, and thinking from a logical point of view are defining features of the strength called judgment. Having a keen thirst for constant improvement by mastering new skills and knowledge gives rise to the strength of love of learning. Understanding the various experiences from a variety of dimensions and points of view is indicative of the perspective strength.

The next virtue is courage. This virtue depicts the determination of achieving the objectives and goals set by the individual by overcoming the obstacles as well as the internal and external conflicts. In all, four strengths are included in this virtue (Niemiec, 2013). The first strength is bravery. Standing fearlessly for the righteous and not backing away from any threat irrespective of its nature is a crucial element of this strength. Perseverance, as the next strength highlights the elements of dedication and

Table 1. List of virtues and character strengths

Virtues	Character Strengths
Wisdom	Creativity Curiosity Judgment Love of learning Perspective
Courage	Bravery Perseverance Honesty Zest
Humanity	Love Kindness Social Intelligence
Justice	Teamwork Fairness Leadership
Temperance	Forgiveness Humility Prudence Self-regulation
Transcendence	Appreciation of beauty and excellence Gratitude Hope Humor Spirituality

sustainment of completing the tasks that were initiated by the individual. Honesty as the next strength under this virtue, is based on the pillars of truth, genuineness and responsible dealings. In other words, the individual possessing this strength will speak the truth and will present himself without any pretense. Apart from this, he will also take ownership of all his activities. The last strength in this virtue is zest. Individuals with this strength are highly active and energetic in all the tasks that they are involved in. They give their best in all the activities as their approach is not halfhearted.

The third virtue is humanity. Love, kindness and social intelligence are the strengths that come under this virtue (Niemiec, 2013). Love as a strength focuses more closely on the intimate relationships that an individual is involved in. Affection, fondness and genuine sentiments are the main pillars of this strength. Kindness as a strength deals with the element of caring for others, being considerate, trying to help the person in need, etc. The last strength in this category of virtue is social intelligence. Being aware of the needs, sentiments and the intentions of oneself as well as others is at the core of this strength.

Justice is the next virtue and it consists of three different strengths (Niemiec, 2013). Teamwork is the first strength. This strength revolves around the facets of accountability, respecting the viewpoints of the team mates, getting along well in a group and being loyal to your team as well as their members. Fairness speaks of being objective in all dealings. In other words, personal bias won't find a place while making a decision if this is an individual's strength. Similarly, this strength also takes into consideration the traits of equality, respecting others and providing a fair opportunity to everyone. Leadership as a strength focuses on motivating and taking each and every individual along with you in accomplishing a task. Goal orientation, planning an array of activities and leading from the front is another important aspect of this strength.

The next virtue is temperance which includes the strengths of forgiveness, humility, prudence and self-regulation in it (Niemiec, 2013). Forgiveness as a strength allows the individual to let go of things without having a slight thought of revenge or vengeance. It allows the individual to forgive others and give them another chance to rectify their mistakes. The strength of humility allows the individual to stay grounded. In other words, the individual's work will speak for himself. He will not boost his success and will be extremely modest in his approach. The next strength is prudence. This strength allows the person to be thoughtful of the choices that he makes. This means that undue risk taking behavior will be avoided. Moreover, every step will be taken in a cautious manner so that later on the chances of regretting the decision will be less. Self-regulation as a strength depicts the strong command and control that the individual holds on his or her sentiments, thought process and overall conduct. Awareness about the strengths and weaknesses, having a disciplined approach towards tasks and decisions is another characteristic feature of this strength.

The sixth virtue is transcendence. This virtue is directed towards the larger meaning of life. It consists of five strengths. They are appreciation of beauty and excellence, gratitude, hope, humor and spirituality (Niemiec, 2013). The first strength under this category is appreciation of beauty and excellence. This is based on the notion of having a keen eye for locating and admiring brilliance in any form. Gratitude deals with having an attitude of being thankful for every small and big experience that the individual comes across. Hope is the next strength. Staying affirmative and optimistic about the present and future is the basis of this strength. Humor deals with the spirit of joy and spreading smiles. Being hilarious, laughing and making others laugh is also one of the features of this strength. Spirituality is the last strength here. These individuals seek a deeper meaning in each of their experiences. They also believe in the presence of an ultimate power that gives them a purpose to shape their lives in a more meaningful way.

The benefits of a character strengths approach are indicated in several researches. By being aware of our strengths and by utilizing it subsequently, improvement in cases of depression has been reported. Similarly, research also indicates that strength based interventions have the potential to enhance the self-efficacy and self-esteem of individuals, including patients with several chronic illnesses (Yan et al., 2020). Strength based interventions have a preventive role against many mental disorders and related challenges (Madden et al., 2020). Satisfaction with life and overall wellness is also enhanced by incorporating a strength based process (Proctor et al., 2011). This approach is equally influential in boosting confidence and optimism among individuals. Strength based interventions are an effective strategy for stress reduction (Drvaric et al., 2015). Family induced stress and related factors like anxiety and depression can also be tackled effectively by this approach (Pollock et al., 2015). Strength based interventions have also proved beneficial in tackling higher level, unpredictable, and sustained stress in environments such as military camps (Boermans et al., 2012). Several studies have also shown that this type of an intervention is effective in dealing with stress across a range of age groups and occupations like children, parents (Waters, 2015), caregivers, counselors (Myers, 2003), individuals with developmental disorders (Steiner & Gengoux, 2018) and across an array of population in emergency situations like a pandemic (Rashid & McGrath, 2020). In the next section, we will explore some simple ways through which strength-based interventions can be utilized for preventing stress and related factors.

DEALING WITH STRESS WITH STRENGTH BASED APPROACHES

If an individual wants to utilize the strength based approach of positive psychology for preventing and reducing stress related problems, then the first important step he should take is to identify his signature strengths. The Value in Action (VIA) survey of 24 character strengths is available freely on the official website. It also gives a detailed report explaining the meaning of the results after the survey is undertaken.

The next important step is to initiate the process of developing the less prominent strengths that the individual possesses. One of the reasons for a potential stressor may be associated with a less developed character strength. For example, whenever an important project is declared by your boss, he does not include you in it. This leads to frustration and acts as a stressor. However, one of the reasons for not including you in the project could also be your less developed strength of teamwork. If you start working on enhancing this lesser developed strength of yours then there are high chances of you being a part of a group project in the future. Thus, the stressor will automatically be eliminated due to your own character strength.

Another helpful strategy can be the utilization of your strengths for responding to a stressor. In simple words, every individual has all the twenty four character strengths but on a different level. Few are dominant, whereas others are less prominent. This means every strength might be utilized smartly to prevent a stressor and its related consequences. In short, we can control our responses to a situation by using our strengths to focus on happiness rather than a stressful state. For example, you are highly disciplined and like to be punctual in your dealings. However, even after leaving the house early for an important meeting, you face heavy traffic on the road. If you start cursing the traffic and lose your temper, then your response is the source of this stressor. Instead, if you deal with this situation by utilizing your signature strengths, then there are high chances that stress will never come into the picture. Say for instance, if justice is your strength, then by utilizing it, you can come to a rational conclusion that this traffic was not in your control. You can ask someone else from your team to attend the meeting on your behalf or maybe use an online meeting tool to mark your virtual presence during the discussion. In this solution, along with justice, the strengths of teamwork and social intelligence have also pitched in to avoid a stressful scenario.

A common source of stress is rigidity or the lack of a tendency to accept criticism. In most cases, people will indulge in the process of overthinking. This will ultimately trigger a stressor that will enforce a series of thought processes and sentiments that are negative in nature. Perceiving an experience from a balanced viewpoint can be another important strategy of a strength based positive psychology approach. This means, utilization of our character strengths can lead us to see good in every situation that we experience. Thus, ultimately preventing the arousal of a stressor to occur. Let's understand this with an example. Pakhi is a renowned speaker. She delivers lectures in big forums and her presentations are always appreciated. During one event, however, a participant criticized her presentation on the basis of the examples given during the presentation. According to the participant, the examples were not relevant to the present era. If Pakhi starts overthinking and feels insulted due to the honest feedback of the participant, she will enter the zone of circumstantial stress. However, if Pakhi looks at this feedback from a balanced point of view, she will avoid stress and will happily take steps to improve her next presentation. The participant did not criticize Pakhi for her overall presentation. This means he appreciates Pakhi for her presentation skills. However, he also wants her to use more relevant examples. This is constructive feedback and is positive. Here, in order to prevent stress, Pakhi is utilizing the character strengths of honesty, self-regulation, judgment, and love of learning.

Acknowledging the behaviors that initiate a wave of positive thoughts and emotions within an individual is also an important strategy of the strength-based approach. For example, if creativity is an individual's strength and he is aware that any creative activity brings joy and happiness to him, then he can utilize this awareness and strength to prevent or reduce stress. Say, for instance, the individual while working on a project, can take a small break and pen a poem or sketch a picture. This joyful activity, which is based on his strength, will allow happiness to freshen up his mind, thus avoiding the outburst of stress.

CONCLUSION

Whether we like it or not, stress has indeed become an inseparable part of every individual's life. The intensity of this stress can vary from a simple headache to a more serious psychological problem. It is thus crucial to use strategies that have the potential of preventing as well as managing stress post its occurrence. Positive psychology and its related approaches is definitely a promising answer to this challenge. It is now time that we start taking the benefits of the science of positive psychology and our character strengths for overcoming stress and other psychological problems.

REFERENCES

Bigham, E., McDannel, L., Luciano, I., & Salgado-Lopez, G. (2014). Effect of a Brief Guided Imagery on Stress. *Biofeedback*, *42*(1), 28–35. doi:10.5298/1081-5937-42.1.07

Boermans, S., Delahaij, R., Korteling, H., & Euwema, M. (2012). Training Resilience for High-risk Environments: Towards a Strength-based Approach within the Military. In International Handbook of Workplace Trauma Support (pp. 313–330). John Wiley & Sons, Ltd. doi:10.1002/9781119943242.ch20

Chaaya, C., Devi Thambi, V., Sabuncu, Ö., Abedi, R., Osman Ahmed Osman, A., Uwishema, O., & Onyeaka, H. (2022). Ukraine – Russia crisis and its impacts on the mental health of Ukrainian young people during the COVID-19 pandemic. *Annals of Medicine and Surgery (London)*, *79*, 104033. doi:10.1016/j.amsu.2022.104033 PMID:35765517

Consolo, K., Fusner, S., & Staib, S. (2008). Effects of diaphragmatic breathing on stress levels of nursing students. *Teaching and Learning in Nursing*, *3*(2), 67–71. doi:10.1016/j.teln.2007.10.003

Csikszentmihalyi, M., & Csikszentmihalyi, I. S. (2006). *A Life Worth Living: Contributions to Positive Psychology*. Oxford University Press.

Drvaric, L., Gerritsen, C., Rashid, T., Bagby, R. M., & Mizrahi, R. (2015). High stress, low resilience in people at clinical high risk for psychosis: Should we consider a strengths-based approach? *Canadian Psychology*, *56*(3), 332–347. doi:10.1037/cap0000035

Fight or Flight Response. (2022). *Psychology Tools*. Retrieved December 16, 2022, from https://www.psychologytools.com/resource/fight-or-flight-response/

Goldstein, D. S., & Kopin, I. J. (2007). Evolution of concepts of stress. *Stress (Amsterdam, Netherlands), 10*(2), 109–120. doi:10.1080/10253890701288935 PMID:17514579

Grossman, P., Niemann, L., Schmidt, S., & Walach, H. (2004). Mindfulness-based stress reduction and health benefits: A meta-analysis. *Journal of Psychosomatic Research, 57*(1), 35–43. doi:10.1016/S0022-3999(03)00573-7 PMID:15256293

Jin, P. (2012). Stress and Learning. In N. M. Seel (Ed.), *Encyclopedia of the Sciences of Learning* (pp. 3202–3205). Springer US. doi:10.1007/978-1-4419-1428-6_203

Lazarus, R. S. (2003). Does the Positive Psychology Movement Have Legs? *Psychological Inquiry, 14*(2), 93–109. doi:10.1207/S15327965PLI1402_02

Liza, V. (2011). Stress management techniques: Evidence-based procedures that reduce stress and promote health. *Health Science Journal, 5*(2), 74–89. https://www.itmedicalteam.pl/

Madden, W., Green, S., & Grant, A. M. (2020). A Pilot Study Evaluating Strengths-Based Coaching for Primary School Students. In *Coaching Researched* (pp. 297–312). John Wiley & Sons, Ltd. doi:10.1002/9781119656913.ch16

McCarty, R. (2016). The Fight-or-Flight Response: A Cornerstone of Stress Research. In G. Fink (Ed.), *Stress: Concepts, Cognition, Emotion, and Behavior* (pp. 33–37). Academic Press. doi:10.1016/B978-0-12-800951-2.00004-2

Monroe, S. M., & Slavich, G. M. (2016). Psychological Stressors: Overview. In G. Fink (Ed.), *Stress: Concepts, Cognition, Emotion, and Behavior* (pp. 109–115). Academic Press. doi:10.1016/B978-0-12-800951-2.00013-3

Myers, J. E. (2003). Coping With Caregiving Stress: A Wellness-Oriented, Strengths-Based Approach for Family Counselors. *The Family Journal (Alexandria, Va.), 11*(2), 153–161. doi:10.1177/1066480702250162

Nguyen, J., & Brymer, E. (2018). Nature-Based Guided Imagery as an Intervention for State Anxiety. *Frontiers in Psychology, 9*, 1–10. doi:10.3389/fpsyg.2018.01858 PMID:30333777

Niemiec, R. M. (2013). VIA Character Strengths: Research and Practice (The First 10 Years). In H. H. Knoop & A. Delle Fave (Eds.), *Well-Being and Cultures: Perspectives from Positive Psychology* (pp. 11–29). Springer Netherlands. doi:10.1007/978-94-007-4611-4_2

Norelli, S. K., Long, A., & Krepps, J. M. (2022). Relaxation Techniques. In *StatPearls*. StatPearls Publishing. https://www.ncbi.nlm.nih.gov/books/NBK513238/

Peterson, C., Park, N., & Sweeney, P. J. (2008). Group Well-Being: Morale from a Positive Psychology Perspective. *Applied Psychology, 57*(s1), 19–36. doi:10.1111/j.1464-0597.2008.00352.x

Pluskota, A. (2014). The application of positive psychology in the practice of education. *SpringerPlus, 3*(1), 147. doi:10.1186/2193-1801-3-147 PMID:24790805

Pollock, E. D., Kazman, J. B., & Deuster, P. (2015). Family Functioning and Stress in African American Families: A Strength-Based Approach. *The Journal of Black Psychology, 41*(2), 144–169. doi:10.1177/0095798413520451

Proctor, C., Tsukayama, E., Wood, A. M., Maltby, J., Eades, J. F., & Linley, P. A. (2011). Strengths Gym: The impact of a character strengths-based intervention on the life satisfaction and well-being of adolescents. *The Journal of Positive Psychology*, *6*(5), 377–388. doi:10.1080/17439760.2011.594079

Rashid, T., & McGrath, R. (2020). Strengths-based actions to enhance wellbeing in the time of COVID-19. *International Journal of Wellbeing*, *10*(4), 4. doi:10.5502/ijw.v10i4.1441

Riley, K. E., & Park, C. L. (2015). How does yoga reduce stress? A systematic review of mechanisms of change and guide to future inquiry. *Health Psychology Review*, *9*(3), 379–396. doi:10.1080/17437199.2014.981778 PMID:25559560

Santos-Ruiz, A., Robles-Ortega, H., Pérez-García, M., & Peralta-Ramírez, M. I. (2017). Effects of the Cognitive-Behavioral Therapy for Stress Management on Executive Function Components. *The Spanish Journal of Psychology*, *20*, 1–30. doi:10.1017jp.2017.10 PMID:28190412

Selye, H. (1950). Stress and the General Adaptation Syndrome. *British Medical Journal*, *1*(4667), 1383–1392. doi:10.1136/bmj.1.4667.1383 PMID:15426759

Steiner, A. M., & Gengoux, G. W. (2018). Strength-Based Approaches to Working with Families of Children with ASD. In M. Siller & L. Morgan (Eds.), *Handbook of Parent-Implemented Interventions for Very Young Children with Autism* (pp. 155–168). Springer International Publishing. doi:10.1007/978-3-319-90994-3_10

Tan, S. Y., & Yip, A. (2018). Hans Selye (1907–1982): Founder of the stress theory. *Singapore Medical Journal*, *59*(4), 170–171. doi:10.11622mcdj.2018043 PMID:29748693

Terjesen, M., Jacofsky, M., Froh, J., & Digiuseppe, R. (2004). Integrating positive psychology into schools: Implications for practice. *Psychology in the Schools*, *41*(1), 163–172. doi:10.1002/pits.10148

Toussaint, L., Nguyen, Q. A., Roettger, C., Dixon, K., Offenbächer, M., Kohls, N., Hirsch, J., & Sirois, F. (2021). Effectiveness of Progressive Muscle Relaxation, Deep Breathing, and Guided Imagery in Promoting Psychological and Physiological States of Relaxation. *Evidence-Based Complementary and Alternative Medicine*, *2021*, e5924040. doi:10.1155/2021/5924040 PMID:34306146

Van der Zwan, J. E., De Vente, W., Huizink, A. C., Bögels, S. M., & de Bruin, E. I. (2015). Physical Activity, Mindfulness Meditation, or Heart Rate Variability Biofeedback for Stress Reduction: A Randomized Controlled Trial. *Applied Psychophysiology and Biofeedback*, *40*(4), 257–268. doi:10.100710484-015-9293-x PMID:26111942

VIA Character Strengths Survey & Character Reports. (n.d.). Retrieved December 21, 2022, from https://www.viacharacter.org/

Waters, L. (2015). The Relationship between Strength-Based Parenting with Children's Stress Levels and Strength-Based Coping Approaches. *Psychology, 6*(6), 6. doi:10.4236/psych.2015.66067

World Health Organization. (2021). *Stress*. Retrieved December 15, 2022, from https://www.who.int/news-room/questions-and-answers/item/stress

Yan, T., Chan, C. W. H., Chow, K. M., Zheng, W., & Sun, M. (2020). A systematic review of the effects of character strengths-based intervention on the psychological well-being of patients suffering from chronic illnesses. *Journal of Advanced Nursing*, *76*(7), 1567–1580. doi:10.1111/jan.14356 PMID:32187708

Yu, B., Funk, M., Hu, J., Wang, Q., & Feijs, L. (2018). Biofeedback for Everyday Stress Management: A Systematic Review. *Frontiers in ICT (Lausanne, Switzerland)*, *5*, 1–22. doi:10.3389/fict.2018.00023

ADDITIONAL READING

Bolier, L., Haverman, M., Westerhof, G. J., Riper, H., Smit, F., & Bohlmeijer, E. (2013). Positive psychology interventions: A meta-analysis of randomized controlled studies. *BMC Public Health*, *13*(1), 119. doi:10.1186/1471-2458-13-119 PMID:23390882

Mongrain, M., & Anselmo-Matthews, T. (2012). Do Positive Psychology Exercises Work? A Replication of Seligman et al. *Journal of Clinical Psychology*, *68*(4), n/a. Advance online publication. doi:10.1002/jclp.21839 PMID:24469930

Oades, L. G., Steger, M. F., Fave, A. D., & Passmore, J. (2016). The Psychology of Positivity and Strengths-Based Approaches at Work. In *The Wiley Blackwell Handbook of the Psychology of Positivity and Strengths-Based Approaches at Work* (pp. 1–8). John Wiley & Sons, Ltd. doi:10.1002/9781118977620.ch1

Ong, L., Linden, W., & Young, S. (2004). Stress management—What is it? *Journal of Psychosomatic Research*, *56*(1), 133–137. doi:10.1016/S0022-3999(03)00128-4 PMID:14987975

Seligman, M. E. P., & Csikszentmihalyi, M. (2000). Positive psychology: An introduction. *The American Psychologist*, *55*(1), 5–14. doi:10.1037/0003-066X.55.1.5 PMID:11392865

Sheldon, K. M., & King, L. (2001). Why positive psychology is necessary. *The American Psychologist*, *56*(3), 216–217. doi:10.1037/0003-066X.56.3.216 PMID:11315247

Vaillant, G. E. (2000). Adaptive mental mechanisms: Their role in a positive psychology. *The American Psychologist*, *55*(1), 89–98. doi:10.1037/0003-066X.55.1.89 PMID:11392869

KEY TERMS AND DEFINITIONS

Character Strengths: The psychological basis that define and give meaning to every virtue is called the character strength.

Positive Psychology: It is an applied branch of psychology that focuses on identifying and understanding human strengths and virtues for making life more productive and progressive.

Strength-Based Interventions: The strategies planned by taking into consideration an individual's character strengths to achieve an objective is referred to as a strength-based intervention.

Stress: It is termed as a feeling experienced by an individual that gets triggered through external or internal challenges.

Stress Responses: These stressors activate a set of biological and psychological responses within the individual that can influence him in a positive or negative way depending on the source and intensity of the stress. These are called stress responses.

Stressors: The challenges or experiences that act as sources of stress are called stressors.

Virtues: The broad pillars which play an important role in the development of a good character are referred to as virtues in positive psychology.

Chapter 9
Read Stress Away:
The Bibliotherapy Way

Aditi Singh Sharma
https://orcid.org/0000-0003-0705-8208
Amity University, Ranchi, India

ABSTRACT

The chapter explores bibliotherapy and its historical background and application as a self-help method to address psychological distress. The author begins by making an evaluative study of how emotions like fear and anxiety lead to stress and the long-term impact of stress mutating into psychological and physiological diseases. The chapter proposes to reposition bibliotherapy as a means of treating distress, boredom, and isolation. The author studies the evolution and development of bibliotherapy. Several studies have been explored to enumerate how bibliotherapy can help individuals overcome distress. The author enumerates the benefits, analysis, and findings of bibliotherapy. The author enumerates how pandemics in the modern digital era are a stimulus that engenders anxiety, depression, and insomnia affecting the global population. The psychological impact can be reduced through bibliotherapy.

INTRODUCTION

The term Bibliotherapy generally refers to the concept of using books or stories as a form of therapy for individuals diagnosed with mental illness, emotional stress or addiction. Bibliotherapy can be applied to all age groups. It can be used in conjunction with other therapy types, such as cognitive behavioral therapy. It can be utilized for the treatment in both individualized and group therapy settings. Bibliotherapy is a systematic intervention that can help people to cope with stress and personal problems through the use of carefully selected reading materials. It is a form of clinical or self-developing therapy, often used in connection to psychotherapy; that includes reading as a part of treatment.

Therapeutic reading can act as a source of appeasement for mental health disorders – anxiety disorders, mood disorders, depressive episodes, phobias, sleep disorders. It can also assist in strengthening psychological health and well-being. It is intended to help bring about personal change through reading. It is often used as a supplementary form of treatment in various psychotherapy approaches and could

DOI: 10.4018/978-1-6684-8565-1.ch009

involve everything from reading in private to discussions in groups. It's natural to feel overwhelmed, alone, or lost when one is going through a big change in life or are experiencing mental health challenges.

One of the ways in which the mind acquires information is the visual form. Reading is one way to transmit information to the brain. The quality and quantity of reading can determine the state of the human mind and how it responds to fear and anxiety and the resultant stress caused. The duration between the emergence of stress and its mutation into full fledged psychological and physiological disorders is critical. In this phase people can be assisted to cope with stress and personal problems through interventions that are not based on medications. Literature - both fiction and nonfiction - might help to develop a higher level of awareness and understanding of motivations and behaviour.

Interventions to decrease stress and enhance resiliency and mindfulness are more likely to be widely implemented. Stress is a ubiquitous problem that is associated with many acute and chronic medical conditions such as cardiac arrhythmia, cardiovascular disease, impaired immune function, and peptic ulcer disease. In moderation, stress is healthily tolerated; excessive stress, however, is associated with poor medical outcomes, unhealthy coping mechanisms and symptoms of anxiety and depression. Stressors are difficult to remove. However, one can enhance one's ability to handle stress, an attribute often called resiliency.

"A word after a word after a word is power," the Margaret Atwood's phrase; aptly connotes the power of how words play a significant role. Many therapists believe in this power so strongly that they use books to aid in patient improvement. The practice called Bibliotherapy is based on the idea that stories can heal, showing how "a word after a word" is truly powerful. It could help learn the "why" behind what one is experiencing through science-based reading. At the same time, it can act a guide with exercises and coping recommendations on hand for easy reference. Through fiction, one could view the scenario through the eyes of a character. In many cases, one might reach an emotional release through that fictional journey before one reaches it in personally. This emotional experience in fiction is what Aristotle referred to as "catharsis" during his own observations on the impact of stories on human emotions.

The power of words on emotions can be immense. Reading the right words can bring tears, laughter, and anger. It can stimulate a drive for self-change. Words can educate and provide insight. At times, words can be a valuable source of comfort. For people navigating through mental well-being challenges, the power of words could be used as a form of treatment called bibliotherapy. Storytelling, creative writing, and reading have long been recognized for their therapeutic potential. The use of literature as a healing method dates to ancient Greece, when Grecian libraries were seen as sacred places with curative powers. In the early nineteenth century, physicians like Benjamin Rush and Minson Galt II began to use bibliotherapy as an intervention technique in rehabilitation and the treatment of mental health issues. During World Wars I and II, bibliotherapy was used to help returning soldiers deal with both physical and emotional concerns.

The therapeutic benefits of reading were first identified by the ancient Romans and Greeks can be found in theories by well-known scholars and thinkers throughout history. In "Poetics", the Greek philosopher Aristotle presented the concept of using literature and drama for healing and purification (catharsis) of negative emotions. The philosopher Friedrich Nietzsche and the neurologist Sigmund Freud referred to Aristotle's idea of catharsis when describing how literature can have a therapeutic effect on negative emotions.

The practice of hospitals maintaining libraries and library services for long-term patients has continued throughout the years and into modern day. It was an established practice that a number of ancient hospitals-maintained libraries for both staff and patients. It was religious texts that came to be the most used literature for early bibliotherapy up until the 19th century. The first known organized form of bibliotherapy in clinical settings can be dated back to thirteenth century Egypt where the hospital staff and the religious leaders at the Al Mansour Hospital in Cairo read the Quran to their parents in addition to medical treatment.

Similar connections between literature and therapy can also be found in the architecture of some of the earliest known libraries. The inscription "The House of Healing for the Soul" was written over the entrance to Ramses II library in Thebes, Egypt around 300 BC. The inscription "apothecary of the soul" can be seen in the medieval library of the Abby of St. Gall in Switzerland. Similarly, Galen of Pergamon kept his personal library at Sanctuary Ascelpion, an ancient Roman therapeutic spa (Lutz, Cora E, 1978).

Inspired by Freud's work, fairytales, symbols and myths became a central theme within the Jungian psychoanalytic context in the mid and late twentieth century. Key publications such as Karl Gustav Jung's, "Man and Symbols", Marie Louis von Franz's, "Interpretation of Fairy Tales", are a few examples of how fairytales and myths can be used for self-development.

Psychologists today theorize that bibliotherapy succeeds because stories offer patients an effective means to process through identification, catharsis, and insight. By following this process, the patient and therapist can interpret the book against the patient's situation, empathize with the fictional character, and productively face mental illness, emotional distress, and addiction.

The transition from stress to severe psychological problems induced by the onset of stress is a gradual process. It is said that the biggest future pandemic the world will soon be dealing with has to do with issues pertaining to mental health. Loneliness has been identified as the predominant cause of several physical and emotional illnesses. The process has been hastened by the COVID-19 pandemic which forced people worldwide into isolation. Although, paradoxically everyone is connected via the powers of the digital world; people seem to be increasingly getting stresses out leading to stress and panic attacks. The one intervention that could slow down or arrest this process at the individual and family level could be the act of getting involved with reading for engagement and self-evolution. For those who are fighting to hang in, it's time to reboot the emotional priorities before it's too late.

BIBLIOTHERAPY

The definition of bibliotherapy has changed throughout history. The word comes for the ancient Greek for book (βιβλίον) and healing (θεραπεία). The practice of prescribing books as a tool for healing has been around since the Middle Ages. Bibliotherapy stems from library science and management. In fact, the oldest known library motto, ψυχῆς ἰατρείον (which translates to "house of healing for the soul") mirrors the basic tenets of bibliotherapy.

Bibliotherapy generally refers to the use of literature to help people cope with emotional problems, mental illness, or changes in their lives (Pardeck, 1994), or to produce effective change and promote personality growth and development (Lenkowsky, 1987; Adderholdt-Elliott & Eller, 1989). By providing literature relevant to their personal situations and developmental needs at appropriate times (Hebert & Kent, 2000), bibliotherapy practitioners attempt to help people of all ages to understand themselves and to cope with problems such as separation and divorce, child abuse, foster care, and adoption.

Freud began utilizing literature in his psychoanalysis practice in the late 19th century. During World War I, the Library War Service helped develop the science of bibliotherapy as they distributed books to patients in military hospitals. The idea of "reading therapy" grew in popularity and, by the 1920's, the

United States began hosting training programs for bibliotherapy at universities. As the concept made its way into academia, the term started popping up in medical journals. Freud, Benjamin Rush, and Minson Galt played a significant role in recognizing bibliotherapy as an intervention technique.

The term 'bibliotherapy" was first coined by Samuel McChord Crothers in the 20th century and it slowly entered the medical lexicon. In a 1916 article published in *The Atlantic Monthly*, Samuel Carothers defined bibliotherapy as the process of using books to teach those receiving medical care about their conditions, In 1941, Dorland's Illustrated Medical Dictionary recognized bibliotherapy as an official mental health treatment. It officially recognized this modality as a form of mental health treatment. Librarians began compiling lists of written material that helped individuals modify their thoughts, feelings, or behaviors for therapeutic purposes. Counselors worked in conjunction with librarians to "prescribe" selected literature for clients experiencing problems.

In the 1950's, Caroline Shrodes published her book – The Conscious Reader. The book explores the impact characters in fiction novels can have on readers who identify with them. This took the field of bibliotherapy to new heights. It was presented as a psychodynamic model by offering a theoretical model based on the idea that story characters can influence readers directly. This provided an explanation for why bibliotherapy might be effective and suggested constructive approaches to implementing the therapy. The 1950s marked the proliferation of research on bibliotherapy in a wide variety of fields – nursing, social work and education in the United States. In 1961, the definition appeared in the Webster International: "bibliotherapy is the use of a set of selected readings as therapeutic tools in medicine and psychiatry; and a way to solve personal problems through directed reading".

The American Library Association issued an official definition in 1966; it was officially introduced into medical vocabulary as the process of using literature to encourage cognitive change. In 1969, The American Library Association adopted an official definition of bibliotherapy and soon after the Association of Poetry Therapy formed as a specific type of bibliotherapy. In the 1970s, librarian Rhea Rubin helped establish clear directions for bibliotherapy by constructing two categories: developmental bibliotherapy (for the classroom) and therapeutic bibliotherapy (for mental health treatment). Her 1978 work, "Using Bibliotherapy: A Guide to Theory and Practice", contributed greatly to developments in the field. In 1983, The International Federation for Biblio/Poetry Therapy was established. (Rubin, Rhea Joyce 1978).

Bibliotherapy –Types

Reading and writing are two vital pillars of education systems and have a significant impact on the intellect and soul. Reading bibliotherapy is receptive and refers to reading, reception, and discussion of the text, as poetry, novels, and short stories. Expressive writing is active and encourages self-expression and sharing of emotions. (Dovey and Ceridwen). Using expressive writing help to identify and explain feelings, reflect on what is read and leads to new insights. It helps to release and get relief from strong or repressed emotions and helps with emotional control.

In its basic conceptual form bibliotherapy was seen as a way for people to solve personal challenges through directed reading. The exact classifications of bibliotherapy vary among scholars but generally fall into two categories split by areas of application:

- Clinical: using literature as a means of creating cognitive change related to psychological needs and therapeutic goals

- Developmental: informational materials used by both medical professionals and other educators to help assist with natural life transitions, such as puberty

Clinical bibliotherapy might be further broken down into subcategories based on the literature that affects the most, the preferred style of learning, and the mental well-being challenges one is facing. Three categories of books used in bibliotherapy are identified. The classical repertoire (novel, poetry, biography, fiction) which often by a process of identification, brings better well-being to the patient. Those whose theme is psychology; that describe a current disorder as well as provide information on specific disorder; aimed to assist readers. The self-help books to be linked to so-called cognitive development publications of personal inspiration, offering a precise methodology to relieve a malaise. (Helliker, K. 2007)

Creative bibliotherapy utilizes imaginative literature—novels, short stories, poetry, plays, and biographies—to improve psychological well-being. Through the incorporation of carefully selected literary works, therapists can often guide people in treatment on a journey of self-discovery. This method is most beneficial when people are able to identify with a character, experience an emotional catharsis as a result of this identification, and then gain insight about their own life experiences. It is often used in groups, and members read books and discuss them in the group. According to research, the brain will react as if experiencing an event when one reads it in a book. When one puts oneself in a character's shoes, one learns to understand the feelings and develop empathy with the characters and other people. (Shechtman, Z. 2009)

Prescriptive bibliotherapy, which is also referred to as self-help, involves the use of specific reading materials and workbooks to address a variety of mental health concerns. Self-help may be conducted with or without the guidance of a therapist. A cognitive behavioral therapist teaching someone deep breathing, and emotion regulation techniques may provide that person with a practice workbook to use at home. Prescriptive bibliotherapy uses nonfiction books and literature intended to offer self-help options at home or with professional treatment. A bibliotherapist will recommend certain books to be read; to help change the way of thinking, feelings, and actions. It can be self-help books on the specific issues being fact or fiction to identify with characters in the same situations. Also called personalized reading, the bibliotherapist recommends books based on what one loves to read or books about problems that need help with. It can be matched to the way one reads – physical books, audiobooks, or eBooks.

Most libraries in the United States carry a set of books from the approved list for this purpose, often providing as a book list on their website. Books on Prescription is a program were reading materials targeting specific mental health needs are "prescribed" by mental health professionals, who might use resources such as the Bibliotherapy Education Project to find the appropriate books. The Carnegie Library of Pittsburg is one such library. Their website also lists books for children, which cover topics like adoption, self-esteem, grief, divorce, and more. (Mckenna, Grainne, et al, 2010)

Through bibliotherapy, children learn essential lessons and values. Through stories, children can reflect on their lives, accept the past, and help them be more optimistic about the future. Stories are a source of comfort, help them connect with others, and they feel less alone. But most important is the way stories give children confidence and a way to use language to ask for help when they struggle to cope by themselves. Stories help them learn about themselves and find their place in the world from within a safe place. (Iaquinta, A., & Hipsky, S. 2006)

Developmental bibliotherapy, primarily used in educational settings, addresses typical childhood and adolescent concerns such as puberty, bodily functions, or developmental milestones. Educators or medical professionals may often encourage parents to use this approach with their children. Therapeutic bibliotherapy takes many forms and can be used in conjunction with many different therapeutic frameworks. Reading has been shown to be able to help people understand the issues they are experiencing, amplify the effects of other treatment, normalize experiences with mental health concerns and care, and offer hope for positive change. Bibliotherapy can also expedite and intensify the therapeutic process by providing one potential format for therapeutic work outside of session. (Afolayan, J. A. 1992)

When making use of fiction, bibliotherapy must be an interactive process. It is not only a matter of reading for enjoyment. But the reader, should identify with a character and its thoughts and emotions. It will also create potential solutions to problems the character needs to solve. Reading how a character overcomes their challenges will inspire to find a solution to problems; when good conquers evil in a novel, it will encourage to keep on fighting this battle in life.

Therapeutic bibliotherapy is often combined with other therapeutic techniques like Cognitive Behavioural Therapy (CBT) to treat psychological issues, like eating disorders, trauma, obsessive compulsive disorder (OCD), Post Traumatic Stress Disorder (PTSD), etc.

Basic Stages in Bibliotherapy

Generally, activities in bibliotherapy are designed to provide information, provide insight, stimulate discussion about problems, communicate new values and attitudes, create awareness that other people have similar problems, provide realistic solutions to problems,

The process goes through four basic stages (Pardeck, 1993): identification, selection, presentation, and follow-up. During the first two stages, the clients' needs must be identified, and appropriate books selected to match their particular problems. The selection process takes skill and insight, as the books must provide correct information about a problem while not imparting a false sense of hope. The books must then be presented carefully and strategically so that the clients are able to see similarities between themselves and the book characters. Once the clients can identify with the main character, they enter the follow-up stage during which they share what they have gained. They express catharsis verbally in discussion or writing, or nonverbal means such as art (Sridhar & Vaughn, 2000), role-playing, creative problem solving, or self-selected options for students to pursue individually (Hebert & Kent, 2000). Once catharsis has occurred, the clients can be guided to gain insight into the problem.

The success of the bibliotherapy program depends largely on how well teachers or counselors play their vital role as facilitator throughout the whole process. Studies provide useful ideas on how teachers can get ready for the process, and what they can do before, during and after reading. Reading is a way of escaping reality and a suspension of self. It is a type of mindfulness and anchors one in the story. Reading for 30 minutes a day helps to improve self-esteem, empathy, and emotional IQ. Reading helps to feel connected to the shared human experience, a critical part of mental well-being. (Sridhar & Vaughn 2000)

BIBLIOTHERAPY – APPLICATIONS

Bibliotherapy is using reading materials for help in solving personal problems or for psychiatric therapy. It uses literature to bridge the gap between what happens in our minds and bodies, to improve lives. Bibliotherapy is a therapeutic process. It helps improve mental health and deal with symptoms related to moods, like depression, grief, and anxiety. Bibliotherapy is applied in many fields. For example, social work, healthcare, counseling, education, and parenting. It is not restricted to literature only. It includes poetry writing, movies, comic books, dance, self-help books, art, songs, journaling, and storytelling. (Pardeck, 1994)

It can be used in two informal ways - Reading fiction and stories for support and guidance. Reading non-fiction for information about topics like mental and health concerns and self-help and self-development.

Bibliotherapy isn't just a mental health term — it's a tool that could be used in many professions to help encourage learning and personal growth. Bibliotherapy could help guide things such as relationships and substance use disorder recovery (Fanner, D. and C. Urquhart, 2008). It could help provide broader scopes of understanding that might help combat negative social constructs, such as racism. Research has shown bibliotherapy could have a positive impact on depression symptoms, stress and anxiety, childhood behavioral challenges, eating disorders, pandemic-related emotional stress, morality development, grief management.

Bibliotherapy practice has varied in approach and focus since it was first used in the 1930s. Traditional bibliotherapy, for example, tended to be more 'reactive' in its approach in that the process focused on getting individuals to react positively or negatively to the reading material. More recent approaches, however, assume that the therapeutic process is actually a more interactive one: the reader becomes part of the unfolding intellectual and emotional process of the story, and in struggling to understand what is being communicated at the deepest levels, the reader responds by making a positive alternation or modification in behavior or attitude (Myers, 1998). In interactive bibliotherapy, participants engage in activities that help them reflect on what they read, such as group discussion and dialogue journal writing (Palmer, et al., 1997; Anderson & MacCurdy, 2000; Morawski & Gilbert, 2000).

In the midst of the First World War, doctors and booksellers at the Alabama Military Hospital in the United States used books to relieve posttraumatic stress disorder for soldiers returning from combat. The underlying premise of bibliotherapy is that clients identify with literary characters similar to themselves, an association that helps the clients release emotions, gain new directions in life, and explore new ways of interacting (Gladding & Gladding, 1991). Teenage readers, for example, may feel relief that they are not the only ones facing a specific problem. They learn vicariously how to solve their problems by reflecting on how the characters in the book solve theirs (Hebert & Kent, 2000).

In clinical bibliotherapy and biblio-counseling, skilled practitioners use therapeutic methods to help individuals experiencing serious emotional problems. Classroom teachers are more likely to use developmental bibliotherapy, which involves helping students in their normal health and development. The advantage of the latter approach is that teachers can identify the concerns of their students and address the issues before problems arise. Students can also be guided through predictable stages of adolescence with knowledge of what to expect and examples of how other teenagers have dealt with the same concerns (Hebert & Kent, 2000).

Whichever approach it involves, bibliotherapy requires careful planning. It seeks to help clients respond directly to the materials they are given, so that change is affected through catharsis (a cleansing of the emotions, primarily through art), insight, or the "copying of character behaviors" (Gladding & Gladding, 1991).

Today, bibliotherapy is still used by some librarians and psychologists, but it has also expanded into several fields including social work, healthcare, education, counseling, and parenting. While originally referring to books alone, bibliotherapy casts a much wider net nowadays, including not only literature, but also poetry writing, self-help books, movies, comic books, art, songs, journaling, dance, and storytelling.

Bibliotherapy is a potentially powerful method for schoolteachers and counselors to use on many levels and in every school grade. In order to establish a strong bibliotherapy program in an institution, practitioners must present the procedure as a non-threatening one, starting by calling the process biblio-guidance, for instance. They must also solicit the input and advice of colleagues, parents, and administrators. In addition, they must always be alert to the limitations of bibliotherapy.

Although bibliotherapy is not recommended in place of more conventional mental health therapies, some cultures utilize bibliotherapy while patients wait to receive conventional therapy. For example, in the United Kingdom—where some patients may wait up to six months for professional treatment—individuals often utilize bibliotherapy during this waiting period, making it a sort of "first step" in mental health treatment.

Other modern examples of bibliotherapy include literature courses aimed at reducing recidivism for prison inmates, the U.S. National Storytelling Network's Healing Story Alliance branch, and the use of therapeutic storytelling for elders with dementia. Although bibliotherapy looks very different today than it did back in the Middle Ages, it's clear that it is still believed that words and art have the power to heal people and improve the society. (Schutt, Russell K., et al, 2013)

Most professionals agree reading is a productive activity that can promote good mental health, as reading has been shown to increase empathy, sharpen the mind, and impact behavior. Anecdotal research suggests bibliotherapy may offer significant benefit in the treatment of mental health issues, and its popularity among mental health professionals further implies positive results. Many therapists believe the inclusion of books in treatment increases participation in therapy and can decrease recovery time, providing more opportunity for insight and behavioral change while also allowing people to take more responsibility in their therapy work. Research on the efficacy of the method has shown it to be a helpful part of the treatment process for those experiencing depression, anxiety, and substance dependency.

BIBLIOTHERAPY – BENEFITS

In modern clinical or developmental settings mental health professionals may prescribe selected fiction or non-fiction materials such as novels, short stories, biographies, dramas, tales, fables and poetry as a part of a patient's treatment. A study by Bruneau and Pehrsson emphasizes the importance of choosing personalized reading materials and encourages bibliotherapists to involve their clients in the selection process as an opportunity to foster self-insight and motivation to read. The growing and increasingly popular self-help books are an additional form of bibliotherapy that can be used in conjunction with cognitive behavioral therapy. Depression, anxiety, posttraumatic stress disorder, panic attacks, insomnia, stress and strokes and their psychological and psychiatric conditions where self-help books have proven to be helpful. (Pehrsson, D. E, Bruneau E.K 2006).

Bibliotherapy has many benefits. Using literature like fiction and non-fiction books has many benefits. It helps one gain a deeper understanding of difficulties and develop plans to cope. These benefits can come from both fiction and non-fiction books. It can also help to develop skills like problem solving and self-awareness. A bibliotherapist assigns a book to read between sessions and gives homework. Reading the book and thinking about how one can relate to the story and its meaning improves the discussions during the therapy session.

Bibliotherapy can help deal with difficult emotions and concerns, for example, depression, anxiety, loss, grief, anger, etc. It can help find solutions to social issues, like shyness, or change the mindset about racism, sexism, etc. Reading helps to better understand the beliefs, desires, and thoughts of other people, even when it is much different to one's own. And through identifying with characters, readers develop higher levels of empathy with others.

Bibliotherapy can also be proactive when one reads books to learn how to cope with likely future challenges. One of the most significant benefits of bibliotherapy is identifying with the character(s) feelings. And see how that character deals with issues one is facing. Reading for pleasure, with no motive to heal, can be deeply therapeutic for many.

Couples can share books and reading interests to get to know each other better, create a shared paradigm, and develop new qualities. It can create opportunities for discussions, help overcome a crisis in a relationship, and have a therapeutic effect.

According to Don Meichenbaum, a leading expert on trauma and violence the habit of reading should be developed in children. He opines that, "More important than therapy, more important than social programs, more important than anything else. The research shows that the single most powerful predictor of their ability to overcome the trauma and survive their circumstances is the ability to read. If they can read, they have a chance to find success in school and overcome all those terrible things in their lives. If they can't, the school will only be another source of pain and failure added to all the other sources of pain and failure. If they can read, they can benefit from therapy and everything else we may try to do for them. If they can't read, all of that is a waste of time." Even though he refers to children in this quote, it is true even for adults. The ability to read might very well be the single most significant factor to overcome trauma or Post Traumatic Stress Disorder (PTSD).

An online survey shows that people who read often feel that what they read have a significant impact on their mental health. Many of these people read books relating to eating disorders. It includes books recommended by others struggling with this issue and recommending books to others. Reading helps them get a new or different perspective about their eating disorder. And gives them helpful, information, motivation, and inspiration from role models. Reading fiction helps to create a kinship with a character. In this way, it distracts one's thoughts *from* fears, loneliness, and discomfort when forming healthier eating habits. It is interesting to note that when reading about eating disorders, the reader's experience was negative about mood, self-esteem and body awareness, diet, and exercise habits. They found the real value in reading other types of fiction, which had a more positive effect on mood. But some people feel guilty when they sit and read (inactive) instead of exercising. So, although bibliotherapy can be beneficial for eating disorders, it should be part of a complete treatment regimen.

Research shows mindfulness related bibliotherapy to lower stress resulted in a significant drop in anxiety and stress, perception of stress, anxiety sensitivity, and life quality. Bibliotherapy provides effective long-term treatment for adults with mild depression, reducing symptoms from three months to three years. According to an online survey, people thought that self-help bibliotherapy is more effective in treating eating disorders than reading fiction books about it. Here, fiction harmed their mood, self-esteem, body image, diet, and exercise habits.

Creative bibliotherapy can help children in three ways - Internal behaviors like anxiety and depression. External behaviors like aggression and social anxiety. Pro-social behaviour, referring to their intentions and attitudes towards others. One study found children who read the *Harry Potter* series were more accepting of certain minority groups, and psychologists from the New School for Social Research determined fiction improved a reader's overall ability to discern and interpret emotion in others.

While this method is not typically recommended instead of a more conventional form of therapy, it is frequently used by individuals in therapy and those who are waiting to receive therapy. In the U.K., where individuals seeking professional mental health treatment may wait up to six months, bibliotherapy is considered a first step in treatment for those who do not need immediate help. Reading can benefit individuals of any age by increasing self-awareness, improving self-esteem, and aiding in the ability to face developmental crises. Studies show reading as a form of therapy to be useful in the treatment of depression, mild alcohol abuse, anxiety, eating disorders, and communication issues.

People in therapy for issues such as family-related challenges, posttraumatic stress, or grief might also benefit from the incorporation of books and reading activities into the approach being used. Books can be incorporated easily into any number of modalities, such as family systems therapy, play therapy, and cognitive behavioral therapy, among others.

A 2011 study that analyzes fMRI brain scans suggests that the brain uses the same brain networks when reading about an experience as when one experience the scenario personally. Other studies revealed that fiction readers, in particular readers of literary fiction, tend to score higher on empathy and social perception tests. These findings seem to align with the theoretical model of identification, catharsis, and insight. Although randomized controlled trials and the neuroscience of empathy offers some insight into bibliotherapy, the truth is, there is need for more research to answer the many questions about bibliotherapy and its effectiveness. What is definitely known, though, is that the practice of bibliotherapy is a testament to the love for books and the belief that they hold real power for one and all.

Recent studies from Sweden and Poland indicate that bibliotherapy can be an efficient complement to therapy and traditional medical interventions. However, more clinical studies are needed to support physicians and psychologists with an evidence based framework for clinical bibliotherapy. Further research may yield more details regarding efficacy and benefits. Presently, bibliotherapy is believed to be one cost-effective and versatile option for the treatment of several mental health issues. Bibliotherapy was originally developed to treat depression. It has also been used among caregivers in recent years. The effectiveness of bibliotherapy for caregivers has been achieved through a series of different studies. The results of these studies suggested that bibliotherapy was effective in improving the care experiences of caregivers of people with psychosis, as well as the resilience of caregivers who care for people with depression.

BIBLIOTHERAPY – ANALYSIS & FINDINGS

In addition to the "how" of conducting bibliotherapy, practitioners also need to be aware of potential benefits and pitfalls associated with this procedure. Bibliotherapy has obvious value in that it provides the opportunity for the participants to recognize and understand themselves, their characteristics, and the complexity of human thought and behavior. It may also promote social development as well as the love of literature in general, and reading in particular (Gladding & Gladding, 1991). It reduces feelings of isolation that may be felt by people with problems.

The effectiveness of bibliotherapy, however, may be limited by the availability of materials on certain topics, as well as the lack of client readiness and willingness to read. Clients may also project their own motives onto characters and thus reinforce their own perceptions and solutions. In addition, participants may be defensive, thus discounting the actions of characters and failing to identify with them, or even end up using them as scapegoats. Some of these limitations can be overcome through the continuation of the process itself, role playing, and the use of group discussions (Gladding & Gladding, 1991). Facilitator limitations are also a challenge: facilitators may have limited knowledge of human development and developmental problems, and inadequate knowledge about appropriate literature. Facilitators thus need to be properly trained and exposed to a repertoire of literature suitable for use in bibliotherapy. One other limitation may lie in the bibliotherapy process itself: for example, clients may be unwilling to discuss areas that are uncomfortable, or facilitators may insist on making a point at the client's expense. The process is also limited if both the client and counselor stay on surface issues. These limitations can be addressed by suspending sessions until both parties are ready and willing to work, by taping and critiquing selected sessions so that facilitators can monitor their own reactions to certain clients or problem areas, and by revisiting issues in stories that have been treated superficially in previous sessions (Gladding & Gladding, 1991).

Literature could be used for both positive and negative outcomes. In fact, experts note that some bibliotherapy could be harmful. Propaganda, which is deliberately skewed or misleading information, is often spread through literature. It could be used to encourage unhelpful or harmful beliefs and viewpoints. A 2020 study suggests that propaganda could be a powerful tool of emotional manipulation.

Bibliotherapy has been ingrained in cultures across the world for years, but it's worth mentioning that many of the ideas it supports are only hypotheses; bibliotherapy has been used widely but without strong scientific evidence of its success. That being said, researchers are beginning to take an interest in the idea that books impact minds. In the last couple decades, scientists have begun utilizing randomized controlled trials to track the effects of this therapy form. Thus far, research finds positive effects of clinical bibliotherapy in those with certain mental illnesses and substance abuse issues. Studies also discovered promising results amongst older patients struggling with depression.

Bibliotherapy is a viable treatment option for people of all ages, but it is not recommended if a person – can't discern between fantasy and reality; has limited cognitive ability or is readily distracted and doesn't enjoy reading.

Generally speaking, bibliotherapy is a safe form of supplemental therapy appropriate for people of all ages and abilities. A healthcare professional might not recommend bibliotherapy if one doesn't enjoy reading, have a short attention span, experience psychosis, doesn't respond strongly to learning through reading. Many other factors could contribute to the decision on whether to include bibliotherapy in the treatment plan.

There is some debate about whether or not bibliotherapy should take place at home, or if we should limit it to clinical settings. Generally, people embrace the idea that art and stories provide an effective way to talk about life situations from a creative third-person perspective. This perspective is meant to offer a productive and less intimidating conversational space for difficult topics. While many therapists work alongside the patient throughout bibliotherapy (in addition to using traditional, clinical mental health therapies), some bibliotherapists are less involved in the active work of therapy. These remote bibliotherapists act similarly to a bookseller, chatting about your reading preferences and the worries you're encountering at that moment in time. These conversations help the bibliotherapists provide a "book list prescription" for their clients.

Stress Management and Resiliency Training (SMART) was developed as a structured and simple program at Mayo Clinic, Rochester to decrease personal stress and enhance resilience. (A.S.V Sood, Darrell Schroeder, Bauer Brent B. Gorman et al 2014) The study was conducted among the Department of Radiology faculty. SMART is an abbreviated version of a therapy called Attention and Interpretation Therapy (AIT). AIT and SMART focus on two aspects of human experience: attention and interpretation. Human attention tends to focus upon threats. These threats, in modern time, may take the form of hurts, regrets, worries and fears that can draw attention away from the present moment and into the domains of the past and the future. These can lead to ruminative thinking, avoidance and ineffective thought suppression. Consequently, untrained attention leads to an increase in perceived stress. SMART teaches learners to focus their attention in the present moment and to defer unrefined judgments. Learners are also taught to cultivate and guide their interpretations by higher-order principles such as forgiveness, acceptance, gratitude, compassion and life's meaning instead of superficial prejudices.

The study conducted on the employees of a large medical center; to assess effectiveness of a self-directed Stress Management and Resiliency Training (SMART) program delivered using only written material for improving stress, resiliency and mindfulness; revealed significant results. A total of 37 employees were recruited under the study and given written material on the SMART program. Subjects were instructed to practice the skills presented in the written materials without any additional training. The skills included education about neuropsychology of stress and resilience, training attention to focus in the present moment and refining interpretations. Primary outcome measures assessed resilience, perceived stress, anxiety and quality of life. Out of the 37 employees; 34 (89%) enrolled subjects completed the study and provided the baseline and follow-up data. A statistically significant improvement in perceived stress, resilience, mindfulness, anxiety and quality of life was observed at 12 weeks. The study demonstrated that a brief, self-directed program to decrease stress and enhance resilience and mindfulness provided excellent short-term effectiveness for enhancing resilience, mindfulness and quality of life; decreasing stress and anxiety.

Bibliotherapy has been in place to treat mental health problems and has been found efficacious by several randomized control trials and meta-analyses to reduce depression and several types of anxiety disorders.

Bibliotherapy – Suggested Readings

Self-help books can come in handy. Self-help books are not a replacement for working with mental health professionals. If one is dealing with a mental illness professional help must be sought. But for situations without a clinical element, a self-help book can make a difference.

When someone finds the right self-help book and puts the time into reading it and doing the work, it can have a number of benefits. One is that they can provide a concrete blueprint for an individual who has identified an issue in their life to navigate addressing it in a healthy manner on their own. In addition to providing a general blueprint for how a person can approach some of their biggest challenges, self-help books can add structure to individuals' day-to-day life. They can motivate individuals to try different strategies and venture into uncomfortable territory. Self-help books can lead to more fluid and healthy communication at work and at home, and many allow individuals to remain introspective and practice self-compassion. It helps individuals identify ways in which they can respond to inevitable stress in a more positive way, and reiterates the fact that they have the power to write their own story and determine their own emotional experience.

"A New Earth: Awakening to Your Life's Purpose" by Eckhart Tolle

This book goes beyond teaching how to live in the moment and helps readers learn how to turn their suffering into peace. All types of suffering are addressed in the book, from anger and grief to jealousy and anxiety. Tolle talks a lot about the ego and how to separate ourselves from it. His examples and recommended exercises really work and are something anyone can do. Whether suffering is rooted in jealousy, anger, grief, sadness, anxiety, or depression, Tolle will help see life from varied perspectives, awakening to life's purpose.

"You Are a Badass" by Jen Sincero

Far too often, fear gets the better of people. Jen Sincero helps readers go beyond that fear in her New York Times best seller "You Are a Badass." What sets this self-help book apart from the others are the engaging end-of-chapter exercises. The exercises also drive home the points Sincero makes through her writing.

"The 7 Habits of Highly Effective Teens" by Sean Covey

Many have read, or at least have heard about, "The 7 Habits of Highly Effective People" by Stephen Covey. Covey's son Sean followed in his footsteps, making a spinoff version for teenagers that uses the same principles to help young adult's master formative areas of their lives. To make this self-help book age-appropriate and downright fun to read, Covey breaks up the text with cartoons, quotes, brainstorming ideas, and stories from real teens to bring the book together. "The 7 Habits of Highly Effective Teens" covers topics like body image, friendships, relationships, goal-setting, peer pressure, bullying, internet safety, and so much more.

"Declutter Your Mind" by S.J. Scott

The subtitle of this book provides great insight into the heart of the book: How to stop worrying, relieve anxiety and eliminate negative thinking. "Declutter Your Mind" is a book that is very hands-on with its reader and full of various exercises to engage your mindset. It discusses the causes of mental clutter, how to change negative thoughts to positive ones, strategies to help with rocky relationships, how to identify what's important, the importance of meditation, how to goal set, and much more. If one is feeling overwhelmed with stress, worry, or anxiety, this powerful book will do its part in offering various techniques, tips, and tricks to cope with an overactive mind.

"Big Magic: Create Living Beyond Fear" by Elizabeth Gilbert

From creating new habits and ridding oneself of old ones to overcoming fear and surrounding oneself with like-minded individuals, Gilbert hits the nail on the head as she dissects the obstacles a creative person may face in pursuing their dreams. Her honest, conversational tone will light a fire in the soul and help to be upfront about what one wants from life. A highlight of this book is the usage of real-life examples from regular men and women across the country who have endured in their creative feats.

"The Wisdom of Sundays" by Oprah Winfrey

Oprah is the queen of interviewing spiritual gurus, world leaders, therapists, doctors, and other thought leaders. "The Wisdom of Sundays" takes the best-of-the-best from these conversations and combines them into one uplifting read. The book has 240 pages full of snippets from what Oprah refers to as "life-changing insights". Authors in The Wisdom of Sundays include Shonda Rimes, Cheryl Strayed, Tony Robbins, Thich Nhat Hahn, Wayne Dyer, and so many more.

CONCLUSION

Bibliotherapy, aka book therapy, is the use of literature to help overcome challenges in everyday life. Whether one is living with a mental health condition or simply going through a natural life change, the right reading material could help increase the intellectual insight - toward self and the people around. While most bibliotherapy in the clinical setting is guided, self-help books and reading literature at home that empowers could also be considered bibliotherapy.

Unfortunately, stressful life experiences, such as loss or bereavement, the divorce of parents, anger, fear, bullying, and feeling diverse or excluded, can enter the life of pupils and students. Aiming at the development of the person as a whole rather than at mere academic success, schools are naturally prone to help, but sometimes lack the means for doing it with care and respect of their primary educational mission.

Bibliotherapy is the activity of using literature to grow towards good emotional health. Offering a responsive interaction with literature, bibliotherapy can assist young people with the challenges of development. It can also offer support in relieving stress, providing successful coping strategies, and helping an individual to express both feelings and ideas about a problem or difficulty.

The modern digital era is defined by instant, constant and universal all-time connectivity. The flow of information is instant and rapid. Unlike in the past when emotions felt by an individual would take time to travel to the other members of the society. It would take time for an emotion to convert into anxiety and further stress leading to psychosomatic and physiological impact. Emotions can now be digitally transmitted from one individual to the other rapidly. Also, significantly the emotion spreads and multiplies rapidly. This creates simultaneous anxiety and stress. Thus when an event occurs anywhere in the world it can be captured and transmitted in a visual form in an instant. This leads to an overflow of emotions and the response to it. The mind seems to react more to the negative emotions more than the positive ones. This helps in accentuating the impact of the event. The impact is immediate, and its duration gets prolonged as it is visually stored and transmitted. The speed at which the emotion engenders anxiety and the resultant stress is rapid and profound. Humans endeavor to manage the emotion – fear and anxiety – to reduce the impact of stress. An individual can undertake several measures to alleviate the impact of stress.

A pandemic such as COVID-19 is often a source of emotional distress. It affects even those who have not been physically affected by the disease. The acknowledgment of the mental health toll of the COVID-19 epidemic has increased considerably as the disease evolved into a pandemic. High prevalence rates of depression, sleep disorders, and post-traumatic stress disorder (PTSD) have been reported. Anxiety, depression, and insomnia are quite prevalent among the general population as a result of self-isolation, social distancing and safety concerns. Symptoms of psychological distress are expected to be long-lasting and have a systemic impact on the global population, warranting the need for evidence-based psychological treatments aimed at relieving immediate stress and preventing the onset of psychological disorders. Mitigating the psychological impact in the post pandemic world for the global population is a major challenge. Mental health professionals may treat patients with increased emotional distress caused by the effects of the pandemic on them, on their families, or on the society. Several recent studies highlight the psychological impact of the COVID-19 and the need for guidelines and increased psychological interventions. Depression, anxiety, and insomnia are some examples of psychological distress found among the general population as a result of the self-isolation, social distancing and safety concerns. This phase is the hardest for the medical professionals in terms of psychological impact.

With new technology and easy access to literature through online libraries and bookshops, bibliotherapy has become an efficient and inexpensive alternative to traditional face-to-face therapy. Self-paced reading with follow-up sessions over the phone, videoconferencing, or being in virtual reality settings enables individuals with economic, geographical, physical, or mental barriers to benefit from bibliotherapy. The new online or telemedicine options for bibliotherapy have the potential to work very well especially in the post pandemic world often connoted by isolation settings.

Despite a call for more evidence-based research about the wider effectiveness of bibliotherapy the reported benefits and zero-harm makes bibliotherapy an effective form of therapy for individuals with mental and personal development issues. Bibliotherapy can be useful for health professionals and physicians.

Even if reading does not replace a session with the psychologist or therapist, scientific studies have proven the many benefits of reading; it reduces stress, improves the quality of sleep, and stimulates emotional intelligence. Even if it is a rather solitary activity, reading can really facilitate human relationships by engendering empathy.

LIMITATIONS

The limitation of this chapter is that it is a subjective review of bibliotherapy rather than statistically sound evaluated findings. The literature for the evidence for the efficacy of bibliotherapy is still heterogeneous. Evidence is homogenous in the field of education. There are some studies in depression but very few well-controlled studies that often include the bibliotherapy as a part of CBT. The effects on mental well-being outcomes are inconclusive due to limited number of studies and this underscores the need for further research. The selection of literary works is also limited to western culture; it can be extended to other cultures.

REFERENCES

Adderholdt-Elliott, M., & Eler, S. H. (1989). Counseling students who are gifted through bibliotherapy. *Teaching Exceptional Children*, *22*(1), 26–31. doi:10.1177/004005998902200106

Afolayan, J. A. (1992). Documentary perspective of bibliotherapy in education. *Reading Horizons*, *33*(2).

Anderson, C. M., & MacCurdy, M. M. (2000). *Writing and healing: Toward an informed practice.* National Council of Teachers of English.

Bibliotherapy. (n.d.). *Good Therapy*. www.goodtherapy.org/learn-about-therapy/types/bibliotherapy

Dovey, C. (n.d.). Can Reading Make You Happier? *The New Yorker*. www.newyorker.com/culture/cultural-comment/can-reading-make-you-happier

Fanner & Urquhart. (2008). Bibliotherapy for mental health service users Part 1: A systematic review. *Health Information & Libraries Journal*, *25*(4). doi:. doi:10.1111/j.1471-1842.2008.00821.x

Gladding, S. T., & Gladding, C. (1991). The ABCs of bibliotherapy for school counselors. *The School Counselor*, *39*(1).

Hebert, T. P., & Kent, R. (2000). Nurturing social and emotional development in gifted teenagers through young adult literature. *Roeper Review*, *22*(3).

Helliker, K. (2007, July 31). *Bibliotherapy: Reading your way to mental health*. Academic Press.

Iaquinta, A., & Hipsky, S. (2006, July). *Bibliotherapy for the inclusive classroom*. Academic Press.

Lenkowsky, R. S. (1987). Bibliotherapy: A review and analysis of the literature. *The Journal of Special Education*, *2*(2).

Lutz, C. E. (1978). The Oldest Library Motto: Ψγxhσ Ἰατρεῖον. *The Library Quarterly*, *48*(1). doi:10.1086/629993

Mckenna, G. (2010). Patients' and Providers' Perspectives on Bibliotherapy in Primary Care. *Clinical Psychology & Psychotherapy*, *17*(6). doi:10.1002/cpp.679

Morawski, C. M., & Gilbert, J. N. (2000). Developmental interactive bibliotherapy. *College Teaching*, *48*(3).

Myers, J. E. (1998). Bibliotherapy and DCT: Co-constructing the therapeutic metaphor. *Journal of Counseling and Development*, *76*(3).

Palmer, B. C., Biller, D. L., Rancourt, R. E., & Teets, K. A. (1997). Interactive bibliotherapy: An effective method for healing and empowering emotionally-abused women. *Journal of Poetry Therapy*, *11*(1).

Pardeck, J. T. (1993). Literature and adoptive children with disabilities. *Early Child Development and Care*, 91.

Pardeck, J. T. (1994). Using literature to help adolescents cope with problems. *Adolescence*, *29*(114).

Pehrsson, D. E., & Bruneau E.K (2006, June). *Benefits of utilizing bibliotherapy with play therapy*. Academic Press.

Rubin, R. J. (1978). *Using Bibliotherapy: a Guide to Theory and Practice*. Oryx Press.

Schutt, R. K. (2013). Using Bibliotherapy to Enhance Probation and Reduce Recidivism. *Journal of Offender Rehabilitation*, *52*(3). doi:10.1080/10509674.2012.751952

Shechtman, Z. (2009, June). *Treating child and adolescent aggression through bibliotherapy*. Academic Press.

Sood, Schroeder, & Gorman. (2014). *Bibliotherapy to decrease stress and anxiety and increase resilience and mindfulness: A pilot trial*. doi:10.1016/j.explore.2014.04.002

Sridhar, D., & Vaughn, S. (2000). Bibliotherapy for all. *Teaching Exceptional Children*, *33*(2).

Chapter 10
Stress in a Crisis Context: Experiences of Portuguese Social Workers in Healthcare During COVID-19

Diana Contente Ferreira
Universidade Lusíada, Portugal

Inês Casquilho-Martins
https://orcid.org/0000-0002-7407-848X
Centro Lusíada de Investigação em Serviço Social e Intervenção Social, Universidade Lusíada, Portugal

ABSTRACT

The emergence of COVID-19 led to a global pandemic framework, decreed in March 2020 by the World Health Organization. This phenomenon led to several changes and restrictions in people's lives, which subsequently questioned many professional practices, namely in social work. This chapter aims to analyze the factors and consequences of stress in the professional activity of social workers, as well as the changes in the health area caused by the pandemic crisis context in Portugal. Social workers' stress levels were affected during the COVID-19 pandemic, while recognizing that there were already present and identified causes of stress before the crisis. Work overload, multiple duties, fatigue, and even a decrease in the quality of professional care were aspects mentioned that need addressing, and since social workers intervene with a vulnerable population in different dimensions, greater attention is required. Therefore, the specificity of stress in social workers is correlated to the responsibility and demands of the professional practice itself.

INTRODUCTION

The COVID-19 pandemic crisis brought about a number of adjustments and limitations in people's lives as well as the examination of institutional and professional procedures. Simultaneously, there was a situation of unprecedented challenges for health professionals, which could lead to high levels of stress and burnout (Monteiro, Cunha, Simões & Relva, 2021; Mendes, Cabral & Melo, 2021). According to

DOI: 10.4018/978-1-6684-8565-1.ch010

Cardoso, Vilar & Casquilho-Martins (2020), the confinement to which the Portuguese population was forced has stimulated social isolation and health fragilities, making the sectors of society that live in precarious situations in terms of health, income, and employment more vulnerable. Thus, it is important the analysis of this pandemic context in light of the new, unpredictable reality that has affected society and the lives of its individuals.

By understanding that the current pandemic is a present reality with medium- and long-term consequences, this research focused on the challenges of social workers in the health area, associated with the dimensions of stress and burnout. This issue emerges as a research problem that has not yet been explored in Portugal and is of relevance to Social Work, both in the field of research and in professional practice. Hence, it was established that it would be significant for the study to deepen the challenges in this field in contemporary times. As for the research objectives, the general aim was to analyze the stress and burnout factors in healthcare social workers during the COVID-19 pandemic. Based on the main intention of this research, the following specific objectives were planned: to characterize the factors and causes of stress in work contexts in the health area, particularly in Social Work during the pandemic; to identify the impacts of stress and burnout on the intervention of social workers in the health area; to systematize strategies for the prevention and management of stress and burnout among social workers in the health area.

The next section presents the theoretical framework focusing on Social Work and the health area, particularly in the pandemic context generated by COVID-19. Attention was also given to the literature review on the conditioning factors of professional activity, such as stress and burnout, and also on the contemporary challenges faced by the health area. Following, the research methodology and procedures are explained, presenting the empirical field, the scientific method used, the sample of this study, and the data collection and processing techniques. Regarding the results to be shared in this chapter, the factors and causes of stress and burnout in social workers in the health area, the consequences of stress and burnout in the intervention of social workers in the health area, the impacts of the pandemic in the professional activity of social workers in the health area, and the strategies for prevention and management of stress in social workers in the health area are mentioned. Finally, it presents the conclusions of the study and the implications for professional practice.

HEALTH SOCIAL WORK: CHALLENGES IN THE PANDEMIC CONTEXT

The spread of the SARS-CoV-2 virus, which originated the disease COVID-19 and resulting pandemic, marked the year 2020. In Portugal, since March 2020, an increase in the number of registered COVID-19 cases was observed, resulting in a worsening of the pandemic situation in Portugal, which required the implementation of urgent measures, including the financial, human, material, and logistic reinforcement of the National Health Service (NHS) (Casquilho-Martins, 2022). The pandemic prompted a set of implications at an individual and collective level, leading to an unprecedented situation in this century (Monteiro, Cunha, Simões & Relva, 2021). One of these challenges was the response of health care, especially in hospital settings. Also, in the field of Palliative Care, the increase in patients with COVID-19 led to a pandemic management model that diverted palliative health professionals to other areas, with problems of human resource allocation occurring even before the pandemic crisis (Comissão Nacional de Cuidados Paliativos, 2021).

As health is a universal right, it is essential for the profession to promote, in its work in this area, fundamental principles and values such as human rights, freedom, human dignity, and social justice, since health is considered as an individual matter and a societal one (Carvalho, 2012). Over time, the concept of health has undergone changes and the practice of Social Work in this field intersects and transforms within the redefinition of this term. Thinking about the definition of health leads to a biopsychosocial view, which needs to be analyzed by also including environmental, social, and behavioral aspects (Santos, 2017; Casquilho-Martins & Ferreira, 2022). Social Work is one profession that integrates multidisciplinary teams in health services since the 20th century, being one of the specific fields of professional action for social workers (Carvalho, 2012). Social work in health is related to the collective nature of health care provision and the configuration of multidisciplinary teams in the health sector, which is linked to the evolutionary path of the profession (Branco & Farçadas, 2012). Given the specificity of health as an area of intervention, Social Work has the role of humanizing services, encompassing a biopsychosocial approach, meaning that, besides considering clinical problems, these professionals consider the possibility of the influence of factors such as psychological and social factors on the users' health status (Santos, 2017). In this sense, professional practice in health care facilities can be regarded as a practice in complex environments, due to the diversity of professions inherent to this system and the interactions between professionals, users, and families (Monteiro, Cunha, Simões & Relva, 2021). According to Carvalho (2012), social workers can develop their professional activity in primary health care, in integrated and palliative continuous care, in family health units, in general or specialized health units, in mental health and community health, and in health promotion with specific groups.

Social workers must ensure citizens' access to their rights, such as security and welfare, as one of their duties. The pandemic accentuated social inequalities and, during the pandemic crisis scenario, social work faced challenging times to meet urgent needs where COVID-19, besides causing physical health concerns, included stress (Mendes, Cabral & Melo, 2021). Still, social workers played an important role, supporting communities, especially the most vulnerable people and groups at risk, being involved from the beginning as key players in combating the lack of information, the scarcity of resources, social isolation, and anxiety in patients and families (Reigada, 2020).

BRIEF LEGAL FRAMEWORK OF THE PORTUGUESE HEALTH LAW

The Constitution of the Portuguese Republic enshrines the protection of health, establishing a set of fundamental values such as human dignity, equity, ethics and solidarity. Health as a fundamental right is promoted through the National Health Service (NHS), tending to be free of charge, in order to minimize economic and social inequalities of citizens in access to this right (Constitutional Law no. 1/2005, Article 64). The first Portuguese Health Law [Lei de Bases da Saúde] (Law no. 48/90) highlighted not only the importance of health as a right, but also the protection of health as a joint responsibility of citizens, society, and the State. The proximity of health services and health protection was reinforced in 1999, with Decree-Law no. 157/99, which established the regime for the creation, organization, and operation of health centers. Within this regulation, social workers are mentioned as members of the multi-professional teams of community care units (Decree-Law no. 157/99, Article 13).

In 2019, the Health Law was amended by Law no. 95/2019, which reinforces the right to health protection as a right of all people at the physical, mental and social level, in articulation with the economic, social, cultural and environmental conditions that contribute to a healthy life, including work and leisure. The right to health is governed by the principles of equality in access to health care and access to information related to it, aiming at the self-determination of citizens regarding the health care offered to them, the promotion of well-being and quality of life during aging. This once again highlights the role of public health as a cornerstone for the population and for the well-being of individuals in the community. As for mental health, Basis 13 of the Portuguese Health Law references this subject, declaring that the State promotes the improvement of mental health of individuals and of society in general, by the means of promoting mental well-being, prevention, and identification of diseases and their associated risks. As such, in Decree-Law No. 113/2021, which establishes the general principles and rules for the organization and functioning of mental health services, the participation of social workers in the National Mental Health Council (Article 7), in the Regional Mental Health Councils (Article 9), in the National Coordination of Mental Health Policies (Article 12), and in the Regional Mental Health Coordination (Article 13), reflects the importance of the profession in promoting and protecting health and ensuring access to this right for all citizens. In this sense, the existence and functioning of the National Health Service in Portugal is a mainstay in the realization of social rights, allowing and facilitating the conditions of access to health care (Casquilho-Martins and Ferreira, 2022).

STRESS AND BURNOUT: CONDITIONING FACTORS FOR PROFESSIONAL ACTIVITY

Work occupies a large part of our time investment in our lives and can influence our well-being, bringing consequences such as stress or burnout. The World Health Organization (WHO) defines mental health as a "state of mental well-being that enables people to cope with the stresses of life, realize their abilities, learn well and work well, and contribute to their community" (World Health Organization, 2022). There is a close relationship between well-being and the work context, as dimensions of analysis, sharing the view of Carrera (2011) who states that for the prevention of stress and burnout it is essential to recognize that it exists and that it is recognized not only by the professionals but also by the organizations where they work and, in a broader sense, by society.

Stress is something that is present in various days or events of our lives, with the work context being no exception. According to Miranda (2011), there is an influence of the conditions and characteristics of the work activity as conditioning aspects of people's feelings and well-being. Gomes & Cruz (2004) refer that the negative effects of stress and burnout have consequences at different levels of individual's health, both at the physical and mental health levels, being reflected in the satisfaction and productivity of professionals.

The concept of workplace stress, according to Colligan and Higgins (2005) can influence the behaviors, emotions, and people's wellbeing. Although it may help to achieve certain goals, it can also cause "emotional distress and physical illness" (p. 90). Goulão (2017) mentions that, in the literature on stress, there are multiple definitions of the concept, focusing on the study of this concept within the work context. Regarding the concept of Burnout, Goulão (2017) states that Burnout was understood as the result of wrong expectations; progressive disappointments, loss of coping strategies, demanding interactions with clients; and lack of reciprocity in relationships with them. (Goulão, 2017, p.22). According to the current classification of the WHO in the 11th revision of the International Classification of Diseases (ICD-11): "Burn-out is a syndrome conceptualized as resulting from chronic workplace stress that has not been successfully managed. It is characterized by three dimensions: feelings of energy depletion or exhaustion; increased mental distance from one's job, or feelings of negativism or cynicism related to one's job; and reduced professional efficacy" (World Health Organization, 2019). The concept of burnout should not be applied to describe experiences in other areas of life, and it refers specifically to phenomena in the occupational context.

METHODS AND PROCEDURES

Considering the scope of the research, this study was exploratory and descriptive in nature, following a predominantly qualitative approach, since data were collected through semi-structured interviews as a data collection technique. The data were processed using categorical content analysis technique. For this purpose, a semi-structured interview script was designed and applied. The interviews were conducted via video call, considering that this would be the most suitable operationalization form for reasons of safety and individual protection, especially when addressing health professionals. As for the data processing of the interviews, a content analysis grid was prepared, which allowed listing the categories and subcategories of analysis for this study. The qualitative approach was the most appropriate for this study. According to Ramos (2005), qualitative methods benefit from the collaboration between the researcher and the research participants, since they can encompass the participants' perspective on the reality being studied, and are also sensitive to the study of the processes that lead to certain results (Flick, 2005; Guerra, 2006).

Considering that we have no information about the total number of social workers working in the health area, the sample of this study is a convenience non-probability, non-representative sampling, according to intentional criteria (Flick, 2005). Since this is a qualitative study, the sample sought to identify privileged participants who could provide detailed information about the problem. It was not the intention of this research to make inferences or generalizations. Thus, the selection of social workers followed the criteria previously defined in the project, namely that: i) they worked in healthcare facilities; ii) they had been working during the pandemic period between 2020 and 2021. It was also a criterion that interviewees had a diversified professional experience in the health area, particularly in hospitals, primary health care, mental health and long-term care, as well as the need to interview professionals from different geographical areas of the country.

In a total of fourteen participants who took part in this study, the study sample was composed mostly of female social workers, with only one male participant. The average age of the participants was 37, ranging from 24 to 64 years old. With reference to the training qualifications in Social Work, namely the undergraduate degree in Social Work - which awards the professional title of social worker in Portugal - the date of graduation is between 1974 and 2019, with the years of professional experience in the health area varying between 2 and 42 years, averaging approximately 13 years of professional experience in the health area in relation to the total number of participants. The coding of the interviewed participants was subject to a random execution, with no specific criteria needed since it does not influence the data treatment. Finally, reference to the municipality where the participants exercised their professional activity was not included so as not to compromise the anonymity of the sources, with professionals from the following geographical areas being chosen: i) Autonomous Region of the Azores, which during the first phase of the pandemic registered a low intensity of cases of COVID-19; ii) Center Region, which during the first phase of the pandemic registered a medium intensity of cases of COVID-19; and iii) the Lisbon Metropolitan Area, which, during the first phase of the pandemic, registered a high intensity of

COVID-19 cases. This choice was intentional, as it was expected that the social workers interviewed could represent distinct areas of the country where there had been a different incidence of positive cases of COVID-19. The largest number of professionals interviewed exercise their professional activity in the geographical zone of lower incidence (6), followed by interviewees in the zone of higher incidence (5) and, finally, interviewees in the zone of medium incidence (3).

According to Batista, Matos & Nascimento (2017) the individual interview is the best choice for research that address sensitive issues, especially issues that could be costly if they were handled in group situations. Thus, the individual interview offers more flexibility in regards to scheduling, time frameworks, setting and location (Batista, Matos & Nascimento, 2017). The interviews were conducted between May and June 2021, with an average duration of 45 minutes, with the longest lasting approximately 90 minutes and the shortest 25 minutes. Interviewees responded to what was asked of them and there were no recorded interruptions or dropouts during the interviews. In addition to completing the informed consent form before the interviews began, permission was sought from the social workers participating in the study to record the interview. All issues relevant to the study were again clarified, being mindful of the principles of ethics and confidentiality that a scientific study is subject to. None of the interviewees objected to the use of recording. Considering the pandemic constraints at that time and the need for these professionals to adopt enhanced individual protection measures, all interviews were conducted by telephone or video call. This opportunity to use distance communication protected both the interviewees and the researcher. Another advantage was that it allowed the researcher to contact professionals from several regions of the country. For data processing, after the interviews were conducted, they were transcribed in full, to allow the creation of detailed content and, subsequently, to acquire knowledge and understanding of the professional experiences described by the interviewees. The data processing was based on the technique of categorical content analysis as the research had an exploratory and descriptive character supported by categories and subcategories of analysis, not favoring the analysis of linguistic expressions since it was not a requirement for obtaining the results.

IMPACTS OF THE PANDEMIC IN HEALTH SOCIAL WORKERS PRACTICE

As seen previously, the pandemic had several consequences on social workers' practice and service provision (Cardoso, Vilar & Casquilho-Martins, 2020). In the Portuguese context, the socio-political transformations created new issues for the Social Work agenda, thus requiring new intervention practices that corresponded to the standards of action applied at the European level. With the emergence of COVID-19, Social Work needed to rethink a way to overcome the discontinuity of social policy orientations (Mendes, Cabral & Melo, 2021). The changes in the functioning of health services during the pandemic throughout the Portuguese territory led to a limitation in the quality of services provided to citizens.

The interviews conducted with the social workers in the context of this study allowed the identification of the main changes in the responses and access to health care, according to the statements of the interviewees. The demand for health services was mainly registered by patients with COVID-19, leading to the perception that patients with symptoms not associated with the new coronavirus avoided using health services. Additionally, due to the overload of health services, COVID-19 patients were given priority over other patients, with implications for social and clinical follow-up.

"In my service (...) initially that they closed right away and suddenly became COVID services. So, it was a readjustment here, a discovery in how I should position myself as a social worker in this new pandemic context" (SW14)

In a period of greater vulnerability, this restriction had an effect on people who could not have contact with their relatives. The limitation and prohibition of hospital visits led to patients feeling more alone and isolated. Similarly, social workers themselves who had direct contact with the patients, experienced limitations in the way they approached and interacted with patients.

In the context of the pandemic crisis, the Health Regulatory Authority had already warned about changes in the activity of health care facilities and in the way health services were provided to users (Conselho Nacional de Saúde, 2020). It is noteworthy that the competencies of social workers during the pandemic sought to fill some gaps that resulted from the pressure and overload of other health professionals due to the urgent response to COVID-19. The interviewees themselves recognize that professionals in the fields of medicine and nursing had a greater exposure to stress and that it was therefore also necessary for social workers to strengthen their relational skills. As direct influence factors on the tasks and actions performed, the interviewees mentioned that the work overload, which increased in degree and intensity during the pandemic, generated delays in responses and conditioned their professional activity.

According to Casquilho-Martins (2022), the response to COVID-19 empowered new forms of contagion prevention, such as the voluntary or mandatory confinement of families, which in several cases did not safeguard the functioning and response of the chronically ill. The resulting interruption and postponement of home and palliative care led to serious consequences in terms of health and quality of life of the patient and their families (Conselho Nacional de Saúde, 2020).

"There was a big impact for healthcare professionals, they were demanding a lot from us. Health professionals couldn't work from home, they couldn't be afraid because they had to keep working. This was in the context of dealing with patients that tested positive for COVID-19. These professionals couldn't do the self-isolation because they were needed, it was very stressful." (SW2)

These challenges reinforce Sakellarides' position that emphasizes the necessity of more fund allocation to the NHS, being equally important the transformation in terms of decentralization, integration, innovation and democratization, as means to put people at the heart of the healthcare system. By eliminating excessive rhetoric, the focus should be on knowledge management, with the implementation of a health governance model that is capable of adapting its strategies (Sakellarides, 2020). One of the main constraints experienced was the lack of social responses that could integrate users after clinical discharge, thus delaying social discharge. With the closure of social services and the reduction of teams, an adaptation was necessary to guarantee the response to citizens and access to primary health care. Regarding the use of digital and remote communication, there has been an increase in creating alternative channels to the formal means of communication, to facilitate contact between professionals, and in order to support telecommuting for some professionals.

Based on the answers collected through the interviews, a summary of the main changes in responses and access to health care is presented: increased spending in the health sector; implementation of periods of prophylactic isolation after admission; prolongation of stays of displaced patients; restrictions in the access of family relationships and of proximity to the patient; absence of external social responses for user referrals; creation of back-up responses for patients who could not return home; creation of alternative projects to ensure care for isolated elderly people; remote monitoring (by phone or email); readaptation of monitoring and contact with family members/multidisciplinary team; opportunities in inter-help and innovation in digital work. Several social workers felt these changes, although they had a greater weight in the territories with higher pandemic intensity due to the elevated number of cases.

The guidelines received by the professionals showed that there was a difference in perception regarding them. In terms of policy orientations, Portuguese social workers in territories with low pandemic density felt less pressure in this domain than professionals who worked in the mainland.

CAUSES AND CONSEQUENCES OF STRESS AND BURNOUT IN HEALTHCARE SOCIAL WORKERS

As social workers are part of multidisciplinary health care teams, it was relevant that the collection of empirical data could give visibility to the reality perceived by social workers in this context. Monteiro, Cunha, Simões & Relva (2021) state that the pandemic caused a position of unprecedented demands and challenges for health professionals; thus, the pandemic brought factors that may lead to high levels of stress and conflict in health professionals. They also mention that these effects may appear at the psychosocial and mental health levels, consequences caused by the episodes experienced by these professionals who were in the front line in fighting the pandemic.

A study conducted on the impact of COVID-19 (Serrão, Duarte, Castro, & Teixeira, 2021) analyzed the role of resilience in depression, anxiety and burnout in health professionals and concluded that most of health professionals show signs of physical or psychological exhaustion and burnout related to the exercise of their profession during the COVID-19 pandemic. To corroborate this idea, Mendes, Cabral & Melo (2021) state that since social workers have an intervention based on professional relationships with other people, they are still involved in solving social, emotional, and physical problems. Thus, when experiencing these situations, they may awaken feelings that are detrimental to their well-being and quality of life.

Many of the stress factors listed by the interviewed social workers are common to each other. The most commonly mentioned stress factors and causes were: lack of time; the increased volume of work; that social work, even more so in a health context, was a profession that dealt directly with problems that would lead to accumulation of stress; pressure demanded of professionals; accumulation of functions; work overload; tiredness; and even the decrease in the quality of professional care, the latter being less mentioned by the interviewees.

"The social worker deals with all that (treatment, clinical diagnosis), deals with the informal network, with the personal problems that the person may have, in short, I think the social worker has an extra [of stress] here" (SW11)

"I have positive stress when I have a new situation that I have to go learn so to know how to respond to and that challenges me, and I have adrenaline, and I call that positive stress. Then I have negative stress, which is caused by all this overload that comes from years and years of buildup, of not having resources, of not having an information system, and the internal and external complications that people sometimes encounter and that make difficult situations. And also, negative stress from the lack of social responses that are inadequate to the population we serve." (SW12)

According to Carrera (2011), the fact that social workers work in vulnerability frameworks characterized by situations of inequality makes this profession and its professionals more prone to stress and burnout, because "if at the beginning there is a great commitment / dedication to work, sometime later they experience a shock with reality" (Carrera, 2011, p.22). With the analysis of this dimension, it was possible to realize that regardless of the level of pandemic incidence, stress factors were common and many of them associated with the working conditions in which social workers in the health area perform their functions. During the pandemic, the interviewees indicated the following stress factors: Emergency in resolving social cases; Increased pressure on social workers; Adaptation to the new reality; Difficulties in transmitting information to the family; Difficulties in finding social answers in the community; Difficulty in effecting hospital discharge; Telework; Excessive work/overtime; Lack of human resources; Fear of disease/emotional distress; Working with vulnerable population; Lack of institutional guidelines. Therefore, one can understand through the data presented that there was an increase in the pressure placed on social workers, a factor that was aggravated with the emergence of the pandemic crisis, but which was already evident and present before COVID-19 appeared. These aspects have also been identified by Cardoso, Vilar & Casquilho-Martins (2020) when they verified a series of difficulties experienced by professionals from different areas and sectors, which restricted the professional practice of social workers during the first phase of the pandemic.

Regarding the consequences, the influence of stress and burnout in professional practice in the health context was due to several factors mentioned above, such as the lack of adequate responses to the users' needs, communication barriers with effects on the relationships established in the professional context, and the insufficient number of professionals and human resources in the health area. Other factors at a more macro-level, such as the lack of information and guidelines for action, as well as limitations in the recognition and appreciation of the profession, were also factors that generated stress.

One aspect mentioned were the changes in the relations among colleagues and how during this period the emotional management was even more demanding due to the physical distance measures imposed, which altered proximity and the relationship created with colleagues, professionals and users. The interviewees stated that stress and burnout impact the relationship with patients, as well as on performing the professional activity itself, being a situation that limits professional skills, both in terms of the more instrumental tasks and in terms of relational skills, which are strongly marked by the fear of the new coronavirus and by demotivation towards work.

"I didn't have moments of crying or anxiety attacks, but I did have moments of questioning whether this was what I wanted for my life, this kind of work, whether I was doing things right. I was demotivated and there were even days when you respond more harshly to colleagues" (SW2)

"If the professional is in a situation of burnout, it is an immense risk both for the professional, because every day they test their limits, and for the user because he will not find the response from someone who is at his full competencies and capacities." (SW13)

Regarding short-term consequences, the accumulation of workload was mentioned in relation to the inability to respond and the difficulty in adequately performing professional activities when experiencing stress or burnout, as well as the isolation from teammates and the lack of initiative or interest in professional activity. When referring to the long-term consequences, the interviewees mentioned further consequences, with more serious effects: exhaustion and fatigue; low productivity; failures in professional activity; professional demotivation and disinterest; and depression and anxiety. Other consequences mentioned were the onset of illnesses, psychological leave, absences from work, personal life problems, difficulty in managing emotions, and hindered relational ability towards others.

As for the manifested symptoms, some social workers shared experiences of stress and burnout that reveal the impacts these have on the professionals' own health and well-being. Some reports do not refer to situations that occurred to the interviewees themselves, but to other social workers with whom they work in the health area. Since the intention of this study was to understand if stress affected the professionals to the point of having a burnout syndrome, the data collected allows to realize that there were indeed professionals who had already felt they were experiencing burnout according to the definition of these concepts. However, none of the professionals reported they had the feeling of burnout after the pandemic started, yet five expressed they had already suffered burnout throughout their professional career. Additionally, the professionals who said they had experienced burnout fit into the three levels of pandemic incidence, which demonstrates that it was not related to the new reality experienced, but rather to the very demands of professional activity in this area of intervention.

Strategies for Prevention and Management of Stress in Healthcare Social Workers

Gomes & Cruz (2004) emphasize that the harmful effects of stress and burnout on the physical and mental health, satisfaction, performance, and productivity of professionals are well known, and it is also important to intervene to prevent them. Regardless of whether the professionals interviewed had reached the point of burnout, it was verified that they felt stress before and during the pandemic in the exercise of their professional activity and that this manifested a set of harmful effects on their well-being and detrimental to the quality of the work performed. One effect mentioned by several social workers was the alteration in their relational capacity and emotional fragility, which was felt to be passed onto their professional performance.

To understand how social workers responded to the stress felt during their professional activity in the pandemic's context, it is important to identify the strategies that were adopted both in relation to the organizational context and in the management of their own professional activity. With regard to the prevention of stress and consequently of an evolution towards a burnout diagnosis, the professional domain strategies mentioned by the sample were more directed towards the self-management of their work plans. Examples were prioritizing tasks to be performed, planning in advance the working day, adapting work according to the needs felt, holding multidisciplinary meetings, asking for help among colleagues and collaborating among colleagues.

"On a professional level, in my opinion, it would be sharing things with colleagues, understanding the different views that exist, right, sharing so that we can solve a problem... also defining work priorities, that's very important." (SW1)

"Outlining your work, organizing it, is up to each one's personal competence, but from my perspective, it's the organization. Sometimes it's difficult, but if there's a common thread, if everything is written down and you see what there is to do, what I've already done and what is a priority, that's a good way of working." (SW3)

Besides strategies with a focus on intrinsic situations or circumstances that can be managed and controlled by the professionals themselves, strategies that could be implemented at a broader level of the organizational structure were also indicated. Thus, regarding the organizational strategies that could be applied to minimize the impact of stress and burnout on their professional activity, the social workers repeated some of the previously mentioned strategies. However, the following were recorded as relevant responses in this domain: the need for professional supervision, the need for a salary increase, more human resources, more regularity of multidisciplinary team meetings, improved organizational leadership, more encouragement to professionals, longer break periods, and flexible working hours.

As a result, a greater investment in the health professionals that integrate the National Health Service is pointed out as a strategy that could prevent stress in the organizational domain. This includes the increase in salaries that would provide professionals with greater satisfaction through monetary compensation for their work, while enhancing the appreciation and recognition of the role of professionals and of the importance of the profession in the health field. On the other hand, the number of social workers assigned to the different services and health teams is clearly insufficient according to the interviewees, which, with the increase of human resources in the area of Social Work, would imply less pressure and less frustration in the existing working staff, tackling the inability to respond due to lack of human resources. More regular multidisciplinary meetings would also be a way for social workers to feel more capable of organizing their work method, since some professionals claim to be dependent on the medical and nursing teams for the signaling of situations that require Social Work intervention. Professional supervision allows for the discussion and critical evaluation of the executed work, thus becoming more efficient and effective. Supervision has contributed to the prevention of work stress, better productivity in the organizations themselves, and to a higher quality in the services provided. Finally, it is noteworthy that the professionals claim to need more rest periods, since they are currently exceeding the contracted working hours and do not have the regulatory breaks to which they are entitled. Professional rest is essential for stress prevention, but often cannot be guaranteed due to the urgency and emergency of the situations in which they intervene. In this sense, it would be important to have more flexible working hours.

In the professional's management capacity domain, regarding strategies that come from the social workers' own initiative as mechanisms for stress prevention, planning in advance the work to be performed each day and prioritizing work tasks are identified as relevant strategies. Planning and prioritization of activities should respect the tasks to be performed, organizing them in accordance with their functions and the needs of the services, contemplating periods for emergency situations. From here, it is also important to practice forms of collaborative work and mutual assistance among professionals, with the cohesion among team members being a fundamental support for well-being in the work context. Finally, it is mentioned that it is necessary to distance oneself from the professional as to not allow a personal level of involvement in the cases that they accompany, since there is an intense emotional stress for those who work in the health area.

The professionals interviewed determined some mechanisms of action and resolution of the impacts of the same stress and burnout in their professional activity. The mechanism most referred to by social workers was the organization and prioritization of work, as had also been demonstrated concerning stress prevention strategies. Accordingly, there is not a very significant difference between what could be implemented as a strategy to prevent stress and burnout, or to mitigate and solve the impacts. However, the results show that there is a greater individualization of the mechanisms mentioned, and therefore, a greater personal accountability in resolving these scenarios.

As for procedures to handle stress and burnout named by the social workers, these professionals ended up adopting practices in order to minimize the impact that stress had or could have in their lives. From the interview excerpts, it is perceived that professionals prioritize well-being actions in their personal lives: relaxation, physical activity, managing emotions, taking breaks during working hours, strengthening teamwork, and, finally, having good family support. It is also understood that the strategies adopted are associated with the lifestyle of each professional and their informal network, while also being dependent on the organizational environment. Finally, it is highlighted that these practices of stress prevention and management are common to many professionals, albeit working in different contexts, in different regions of the country and with different levels of pandemic incidence.

CONCLUSION

In contemporary times, the social worker profession is progressively faced with more challenges, that can lead professionals to assume more visible positions before organizational bodies in the search for the improvement of citizens' living conditions and reality (Santos, 2017). These challenges refer to deontological and ethical aspects that should be anchored in their objectives, aiming at change and development, as well as promoting human relationships and the strengthening of people's empowerment and well-being (Sousa, 2015).

During the pandemic crisis, social inequalities were accentuated and the need to meet the urgent needs that arose led to challenging times. Besides the fact that social workers were already exposed to stressful activities, the pandemic brought some factors that can lead to high levels of stress and internal and external conflicts, such as the emergence of consequences that can arise at the psychosocial and mental health level of professionals working in health care. The effects of the pandemic crisis on the professional activity of social workers in health care caused changes in the work dynamics of health services and led to negative impacts. These impacts included the existence of internal conflicts and the difficulty of articulation with other social responses in the community, since many were subject to closure and others continued without full response capacity. The pressure felt by social workers to resolve cases, namely for social discharges and to refer users to the appropriate responses in the community, was always present as a major stressor, with the pandemic exacerbating this issue. Therefore, the specificity of stress in social workers is due to the responsibility and demands of the professional practice itself, which allowed the characterization of the factors and causes of stress in health work contexts, namely in Social Work during the pandemic.

In this way, it becomes clear that stress and burnout in professionals is defined by different factors that, in an uncertain context such as the one experienced due to COVID-19, can generate impacts directly on health professionals, particularly social workers, and consequently on the quality of the services they provide. It becomes, therefore, important to reflect on the challenges listed here to provide a better service to citizens and safeguard mental health of professionals.

REFERENCES

Batista, E. C., Matos, L. A. L., & Nascimento, A. B. (2017). A entrevista como técnica de investigação na pesquisa qualitativa. *Revista Interdisciplinar Científica Aplicada*, *11*(3), 23–38.

Branco, F., & Farçadas, M. (2012). O Serviço Social nos cuidados de saúde primários: contexto, perspetivas e desafios. In M. I. Carvalho (Ed.), *Serviço Social na Saúde* (pp. 1–24). Pactor.

Cardoso, J., Vilar, D., & Casquilho-Martins, I. (2020). Desafios ao Serviço Social no contexto da COVID-19. *Intervenção Social, 55/56*, 9–87. doi:10.34628/9y57-1x20

Carrera, J. F. G. F. (2011). *Stress e Burnout: um estudo de caso de assistentes sociais que trabalham com idosos em IPSS's* [Master's Thesis, Instituto Superior de Ciências Sociais e Políticas]. http://hdl.handle.net/10400.5/3097

Carvalho, M. I. (Ed.). (2012). *Serviço Social na Saúde*. Pactor.

Casquilho-Martins, I. (2022). Consequences of COVID-19: Limitations to the Quality of Palliative Care and Social Work Intervention. *Journal of Social Work in End-of-Life & Palliative Care, 18*(3), 195–198. doi:10.1080/15524256.2022.2050338 PMID:35333687

Casquilho-Martins, I., & Ferreira, S. (2022). Migrants' Health Policies and Access to Health Care in Portugal within the European Framework. *Societies (Basel, Switzerland), 12*(2), 55. doi:10.3390oc12020055

Comissão Nacional de Cuidados Paliativos. (2021). *Plano Estratégico para o Desenvolvimento dos Cuidados Paliativos 2021–2022*. http://www.acss.min-saude.pt/wp-content/uploads/2017/01/PEDCP-2021_2022.pdf

Conselho Nacional de Saúde. (2020). *Portugal e a resposta à covid-19 a posição do Conselho Nacional de Saúde e o contributo das entidades que o constituem*. https://www.cns.min-saude.pt/wp-content/uploads/2020/10/CNS_Reflexao-Conselho-Nacional-Saude-resposta-COVID-19.pdf

Flick, U. (2005). Métodos Qualitativos na Investigação Científica. *Monitor (Charlottetown)*.

Gomes, A. R., & Cruz, J. F. (2004). A experiência de stresse e "burnout" em psicólogos portugueses: Um estudo sobre as diferenças de género. *Psicologia: Teoria, Investigação e Prática, 9*(2), 193–212.

Goulão, M. P. de L. M. S. (2017). *Efeitos do clima de comunicação organizacional no "stress", "work" "engagement" e comportamentos extra-papel* [Doctoral Thesis, Iscte – Instituto Universitário de Lisboa]. http://hdl.handle.net/10071/15427

Guerra, I. C. (2006). *Pesquisa qualitativa e análise de conteúdo. Sentido e formas de uso*. Principia Editora.

Mendes, J., Cabral, H., & Melo, F. (2021). Burnout em profissionais de Serviço Social durante a pandemia de COVID. *Revista Portuguesa De Investigação Comportamental E Social, 7*(1), 25–40. doi:10.31211/rpics.2021.7.1.204

Miranda, S. C. C. (2011). *Stress ocupacional, burnout e suporte social nos profissionais de saúde mental* [Master's Thesis, Universidade Católica Portuguesa]. http://hdl.handle.net/10400.14/8796

Monteiro, A. P., Cunha, P., Simões, M., & Relva, I. (2021). Conflitos Psicossociais e saúde mental em período de pandemia. In P. Cunha & A. P. Monteiro (Eds.), *Gestão de conflitos na saúde* (pp. 197–212). Pactor.

Ramos, M. A. S. (2005). *Crianças, tecnologias e aprendizagem: contributo para uma teoria substantiva* [Doctoral Thesis, Universidade do Minho]. https://hdl.handle.net/1822/6914

Reigada, C. (Ed.). (2020). *Boas Práticas do Assistente Social COVID-19 (Perspetiva: grupo de Assistentes Sociais de Cuidados Paliativos).* https://drive.google.com/file/d/1ZMw0_KaeaDf2fkVOgLhS4p5gsAOwWgc5/view

Sakellarides, C. (2020). National Health Service: Responding to Current Challenges Through Necessary Transformations. *Acta Medica Portuguesa, 33*(2), 133–142. doi:10.20344/amp.12626 PMID:32035499

Santos, M. F. J. (2017). *A Prática Profissional Do Assistente Social Em Contexto De Cuidados De Saúde Primários Infantojuvenis* [Master's Thesis, Instituto Superior de Serviço Social do Porto]. http://hdl.handle.net/10400.26/22393

Serrão, C., Duarte, I., Castro, L., & Teixeira, A. (2021). Burnout and Depression in Portuguese Healthcare Workers during the COVID-19 Pandemic—The Mediating Role of Psychological Resilience. *International Journal of Environmental Research and Public Health, 18*(2), 636. doi:10.3390/ijerph18020636 PMID:33451083

Sousa, I. (2015). Serviço Social em debate: Que referenciais genéricos? *Intervenção Social, 42/45*, 11–23.

World Health Organization. (2019). *Burn-out an "occupational phenomenon": International Classification of Diseases.* https://www.who.int/news/item/28-05-2019-burn-out-an-occupational-phenomenon-international-classification-of-diseases

World Health Organization. (2022). *Mental health: Strengthening our response.* https://www.who.int/en/news-room/fact-sheets/detail/mental-health-strengthening-our-response

Chapter 11
Work and Life Balance Post COVID-19

Aditi Singh Sharma
https://orcid.org/0000-0003-0705-8208
Amity University, Ranchi, India

ABSTRACT

The chapter explores the issue of work-life balance and its importance to the individual and the organization. The work-life balance issue is defined and looked at from all perspectives. The chapter will study the major components that affect work-life balance. The chapter will make an evaluative study of the way individuals and organizations have tried to approach the issue of work and life balance post COVID-19. Next, the chapter will explore the emerging challenge for people to balance work and home post COVID-19 after working from home for over two years. The emergence of digital technology and how it has impacted the global work and life balance will be discussed. Further, it elaborates how the COVID-19 pandemic has impacted the global workplace and why striking the right work and life balance is a challenge for humankind like never before. Finally, the chapter will conclude by looking into how people and organizations achieve the right balance in the new post-COVID-19 paradigm.

INTRODUCTION

The quest for all human endeavours is enduring joy and happiness. Every individual tries to achieve a state of abundant happiness for self and family. Throughout history the concept of nurturing self and family has been the over-riding thought that has led people to engage in various activities. People looked for sustainable sources of livelihood to provide for the families. In their quest for livelihood the nature and tenor of activities kept changing. The responsibility of fending for the family was pretty much on the man of the house. Women were involved in nurturing and taking care of men and children in the family. The roles were pretty well defined and it was an unwritten code that was accepted by all societies across the world. There doesn't seem to be much differentiation to be seen across the continents.

The concept of workplace was not delineated as the primary task was to take up activities in the field of food production. People were engaged in primary activities and men and women both contributed

DOI: 10.4018/978-1-6684-8565-1.ch011

in the agriculture and allied activities. Majority of households earned their livelihood through farming and other household based activities. People lived in small, rural communities and there was not much travel involved for work. Families were large with several members living together in small communities. Work essentially was of localized nature and did not involve much dislocation.

The first significant alterations to this way of life can be seen around 200 years ago starting from Europe primarily Britain. The advent of the Industrial Revolution in the 18th century left a profound impact on how people lived and the way the world of organizations evolved. The development of the mechanized production systems led to the establishment of factories and the modern cities of today. Wage employment gradually became an alternative source of income apart from the families' traditional sources of livelihood. People began working for companies. Often the working conditions and wages were not as desired. However, working for such businesses still paid a better living than farming.

Across the rest of the world the 19th Century saw the emergence of the work for wage employment. The colonial powers used the large population to create a labor force and set up manufacturing bases in far away countries. The 20th Century saw the acceleration of this process. These changes altered the fabric of human life and endeavours. Working people were engaged in leaving their small communities and seek employment in places away from their parental homes. The gradual shift from the agrarian to the industrial economies brought about significant changes to the lifestyles of people. The evolution of the human resource movement started looking into the conditions at the workplace. The concept of valuing the individual as a critical resource probably led to the emergence of the concept of work and life balance.

The concept of human as a resource emerged. This led to the development of the concept of human resource management; to deal with the issues pertaining to the human at the work place. The academic world was also involved in conducting surveys, studies and research to assist and manage the vast multitude of the workforce. Several studies were conducted to study the human behavior at work looking into issues pertaining to achieving good work-life balance.

As the 21st century dawned with the power of digital technology; the employment opportunities in the services sector have evolved at a rapid pace. This trend has significantly altered the lifestyle and family patterns. The work and life balance debate increased in significance as family patterns were affected. Several studies and research have proven and recognized that the people coming to work are emotional beings connected to family and society. So every worker is trying to strike the optimum balance between the responsibilities of the family, society and organization. Since there are only 24 hours in a day the appropriate apportioning had to be done as per the individual preferences and choices.

Any discussions about the work and life balance conundrum will be lop-sided without the consideration of the fact that men and women have to be studied differently. Over the last century the number of women taking up wage employment has significantly increased. Men and women could perform the same tasks with equal elan without the element of physical differentiation. This has led to a rapid rise in the women workforce across the globe. This is another factor that has led to the concept of work and life balance debate taking centre-stage in recent times. Organizations are now waking up to the reality that the work-and-life balance is an essential part of why employees stay where they are, so knowing how to give them a good work-and-life balance is crucial today. Many organizations have faced the challenge of people giving up jobs to achieve balance in the pursuit of happiness.

The issues at the work environment are more impactful on the work-life imbalance than the family environment. Work involves time to be dedicated to completing the task at hand on a daily, weekly, and monthly basis at the workplace. It involves long working hours, work intensity, and fulfilling organizational targets. High work intensity or work pressure may result in fatigue, anxiety, or other physiological consequences that affect the quality of home and family life. Since there is limited time in which people have to perform many other activities other than their jobs; striking the right time balance between work and family or personal time becomes stressful even in normal times; leave alone the challenges unleashed by the COVID and the post-COVID era. Striking the right balance between work responsibilities and family responsibility becomes a matter of emotional discord affecting all aspects of life. For those who think that the main objective in life is to work; their career becomes the core of life. Individuals have family responsibilities e.g., looking after the old members, children. Further, people find time to engage in relaxation, vacations, sports, and personal development programs. Work and life balance is not the allocation of time equally among work, family, and personal demands. It is s also emphasized that work and life balance is a subjective phenomenon that changes from person to person. In this regard, work and life balance should be regarded as allocating the available resources like time, thought, and labor wisely among the elements of life. While some adopt the philosophy of "living to work"; see work as the principal objective. Others consider "working to live", focusing on family and personal life on an equal measure.

WORK AND LIFE BALANCE

Any attempt at defining what work and life balance means is a difficult task as there is multitude of variables involved. There is no perfect, one-size fits all, work-life balance that can be defined. At best work-life balance is different for each individual because everyone has different priorities. The work-life balance for an individual will vary over time. The right balance for when a person is single will be different from when the person gets married; or if they have children. Work-life balance will have different connotations when a person is starting a new career. Similarly the balance will vary for those in the middle of their career or nearing retirement. The notion of work-life balance will vary from men to women even within the same organization, social or cultural settings.

Researchers are divided in their opinion about work-life balance. Generally they agree that work-life balance translates to satisfaction with one's entire life - professional and personal. Work-life balance does not mean an equal balance between work and life. Trying to schedule an equal number of hours for work and personal activities is practically next to impossible. The connotations will change depending upon the socio-economic and cultural settings. Thus, work-life balance for an American will be vastly different from that of the Japanese. Similarly, it will mean different things for an Indian as compared to a European individual.

However, despite these variations the concept of work–life balance can be looked at as establishing the right mix between professional and personal life. Identifying and setting up the right priorities for professional as well as personal life. The time spent at work compared with the time spent with the managing responsibilities in the family and doing things that one can enjoy. Work-life balance can be viewed as establishing a relative state of equilibrium between peoples' primary priorities of their responsibilities at work and their private lifestyle. Majority of the psychologists agree that the demands of an individual's career should not overwhelm the individual's ability to enjoy a satisfying personal life. Creating and establishing the right work-life balance lies not only in carefully defining how one wants to spend time, but in making sure that there is the right adjustment made when needs change. Sometimes even small changes can make a difference. A sudden change in schedule or out of control home life can lead to stress and depression, poor performance at work, and conflict within the family.

The concept of work-life balance took centre-stage around the 1980's. The policies and programs set up by an organization with the goal to enable employees to efficiently do their jobs and at the same time provide flexibility to handle personal concerns or problems on their family front. The emergence of the dual-wage-earning families brought about significant alterations to the circumstances under which men and women tried to strike the right work-life balance. A balanced work and life is supposed to exist when there is a proper functioning at work and at home with a minimum of role conflict. Consequently, the incompatibility between the demands from the work and non-work environments gives rise to conflict and consequently, people experience a lack of work-life balance. There is confirmation of the fact that people entering the workforce today are laying emphasis on the importance of work-life balance more than their predecessors. In spite of this, the extent to which this balance is being achieved is far less than what is desired. In fact, researches bring to mind that graduates are being drawn into situations where they have to work for progressively longer hours and so experience an increasingly unsatisfactory balance between home life and work-life.

It is a general notion that employees need to work long hours and deal with difficult and complex issues. Some days on the job are likely to be filled with fun and positive and other days are tension-filled and stressful. A major dilemma for many people is how they manage all of the competing demands in work and life and avoid letting any negative effects of work spill over into their personal lives.

Research has in fact shown that employees who believe they do not have time for the personal life feel drained and distracted while they are at work. In addition, the spillover of negative aspect of work into an employee's personal life can lead to job exhaustion, disruption of relationships with family and friends, loss of enjoyment, and increased stress. Work-life balance is about creating and maintaining supportive and healthy work environments, which will enable employees to have balance between work and personal responsibilities and thus strengthen employee loyalty and productivity.

"Eight hours to work, Eight hours to play, Eight hours to sleep, Eight bob a day. A fair day's work, for a fair day's pay." This mantra was intoned by stonemasons who walked off their jobsite at Melbourne University in 1856. According to Franklin (2010), these skilled workers were among the first in the world to achieve an 8-hour working day. The nineteenth-century movement for a 40-hour working week recognized the rights of humans for lives that included work, recreation, family, and recuperation and effectively preempted and sculpted the shape of the modern concept of work–life balance. Initially a simple formula in an era when the workforce was predominantly male, the concept has remained difficult to define and operationalize (Kalliath and Brough 2008). This could largely be due to paradigms suggesting that balance was about portions of time and the domains of work, home, and social life were separate entities. Kanter (1977) challenged any notion of such separation, tendering that the different domains of workers' lives were permeable and interconnected. In addition, societal changes precipitated by the entrance of large numbers of women into the workplace, simulating consequent changes in traditionally socially predetermined gender roles balanced against organizational imperatives for productivity gains, have also exacerbated the importance of the work–life interface (Brough et al. 2007; Lappegard et al. 2017)

Within the last 20 years, scholars have attempted to provide a more integrated view of the work–family interface, and work–life balance has been a dominant concept reflecting this perspective. However, while the term work–life balance is commonly coined, it is "a concept whose popular usage has outpaced its theoretical development" (Valcour 2007, p. 1513). Across the literature, there is still not a clear consistency in terms used to articulate the construct, and the themes that underpin conceptualizations of the construct are varied. Initial attempts to operationalize work–life balance drew upon the two primary perspectives in the extant literature, that is, role conflict and role enrichment. Within these approaches, work–life balance was commonly represented by an absence of work–family conflict coupled with high levels of work–family enrichment (Duxbury and Higgins 2001; O'Driscoll et al. 2006). Other early conceptualizations of work–life balance focused on the notion of equal distribution of resources across work and family or other life roles. Following this approach, Kirchmeyer (2000) suggested that balance is achieved when an individual's time, energy, and commitment are evenly distributed across life roles. Meanwhile, Marks and MacDermid (1996) defined role balance as being fully engaged across all life roles. Greenhaus et al. (2003) also progressed the equality approach, suggesting that work–life balance is "the extent to which an individual is engaged in and equally satisfied with his or her work role and family role"

Components of this definition include equal time, involvement, and satisfaction across an individual's work and non-work roles. The equality approach, however, has received criticism, with researchers suggesting that it fails to account for an individual's role preferences or their subjective sense of balance (Brough et al. 2007). For example, Kalliath and Brough (2008b) described balance as the extent to which investment in roles is consistent with the importance or salience an individual places on a role. Similarly, work–life balance has been described as the extent to which an individual's needs for autonomy, competence, and connection with others are met. While, Voydanoff (2002) focused on the fit with available resources, suggesting that work–life balance is achieved when personal resources are adequate to meet demands in work and family roles, thereby enabling effective participation in each domain.

Establishing a harmonious balance between work and personal life is critical to creating a healthy and stress-free environment and allowing employees to unleash their full potential. However, striking a good work-life balance is a challenge for most workers. It is also believed that creating a flexible and family friendly workplace can help to improve the well-being of the workforce.

FACTORS IMPACTING WORK-LIFE BALANCE

People who see work and non-work as two separate spheres tend to get frustrated when they conflict with one another. A coping mechanism might be to view life holistically, where everything is a part of the work - life balance. If the employees don't have a good work-life balance, they may not feel as happy with their job and want to leave. A poor work-life balance can also negatively affect employee's health and overall work output. In fact, studies show working over 55 hours a week can increase a person's risk of heart attack and stroke. According to Lowe, work and life imbalance affect the overall well-being of the individual causing such problems as dissatisfaction with life, prolonged sadness, and using drugs or alcohol.

Two American cardiologists Rosenman and Friedman determined two different types of personality depending on heart disorders and individual behaviors: type A and type B. Type A express someone who is more active, more work-oriented, more passionate, and competitive, while Type B is calm, patient, balanced and right-minded. It can be argued that since type A is more work-oriented, there will be a negative reflection of its work and life balance. Work-a-holism, which is considered an obsessive behavior, is another thing that destroys work and life balance. When work-a-holism connotes addiction to work, being at work for a very long time, overworking, and busy with work at times out of work. Since life is not only about work, work-a-holics suffer from alienation, family problems, and some health problems. It is assumed that workaholics neglect their families, friends, relations, and other social responsibilities.

Stress–based conflict occurs when one of the roles of the individual at work or in the family causes stress on the individual and this stress affects the other roles of the individual. Behavior stress occurs when the behavior at work and out of work is dissonant and conflicting.

The organization expects individuals to allocate more time for their work while at the same time the family wants them to perform their responsibilities too. Those who can't sustain a work-life balance are bound to experience many problems in their families such as lower family satisfaction, decreased involvement in family roles, etc. Those whose demands of the family and one's social interest are not met duly naturally prefer sacrificing their working hours and carrying out their personal needs.

To decrease the negative consequences of work and family conflict on working individuals, family-friendly organizational culture and human resources applications have recently been on agenda of the executives. The components of the organizational strategy are flexible working hours, child care and elderly care scheme, home working, and job sharing.

Supportive programs for the family life of employees in an organization contribute to providing work-life balance. Thanks to these programs, the employees will be encouraged, their attendance will be supported and their efficiency will increase. Flexible working hours are one of the methods used to maintain work-life balance. For example employees with flexi-time will have to fulfill a certain amount of time weekly. Another thing that can be done is to allow employees to work at home away from the traditional work environment.

If one has managed to allocate the required time for every aspect of life duly and not to reflect the problems in one part of life to another it means that he has been able to achieve a work-family balance. Life as a whole is composed of many other aspects along with work. Those who have achieved a balance among these aspects are sure to achieve a life balance, which does away with any imbalance.

Job resources are the physical, psychological, social, or organizational aspects of the job that facilitate the achievement of work goals. In general, employees strive to protect their current resources and acquire new resources, which enable them to cope with their job demands (Halbesleben et al. 2014). Similar to job demands, job resources are also categorized as time-based resources (e.g., job flexibility and alternative work schedules), cognitive resources (e.g., mental resilience and attention), emotional resources (e.g., mood and optimism), or physical resources (e.g., strength and skills). Evidence is consistent that job resources have a positive impact on work–life balance. For example, Hill et al. (2001) found that job flexibility in terms of timing (flextime) and work location (flexiplace) generated a positive spillover effect from work to home, helping employees to achieve work–life balance. Similarly, Ferguson et al. (2012) demonstrated that both co-worker and partner support reinforced positive experiences facilitating work–life balance. Finally, both Greenhaus et al. (2012) and Brough et al. (2005) also showed that having a supervisor who was supportive of an employee's family demands was positively related to the employee's levels of work–life balance

Less attention has been focused on the family-related antecedents of work–life balance. The associations between family-related antecedents and work–life balance are generally weaker than compared to the associations between work-related antecedents and work–life balance. Alongside partner support (Ferguson et al. 2012), other specific family resources demonstrating an influence for work–life balance include family support (Russo et al. 2016), family-to-work enrichment (Chan et al. 2016), spending quality time with children (Milkie et al. 2010), partner's work–life balance satisfaction (Stock et al. 2014), and home-based business (Walker et al. 2008). Interestingly, these family resources have been found to benefit female employees more than male employees. Family demands which have been examined in relation to work–life balance include family involvement (Aryee et al. 2005; Stock et al. 2014) and caring for children and/or aging parents and relatives (Brough and O'Driscoll 2005; Neal and Hammer 2017). Family demands predominately affect employees juggling both work and family commitments and generally hinder an individual's ability to achieve their desired level of work–life balance (Chan et al. 2017).

Job security and the consequent financial stability is an important factor for work-life balance optimization. The overall socio-economic condition leads to emergence and growth of stable organizations. These factors have a positive impact on the work-life balance. People with stable jobs and financial security have a balanced work-life equation. Those with job and financial insecurity are liable to struggle with work-life balance.

Another important factor that impacts work-life balance is the age of the work-force. On the whole people in the middle-aged working population are more challenged with the issues pertaining to work-life balance. In most cases the responsibility of managing and running a family conflicts with the responsibilities at work. The pressures on time will be felt more by those managing both work and family. Those young in age are part of the younger work-force; are relatively free from the pressures on time due to family responsibility. Those who are married will have to work out the work-life balance as compared to those who are unmarried. Issues concerning and related to marriage have been a significant factor in determining work-life balance. The significant rise in the number of the Double-Income-No-Kids (DINK) families in Japan can be seen as a direct consequence of families dealing with the work-life conundrum. This is a global trend as the size of the families with reduced number of children can be seen across all major societies,

Another perspective worth noting is the fact that in the latter half of the 20th century; the transition from the colonial societies to the emergence of the independent nation states made a significant impact on the issues concerning work-life balance. The dynamic socio-economic factors played a significant role. The same period saw the emergence of the multi-national corporations defining the norms and standards for managing the global work-force. It was assumed that the people irrespective of their social background will try to achieve the same work-life balance. Several governments made legal and regulatory provisions to deal with the issues of work-life balance. Thus we see that most of the laws framed from time to time have tried to address the issues and factors impacting the work-life balance. Most significant amongst those have been the regulations made to protect the work-life balance for the women workforce.

WORK-LIFE BALANCE ACROSS SECTORS

Issues concerning work – life balance vary from sector to sector. Millions of employees have had to figure out how to divide work and home time. Before the COVID-19 pandemic hit it was easier for employees to separate their work and personal lives.

In the primary agricultural sector people are mostly engaged in their own activities. There is very little in terms of regular wage employment. Whatever labor is involved is pretty much engaged on a daily wage basis. So it is next to impossible to map issues concerning work-life balance for those in this sector. Rural or cottage based small industries are run on an ownership basis with very little organized workforce. People are engaged in various work and non-work activities and there seemingly is no pressure in terms of work hours. The flexibility available to people probably helps balance out the work – life conundrum. Further, the rural societies across the world is engaged in lots of non-work activities that gives people a semblance of satisfaction and happiness. People are not stressed out and have the ease of life not available to those in the urban areas. The COVID pandemic has not altered the working patterns of people engaged in the primary sector.

The industrial sector on the other hand has dominated the employment opportunities generated across the world over the last century. It has been a principal factor for the growth of the modern cities in every country. It has caused large scale migration of people seeking employment and business opportunities. The working style involved lot of traveling to and from work adding to the pressure on time available on a per day basis.

A forty hour work week was the accepted norm for the industrial workforce. Organizations structured their human resource management around the concept that people will be asked to work in regimented shifts. Over-time was well defined. Several nations created regulations and laws to be implemented to manage the organizations and their workforce. People could devote ample time outside the work hours for family and personal life. For much of the pre-COVID era it was the established norm and those working found out ways and means to balance the work-life conundrum. The COVID pandemic has brought about large-scale impact. Initially the entire workforce was affected due to the lockdowns. Subsequently, several industries were put out of business due to the prolonged economic impact. People who were struggling to balance out the work – life equation were provided the time to rethink and reorient their lives.

The last decade of the 20th century and the first two decades of the 21st century have seen a major shift with the growth of the services sector across the world. It is significant to note that the internet and digital era created opportunities for a large employment seeking population. Man-hours and man days were created as work involved 24/7 working. The global connectivity facilitated opportunities for the growth of the Business Process Outsourcing and other similar industries. The penetration of the digital mobile services into the rural heartlands across the world facilitated employment generation. Thus, a large number of people have entered the global workforce. In the five years preceding the COVID pandemic concepts like work from anywhere, flexi-working hours, remote working gained acceptance. People could work out of their homes and could feel a sense of satisfaction as the travel to and from work component was taken out of the work-life balance equation. Organizations were divided on their opinions and choices to let employees work without coming to office. The COVID pandemic forced a complete shutdown of the office space. There was virtual working possible and organizations quickly adopted this model to keep the business going. Post-COVID most organizations continued to give their employees the option of working from locations. However, those engaged in the sector are working way beyond the forty hour work week which was the norm earlier. Many employers moved to virtual work when the COVID-19 pandemic hit. Having to work from home blurred the line between professional and personal life and made it harder for many employees to maintain a work-life balance. When they left the office, they could leave their work there and not bring it home with them. But, remote work makes this separation harder. If there is one sector that has faced the brunt of the COVID pandemic – it is the caregivers in the medical profession.

Recalling pre COVID-19 pandemic life, for decades working in an assigned workspace has been a standard pattern of work in many countries, while conversely, before the pandemic struck, work from home (WFH) was considered as a privilege for certain employees. The COVID-19 pandemic became an unexpected catalyst for remote work and forced a reconsideration of work in terms of the designated workplace location and workplace practices (de Lucas Ancillo et al., 2020; Kniffin et al., 2021; Ratten, 2020; Savi´c, 2020) on a global scale never seen before. It is worth pointing out that many of workers worldwide had never worked from home before. Although there was a slow but gradual increase in the number of remote workers before the pandemic, the world of work has fundamentally changed because of the COVID-19 pandemic: WFH in has become commonplace and meeting virtually is increasingly mainstream.

In the days when Severe Acute Respiratory Syndrome (SARS) swept across the globe in 2003, home working was not an option for most workers worldwide, as the majority of them did not have access to essential devices and equipment to carry out their work at home. This is quite different from working in and after the COVID-19 pandemic era, with technology now providing more options for work practices. In Hong Kong, for example, WFH was not an option for the workforce during SARS. However, in the midst of the ongoing coronavirus disease pandemic, such work arrangements were adjusted based on the severity of the local epidemic situation. Now more than two years into the post-pandemic era, companies worldwide are still pondering the workplace practice that best suits their own needs, and there is no doubt that the lively debate on remote working will continue. Yet this trial run of remote working has shed some light on the future of the workplace, ranging from the tele-work capacity of the economy to the public attitudes toward remote working. All this is owing to the pandemic as an impetus for a massive and unprecedented change. The pandemic has caused an early arrival of the future of work that was initially envisioned by policymakers around the world. All this is affecting the work-life balance conundrum in a significant manner.

IMPACT OF COVID-19 ON WORK-LIFE BALANCE

The COVID pandemic altered everything. The entire world went through the phases of the pandemic which involved periodic lockdowns and isolation to be maintained. The concept of shut down of the workplace forced organizations to explore new avenues to get work done. The digital technology came in handy as people could work from anywhere using the digital tools.

The COVID-19 pandemic has significantly altered the labor markets, triggering major series of experimentations with flexible work arrangements and new relationships to centralized working environments. The new arrangements, especially flexible work arrangements, have challenged traditional relationships with employees and employers, work time and working hours, the work–life balance; and the relationship of individuals to work. There is a clear evidence that hybrid and remote working would be more popular in the post-COVID era for non-manual work, it will not be "one size fits all" solution. Traditional work practices are getting back to the pre-COVID normal and offices have gradually opened up.

The pandemic has affected occupations and segments of the labor market differentially according to the studies and reports emanating from the International Labour Organization (ILO). White-collar workers in particular have been affected by the pandemic, experiencing significant changes in working practices. Work-from-home arrangements have been widespread, with various repercussions in terms of productivity, locality, working hours, and the traditional separation of work and home environments. The home environment is the one that allows the stresses of work to melt away. It permits workers to enjoy time with family separated from work pressures or activities. The conversion of the home environment into a work environment has tended to corrupt the sanctity of the home, with job-related issues fusing into the home and time previously free of work. Firmly demarcated work hours - which begin and end with arriving at and departing from a physical workplace - have disappeared, making it easy to carry on working out of hours and disrupt the home life and Work-Life Balance. In contrast, work and work conditions for blue-collar workers have largely remained unchanged outside of social distancing, sanitation, and related health measures. However, the focus here must not be on how the job has changed, but rather on the implications of continuing to work through the pandemic. Blue-collar workers have been forced to face the health dangers of continued social contact, risking sickness with every interaction. The demands of the job mean that those more vulnerable than others have no alternative safer option. For these workers, sitting at home means being unable to work, adding to the financial strain. Further, continuing to work outside the home may cause tension at home due to the workers being at risk of bringing the virus back and infecting loved ones. Both white-collar and blue-collar workers have been impacted; however, their work practices have changed in different ways because of the COVID-19 pandemic.

The biggest impact of the COVID-19 pandemic is the instability and financial insecurity unleashed by the lockdowns and prolonged shut-down of the workplace. This was most accentuated in the industrial and manufacturing sector. Several organizations have not survived the economic downturn unleashed by the COVID-19 pandemic. People have been consequently forced out of jobs and rendered without job stability. The uncertainty with respect to the future has caused a severe impact on the work-life balance.

In the post-COVID era there is a new norm. The concept of work from anywhere is now a reality. Especially in the services based sector work can be completed in the digital mode. There is also the emergence of the digital corporations – organizations that operate entirely in the digital space of the internet. Also, there is now talk of the meta-physical world and working in the meta space.

The pandemic gave a lot of workers time to re-think and reconsider what they wanted out of their work situations. This reflection led to what emerged as a global trend that has come to be known as the Great Resignation, where many people left their jobs for new opportunities. The truth is - most people didn't leave their job only because of wage or benefits issues. Many also left in pursuit of what is known in Greek as "eudaimonia." The pandemic gave many employees a taste of what their work-life balance could look like, and it's not an experience they'll be quick to forget. This means it's crucial to listen to their feedback and improve the areas of concern in your workplace.

Work and Life Balance has recently taken a centre stage across the globe in the post-COVID era. People have been exposed to new ways of working leading to increased levels of distress and anxiety, particularly as a result of social isolation. Many are facing challenges that can be stressful and overwhelming.

A new approach applied by organizations involves the concept of workplace flexibility. The post-COVID era has shown that flexible working is actually relatively widespread, although this varies at different levels and between sectors. There are examples which show how flexible working arrangements can contribute to managing work and family effectively and also to facilitating employment progression. However, it is to be highlighted that the conflicts between work and care; although women appeared to access fairly widespread flexibility, the extent to which this addressed work-life balance in any tangible way is highly variable. There is ample evidence of such conflicts at all levels and modes of working and highlight how a variety of factors both inside and outside the workplace can affect work-life balance.

Many workers now work from their "workspace" of choice which includes home, office, and co-working spaces. Workers may thereby see better outcomes for their health, family, and overall well-being. While many have adjusted to and enjoyed this change, others have had challenges in drawing a line between working and non-working hours. The likelihood is high for a number of employees to experience increased working hours, as well as increased work-life conflict. For example, in today's hyper-connected world, many remote working employees are expected to respond to urgent tasks as well as after-work emails, resulting in a blur between work and leisure. A recent study revealed that employees working from home (WFH) during the COVID-19 pandemic experienced an increase in work-related fatigue and overlap between work and non-work-life. Different scholars have different views on the impact of remote working on the work-life balance of workers. Some believe that WFH has positive impact on the work-life balance. In contrast, there are adverse effects found in studies where a blur between work-life and personal life is visible and it seems that home-based working may negatively impact work-life balance. However, employees often are not able to balance their work and personal time as their working environment might be flexible, but their hours are increased. It has also been found that working from home or working remotely at least one day a week gave employees a better work-life balance. The trend seems to favour hybrid working over a completely remote working environment.

The COVID-19 pandemic has unleashed key trends that will manifest themselves in the future. Accelerating digital transformation is critical for the workplace. Hybrid work is the new normal at work in the post-pandemic era. Despite this, some work practices will not be eliminated. The existence of the "office" albeit in a modified form. There are induced changes in organizational infrastructure and labor mobility. There is potential exacerbation of existing inequalities. All these trends are significantly affecting the work-life balance. Several organizations have attempted to reduce their working costs by large-scale retrenchment and lay-offs adding to the uncertainty. There is a trend to move from regular work-force to contractual work-force in order to reduce costs and burden. This trend has affected the overall work-life balance negatively.

As the trend seems to favor hybrid working over a completely remote working environment, whole or partial renegotiation and reorganization will be essential. Managers and HR will have to accommodate the changes in organizational strategies as well as in HR policies. People in higher education institutions employees revealed that supervisor support during coronavirus disease helped employees enhance their living quality. Similar it has been reemphasized in coronavirus disease times that supervisors' or managers' support can help employees achieve a good work-life balance. Alternatively, governments may opt to implement specific policies in this regard. One notable example would be to adopt the "right-to-disconnect" law similar to that which is enforced in the Philippines and France, where employees have the right not to respond to work-related engagements and demands during non-working hours. Encouraging healthy work practices such as working within regular hours and taking regular breaks will help employees to draw a firm line between work and non-work activities.

CONCLUSION

The pursuit of happiness is a global phenomenon for all people and societies. Work-life Balance is a significant factor that impacts the happiness quotient from all perspectives. People endeavour to strike the right balance to make the most out of work and life. The two components are like two sides of the coin. The overall demeanour of the society depends upon how well people have been successful at striking the right balance on the work-life balance equation.

Any attempt at defining work-life balance is challenging because of the multiple variables involved. These variables keep changing from one society to the other. Through the ages the work-life balance connotation has changed too because of the dynamic socio-economic factors. Further, the overall work situation has kept changing with the changing times. The most significant changes were seen in the latter half of the 20th century. There are laws and regulations in every country to help manage the work-force and consequently its work-life balance.

Although the work-life balance issue is gender neutral; it is a given fact that the matter and issues concerning work-life balance has been put under critical scrutiny with the rise in the number of women joining the organized work-force. Major provisions have been implemented to help achieve the right balance for the working women as they are significant to the overall management of the family responsibility. For most women who attempt to rise up the corporate ladder; it's always at the cost of compromises with respect to personal life and family. Work-life balance is achieved through the help and support of the other members of the family.

The COVID-19 pandemic affected the global working patterns. To start with people enjoyed the convenience offered by the flexible working options. Work from home and flexible working options gained greater acceptance. There was a semblance of people achieving the right work-life balance. However, this impact was seen more in the sectors that were based on digital functioning. The industrial sector was the worst affected due to the COVID-19 pandemic. Over the last couple of years organizations have been able to get back to the pre-pandemic working mode. There has however been a major transition period for the manufacturing sector as there are new protocols in place to manage another outbreak of the pandemic.

Several people are faced with insecurities with respect to jobs. The consequent financial instability has left a severe impact on the work-life balance equation. The change in the nature of the workplace from the physical to the digital or in many cases phygital – both physical and digital; has caused severe disruptions to the work-life balance. The future uncertainties and financial strain has forced several people to take up multiple jobs simultaneously. This new trend called moonlighting seems to be a new challenge that the organizations are trying to deal with.

Organizations are altering the workplace by changing from regular employment to contractual force. There is also an attempt to bring in fresh young talent with adequate new age skills. This has impacted the work-life balance of the middle-aged working population. There is immense pressure to re-invent under trying circumstances adding to the insecurity and a negative impact on the work-life balance. Those in the middle-aged working population feel the pressure of balancing the time to attend to responsibilities at work and the responsibilities of the family. The younger unmarried work-force is relatively free from the work-life conundrum.

The Post-COVID-19 pandemic era has thrown up new challenges with respect to the issues concerning work-life balance. There appears to be no demarcation between working and non-working hours. Most people were comfortable to start with; however, there are significant reports of people being over-stressed and fatigued. The overall happiness index seems to have been impacted as the digitally wired work-force seems to be on the job 24 hours of the day. The time available to carry out non-work-related activities that somehow balance and helps manage the pressures emanating out of the work-related activities is significantly reduced.

All said and done the COVID-19 pandemic seems to have left a severe long-term impact on the work-life balance. Most of the tremors felt have created a negative impact. There are a few positive trends. Flexi-working and anytime anywhere working are significant factors that will play major role in striking the right work-life balance in the future.

Optimizing the personal and work-life is not easy when adopting a "new normal" working model. Employees need to be disciplined and well-organized in their work and personal life management. In order to attain a work-life balance in the post COVID-19 world, employers may need to consider and plan a way forward such as providing clarity to employees and a variety of programs to support employees in their well-being as well as fostering a "trust- and outcome-based working culture". Employers' attention to employees' work-life balance will assist in keeping employees motivated and maintaining their performance. Therefore, work-life balance in the post-pandemic times is being brought to both employers' and employees' attention and is being considered when developing a plan for policy changes that would benefit both companies and employees.

REFERENCES

Allen, T. (2013). The work-family interface: a synthesis of research from industrial and organizational psychology. In I. Weiner (Ed.), Handbook of psychology (2nd ed., Vol. 12, pp. 698–718). Wiley.

Allen, T. D., & Kiburz, K. M. (2012). Trait mindfulness and work–family balance among working parents: The mediating effects of vitality and sleep quality. *Journal of Vocational Behavior*, *80*(2), 372–379. doi:10.1016/j.jvb.2011.09.002

Aryee, S., Srinivas, E. S., & Tan, H. H. (2005). Rhythms of life: Antecedents and outcomes of work–family balance in employed parents. *The Journal of Applied Psychology*, *90*(1), 132–146. doi:10.1037/0021-9010.90.1.132 PMID:15641894

Brough, P., & O'Driscoll, M. (2005). Work-family conflict and stress. In A. Antoniou & C. Cooper (Eds.), *Research companion to organizational Health Psychology* (pp. 346–365). Edward Elgar Publisher. doi:10.4337/9781845423308.00032

Brough, P., O'Driscoll, M. P., & Kalliath, T. J. (2007). Work-family conflict and facilitation: achieving workfamily balance. In A. I. Glendon, B. M. Thompson, & B. Myors (Eds.), *Advances in organisational psychology* (pp. 73–92). Australian Academic Press.

Carlson, D. S., Kacmar, K. M., Wayne, J. H., & Grzywacz, J. G. (2006). Measuring the positive side of the workfamily interface: Development and validation of a work-family enrichment scale. *Journal of Vocational Behavior*, *68*(1), 131–164. doi:10.1016/j.jvb.2005.02.002

Carney, T., & Stanford, J. (2018). *The dimensions of insecure work: A factbook*. Retrieved from Canberra: https://www.tai.org.au/sites/default/files/Insecure_Work_Factbook.pdf

Chan, X. W., Kalliath, T., Brough, P., Siu, O. L., O'Driscoll, M. P., & Timms, C. (2016). Work–family enrichment and satisfaction: The mediating role of self-efficacy and work–life balance. *International Journal of Human Resource Management*, *27*(15), 1755–1776. doi:10.1080/09585192.2015.1075574

Duxbury, L., & Higgins, C. (2001). *Work–life balance in the new millennium: Where are we? Where do we need to go?* CPRN.

Ferguson, M., Carlson, D., Zivnuska, S., & Whitten, D. (2012). Support at work and home: The path to satisfaction through balance. *Journal of Vocational Behavior*, *80*(2), 299–307. doi:10.1016/j.jvb.2012.01.001

Franklin, N. (2010). The rise and fall of the 8 hour day: part one. In Hindsight. Australian Broadcasting Commission.

Greenhaus, J. H., Collins, K. M., & Shaw, J. D. (2003). The relation between work–family balance and quality of life. *Journal of Vocational Behavior*, *63*(3), 510–531. doi:10.1016/S0001-8791(02)00042-8

Halbesleben, J. R., Neveu, J. P., Paustian-Underdahl, S. C., & Westman, M. (2014). Getting to the "COR" understanding the role of resources in conservation of resources theory. *Journal of Management*, *40*(5), 1334–1364. doi:10.1177/0149206314527130

Hill, E. J., Hawkins, A. J., Ferris, M., & Weitzman, M. (2001). Finding an extra day a week: The positive influence of perceived job flexibility on work and family life balance. *Family Relations, 50*(1), 49–58. doi:10.1111/j.1741-3729.2001.00049.x

Kalliath, T., & Brough, P. (2008a). Work–life balance: A review of the meaning of the balance construct. *Journal of Management & Organization, 14*(3), 323–327. doi:10.5172/jmo.837.14.3.323

Kalliath, T., & Brough, P. (2008b). Achieving work-life balance. *Journal of Management & Organization, 14*(3), 224–226. doi:10.5172/jmo.837.14.3.224

Kanter, R. M. (1977). *Work and family in the United States: a critical review and agenda for research and policy*. Russell Sage Foundation.

Kirchmeyer, C. (2000). Work–life initiatives: greed or benevolence regarding workers' time? In C. L. Cooper & D. M. Rousseau (Eds.), *Trends in organizational behavior: time in organizational behavior* (Vol. 7, pp. 79–94). Wiley.

Lappegard, T., Goldscheider, F., & Bernhardt, E. (2017). Introduction to the special collection on finding work-life balance: History, determinants, and consequences of new breadwinning models of the industrialized world. *Demographic Research, 37*(26), 853–865. doi:10.4054/DemRes.2017.37.26

Marks, S. R. (1977). Multiple roles and role strain: Some notes on human energy, time and commitment. *American Sociological Review, 42*(6), 921–936. doi:10.2307/2094577

Marks, S. R., & MacDermid, S. M. (1996). Multiple roles and the self: A theory of role balance. *Journal of Marriage and Family, 58*(2), 417–432. doi:10.2307/353506

Milkie, M. A., Kendig, S. M., Nomaguchi, K. M., & Denny, K. E. (2010). Time with children, children's Wellbeing, and work–family balance among employed parents. *Journal of Marriage and Family, 72*(5), 1329–1343. doi:10.1111/j.1741-3737.2010.00768.x

Neal, M. B., & Hammer, L. B. (2017). *Working couples caring for children and aging parents: effects on work and Well-being*. Psychology Press. doi:10.4324/9781315083865

O'Driscoll, M., Brough, P., & Kalliath, T. (2004). Work-family conflict, psychological Well-being, satisfaction and social support: A longitudinal study in New Zealand. *Equal Opportunities International, 23*(1/2), 36–56. doi:10.1108/02610150410787846

O'Driscoll, M., Brough, P., & Kalliath, T. (2006). Work-family conflict and facilitation. In F. Jones, R. J. Burke, & M. Westman (Eds.), *Work-life balance: A psychological perspective* (pp. 117–142). Psychology Press.

Russo, M., Shteigman, A., & Carmeli, A. (2016). Workplace and family support and work–life balance: Implications for individual psychological availability and energy at work. *The Journal of Positive Psychology, 11*(2), 173–188. doi:10.1080/17439760.2015.1025424

Stock, R. M., Bauer, E. M., & Bieling, G. I. (2014). How do top executives handle their work and family life? A taxonomy of top executives' work–family balance. *International Journal of Human Resource Management, 25*(13), 1815–1840. doi:10.1080/09585192.2013.860383

Valcour, M. (2007). Work-based resources as moderators of the relationship between work hours and satisfaction with work–family balance. *The Journal of Applied Psychology*, *92*(6), 1512–1523. doi:10.1037/0021-9010.92.6.1512 PMID:18020793

Voydanoff, P. (2002). Linkages between the work-family interface and work, family, and individual outcomes: An integrative model. *Journal of Family Issues*, *23*(1), 138–164. doi:10.1177/0192513X02023001007

Walker, E., Wang, C., & Redmond, J. (2008). Women and work-life balance: Is home-based business ownership the solution? *Equal Opportunities International*, *27*(3), 258–275. doi:10.1108/02610150810860084

Chapter 12
Work-Life Balance and Role Outcomes Expectations:
Buffering Effect of Anasakti Among Female University Teachers

Sandhya Gupta
Banasthali Vidyapith, India

Chandra Kumari
Banasthali Vidyapith, India

ABSTRACT

For university professors, qualities like maintaining well-being, striking a work-life balance, and roles result expectations are all psychologically taxing. It partially depends on how one perceives and interprets the situations and events that one encounters in life. Using concepts like "anasakti," Indian psychologists have attempted to understand the usefulness and significance of Indian metaphysical notions in dealing with difficult situations. In light of the COVID-19 crisis, this study examined the relationship between work-life balance, roles and outcomes expectations, anasakti, mental health, and life happiness among university professors. Anasakti was found to be a highly significant predictor of life satisfaction, mental health, and work-life balance.

INTRODUCTION

The academic world has never experienced a pervasive epidemic that called for a complete shift to virtual classrooms. University professors' well-being might be harmed as a result of changes to the working environment. Female professors believe that because of their responsibilities at home, they face more limitations and struggle to strike a balance between their employment and raising a family in COVID 19. This chapter attempts to explore the relationship among work-life balance, anisakis, roles outcome expectations, mental health, and life satisfaction.

DOI: 10.4018/978-1-6684-8565-1.ch012

BACKGROUND

Academic work, classroom instruction, expert service, and other demanding tasks are all performed by university faculty members. Normal circumstances for faculty members include considerable stressful situations related to their workload as educators (Cladellas-Pros et al., 2018; Carrillo-Gonzalez et al., 2021). In academic circles, teleworking (home-based teaching) is not exactly a new phenomenon (Almhdawi, 2022). However, the academic world has never experienced a pervasive epidemic that called for a complete shift to virtual classrooms. University instructors may experience lesser physical work, lower living quality, and higher emotional difficulties during lockdowns (Brailovskaia et al., 2021; Redondo-Fl'orez, 2020; Barkley, 2020).

University professors' well-being might be harmed as a result of changes to the working environment. It appears that elements of the educational work environment, such as being unable to spend additional time with students to address their problems and having poor task management, are related to stress and job satisfaction (Sirajudeen et al., 2018). Furthermore, female professors believe that because of their responsibilities at home, they face more limitations. Furthermore, there is a perception that commitments to one's family impede career advancement and residual growth. As per Monk-Turner and Fogerty (2010), women in academia struggle to strike a balance between their employment and raising a family in COVID 19.

WORK-LIFE BALANCE

The concepts of "work-life balance" and "work-personal life reconciliation" are frequently used to emphasise which facets of life should be assimilated and harmonised, dividing working from non-working life, and emphasising that peaceful settlement is essential not only for work and home life but also for endeavours linked to faith, civic engagement, instructional practices, and many other activities (Korpa, 2012). According to scientific and practical research (Galvez et al., 2020; Uresha, 2020; Cartmill, 2020), telecommuting is one of the tools for work-life balance. However, it should be kept in mind that the COVID-19 crisis for workers with dependent kids changed the regular activities of the personal sphere, commitments, and timeframe (Power, 2020; Eurofound, 2017). Regardless of the sort of work they do or the number of hours they put in, it is crucial to allow employees to balance their professional and personal lives given that the current crisis has increased the use of telecommuting (Lonska et al., 2021).

The majority of institutions and organisations in India decided to continue operating from their homes throughout the lockdown. Although the crackdown allowed for more time spent together as a family, it also made it more difficult to manage home responsibilities. The limitations on outside mobility altered peoples' way of life. The crackdown has an adverse effect on household helpers' amenities. In the aforementioned scenario, the majority of employed people are weighed down by domestic responsibilities that consume their time and energy and exhaust them (Bhumika, 2020). According to the boundary theory, it is theorised that because professionals were working remotely throughout the crackdown, they may have fought to maintain equilibrium between their personal and professional lives by trying to establish and maintain time and space, physical, and mental boundary lines. The possibility of a conflict between work and family life, or a conflict between work and home life, or both, cannot be ruled out while working from home. Due to the clash between personal and professional life during the shutdown, employees may have felt emotionally worn out.

The task of balancing work and life would evolve over time, depending on the stages of a person's life and profession as well as their value systems, aspirations, and goals. According to literature, rebalancing work and life is largely determined by themes like mindful interaction in multiple or numerous roles, attempting to manage time and involvement across all the countless distinctive roles, finding contentment along all varied spheres, and attaining equal and fair involvement and fulfilment across all spheres of life (Sirgy & Lee, 2018). A person will feel balanced if their role expectations and effectiveness are in line with their present life choices (Greenhaus & Allen, 2011).

ROLES OUTCOME EXPECTATIONS

The capability of women to handle several responsibilities and their perception of this ability may have an impact on their psychological health, general wellbeing, and career success (Ahrens & Ryff, 2006). People typically play a variety of roles depending on the relationships they have and the positions they have. The partner role, which represents the relationship with a significant other, the parent role, which represents the relationship(s) with one's children, and the work role, which represents one's position and associated duties in the professional sphere, are prevalent supplemental roles among adult women. Although not all women develop the combination of mother, partner, and worker roles, a review of the literature analyzing the effect of numerous roles reveals they are frequently evaluated roles (Thoits, 1986).

Various roles have an influence on both men and women, and as they prepare to join the workforce, they may take into account their capacity to manage such multiple roles (Amatea, Cross, Clarke, & Bobby, 1986). The current study was particularly interested in women's abilities to handle these numerous responsibilities since it may provide insight on the widespread cultural expectations of women as partners and moms. The expectation that women will take on partner and mother roles is partly founded on the idea that women are more fitted to handle the duties associated with family obligations. A focus on specialized responsibilities related to the house, even among women for whom these roles have been formed, may make managing a profession difficult and burdensome for women, even while the establishment of these family and mother roles is not universal. For instance, Tal (2006) cited the combination of a profession and family responsibilities as one of the biggest issues working women face today. Additionally, single mothers may face new difficulties and obligations as they attempt to balance the demands of motherhood and professional activities.

Nevertheless, there are various viewpoints in the research addressing how numerous roles affect a person's wellbeing. According to some studies, playing too many roles can significantly affect a woman's health and wellbeing to the point that she feels overburdened and unable to perform the duties entailed with her different positions (Adelmann, 1994; Goode, 1960; Marks, 1977). Additional research emphasizes the protective effect of playing numerous roles since roles in some contexts can balance out problematic situations or features of roles in other contexts in which a woman may be grappling (Barnett & Hyde, 2001). Despite the likelihood of role saturation brought on by these numerous roles, research examining this latter perspective has identified a woman's capacity to handle multiple roles as something that can help avoid the sense of overload from forming (Barnett & Hyde, 2001; Sieber, 1974). Thus, whether playing many roles has a beneficial or negative impact on an individual seems to depend on their subjective view of their capacity to do so. If women are more capable of managing multiple roles, this may mean that role overload is less likely to occur.

MENTAL HEALTH

In addition to having an impact on students' mental health, the pandemic has put educators under a lot of stress since it first started (Cachón-Zagalaz et al., 2020). According to recent studies, instructors experience stress and strain during the shutdown period due to the need to quickly acclimatise in order to deliver digital lessons (Besser et al., 2020). In several research, it was determined that women were more likely than men to have stress symptoms and anxiety (Zhou & Yao, 2020; Li et al., 2020). Confusion (UNESCO, 2020a), a muddled work-life balance (Jakubowski & Sitko-Dominik, 2021), domestic abuse and divorce (Al Lily et al., 2020), the perspective of a poor quality of life (Lizana et al., 2021), sleep disruption, issues with interpersonal interaction, inadequate training and employment apprehensions (Perez, 2003), psychosomatic issues, tiredness and elevated workload are factors interfered in their ability to instruct. Additionally, previous studies have shown that using ICT while working remotely can cause emotions of tension, anxiety, fatigue, and decreased job satisfaction (Cuervo et al., 2018), and in the event of a global epidemic, these have been the only tools or gadgets available to instructors.

According to studies by Arias et al. (2019), Puertas-Molero et al. (2018), and Malik et al. (2017), university teachers suffer psychological symptoms. There are many different elements to take into account, including remuneration, interactions with students, and relationships with other students (Prieto & Bermejo, 2006). Another important factor is the current global economic downturn (Torres & Fernández, 2020). By leading to additional layoffs and instability, COVID-19 alone has exacerbated the problem (Aunión & Romero, 2020; La Vanguardia, 2020).

Anasakti

The maintenance of well-being, striking a balance between job and family, and role result expectations are all psychologically taxing for women. It somewhat depends on how one perceives and interprets the situations or events they encounter in life. Using concepts like "asakti" and "anasakti," Indian psychologists have endeavoured to understand the relevance and significance of Indian metaphysical principles in dealing with difficult situations. Asakti and Anasakti are the two emotional/affective factors that make up Anasakti Yoga. Anasakti denotes non-attachment, while Asakti denotes attachment (Singh & Raina, 2015).

Multiple works of Indian literature, including the Vedas, Yoga Sutras, and Upanishads, extol non-attachment. On the contrary hand, Hindu scriptures like the Bhagvad Gita went on to elucidate in great detail about Anasakti (non-attachment). The fundamental idea behind this construct is that in order to achieve a stable mental state that results in a profound sense of contentment, one must distance themselves from earthly cravings and pleasures. According to the Bhagvad Gita, practising non-attachment makes it possible to live a purposeful and fulfilling life in the physical domain (Bhagvad Gita, 3.7). In actuality, this worldview is acceptable for people in all stages of life and resonates to them. Anasakti is defined as the attainment of a state of yoga (Bhagvad Gita, 2.48) or mental equilibrium.

The events or people in an Anasakt's environment have no effect on his or her ego. Regardless of whether his or her actions result in enjoyment or discomfort, honour or respect, or dishonour, he or she consistently works hard but evenhandedly toward his or her goals (Bhagvad Gita, 2.51). With this constant intellect, one may perceive all events and individuals objectively and without bias, which is likely to lead to emotional consistency. In actuality, an individual maintains emotional equilibrium in the early aftermath of any kind of event, and his or her objective perspective on events aids him or her

in effectively coping with life situations, improved adaptation (Agrawal, 2019), and fulfilling existence (Banth & Talwar, 2012).

Because they believe that everything originates from a same source, Anasakts see unity and inclusion in all living things (Bhagvad Gita, 6.10). In reality, he or she responds to the happiness and grief of individuals around him or her with empathy and heartfelt caring. Anasakt develops coping mechanisms or the ability to reframe a difficult situation. Anasakt responds to practically any situation with symphony, balance, and serenity because of his or her strong belief in the higher authority. He knows that in the end, everything will be okay. He or she is unaffected by both positive and negative events that happen on the path to job completion. The development of an additional resource base for embracing and surviving a terrible event, it seems, is facilitated by anasakt action. As per researches, a person's ability to recover from a negative life event is thus influenced by how they perceive (Rajeev & Hebbani, 2020), acknowledge, and deal with the challenges they face in life (Moreira-Almeida, Neto, & Koenig, 2006). With these coping resources in place, individuals can keep pursuing their goals with greater clarity and tenacity, regardless of unrest. In addition, it invariably results in feelings of joy, well-being, and contentment in life (life satisfaction).

LIFE SATISFACTION

The COVID-19 pandemic's unexpected emergence (Holgun, 2021) has had consequences on worldwide community wellbeing and crucial facets (Randall et al., 2021) including higher education (The Lancet, 2020). For university professors, such a situation has structured a substantial dilemma and shift (Kecojevic et al., 2020). In this context, universities all over the globe had to make adjustments to new circumstances and instruct online courses in order to maintain the instructional and learning process moving forward (Berry, 2020; Mishra et al., 2020). In this particular circumstance, faculty members stand out as leading people who are anticipated to be ready to instruct digitally and facilitate learning even during pandemic, as demonstrated by the requirement for a reorganisation of educators' presence and learning task throughout the health emergency (Rapanta et al., 2020). Female educators, on the contrary, warrant special attention because they have to deal with the monetary, economic, household and social consequences of the corona virus (Chang, 2020).

It's interesting to note here that throughout the health crisis, female university lecturers were forced to make adjustments to digital classes by converting their residences into workplaces, study rooms, and online educational centres (Sahu, 2020; Konig et al., 2020). As a result, it was challenging for them to concentrate solely on their task because they also had to deal with house chores, care for children and older adults (Esteban et al., 2021). It has considerably improved their emotional toll, had a deleterious effect on their mental health, and had a significant influence on their level of life satisfaction (Malisch et al., 2020).

In respect of life satisfaction, the evidence strongly suggests that this concept can be described as an individual's hopeful and positive evaluation of one's life in specific areas like household, education, labor, fitness, friends, and spare time (Merino-Soto & Ruiz-del Castillo, 2018). In this respect, a few researchers have discovered that university lecturers who are satisfied with their lives have greater levels of prosocial behaviour as assessed by pupils (Braun et al., 2020). Another team of investigators, on the contrary, attempted to analyze the professors' life satisfaction using socio-demographic factors (Türko g lu et al., 2014), social support (Yuh & Choi, 2017), conditions of labor (Sahito & Vaisanen, 2020),

technostress (Penado-Abilleira et al., 2021), stress (Hasan et al., 2020; Song et al., 2020), anxiety and depression (Ozamiz-Etxebarria et al., 2021a), negative/positive emotionality (de la Fuente et al., 2021), motivational variables (de la Fuente et al., 2017), strategies of coping (de la Fuente et al., 2020a), reaction towards academic stress (de la Fuente et al., 2020c) and job satisfaction (Bhatia & Mohsin, 2020). According to some research findings, university lecturers encounter professional exhaustion or burnout as a result of their dual obligations at residence and at workplace (Gaxiola-Villa, 2014). It is in line with current research results that teaching is among the most difficult and stressful jobs (Bhatia & Mohsin, 2020).

There have been studies in the literature that show a link midst mental distress and life satisfaction. According to a research, emotional pain was linked to stressful events, preventing a reasonable level of life satisfaction (Arvidsdotter et al., 2016). A few other studies found that fear and depression was negatively correlated related to optimism in female educators (Stachteas & Stachteas, 2020); such a scenario was repetitive triggered by social restrictions and isolation, which affected their mental health (Gao & Sai, 2020). Such findings are compatible with earlier researches showing that a laborer's emotions have an immediate effect on one's level of life satisfaction (Moreta et al., 2018). Work saturation is widely recognized to have a deleterious impact on life satisfaction (De Simone et al., 2014; Erdogan et al., 2012; Nastasa et al., 2020). Work overburden is the second highest threat among university faculty, according to new findings (Pace et al., 2021). Finally, putting the focus on a gender-based assessment, a few researchers claim that women are a susceptible group when it comes to volume of work, which is really a component that lowers their level of life satisfaction (Kuhn et al., 2021). Furthermore, while a few little research findings demonstrate that men are much more discontented with their lives than women (Dutot, 2020). Similarly, Clark et al. (2021) found that working mothers were more severely affected by COVID-19 as compared to men, exploring new problems with respect to their well-being. In addition, mental distress and heavy workload are noted to be the constructs that have a straightforward influence on life satisfaction (Moreta-Herrera et al., 2018).

According to the preceding overview of literature, it will be intriguing and informative to assess university teachers' mental health, life satisfaction and work-life balance as their work responsibilities and circumstances altered as a result of continuing to work entirely from residence. Though voluminous research work has been initiated on work-life balance before and after COVID 19 situation but there is dearth of studies that explored university teachers' work-life balance in conjunction with roles outcomes expectations, life satisfaction, mental health and anasakti in the wake of COVID 19 situation.

Participants

With the use of random sampling, 102 married female university teachers belonged to middle class, with more than five years of teaching experience and ages 35 to 55 were selected as the study's sample. In the Rajasthan's private universities, an online survey was undertaken.

TOOLS

General Health Questionnaire (GHQ 12)

By Goldberg, the questionnaire was created (1988). This is done to assess someone's mental health. Less than usual, no more than usual, somewhat more than usual, or much more than usual were the four possible grades for each question on the survey. As a consequence, based on the possible answers, statements were evaluated as 0, 0, 1, or 1. The range of possible total scale scores with this scoring method is 0 to 12. The scale's psychometric qualities are strong.

Multiple Roles Outcome Expectations Questionnaire (2006)

Kirby was responsible for creating this survey. It has 24 items that evaluated the advantages and disadvantages of being a working mother with a spouse. Each item on the measure asked respondents to reflect how much they identified with it. A ten-point Likert scale with response options ranging from 1 to 10 was offered to the respondents. Higher scores indicated greater concurrence with the items. The scale's psychometric qualities are strong.

Life Satisfaction Scale (1985)

Diener, Emmons, Larsen, and Griffin created the scale. A five-item scale developed to assess one's overall cognitive decisions of life satisfaction. Participants rate how often they disagree or agree with each of the five items on a seven-point scale ranging from seven (strongly agree) to one (strongly disagree) (strongly disagree). The scale has good psychometric properties.

Work-Life Balance Scale (2005)

Hayman was the one who created the scale. A 5-point Likert scale with the end nodes of 1 = strongly disagree and 5 = strongly agree was used to evaluate WLB. The scale has good psychometric qualities.

Anasakti Scale (2015)

Singh and Raina created the scale. It consists of 22 items, each of which is assessed on a 5-point Likert scale from 1 (never) to 5 (always). It comprises of six subscales – faith in God, outcome vulnerability, empathy, persistence and fortitude, frustration tolerance and emotional equipoise. The scale had a reliability of.70. The six subscales' Cronbach alpha scores varied from 0.40 to 0.81 and had good convergent validity.

RESULTS

Table 1. Correlation matrix

Variables	FG	OV	EM	PF	FT	EE	ROE	WLB	MH	LS
FG	1									
OV	0.33**	1								
EM	0.30**	0.31**	1							
PF	0.39**	0.20*	0.41**	1						
FT	-0.05	-0.04	-0.08	0.10	1					
EE	0.29**	0.19	0.23*	0.46**	0.09	1				
ROE	-0.47**	-0.50**	-0.53**	-0.34**	0.09	-0.20*	1			
WLB	0.65**	0.73**	0.75**	0.43**	-0.05	0.32**	-0.68**	1		
MH	0.30**	0.40**	0.46**	0.21*	-0.01	0.13	-0.38**	0.56**	1	
LS	0.42**	0.47**	0.60**	0.46**	0.23*	0.23*	-0.49**	0.68**	0.48**	1

*Value of correlation significant at 0.05 level
** Value of correlation significant at 0.01 level
FG – Faith in God OV – Outcome Vulnerability
EM – Empathy PF – Persistence and Fortitude
FT – Frustration Tolerance EE – Emotional Equipoise
ROE – Roles Outcome Expectations WLB – Work-Life Balance
MH – Mental Health LS – Life Satisfaction

Table 1 exhibits that faith in God is significantly and positively associated with outcome vulnerability (r = 0.33, p< 0.01), empathy (r = 0.30, p< 0.01), persistence and fortitude (r = 0.39, p< 0.01), emotional equipoise (r = 0.29, p< 0.01), work-life balance (r = 0.65, p< 0.01), mental health (r = 0.30, p< 0.01), life satisfaction (r = 0.42, p< 0.01)and negatively related with roles outcome expectations (r = -0.47, p< 0.01).

Similarly, outcome vulnerability is significantly and positively associated with empathy (r = 0.31, p< 0.01), persistence and fortitude (r = 0.20, p< 0.05), work-life balance (r = 0.73, p< 0.01), mental health (r = 0.40, p< 0.01), life satisfaction (r = 0.47, p< 0.01) and negatively related with roles outcome expectations (r = -0.50, p< 0.01).

Empathy is significantly and positively associated with persistence and fortitude (r = 0.41, p< 0.01), emotional equipoise (r = 0.23, p< 0.05), work-life balance (r = 0.75, p< 0.01), mental health (r = 0.46, p< 0.01), life satisfaction (r = 0.60, p< 0.01) and negatively related with roles outcome expectations (r = -0.53, p< 0.01).

Persistence and fortitude is significantly and positively associated with emotional equipoise (r = 0.46, p< 0.01), work-life balance (r = 0.43, p< 0.01), mental health (r = 0.21, p< 0.05), life satisfaction (r = 0.46, p< 0.01) and negatively related with roles outcome expectations (r = -0.34, p< 0.01).

Frustration tolerance is significantly and positively related with life satisfaction (r = 0.23, p< 0.05). Likewise, emotional equipoise is significantly and positively associated with work-life balance (r = 0.32, p< 0.01), life satisfaction (r = 0.23, p< 0.05) and negatively related with roles outcome expectations (r = -0.20, p< 0.05).

Roles outcome expectations is significantly and negatively correlated with work-life balance (r = -0.68, p< 0.01), life satisfaction (r = -0.49, p< 0.01) and mental health (r = -0.38, p< 0.01).Work-life balance is significantly and positively correlated with life satisfaction (r = 0.68, p< 0.01) and mental health (r = 0.56, p< 0.01). Mental health is significantly and positively correlated with life satisfaction (r = 0.48, p< 0.01).

Multiple Regression Analysis

In order to assess the cause-effect relationship, stepwise multiple regression analysis was computed. The predictor variables are anasakti (faith in God, outcome vulnerability, empathy, persistence and fortitude, frustration tolerance and emotional equipoise) and roles outcome expectations were predictor variables and work-life balance, life satisfaction and mental health were criterion variables –

Anasakti Predicted Work-Life Balance

Table 2. Stepwise regression analysis for work-life balance

Model	R	R Square	Adjusted R square	R Square Change	F change	Sig. F Change	Beta
1 Empathy	0.75	0.57	0.56	0.57	130.70	.000	0.75
2 Empathy & Outcome Vulnerability	0.92	0.84	0.84	0.27	169.23	.000	0.58 0.55
3 Empathy, Outcome Vulnerability & Faith in God	0.97	0.94	0.94	0.10	174.76	.000	0.51 0.46 0.35

The above table exhibits the results of multiple regression analysis when criterion variable was work-life balance. A positive relationship exists, model 1, between empathy and work-life balance (0.75). That is, there exist 75% chances that empathy would enhance work-life balance. Similarly, both empathy and outcome vulnerability (model 2) have positive relationship with work-life balance (0.92). Their combined effect has a 92% chance of increasing work-life balance. Empathy, outcome vulnerability and faith in God (model 3) have positive relationship with work-life balance (0.97). Their combined effect has a 97% chance of increasing work-life balance. Value of R square, in model 1, is 0.57, i.e., 57% of the change or variation in work-life balance is accounted for by empathy. Likewise, in model 2, 84% of the changes in work-life balance are accounted for by both empathy and outcome vulnerability. In model 3, 94% of the variations in work-life balance are accounted for by empathy, outcome vulnerability and faith in God. Moreover, persistence and fortitude, frustration tolerance, emotional equipoise and roles outcome expectations added no change to the study model.

Each of the predictors (empathy, outcome vulnerability and faith in God) added with the exception of persistence and fortitude, frustration tolerance, emotional equipoise and roles outcome expectations improved the model. Therefore, adjusted R square is increased. That is, 56%, 84% and 94% of the variations in work-life balance are explained by empathy, empathy and outcome vulnerability (both) and empathy, outcome vulnerability and faith in God (all three together) respectively. Moreover, when outcome vulnerability is added to empathy (model 2), the change in R square is 0.27. This means that outcome vulnerability contributed 27% of the variation in work-life balance. In addition, when faith in God is added to empathy and outcome vulnerability (model 3), the change in R square is 0.10. This means that faith in God contributed 10% of the variation in work-life balance. Thus, these values of R square change are significant as the values of F change (169.23) and (174.76) respectively are significant at a p-value of 0.05. This means that the variables, outcome vulnerability (added in model 2) and faith in God (model 3) are significant. It implies that outcome vulnerability as well as faith in God influences work-life balance. So, it can be inferred that the variables added (outcome vulnerability and faith in God) significantly improves the model prediction.

Model 1 shows that every unit increase in empathy led to an increase in work-life balance scores by its respective coefficient of 0.75. Similarly, model 2 implicates that for every unit increase in both empathy (0.58) and outcome vulnerability (0.55) collectively led to increase in work-life balance scores. Also, model 3 implicates that for every unit increase in all the three variables collectively, viz, empathy (0.51), outcome vulnerability (0.46) and faith in God (0.35), led to increase in work-life balance scores.

Anasakti Predicted Mental Health

Table 3. Stepwise regression analysis for mental health

Model	R	R Square	Adjusted R square	R Square Change	F change	Sig. F Change	Beta
1 Empathy	0.45	0.20	0.19	0.20	24.76	.000	0.46
2 Empathy & Outcome Vulnerability	0.53	0.28	0.26	0.08	10.68	.000	0.35 0.29

Perusal of table 3 revealed the results of multiple regression analysis when criterion variable was mental health. A positive relationship exists, model 1, between empathy and mental health (0.45). That is, there exist 45% chances that empathy would enhance mental health. Similarly, both empathy and outcome vulnerability (model 2) have positive relationship with mental health (0.53). Their combined effect has a 53% chance of increasing mental health. Value of R square, in model 1, is 0.20, i.e., 20% of the change or variation in mental health is accounted for by empathy. Likewise, in model 2, 28% of the changes in mental health are accounted for by both empathy and outcome vulnerability. Moreover, persistence and fortitude, frustration tolerance, emotional equipoise and roles outcome expectations added no change to the study model.

Each of the predictors (empathy and outcome vulnerability) added with the exception of persistence and fortitude, frustration tolerance, emotional equipoise and roles outcome expectations improved the model. Therefore, adjusted R square is increased. That is, 19% and 26% of the variations in mental health are explained by empathy, empathy, and outcome vulnerability (both) respectively. Moreover, when outcome vulnerability is added to empathy (model 2), the change in R square is 0.08. This means that outcome vulnerability contributed 8% of the variation in mental health. Thus, this value of R square change is significant as the value of F change (10.68) is significant at a p-value of 0.05. This means that the variable, outcome vulnerability, added in model 2, is significant. It implies that outcome vulnerability influences mental health. So, it can be inferred that the variable added (outcome vulnerability) significantly improves the model prediction.

Model 1 shows that every unit increase in empathy led to an increase in mental health scores by its respective coefficient of 0.46. Similarly, model 2 implicates that for every unit increase in both empathy (0.35) and outcome vulnerability (0.29) collectively led to increase in mental health scores.

Anasakti Predicted Life Satisfaction

Table 4. Stepwise regression analysis for life satisfaction

Model	R	R Square	Adjusted R square	R Square Change	F change	Sig. F Change	Beta
1 Empathy	0.60	0.36	0.36	0.36	56.51	.000	0.60
2 Empathy & Outcome Vulnerability	0.67	0.45	0.44	0.09	15.31	.000	0.51 0.31
3 Empathy, Outcome Vulnerability & Frustration Tolerance	0.73	0.53	0.51	0.08	16.52	.000	0.53 0.31 0.28
4 Empathy, Outcome Vulnerability, Frustration Tolerance & Faith in God	0.75	0.56	0.54	0.07	14.40	.000	0.48 0.26 0.29 0.20

The above table shows the results of multiple regression analysis when criterion variable was life satisfaction. A positive relationship exists, model 1, between empathy and life satisfaction (0.60). That is, there exist 60% chances that empathy would enhance life satisfaction. Similarly, both empathy and outcome vulnerability (model 2) have positive relationship with life satisfaction (0.67). Their combined effect has a 67% chance of increasing life satisfaction. Empathy, outcome vulnerability and frustration tolerance (model 3) have positive relationship with life satisfaction (0.73). Their combined effect has a 73% chance of increasing life satisfaction. Moreover, empathy, outcome vulnerability, frustration tolerance and faith in God (model 4) have positive relationship with life satisfaction (0.75).Their combined effect has a 75% chance of increasing life satisfaction.

Value of R square, in model 1, is 0.36, i.e., 36% of the change or variation in life satisfaction is accounted for by empathy. Likewise, in model 2, 45% of the changes in life satisfaction are accounted for by both empathy and outcome vulnerability. In model 3, 53% of the variations in life satisfaction are accounted for by empathy, outcome vulnerability and frustration tolerance. In model 4, 56% of the variations in life satisfaction are accounted for by empathy, outcome vulnerability, frustration tolerance and faith in God. Moreover, persistence and fortitude, emotional equipoise and roles outcome expectations added no change to the study model.

Each of the predictors (empathy, outcome vulnerability, frustration tolerance and faith in God) added with the exception of persistence and fortitude, emotional equipoise and roles outcome expectations improved the model. Therefore, adjusted R square is increased. That is, 36%, 44%, 51% and 54% of the variations in life satisfaction are explained by empathy, empathy and outcome vulnerability (both), empathy, outcome vulnerability and frustration tolerance (all three together) and empathy, outcome vulnerability, frustration tolerance and faith in God (all four together) respectively. Moreover, when outcome vulnerability is added to empathy (model 2), the change in R square is 0.09. This means that outcome vulnerability contributed 9% of the variation in life satisfaction. In addition, when frustration tolerance is added to empathy and outcome vulnerability (model 3), the change in R square is 0.08. This means that frustration tolerance contributed 8% of the variation in life satisfaction. Likewise, when faith in God is added to empathy, outcome vulnerability and frustration tolerance (model 4), the change in R square is 0.07. This means that faith in God contributed 7% of the variation in life satisfaction. Thus, these values of R square change are significant as the values of F change (56.51), (15.31), (16.52) and (14.40) respectively are significant at a p-value of 0.05. This means that the variables, outcome vulnerability (added in model 2), frustration tolerance (model 3) and faith in God (model 4) are significant. It implies that outcome vulnerability, frustration tolerance as well as faith in God influences life satisfaction. So, it can be inferred that the variables added (outcome vulnerability, frustration tolerance and faith in God) significantly improves the model prediction.

Model 1 shows that every unit increase in empathy led to an increase in life satisfaction scores by its respective coefficient of 0.60. Similarly, model 2 implicates that for every unit increase in both empathy (0.51) and outcome vulnerability (0.31) collectively led to increase in life satisfaction scores. Also, model 3 implicates that for every unit increase in all the three variables collectively, viz, empathy (0.53), outcome vulnerability (0.31) and frustration tolerance (0.28), led to increase in life satisfaction scores. In the same manner, model 4 implicates that for every unit increase in all the four variables collectively, viz, empathy (0.48), outcome vulnerability (0.26), frustration tolerance (0.29) and faith in God (0.20), led to increase in life satisfaction scores.

DISCUSSION

The COVID 19 time frame was preceded by an emergency shutdown and prolonged social isolation, which led to emotional turmoil, stress, anxiety, depression, and other problems with mental and physical wellness. The situation was made bleaker by the deaths of close friends and family members as well as the challenges that come with working from home. And in the light of the current study, this appears even more pertinent. The results of this study indicated that Anasakti's factors (empathy, outcome vulnerability, frustration tolerance, and faith in God) predicted work-life balance, mental health, and life satisfaction for female teachers who worked or taught at the university level via virtual mode during the COVID 19 era.

Female teachers changed their teaching process during the epidemic from one-on-one engagement to virtual format from residence. If the responsibilities of the job make it difficult to meet domestic obligations, especially for employees, this could result in a work-home conflict (Kelly et al., 2008). According to the conflict theory of work-life balance, career and family role problems can potentially be mutually exclusive in some aspects, meaning that taking on a professional position can make taking on a family role more difficult (Greenhaus & Beutell, 1985), and the other way around (Frone et al, 1992). Here, a person's perspective or attitude toward the situation influences how she behaves. People who are non-attached (Anasakti), calm, and intelligent are better able to cope with stress and misfortune. According to the study 's conclusions, university professors in the COVID 19 scenario put in a lot of effort toward a goal without thinking about the results (a practise known as "Niskamakarma" — impartial involvement in the process of accomplishing a goal). Faculty members have a non-partisan, emotionless perspective on all other people and events as a result of their sustained intelligence, which leads to emotional maturity. The academic staff was actually able to maintain emotional and internal balance in the wake of any kind of event, so by ignoring role-conflict, she is able to deal with life's conditions effectively and attains contentment and constructive functioning at home and at work (Bhumika, 2020; Clark, 2000). Presumably, dividing up one's time, energy and devotion among several life areas, results in a sense of contentment in all of them, making work-life balance simpler to accomplish (Kirchmeyer, 2000). The enrichment hypothesis of work-life balance can also be used to understand this advantageous feature of balancing professional and family obligations. In other words, action in one realm might enhance the subjective experience in another sector as opposed to depleting it. For instance, career-family facilitation is a form of cumulative impact in which assets from one function, such as emotion, abilities, and self-esteem, ultimately make it easier to participate in another one (Wayne et al., 2004).

However one such state of mind, as stated in the Bhagvad Gita, may only be obtained by developing a firm belief in a higher power or Deity (Bhagvad Gita, 6.7). An anasakt acknowledges the unity and inclusivity of all living beings because she sincerely believes that everything has a single origin (Bhagvad Gita, 6.10). She thus responds with empathy, compassion, and great care to the joy and annoyance of individuals around her.

Anasakt action is required to handle life's difficulties (Pande & Naidu, 1992). Such resources and adaptability are available to Anasakt, along with the skill to view a stressful situation from a different perspective. Because of her strong faith in the higher power, Anasakt responds to every situation with composure and calm. She is utterly unaffected by both positive and negative events that occur on the way to job completion because she is persuaded that everything is happening for the best. It helps to build up greater resources for accepting and tolerating a distressing incident. Findings show that a person's ability to bounce back from a negative life experience depends on how they view, acknowledge, and deal with adversity (Moreira-Almeida, Neto, & Koenig, 2006). A person who has mastered these adaptive skills is able to keep their composure and intelligence under pressure. This results in enhanced life happiness and better mental health. Anasakti is connected to happiness, life satisfaction and wellbeing, according to a few researchers (Singh & Raina, 2015). These findings are supported by the transactional theory of stress (Lazarus & Folkman, 1984).

CONCLUSION

To conclude, educators are the proactive and responsible forces behind a system of education. Their general perspective and method of handling situations would change into their instructional strategy, enhancing the calibre of instruction. Teachers who practise anasakti, or non-attachment, have greater adaptive skills and a higher sense of self, which empower them to carry out their obligations and responsibilities. They also have a tendency to work more rigorously toward a target without worrying about the outcome. With general, it would aid them in pupil's grooming.

LIMITATIONS

This study sheds light on the meaning of the Indian concept of "Anasakti" and explores how it relates to other concepts like mental health, life satisfaction, and happiness orientation. Additionally, it creates possibilities for additional studies in this area to fully understand the concept and prepare module for teachers to practise anasakti.

REFERENCES

Adelmann, P. K. (1994). Multiple roles and psychological well-being in a national sample of older adults. *The Journals of Gerontology. Series B, Psychological Sciences and Social Sciences*, *49*(6), S277–S285. PMID:7963284

Agrawal, S. (2019). Anasakti and Adjustment. *Journal of Indian Council of Philosophical Research*, *36*(1), 39–51. doi:10.100740961-018-0155-9

Ahrens, C. J. C., & Ryff, C. D. (2006). Multiple roles and well-being: Socio-demographic and psychological moderators. *Sex Roles*, *55*(11-12), 801–815. doi:10.100711199-006-9134-8

Al Lily, A. E., Ismail, A. F., Abunasser, F. M., & Alhajhoj, R. H. (2020). Distance education as a response to pandemics: Coronavirusand Arab culture. *Technology in Society*, *63*, 101317. doi:10.1016/j.techsoc.2020.101317 PMID:32836570

Almhdawi, K. A. (2022). Influencing Medical Students' Knowledge and Attitudes Related to Disability: A Randomized Controlled Trial. *American Journal of Physical Medicine & Rehabilitation*, *101*(2), 113–118. doi:10.1097/PHM.0000000000001740 PMID:33657029

Amatea, E. S., Cross, E. G., Clarke, J. E., & Bobby, C. L. (1986). Assessing the work and family role expectations of career-oriented men and women: The Life Role Salience Scales. *Journal of Marriage and Family*, *48*(4), 831–838. doi:10.2307/352576

Arias Gallegos, W. L., Huamani Cahua, J. C., & Ceballos Canaza, K. D. (2019). Burnout Syndrome in School Teachers and University Professors: A Psychometrical and Comparative Analysis from Arequipa City. *Journal of Educational Psychology-Propositos y Representaciones*, *7*(3), 92–113.

Arvidsdotter, T., Marklund, B., Kylén, S., Taft, C., & Ekman, I. (2016). Understanding persons with psychological distress in primary health care. *Scandinavian Journal of Caring Sciences*, *30*(4), 687–694. doi:10.1111cs.12289 PMID:26463897

Aunión, J. A., & Romero, J. M. (2020). *Educación: cómoreparar los destrozos*. Madrid: El País. Available online at: https://elpais. com/ideas/2020-09-05/educacion-como-reparar-los-destrozos. html

Banth, S., & Talwar, C. (2012). Anasakti, the Hindu ideal, and its relationship to well-being and orientations to happiness. *Journal of Religion and Health*, *51*(3), 934–946. doi:10.100710943-010-9402-3 PMID:20953711

Barkley, J. E., Lepp, A., Glickman, E., Farnell, G., Beiting, J., Wiet, R., & Dowdell, B. (2020). The acute effects of the COVID-19 pandemic on physical activity and sedentary behavior in university students and employees. *International Journal of Exercise Science*, *13*(5), 1326. PMID:33042377

Barnett, R. C., & Hyde, J. S. (2001). Women, men, work, and family. *The American Psychologist*, *56*(10), 781–796. doi:10.1037/0003-066X.56.10.781 PMID:11675985

Berry, S. (2020). *An Assessment of Acne, Stress, and Psychological Symptoms in College Students: A Daily Diary Study*. Academic Press.

Besser, A., Lotem, S., & Zeigler-Hill, V. (2020). Psychological stress and vocal symptoms among university professors in Israel: Implications of the shift to online synchronous teaching during the COVID-19 pandemic. *Journal of Voice*. PMID:32600872

Bhatia, A., & Mohsin, F. (2020). Determinants of college teachers' hapinness- A comprehensive review. *J.Crit. Rev.*, *7*(9), 9–17.

Bhumika. (2020). Challenges for work-life balance during COVID-19 induced nationwide lockdown: exploring gender difference in emotional exhaustion in the Indian setting. *Gender in Management, 35*(7-8), 705-718.

Brailovskaia, J., Cosci, F., Mansueto, G., Miragall, M., Herrero, R., Baños, R. M., Krasavtseva, Y., Kochetkov, Y., & Margraf, J. (2021). The association between depression symptoms, psychological burden caused by Covid-19 and physical activity: An investigation in Germany, Italy, Russia, and Spain. *Psychiatry Research*, *295*, 113596. doi:10.1016/j.psychres.2020.113596 PMID:33261924

Braun, S.S., Schonert-Reichl, K.A., & Roeser, R.W. (2020). Effects of teachers' emotion regulation, burnout, and satisfaction with life on student well-being. *J. Appl. Dev Psychol. 69*, 1–13.

Cachón-Zagalaz, J., Sánchez-Zafra, M., Sanabrias-Moreno, D., González-Valero, G., Lara-Sánchez, A. J., & Zagalaz-Sánchez, M. L. (2020). Systematic review of the literature about the effects of the COVID-19 pandemic on the lives of school children. *Frontiers in Psychology*, *11*, 2457. doi:10.3389/fpsyg.2020.569348 PMID:33162910

Carrillo-Gonzalez, A., Camargo-Mendoza, M., & Cantor-Cutiva, L. C. (2021). Relationship between sleep quality and stress with voice functioning among college professors: A systematic review and meta-analysis. *Journal of Voice*, *35*(3), 499–e13. doi:10.1016/j.jvoice.2019.11.001 PMID:31866075

Cartmill, C. (2020). New survey shows 87% of staff wish to work from home in post lockdown world. *Belfast Newsletter, 28*.

Chang, W.-H. (2020). Understanding the COVID-19 pandemic from a gender perspective. *Taiwanese Journal of Obstetrics & Gynecology*, *59*(6), 801–807. doi:10.1016/j.tjog.2020.09.004 PMID:33218392

Cladellas-Pros, R., Castelló-Tarrida, A., & Parrado-Romero, E. (2018). Satisfaction, health, and work-related stress of the university professorship according to their contractual status. *Revista de Salud Publica (Bogota, Colombia)*, *20*(1), 53–59. PMID:30183885

Clark, S., McGrane, A., Boyle, N., Joksimovic, N., Burke, L., Rock, N., & O' Sullivan, K. (2021). You're a teacher you're a mother, you're a worker. In Gender Inequality during COVID-19 in Ireland. Academic Press.

Clark, S. C. (2000). Work/family border theory: A new theory of work/family balance. *Human Relations*, *53*(6), 747–770. doi:10.1177/0018726700536001

Cuervo, T. C., Orviz, N. M., Arce, S. G., & Fernández, I. S. (2018). Technostressin Communication and Technology Society: Scoping Literature Review from the Web of Science. *Archivos de Prevencion de Riesgos Laborales*, 18–25. doi:10.12961 / aprl.2018.21.1.04

de la Fuente, J. (2017). Theory of self- vs. externally-regulated learning: Fundamentals, evidence, and applicability. *Frontiers in Psychology*, *8*, 1675. doi:10.3389/fpsyg.2017.01675 PMID:29033872

de la Fuente, J., Amate, J., González-Torres, M. C., Artuch, R., García-Torrecillas, J. M., & Fadda, S. (2020a). Effects of levels of self-regulation and regulatory teaching on strategies for coping with academic stress in undergraduate students. *Frontiers in Psychology*, *11*, 22. doi:10.3389/fpsyg.2020.00022 PMID:32082213

de la Fuente, J., Pachón-Basallo, M., Santos, F. H., González-Torres, M. C., Artuch Garde, R., Peralta-Sánchez, F. J., ... Gaeta, M. L. (2021). How has the COVID-19 crisis affected the academic stress of university students? The role of teachers and students. *Frontiers in Psychology*, *12*, 1554. doi:10.3389/fpsyg.2021.626340 PMID:34140911

de la Fuente, J., Peralta-Sánchez, F. J., Martínez-Vicente, J. M., Sander, P., Garzón-Umerenkova, A., & Zapata, L. (2020c). Effects of Self-Regulation vs. External Regulation on the Factors and Symptoms of Academic Stress in Undergraduate Students. *Frontiers in Psychology*, *11*, 1773. doi:10.3389/fpsyg.2020.01773 PMID:32982819

Dutot, V. (2020). A social identity perspective of social media's impact on satisfaction with life. *Psychology and Marketing*, *37*(6), 759–772. doi:10.1002/mar.21333

Erdogan, B., Bauer, T. N., Truxillo, D. M., & Mansfield, L. R. (2012). Whistle while you work: A review of the satisfaction with life literature. *Journal of Management*, *38*(4), 1038–1083. doi:10.1177/0149206311429379

Esteban, R. E. C., Mamani-Benito, O., Chaparro, J. E. T., Lingan-Huaman, S. K., & Pajares, A. E. (2021). Psychological distress and workload as predictors of satisfaction with life in Peruvian female university professors with a family burden. *Heliyon*, *8*, 2022. PMID:35071805

Eurofound, I. L. O. (2017). Working anytime, anywhere: The effects on the world of work. Author.

Frone, M. R., Russell, M., & Cooper, M. (1992). Antecedents and outcomes of work-family conflict: Testing a model of work-family interface. *The Journal of Applied Psychology*, *77*(1), 65–78. doi:10.1037/0021-9010.77.1.65 PMID:1556042

Gálvez, A., Tirado, F., & Martínez, M. J. (2020). Work–life balance, organizations, and social sustainability: Analyzing female telework in Spain. *Sustainability*, *12*(9), 3567. doi:10.3390u12093567

Gao, G., & Sai, L. (2020). Towards a 'virtual' world: Social isolation and struggles during the COVID-19 pandemic as single women living alone. *Gender, Work and Organization*, *27*(5), 754–762. doi:10.1111/gwao.12468 PMID:32837008

Gaxiola-Villa, E. (2014). Bienestar psicol_ogico y desgaste profesional [DP] en amas de casa docentes universitarias. *J. Behav. Health Soc.*, *6*(1), 79–88.

Goode, W. J. (1960). A theory of role strain. *American Sociological Review*, *25*(4), 483–496. doi:10.2307/2092933

Greenhaus, J. H., & Allen, T. D. (2011). Work-family balance: A review and extension of the literature. In J. C. Quick & L. E. Tetrick (Eds.), Handbook of occupational health psychology (2nd ed.). Washington, DC: American Psychological Association.

Greenhaus, J. H., & Beutell, N. (1985). Sources of conflict between work and family roles. *Academy of Management Review*, *10*(1), 76–88. doi:10.2307/258214

Hasan, A. H., Sultana, S., Hossain, S., Hasan, M., Ahmed, H. U., & Sikder, T. (2020). The impact of COVID-19 pandemic on mental health & wellbeing among home-quarantined Bangladeshi students: A cross-sectional pilot study. *Journal of Affective Disorders*, *277*, 121–128. doi:10.1016/j.jad.2020.07.135 PMID:32818775

Holguín, E. C. (2021). Implicaciones de la pandemia por COVID-19 en la salud docente. Revisión sistemática. *Temas sociológicos*, (28), 113-142.

Jakubowski, T. D., & Sitko-Dominik, M. M. (2021). Teachers' mental health during the first two waves of the COVID-19 pandemic in Poland. *PLoS One*, *16*(9), e0257252. doi:10.1371/journal.pone.0257252 PMID:34555049

Kecojevic, A., Basch, C. H., Sullivan, M., & Davi, N. K. (2020). The impact of the COVID-19 epidemic on mental health of undergraduate students in New Jersey, cross-sectional study. *PLoS One*, *15*(9), e0239696. doi:10.1371/journal.pone.0239696 PMID:32997683

Kelly, E. L., Kossek, E. E., Hammer, L. B., Durham, M., Bray, J., Charmack, K., Murphy, L. A., & Kaskubar, D. (2008). Getting there from here: Research on the effects of work-family initiatives on work-family conflict and business outcomes. *The Academy of Management Annals*, *2*(1), 305–349. doi:10.5465/19416520802211610 PMID:20589229

Kirchmeyer, C. (2000). Work–life initiatives: greed or benevolence regarding workers' time. In C. L. Cooper & D. M. Rousseau (Eds.), *Trends in Organisational Behaviour* (pp. 79–93). John Wiley and Sons.

Konig, J., Jager-Biela, D. J., & Glutsch, N. (2020). Adapting to online teaching during COVID-19 school closure: Teacher education and teacher competence effects among early career teachers in Germany. *European Journal of Teacher Education*, *43*(4), 608–622. doi:10.1080/02619768.2020.1809650

Korpa, V. (2012). *DarbaunģimenesdzīvesSaskaņošanaPrivātāSektoraOrganizāci jās* [Reconciliation of Work and Family Life in Private Sector Organizations] [Ph.D thesis]. Available online at: https://www.szf.lu.lv/fileadmin/user_upload/szf_faili/Petniecciba/promocijas_darbi/Viola_Korpa_2012.pdf

Kuhn, U., Klaas, H.S., Antal, E., Dasoki, N., Lebert, F., Lipps, O., Voorpostel, M. (2021). Who is most affected by the Corona crisis? An analysis of changes in stress and wellbeing in Switzerland. *Eur. Soc.*, *23*(sup1), S942–S956.

La Vanguardia. (2020). *USOC y UGT advierten de despidos de profesoresen lasescuelasconcertadas*. Barcelona: La Vanguardia. Available onlineat: https://www.lavanguardia.com/vida/20200408/48387012784/usoc-y-ugtadvierten-de-despidos-de-profesores-en-las-escuelas-concertadas.html

Lazarus, R. S., & Folkman, S. (1984). *Stress, appraisal, and coping*. Springer.

Li, Q., Miao, Y., Zeng, X., Tarimo, C. S., Wu, C., & Wu, J. (2020). Prevalence andfactors for anxiety during the coronavirus disease 2019 (COVID-19) epidemic among the teachers in China. *Journal of Affective Disorders*, *277*, 153–158. doi:10.1016/j.jad.2020.08.017 PMID:32828002

Lizana, P. A., & Vega-Fernadez, G. (2021a). Teacher teleworking during the covid-19 pandemic: Association between work hours, work–family balance and quality of life. *International Journal of Environmental Research and Public Health*, *18*(14), 7566. doi:10.3390/ijerph18147566 PMID:34300015

Lizana, P. A., Vega-Fernadez, G., Gomez-Bruton, A., Leyton, B., & Lera, L. (2021). Impact of the COVID-19 Pandemic on Teacher Quality of Life: A Longitudinal Study from before and during the health Crisis. *International Journal of Environmental Research and Public Health*, *18*(7), 3764. doi:10.3390/ijerph18073764 PMID:33916544

Lonska, J., Mietule, I., Litavniece, L., Arbidane, I., Vanadzins, I., Matisane, L., & Paegle, L. (2021b). Work–Life balance of the employed population during the emergency situation of COVID-19 in Latvia. *Frontiers in Psychology*, *12*, 1–15. doi:10.3389/fpsyg.2021.682459 PMID:34421734

Malik, N. A. A., Björkqvist, K., & Österman, K. (2017). Factors associated with occupational stress among university teachers in Pakistan and Finland. *Journal of Educational, Health and Community Psychology*, *6*(2), 1–14. doi:10.12928/jehcp.v6i2.7047

Malisch, J. L., Harris, B. N., Sherrer, S. M., Lewis, K. A., Shepherd, S. L., McCarthy, P. C., & Deitloff, J. (2020). Opinion: In the wake of COVID-19, academia needs new solutions to ensure gender equity. *Proceedings of the National Academy of Sciences of the United States of America*, *117*(27), 15378–15381. doi:10.1073/pnas.2010636117 PMID:32554503

Marks, S. R. (1977). Multiple roles and role strain: Some notes on human energy, time, and commitment. *American Sociological Review*, *42*(6), 921–936. doi:10.2307/2094577

Merino-Soto, C., & Ruiz-del Castillo, C. G. (2018). Explorando el vínculo de la inteligencia emocional y la satisfacci_on con la vida en adultos peruanos. *Ansiedad y Estrés*, *24*(2–3), 140–143. doi:10.1016/j.anyes.2018.03.004

Mishra, L., Gupta, T., & Shree, A. (2020). Online teaching-learning in higher education during lockdown period of COVID-19 pandemic. *Int. J. Educ. Res. Open*, *1*, 1–8. doi:10.1016/j.ijedro.2020.100012 PMID:35059663

Monk-Turner, E., & Fogerty, R. (2010). Chilly environments, stratification, and productivity differences. *The American Sociologist*, *41*(1), 3–18. doi:10.100712108-009-9083-0

Moreira-Almeida, A., Neto, F. L., & Koenig, H. G. (2006). Religiousness and mental health: A review. *RevistaBrasileira de Psiquiatria*, *28*(3), 242–250. PMID:16924349

Moreta, R., Lopez, C., Gordon, P., Ortiz, W., & Gaibor, I. (2018). Satisfaction with life, psychological and social well-being as predictors of mental health in Ecuadorians. *Actualidades en Psicología*, *32*(124), 111–125.

Nastasa, M., Golu, F., Buruiana, D., & Oprea, B. (2020). Teachers' work – home interaction and satisfaction with life: the moderating role of core self- evaluations life: The moderating role of core self-evaluations. *Educ. Psychol*, 1–16.

Ozamiz-Etxebarria, N., Dosil Santamaría, M., Idoiaga Mondragon, N., & Berasategi Santxo, N. (2021a). Estado emocional del profesorado de colegios y universidades en el norte de España ante la COVID-19. *Revista Espanola de Salud Publica*, *95*(1), e1–e8.

Pace, F., D'Urso, G., Zappulla, C., & Pace, U. (2021). The relation between workload and personal well-being among university professors. *Current Psychology (New Brunswick, N.J.)*, *40*(7), 3417–3424. doi:10.100712144-019-00294-x

Pande, N., & Naidu, R. K. (1992). Anāsakti and health: A study of non-attachment. *Psychology and Developing Societies*, *4*(1), 89–104. doi:10.1177/097133369200400106

Penado Abilleira, M., Rodicio-García, M. L., Ríos-de Deus, M. P., & Mosquera-González, M. J. (2021). Technostress in Spanish university teachers during the COVID-19 pandemic. *Frontiers in Psychology*, *12*, 496. doi:10.3389/fpsyg.2021.617650 PMID:33732187

Pérez, V. M. O. (2003). Estrés y ansiedad en los docentes. *Pulso: revista de educación*, (26), 9-22.

Power, K. (2020). The COVID-19 pandemic has increased the care burden of women and families. *Sustainability: Science, Practice and Policy*, *16*(1), 67–73.

Prieto, M., & Bermejo, L. (2006). Contextolaboral y malestardocente en unamuestra de profesores de Secundaria.*Rev. Psicol. TrabajolasOrganiz.*, *22*, 45–73.

Puertas-Molero, P., Zurita-Ortega, F., Chacón-Cuberos, R., Martínez-Martínez, A., Castro-Sánchez, M., & González-Valero, G. (2018). An explanatory model of emotional intelligence and its association with stress, burnout syndrome, and non-verbal communication in the university teachers. *Journal of Clinical Medicine*, *7*(12), 524. doi:10.3390/jcm7120524 PMID:30544532

Rajeev, A., & Hebbani, S. (2020). Anasakti and resilience in older adults in south India: a correlation study. *International Journal of Indian Psychology, 8*(4), 1534-1544. DOI: doi:10.25215/0804.166

Randall, K., Ford, T. G., Kwon, K.-A., Sisson, S. S., Bice, M. R., Dinkel, D., & Tsotsoros, J. (2021). Physical activity, physical well-being, and psychological well-being: Associations with life satiscfaction duing the COVID 19 pandemic among early childhood educators. *International Journal of Environmental Research and Public Health*, *18*(18), 9430. doi:10.3390/ijerph18189430 PMID:34574354

Rapanta, C., Botturi, L., Goodyear, P., Guàrdia, L., & Koole, M. (2020). Online university teaching during and after the covid-19 crisis: Refocusing teacher presence and learning activity. *Postdigital Sci. Educ.*, *2*(3), 923–945. doi:10.100742438-020-00155-y

Redondo-Fl´orez, L., Fern´andez-Lucas, J., & Clemente-Suarez, V. (2020). *Cultural differences in stress-related psychological, nutrition, physical activity, and oral health factors of professors*. Academic Press.

Sahito, Z., & Vaisanen, P. (2020). A literature review on teachers' job satisfaction in developing countries: Recommendations and solutions for the enhancement of the job. *Review of Education*, *8*(1), 3–34. doi:10.1002/rev3.3159

Sahu, P. (2020). Closure of universities due to coronavirus disease 2019 (COVID-19): Impact on education and mental health of students and academic staff. *Cureus*, *12*, e7541. doi:10.7759/cureus.7541 PMID:32377489

Sieber, S. D. (1974). Toward a theory of role accumulation. *American Sociological Review*, *39*(4), 567–578. doi:10.2307/2094422

Singh, K., & Raina, M. (2015). Development and validation of a test on Anasakti (non-attachment): An Indian model of well-being. *Mental Health, Religion & Culture*, *18*(9), 715–725. doi:10.1080/13674676.2015.1084612

Sirajudeen, M. S., Alaidarous, M., Waly, M., & Alqahtani, M. (2018). Work-related musculoskeletal disorders among faculty members of college of Applied Medical Sciences, Majmaah University, Saudi Arabia: A cross-sectional study. *International Journal of Health Sciences*, *12*(4), 18. PMID:30022899

Sirgy, M. J., & Lee, D. J. (2018). Work-life balance: An integrative review. *Applied Research in Quality of Life*, *13*(1), 229–254. doi:10.100711482-017-9509-8

Song, K., Xu, R., Stratton, T. D., Kavcic, V., Luo, D., & Hou, F. (2020). (Preprint). Sex differences and psychological stress: Responses to the COVID-19 epidemic in China. *MedRxiv*. Advance online publication. doi:10.1101/2020.04.29.20084061

Stachteas, P., & Stachteas, C. (2020). The psychological impact of the COVID-19 pandemic on secondary school teachers. *Psychiatriki*, *31*(4), 293–301. doi:10.22365/jpsych.2020.314.293 PMID:33361059

Tal, A. I. (2006). *Pregnant women's self-efficacy for integrating multiple roles* [Unpublished doctoral dissertation]. Fordham University.

The Lancet. (2020). Research and higher education in the time of COVID-19. *Lancet, 396*(10251), 583.

Thoits, P. A. (1986). Multiple identities: Examining gender and marital status differences in distress. *American Sociological Review*, *51*(2), 259–272. doi:10.2307/2095520

Torres, R., & Fernández, M. J. (2020). La políticaeconómicaespañola y el COVID-19. *Funcas. Cuadernos de InformaciónEconómica*, *275*, 1–7.

Türkoglu, D., Ozbey, S., & Büyüktanir, A. (2014). Analysis of the satisfaction with life of preschool prospective teachers according to some variables. *Procedia: Social and Behavioral Sciences*, *116*, 4175–4181. doi:10.1016/j.sbspro.2014.01.912

Uresha, K. I. (2020). Influence of telecommuting on work-life balance and employee happiness: An empirical study of Sri Lankan employees. *Int. J. Manag. Excell*, *15*, 2234–2243.

Wayne, J., Musisca, N., & Fleeson, W. (2004). Considering the role of personality in the work-family experience: Relationship of the Big Five to work-family conflict and facilitation. *Journal of Vocational Behavior*, *64*(1), 108–130. doi:10.1016/S0001-8791(03)00035-6

Yuh, J., & Choi, S. (2017). Sources of social support, job satisfaction, and quality of life among childcare teachers. *The Social Science Journal*, *54*(4), 1–8. doi:10.1016/j.soscij.2017.08.002

Zhou, X., & Yao, B. (2020). Social support and acute stress symptoms (ASSs) during the COVID-19 outbreak deciphering the roles of psychological needs and sense of control. *European Journal of Psychotraumatology*, *11*(1), 1779494. doi:10.1080/20008198.2020.1779494 PMID:33062202

Chapter 13
Maintaining Work-Life Balance in Remote Work in COVID-19

Nikita Jain
Maharshi Dayanand University, Rohtak, India

Deepa Bhardwaj
Maharshi Dayanand University, Rohtak, India

Rekha Dhingra
Maharshi Dayanand University, Rohtak, India

ABSTRACT

COVID-19 rapidly spread over the world by the end of 2019 and the commencement of 2020. Therefore, organizations suddenly transitioned to fully digitalized virtual organizations that allowed for remote work from home. The workers connected to a remote computer site utilizing communication tools while working from home. A flexible work schedule necessitates modification. For a better work-life balance, employees spend time working from home. Therefore, the study aims to understand the opportunities and challenges associated with remote work. In addition, it focuses on exploring the factors that influence the work-life balance in remote work and suggesting ways to maintain work-life balance in remote work.

INTRODUCTION

The use of communication and information technology (ICT) in the 21st century, particularly smart phones and Internet technology, has allowed for the creation of virtual organizations that can operate autonomously and remotely from any location at any time. The "COVID-19" had quickly spread over the world by the end of 2019 and the beginning of 2020. Due to the COVID-19 epidemic created an unexplored space for remote work (Das & Mishra, 2016). Further numerous employees managed their duties and this promoted at-home learning at the same time (Rao et al., 2019). Consequently, organizations embrace a virtual organization that is fully digital and allows for remote working from home.

DOI: 10.4018/978-1-6684-8565-1.ch013

Moreover, businesses used remote work choices to bring and keep talent (Morgan 2014) and on the way to improve "work-life balance" for their employees (Prasada et al., 2020). Presenting flexible "work schedules" can signify a company's willingness to change in response to workers' requirements (Johari et al., 2018). Employees might also consider it as facilitating a greater connection linking themselves and workplace, which is a feature of positive work role adjustment (Muralidhar et al., 2020). In addition, now-a-days offices support remote work; being family-friendly alternative to improve "work-life balance" (Robertson et al., 2017). Thus, remote workers believe their companies are sympathetic towards their happiness (Danna and Landry 2011) and on the other hand remote work is supported by organizational leaders who recognize its importance in building the relationship between workforce and business.

Given that extreme contexts make it easier to get insight into "best and worst" circumstances, where presumptions may be questioned and common wisdom fails, the pandemic presents a fantastic chance to consider the following:

- Is the concept that working remotely is a preferable option been contested?
- What can be inferred from the prevalent instinctive distant work that workforce are subjected to?

The pandemic's effects on work life balance and distant work offers a special opportunity to research a phenomenon that is difficult to observe (Songsangyos & Iamamporn, 2020). This study considered the academic publications on work-life balance and isolated work to provide answers to these concerns. The "remote working" which suggests employee the chance to work from home or nearby office may offer flexibility to work which ultimately raise employee morale, lower absenteeism and fatigue and improve the worker's quality of life (Arvanitis, 2005). To begin with, let's comprehend the meaning of "remote work" and "work-life balance".

REMOTE WORK

"The act of an employee working remotely, apart from the employer's main office, is known as remote work." It includes a worker's home, common area, co-working area, or any other place other than the classic corporate workplace building could be considered such places. Remote work is becoming more common since it helps both employers and employees. The COVID-19 epidemic compelled many firms to immediately move from a conventional face-to-face work setting to a entirely "remote workforce".

Distant working requires amalgamation of the proper technology, culture and processes which is intended to let virtual team to work effectively from anyplace. To have a thriving distant working requires a moving premise that individuals or teams will commonly work distantly. A constructive distant employee generally has the following traits:

1. **Robust, stable connectivity**: Fast internet and mobile technology that can withstand intensive use are essential for virtual teams.
2. **Tools for communication and collaboration**: To facilitate collaboration the workforce must be there in one place. It requires the technologies like chat, file sharing, videoconferencing, isolated desktops, and additional business supplies, which necessitate secure and premium quality platform.
3. **Healthy work atmosphere**: Virtual teams that perform well have surroundings that give importance to collaboration and outcomes over "face time" or workplace hours. A work culture further

includes encouraging administration which believes in this approach and supports personnel and teams to be successful in this type of work.

Working from home and enhanced employee allows for flexibility leads to more productive work with fewer interruptions. Better work-life balance, and improved employees control over resources all add to better employee performance. Employee performance was improved by eliminating travel and allowing for flexible scheduling (Raghavendra & Raghunandan, 2018). Working remotely to fulfill an organization's objectives, vision, and mission is what telecommuting is all about, and its accomplishment depends on the level of confidence between worker and company.

WORK LIFE BALANCE

It means balancing between the work and private life and feeling satisfied with equal work and non-work commitment. It is the balance between private and specialized life. In 1986 the term "work life balance" was used but the use of the term work life balance is in the daily language is occasional for many years, various work life balance programs were seen around 1930 (Suresh, V Kandaswamy SharmaDr. Beulah & Assistant, 2018).

"Work-life balance" includes the situation of stability among the responsibilities of work and life. A worker will comprise work-life balance in their private and professional lives if they place equal attention on both family life and office work and manage to strike a good balance with the appropriateness of both employee and family responsibilities.

The work and non-work activities are distributed in three types of balances: (i) first one is time balance that is the participation of time in both job and personal life; (ii) second one is involvement balanced that is distribution of psychological involvement in between job and personal life; and (iii) the third is the satisfaction balance that is the satisfaction between job and personal life (Bhandari & Soni, 2015). Work life balance was influenced by the number of factors that is dependent care, role overload, health issues, social support and time management (Purohit, 2013). A study found that the 90% of the working adult are not able to spend the proper time with their families (Prasada et al., 2020). In a person life there is a lots of roles, when a person is in capable of involve in these multiple role at a satisfactory level is defined as a work life balance (Mas-Machuca et al., 2016).

During the 1960 and 1970 employer consider that the women with children are face problem about the work life balance. In 1980's due to contribution of women in the organization some of the employer such as Merck, Deloitte and IBM began to change policies and programs for the women employees like they provided with the benefit of the maternity leave, employee assistance program, flexible time and childcare. But after that men also start voicing about the work life balance problem at the end of decade it is a problem of men women, families, and organizations too.

The work-life balance is a topic that frequently comes up in board meetings today and is of great importance to managers and HR specialists. Even though the workplace is a paid profession, and the personal life is private time, work-life balance is still required. Work-life balance increases productivity and raises employee performance. Work-life balance has a favorable influence on growth and productivity, lowers health care expenses, improves employee engagement, and improves talent management.

The goal of this paper is to give a concise review of telework research and practice so that readers can better understand of this innovative approach to working. Additionally, it also focuses on examining the ways to maintain "work-life balance" in remote working. It begins with a description of its rising popularity before reviewing some important findings from earlier studies, focusing on work-life balance.

LITERATURE REVIEW

A "remote worker" work for a corporation but works outside the conventional workplace setting, whether from home, a nearby co working space, or any other city in the world. To obtain peer approval, employees might create a remote work case (Mas-Machuca et al., 2016). Due to COVID-19, the concept of remote working has become the norm everywhere. The accessibility of tools such as zoom, team viewer, Microsoft teams, Microsoft remote desktop and communication tools are necessary for working. It also includes "task prioritization reports", as well as the solutions provided by (Johari et al., 2018). According to Economic Time, the SCIKEY MindMatch (2020) research found that 99.8% of IT workers are unable to operate remotely.

It lists the following three generations of teleworkers.

- The first generation, known as "**home offices**" in the 1970s and 1980s, used desktop computers stationary and fixed telephones in the workers' houses to interact. It was a stand-in for "telecommuting," or working remotely.
- The second generation is referred to as "**the mobile office**". This allowed employees to work both at the office and at home. At this point, telework was serving as a partial replacement for office work.
- The third generation of telework, known as "**virtual office**," is made possible by the Internet's rapid expansion and the fact that it can now be accessed on smaller, more capable devices like smart phones and tablets. Due to mobile devices, modern ICTs allow employees to work whenever and wherever they choose.

The performance of the organization is most influenced by the employees who have a better work-life balance since an effective and efficient workforce enables the business to offer better customer service. Single-parent family, nuclear families,, dual-working parents are just a few examples of how alteration in the family surroundings have impacted people's "work-life balance" in the modern era (Johari et al., 2018).

In the remote working the workers connect to a remote computer site from their homes using communication methods such a smart phone, videoconference, email, or Line. A flexible work arrangement allows for improved "work-life balance" by adjusting functioning hours and locations. "Work-life balance" (WLB) is described by Davis and Francis (Muralidhar et al., 2020) as "an overall level of contentment arising from an appraisal of one's degree of success at fulfilling work and family role expectations." In contrast, "work-family conflict" (WFC) arises is a situation of conflict among the role played in the distinct spheres of family and job.

Progressing on these thoughts, Muralidhar et al. (2020) presented a study investigating the relationship between "job stress, job satisfaction and work-life balance". The study was conducted on the teacher of the University concerning the Gujarat. A section of teachers was chosen from "Hafiz Hayat campus of University of Gujarat". To collect the data random sampling technique was used. The finding reveals strong association connecting work-life balance and job satisfaction.

Moreover, it was initiated that female employees are more satisfied as compared to male employees in terms of job satisfaction due to the lack of paternity leave, according to (Das & Mishra, 2016). Paternity leave was recently added by certain employers to improve motivation and work-life balance. It benefits both individuals and organizations. A harmonious bond between the worker and the company for their mutual benefit is supported for successful work-life balance programs. Human resources that are more competent at managing their time demands are happier and more content. They can so perform better.

Later, Robertson et al. (2017) has observed the relationship between perceived organizational support, marital status and stress coping strategies related to the "work-life balance". A sample of 254 bank workers is used for the data analysis. The results of the study revealed that perceived organizational support and coping strategies are a predictor of work-life balance but marital status according to the results is not a forecaster of the "work-life balance".

Raghavendra & Raghunandan (2018) surveyed teachers in public schools in Malaysia to investigate the effects of autonomy, workload, and work-life balance on performance of employees. The results indicate that "work-life balance" has a major influence on employees' job performance. The investigator added that the current theory only offers an incomplete picture of the needs of workers in terms of their "work-life balance" and that there is a need to expand this idea beyond the workforce to include other social groupings.

Songsangyos & Iamamporn (2020) cited statistics from "Gallup Research", distant work boosts trade results, draws an engaged workforce and talent produces the best financial results. According to the study, a remote worker's experience with workplace isolation will be impacted by a lack of organizational knowledge and management skills needed to create and implement strategies for policies and practices governing remote work.

From literature review it can be concluded that the majority of researchers concentrated their research on the effects of planned distant employees based at home before the pandemic (Purohit, 2013); however, hardly any have looked at the results of unplanned distant work circumstances (Suresh, V Kandaswamy Sharma, Beulah & Assistant, 2018). An additional common subject in the previous studies is that managers might use "remote work" to create monitoring and surveillance techniques (Bhandari & Soni, 2015). Thus, this study aims to study the perceived benefits and drawbacks of working from home during pandemic and how to create a balance between the work and life.

OBJECTIVES OF THE STUDY

1. To analyze the factors that affect work-life balance during remote work.
2. To understand the opportunities and challenges related with distant working during the COVID-19 period.
3. To make recommendations for improving "work-life balance" while working distantly.

CONTENT OF REMOTE WORKING

To get the full benefits of remote working, it should include people, processes, and technology, as illustrated in Figure 1.

Figure 1. Content of remote working
Source: Muralidhar et al. (2020)

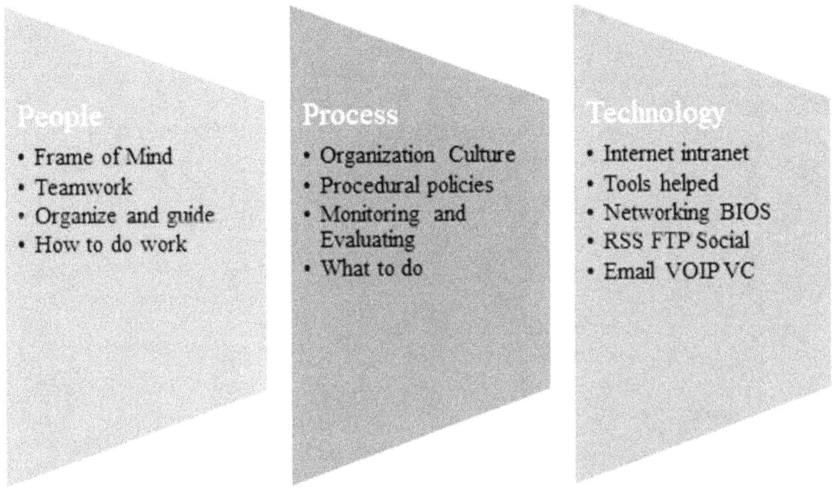

Muralidhar et al. (2020) stated that "**people, process and technology**" collectively vital in adoption of "remote working". The people must have a mind frame or mental outlook to perform the task successfully. Moreover the employee must understand the importance of teamwork to complete the work well. Process first of all, comprise organization culture. The "**organization culture**" includes the compilation of "beliefs, principles and thoughts" that guide the actions of the workforce and have an effect on their behavior. It helps the employee to understand the expectation of organization from their employees, so that they can work on it. Process also includes monitoring and evaluationg continuosly to help orgainzation achieving their targets. Moreover policies which serves as a guides are also also communicated so that there must be clearity regarding their task. Thus process includes providing a "**good organization culture**", communicating policies and monitoring the employees to achieve desred results. Next, the technology includes "**internet connection**", "**work station**" and other tools neceesary to set up for "remote working". To work effectively, high speed internet connection is mandatory along with the PC or a laptop is required.

FACTORS WHICH AFFECT WORK-LIFE BALANCE DURING REMOTE WORK

Productivity when "working from home" during in the COVID-19 epidemic is impacted by a several factors. The following primary aspects affect an employee's ability to manage their work and personal lives during distant working. Prasada et al. (2020), Rao et al. (2019) provided recommendations on remote work, job stress, and coping as shown in Figure 2. It includes **social, psychological, technology related and work-related factors.** Social factors include factors related to surroundings i.e., family and society. Next comes, physiological factors include factors related to health i.e., ergonomics, stress and emotional tiredness. Next comes, work related factors include factors associated with the work i.e., working too much and work schedules. Lastly, technology related factors include factors such as infrastructure, additional cost, and digital assets.

Figure 2. Four key aspects affecting work-life balance in distant working
Source: Prasada et al. (2020)

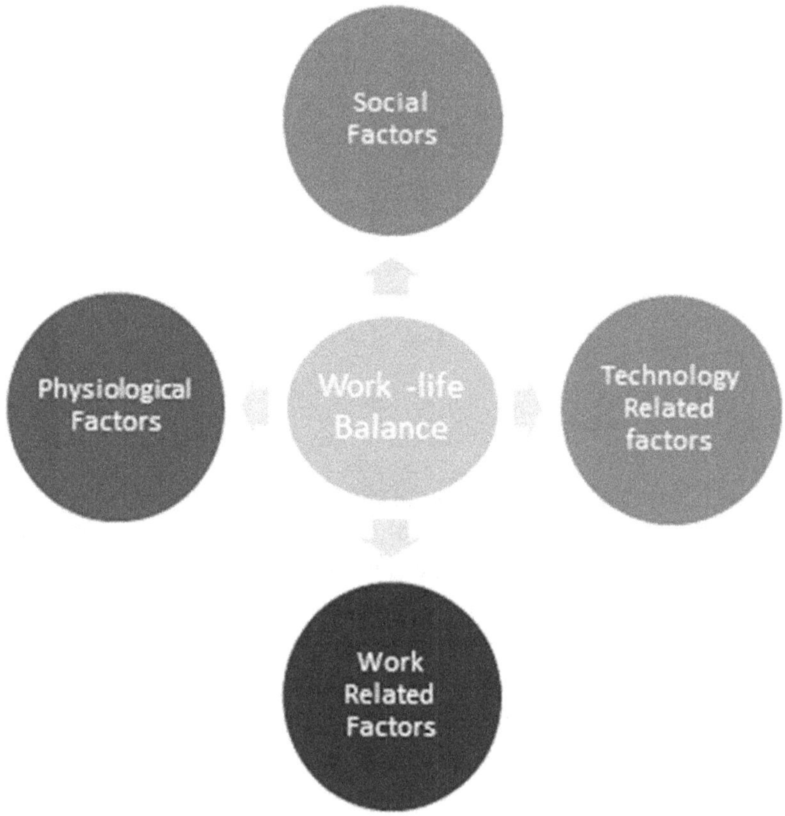

Social Factors

- *Family disturbance:* During "distant working" the employees work from home. Although it has given the family extra time together and freedom in managing work and family obligations, employees has to face family or social disturbance during work which affect the work life balance. It serves as a biggest distraction of "working from home".
- *Lack of guidance:* In the distant working the employees as well as managers frequently express concern about the loss of face-to-face interaction. Supervisors are concerned that workers didn't bring in as much effort or be as productive. On the other side, many workers struggle with a lack of communication and assistance from management. In that case, it is difficult to manage work and personal life.

Physiological Factors

- *Ergonomics:* Sitting in an uncomfortable position or maintaining the same position for extended periods of time is called ergonomics. As a result of bad posture, prolonged sitting, extended wrists, and relying on laptop screens for remote work, many employees nowadays have new aches and pains. It affects the working life of an employee.
- *Affects personal health:* Greater emotional tiredness and cognitive stress were observed in those who worked more days from home, and this was associated with a decline in the social support they received from their peers. Due to this, it is difficult for an employee to work effectively and efficiently in "remote working".

Work Related Factors

- *Work Schedules:* Employees in the "remote work" generally find it difficult to stick to their work schedules. The main reason behind this is absence of typical office setting and improper supervision. Consequently, due to the social and family disturbances employee cannot focus on work, which affect their "work-life balance".
- *Working too much:* As per research, "remote workers" are working longer hours, attending further meeting, and running additional communication channels. According to a survey of 2,800 workers conducted by Los Angeles-based staffing business Robert Half, nearly 70% of professionals who switched to remote work as a result of the pandemic say they now work on the weekends, and 45% say they typically put in more hours during the week than they did previously. Thus, it is difficult for the employees to manage their professional and personal life.

Technology Related Factors

- *Dependent on Infrastructure:* If your workforce lacks the resources necessary to carry out their tasks efficiently, their productivity will suffer. Although your workers may be well-prepared for success at the office, if your business isn't currently set up to allow remote work, you will probably need to make a few infrastructure adjustments. Thus distant working makes employees dependent on infrastructure which affects their work.
- *Securing the digital assets of your business:* Employees who work from home probably need to access company resources remotely, such as internal networks or confidential information. Thus in "remote working" businesses have to communicate with MSSP (managed security services provider) to help business migrate and keep their digital assets safe both during and after the change. In case of negligence the company key information can be disclosed, this can influence the company image and its operations.
- *Additional Cost:* "Remote work" makes a worker reliant on technology, in case of absence of which influence the work. It requires employees to incur additional cost on the following basic requirements:
    - A dependable internet connection, such as a commercial broadband plan with unlimited data or a cellular backup based on a mobile router.
    - An electronic device such as a laptop or computer, as well as extra hardware like a laptop riser, an external keyboard and mouse, and a second (or third) display.

- Specialized software, as well as effective communication and teamwork, to complete your work.
- Proper furniture: Use an ergonomic chair to set up your workstation so that you may work comfortably.

OPPORTUNITIES OF REMOTE WORKING

Due to several obvious advantages that remote work has over conventional on-site work, both individuals and organizations frequently choose it. These comprise of (i) reduced or eliminated travel: Distant workers usually spend a smaller amount time getting to and from work. This often entails that a remote worker regains a considerable time every week. "Working from home" would allow somebody who would normally travel for 20-30 minutes each way to save many hours per week further saving funds on conveyance. Thus, the remote workers can then schedule their jobs at a specified time or have extra time. Distant workers are more expected to obtain less sick days than traditional employees since they can take care of themselves, (ii) talent pool: When choosing remote employees, business owners have more options. Depending on the hiring location's time zone, employees may be located anywhere in the world. As a result, there is a better chance of finding employees with specific talents and avoiding the need for training. The organization does not incur relocation expenses, which can be thousands of dollars, which is another advantage of hiring remote labor. As a result of having grown up with technology that makes working remotely possible, today's millennials almost expect to receive this option, (iii) improvements to business continuity: Due to the fact that virtual teams can work from different locations, they are often naturally adaptable. Where personnel would suddenly be unable to work in conventional office setting, it might be very helpful for continuous business scheduling, especially in any unanticipated or crisis conditions, (iv) reduced demand for corporate office space: Businesses that make use of a large number of distant workers usually need less office space, resulting in savings and longer-term elasticity, (v) advantages of hiring and recruiting: Because candidates do not have to be local or the company does not have to provide expensive relocation packages, hiring for a remote workforce can significantly increase a manager's pool of potential candidates. Any recruiter or hiring manager working in a highly competitive local labor market or experiencing a skills gap for specific roles can benefit greatly from this, (vi) reduced absenteeism: When working from home, an individual is more inclined to keep going even if they are experiencing a little unwell. They are not compelled to travel when feeling unwell and can take a break if they need to. There is a high probability that someone with a long commute is much more likely to call in sick than someone who only needs to travel a short distance between rooms. This also covers time off for events or appointments. If an employee can schedule their day around their job, they won't take extra time off, (vii) rise in productivity: The rise in productivity is experienced by staff members who are permitted to work from home (WFH) or remotely. (Prasada et al., 2020), conducted an experiment regarding "work from home" on employees in Chinese corporation, which states that "work from home" led to a 13% improvement in performance. This was brought on by two main causes: Firstly, on a monthly average, employees were able to work longer shifts thanks in large part to fewer breaks and sick days. Secondly, the remote workers were capable to perform the job in an additional constructive setting which allowed them to concentrate better and complete additional related activities in the similar amount of time, (viii) politics in the workplace: Workplace politics is a part of working life. Everyone has to face it whether it is a small business or a multi-millionaire business. In this a person or a group continuously cause or face difficult situations. In an office, there always exist persons with different likes and dislikes. It is the responsibility of the managers and human resources team to find the solution of these issues for the benefit of the business. Workforce is more fruitful and less concerned about whether A spent 10 to 15 minutes chatting with B at the vending machine when workplace politics aren't present.

Challenges of Remote Working

When best practices and basic concepts of how remote teams work are not followed, problems with remote working arise. This presents difficulties like: (i) **Impact on efficiency:** Employees might become detached and work less efficiently in due to lack of clear set of laws and conventions. (ii) **Micromanagement and lack of trust:** Low morale and increased anxiety can result from micromanagement, which is the psychological counterpart of watching someone's back to make sure they are performing their job. (iii) **Improper technology:** Remote workers will rely entirely on technology; therefore it must be ensured that everyone is immediately approachable via ICTs such as email, smartphone, and so on. For virtual teams, using insufficient tools and technologies can kill productivity and morale. Ineffective broadband connections, unstable software, and old hardware can all frustrate users and significantly reduce outcomes. (iv)**The resistant remote workforce:** When an employer or employee chooses not to work remotely as a deliberate decision or plan, there may be even another difficulty. The best candidates for remote work are those that actively seek it out for themselves and their employers. (v) **Easy Distraction:** The remote workers generally face distraction like children, TV shows. Moreover, they have full access to websites and social media, which affects their productivity and ability to complete responsibilities. (vi) **Difficult to build culture:** Business may find difficult to build a culture that recognize and supports "remote work", as it can be counterproductive to maintain efforts because it can affect employee motivation and happiness. Additionally, it can be challenging for a company to keep track of exactly who is working remotely, when they do it, and how they do it, especially when the practice is more casual. (vii) **Limited Learning:** Notably, there is no teamwork or knowledge sharing when working remotely. Therefore, no one can become more skilled by studying the work of others or specialists. (viii) **No Proper Supervision:** Since no one is always watching over our work remote employees need to be highly motivated, organized, and self-sufficient. Even though it can be tough for all employees to maintain a plan and manage their to-do lists, remote employees who have more flexible, free-form schedules and managers who are located elsewhere in the world often find it particularly difficult.

Thus, after understanding the complexity of the situation, the study provides practical suggestions to improve "work-life balance" in the "remote work".

SUGGESTIONS TO IMPROVE "WORK-LIFE BALANCE" IN THE "REMOTE WORK"

1. Creating the work zone: To focus on the task at hand, create a discrete workstation area from the rest of the house. If there isn't a designated workstation in the home, try to identify a spot or corner and utilize furniture to divide it up into a workspace. Additionally, let the family members know that this is a quiet area for working.
2. Avoid distracting surroundings: Regardless of the numerous noises, such as the sound of parents watching TV, light music headphones will help in improving concentration of the employees while

working. Additionally, let the family members know they shouldn't phone or visit during business hours. In this way, there won't be a clash between work and family.

3. Compliance to the working plan in detail: Discipline is essential when working from home. It involves spending the same amount of time each day in front of the computer at home. Thus for improving work life balance a detailed work schedule is required that includes rest periods. It is a great method to keep to a schedule similar to that of an office job.
4. Get ready to interact with the group: Stress and loneliness may result from working from home. The employees collaborate with coworkers via videoconference services like Zoom or a group chat line to support and share ideas on work. Additionally, effective remote communication can help workers to keep relationship with their coworkers, and managers.
5. Exit once you've finished working: The lack of distinction between personal and professional environment is a drawback of working from home. It results in people experiencing stress at work. Thus, after spending a long time at the computer, turn off all the work-related items. Then engage in other activities to relieve tension, regain energy, and get ready for work the following day.
6. Use leisure time to run individual assignment or engage in other activities: In "remote working", employees can use leisure time to run individual assignment or engage in other activities. Employees must take a little break from your desk or computer in order to maintain a healthy balance between work and life. In this manner employees can take breaks from work that are still beneficial and facilitate doing personal duties.
7. Avoid rescheduling or cancelling any of your meetings: Personnel may even be inclined to reschedule meetings so that he/she can attend them in the office. But if work schedule is ignored, that could actually make next day at work more difficult. Instead, arrange live meetings using video conferencing solutions from your house to ensure that you can complete your task even if you want to work from home.
8. Use of various applications for effective working: To assist working from home, there are numerous applications. The following applications are suggested as beneficial:
    - Everyone has the most widely used program, Line, installed on their smartphone or computer. Line is great for discussion, keeping track of actions, or making notes, generally in the form of "group lines."
    - Full videoconference services are offered by Zoom. It serves as a communication tool for a variety of enterprises. Particularly the Zoom Meetings and Chat service, which offers both audio and video calling capabilities. Zoom makes voice calls and video conferencing more practical and simple. It helps a small team's work in the free service model.
    - Once the work is complete, the use of Dropbox app is advised for transmitting information to the manager or staff. This program is a very practical cloud-based data management service. Others can browse or download up to 2TB of files for free using its file-sharing feature.
    - In remote work, Google Drive is useful. Due to a number of features, it performs better than comparable drives and function flawlessly on Mac computers. Users must be connected to the internet in order to utilize Google Drive and Google Docs. Additionally, Google Drive enables users and coworkers to collaborate on the same document or spreadsheet calculation program in real-time, allocate all participants to observe the modification and leave comments on the document.

- Word, Excel, PowerPoint, Outlook, OneNote, Access, and Publisher are all included in the Office 365 suite, to put it simply. It offers a variety of services and features and is a fully complete Office solution. Up to 6 persons can utilize Office 365 Home.

CONCLUSIONS AND RECOMMENDATIONS

In response to the unpredictable environment brought on by the COVID19 pandemic, Prasada et al. (2020) indicated that more and more businesses have noticed an increase in the number of their remote employees in recent years, and this trend will only continue. Under these considerations, the study set out on a search to discover and collect all the insightful information that was already available in the literature, intending to contribute to a better knowledge of a pervasive phenomenon and its improvement in the upcoming months and years. This study is a relevant contribution to our knowledge of remote work, which has been more common since the COVID-19 pandemic's onset. As a result, we deepen our understanding of how remote workers feel work-life balance and provide fresh viewpoints that may be crucial in promoting remote workers' wellbeing.

The workers connect to a remote computer site utilizing communication tools while working from home. A flexible work schedule allows employees to change their working hours at home for an improved employee balance. Work-family conflict, on the other hand, arises when there is conflict and stress between the significant role played in the two distinct domains of work and family. People, processes, and technology should all be present when working remotely. The benefits of remote work include reduced travel expenses and time savings from home to the workplace and back again. Additionally, the organization's resources, such as its use of water and electricity, are conserved by this distant operation. These are the drawbacks of working remotely. Using ICTs will be essential for remote workers. Due to an increase in Internet usage, things won't be as usual.

Therefore, the company should encourage workers to work from home by, for instance, providing them with an additional payment for Internet use, allowing them to borrow a computer and other equipment, or both. Importantly, there may be work-family tension when working from home. Employers have successfully embraced remote work, in addition to employees. The supervisor must be conscious of the factors that affect task completion, have a solid strategy, offer accessibility and adaptability of work, and be engaged in the goal. Some workers might choose to only work during regular business hours. The others, however, may schedule their time as convenient. Then, the milestones are utilized to monitor if the tasks will be completed on time.

Thus due to this pandemic, practically all firms now have the chance to abruptly transition to working online as virtual or digital businesses. However, once the pandemic has passed, the expense of adopting remote working may need to be covered by the organizations. Then, working remotely will be an addition to or a replacement for doing office job.

Moreover, Muralidhar et al. (2020) specified that technology, people and process plays an important role in the effective implementation of "remote working" by the employees as shown in Fig 1. For its execution high quality internet with workstation is required. Thus, company adopting it must ensure it.

Several companies like Google, Microsoft, and General Electronic used these methods and made a lot of benefits and not only fulfilled the organization goals but also enhanced the cooperation between organization and worker (Harris, 2007). Moreover, human resource managers use various types of FWA practices to face competitions and lots of challenges like rapid development in technology, price wars, and changes in the financial capital market (Arvanitis, 2005, Kauffeld, 2004).

The research demonstrates that remote working is, overall, advantageous to businesses and employees, despite these limitations and several high-profile employer U-turns. It also implies that, despite the lack of a full-fledged revolution, the separation of labor from place is unquestionably a crucial part of how work is changing in the twenty-first century. Therefore, those who are reading and writing for periodicals like New Technology, Work and Employment should pay great attention to this theme.

REFERENCES

Arvanitis, S. (2005). Modes of labour flexibility at firm level: Are there any implications for performance and innovation? Evidence for the Swiss economy. *Industrial and Corporate Change*, *14*(6).

Bhandari, K., & Soni, H. (2015). Impact of Gender, Age and Work Experience on Satisfaction towards Work Life Balance (with special reference to Bank of Baroda, Udaipur). *IOSR Journal of Business and Managemen*, *17*(3). doi:10.9790/487X-17324853

Das, S. S., & Mishra, S. A. (2016). A Study on Work Life Balance of Women Working in IT Sectors of Mumbai City. *International Journal of Humanities and Social Science Invention*, *5*(9), 43–47. www.ijhssi.org

Harris, P. (2007). Flexible work policies-means business. *T+D Journal*, 32-36.

Johari, J., Yean Tan, F., & Tjik Zulkarnain, Z. I. (2018). Autonomy, workload, work-life balance and job performance among teachers. *International Journal of Educational Management*, *32*(1), 107–120. doi:10.1108/IJEM-10-2016-0226

Kauffeld, S., Jonas, E., & Frey, D. (2004). Effect of a flexible work-time design on employee-and company – related aims. *European Journal of Work and Organizational Psychology*, *13*(1), 79–100. doi:10.1080/13594320444000001

Mas-Machuca, M., Berbegal-Mirabent, J., & Alegre, I. (2016). Work-life balance and its relationship with organizational pride and job satisfaction. *Journal of Managerial Psychology*, *31*(2), 586–602. doi:10.1108/JMP-09-2014-0272

Muralidhar, B., Prasad, K., & Rao Mangipudi, M. (2020). Association Among Remote Working Concerns and Challenges on Employee Work-Life Balance: An Empirical Study Using Multiple Regression Analysis With Reference To International Agricultural Research Institute, Hyderabad. *International Journal of Advanced Research in Engineering and Technology*, *11*(6), 281–297. doi:10.34218/IJARET.11.6.2020.025

Prasada, K. D. V., Vaidyab, R. W., & Mangipudic, M. R. (2020). Effect of occupational stress and remote working on psychological well-being of employees: An empirical analysis during covid-19 pandemic concerning information technology industry in Hyderabad. *Indian Journal of Commerce & Management Studies*, *XI*(2), 1. doi:10.18843/ijcms/v11i2/01

Purohit, M. (2013). a Comparative Study of Work Life Balance in Various Industrial Sectors in Pune Region. *International Journal of Marketing, Financial Services & Management Research*, *2*(3), 198–206.

Raghavendra, H. K., & Raghunandan, M. V. (2018). Women engineers and work life balance a case study of women working in manufacturing industries in Mysuru city. *International Journal of Mechanical Engineering and Technology*, *9*(1), 752–755.

Rao, M., Prasad, K. D. V., & Vaidya, R. (2019). Employee competencies as the predictors of the performance management system: An empirical study in IT enabled service companies around *Hyderabad. International Journal of Management*, *10*(6), 33–44. doi:10.34218/IJM.10.6.2019.004

Robertson, S. L., Robinson, M. D., & Reid, A. (2017). Electronic Health Record Effects on Work-Life Balance and Burnout Within the I3 Population. *Collaborative Journal of Graduate Medical Education*, *9*(4), 479–484. doi:10.4300/JGME-D-16-00123.1 PMID:28824762

Songsangyos, P., & Iamamporn, S. (2020). Remote Working with Work-life Balance. International. *Journal of Applied Computer Technology and Information Systems*, *9*(2), 85–88.

Suresh, Sharma, & Beulah. (2018). A Conceptual Analysis on Work Life Balance. *Journal of Management*, *5*(4), 97–100.

workforce in IT sector incapable of remote working: Study. (n.d.). Retrieved from https://economictimes.indiatimes.com/tech/ites/99-8pc-workforcein-it-sector-incapable-of-remote-working-study/articleshow/75080948.cms

Chapter 14
Exploring the Interplay Between Stress Management and Work-Life Balance for Employees

Shweta Saini
https://orcid.org/0000-0001-8639-9339
Maharshi Dayanand University, India

Rohit Bansal
https://orcid.org/0000-0001-7072-5005
Vaish College of Engineering, India

ABSTRACT

Stress at the workplace has become a predominant issue. Numerous people's lifestyles are seriously impacted by the influence of longer workdays, which eventually impacts their social and psychological well-being. And because of this, the idea of work-life balance is becoming increasingly important in a workplace that is always changing. This study aims to discover the techniques to manage stress to ensure work-life balance in today's world. Data were collected from various secondary sources, such as journals, books, websites, etc., using different search engines such as Google Scholar and Scopus. The findings reveal that stress management is helpful for all the employees at the workplace as it helps employees to balance their work-life and improve their morale. The techniques to manage stress also allow the human resource to take the initiative for their employees to facilitate better work-life balance options.

INTRODUCTION

At the whirlwind, the nature of employees is changing. And as a result, stress is a worldwide issue that affects not just the health and happiness of workers but also the productivity of businesses. When something feels too much, when someone is overburdened and doesn't feel like they can handle all the expectations and obstacles that are being placed on them, that is when they say they are stressed. Stress has varied meanings for different people. When employees struggle to handle the demands and other

DOI: 10.4018/978-1-6684-8565-1.ch014

problems, they become stressed. Although stress is not a disease, it can nonetheless make you ill. The answer seems to lie in how individuals can cope, with it, since stress can occasionally inspire, revitalize, and help them to achieve more. Therefore, the aim of this chapter is to discover the techniques to manage stress to ensure work-life balance in today's world.

LITERATURE REVIEW

Kalliath & Brough (2008) evaluated six popular conceptions of work-life balance and pinpoints the key characteristics that seem to best capture the concept of work. The research identified six conceptualizations of numerous roles: perceived control between multiple roles, equity across multiple roles, satisfaction between multiple roles, fulfilment of role salience between multiple roles, and a relationship between conflict and facilitation.

Rao (2016) Describes numerous aspects of stress and draws a distinction between it and burnout. Sound sleep, exercise, and a healthy appetite, according to the author, are the three signs of excellent health. As long as a person is in excellent health, manages their stress, and leads a fulfilling life.

Appiah et al. (2013) studied the work-life balance policies and practices in some of Ghana's banking institutions and how they affected some employees. For primary data, a quantitative approach was employed in conjunction with descriptive statistics. According to research, there are no cultures that effectively support work-life balance and improve employees' performance at work and at home.

Atheya & Arora (2014) demonstrated that stress has an impact on how well an organization works. People must examine their values and goals to determine what they want from work and life. They must then devise effective methods for juggling the two, as well as take action to lessen stress and burnout. "Employers should educate staff members on work-life balance and stress-reduction initiatives. Even while organizations offer employee assistance programs" like stress-management and flexible work-schedules, the complex nature of stress still seems to have a negative impact on health and work-life balance.

Wafula & Nyaboga (2019) studied the effects of psychotherapy on stress management and employee performance. Purposive sampling and survey research design were employed. Data collection involved the use of questionnaires. According to the findings, stressors undoubtedly have a bad effect on one's mental state, affecting how well one performs at work.

WORK-LIFE BALANCE

A specific collection of corporate practices, policies, initiatives, and a philosophy known as "work-life balance" actively supports efforts to aid people in being successful at both work and home (Bansal, R., & Pruthi, N. 2021). While attempting to schedule an equal amount of hours for each of your interests is typically difficult and unsatisfying, work-life balance does not require an equal balance. Because everyone has various objectives and lives, the significance of work-life balance varies from person to person (Asamoah-Appiah, W., & Aggrey-Fynn, I 2017).

STRESS MANAGEMENT

People deal with a lot of pressure in daily life, which negatively affects them. Stress is a negative response that someone has to being under a lot of strain. We are said to feel "stressed" when we believe the situation is beyond our capacity for handling it. Workplace stress issues have a negative impact on both employee health and corporate productivity. It can cause a variety of issues, including poor job performance, drunkenness, job unhappiness, and absenteeism (Asiedu-Appiah, F., Dufie-Marfo, I., & Frempong, E. 2016). The level of job stress has grown to frightening proportions and is now a significant problem for businesses. Stress can both benefit and harm a person. Good stress inspires someone, gives their lives a little extra flavor, and gives them a lethal charge. However, stress turns damaging and causes distress or unpleasant stress when it is protracted or irritating.

Figure 1. Common Causes of Stress at Workplace
Source: Evolveinc.io

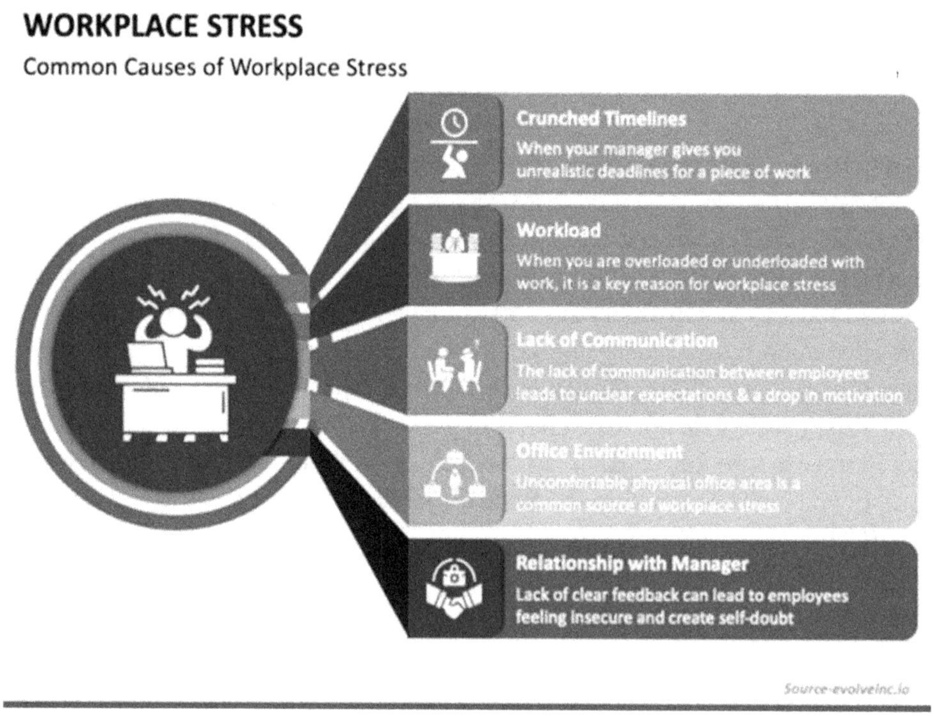
WORKPLACE STRESS
Common Causes of Workplace Stress
Crunched Timelines
When your manager gives you unrealistic deadlines for a piece of work
Workload
When you are overloaded or underloaded with work, it is a key reason for workplace stress
Lack of Communication
The lack of communication between employees leads to unclear expectations & a drop in motivation
Office Environment
Uncomfortable physical office area is a common source of workplace stress
Relationship with Manager
Lack of clear feedback can lead to employees feeling insecure and create self-doubt
Source-evolveinc.io

Techniques To Manage Stress

Avoid Unnecessary Stress

While delaying a problem that needs to be tackled is unhealthy, not all stress can be avoided. You might be surprised by how many stressors you can get rid of, though. Get good at saying "no" Recognize your limits and respect them. In your personal or professional life, don't accept more responsibilities when you're about to finish them (Bansal, R., Masood, R., & Dadhich, V. 2014). Stress will only result from trying to take on more than you can bear. Avert stressful individuals - You should either limit your time with them or end the relationship entirely if a person consistently adds stress to your life and you are unable to improve the relationship. Control your environment by turning off the TV if the nightly news gives you anxiety. Take a longer, less-traveled route if traffic is making you anxious. If visiting the market is a pain, order your groceries online. Stop bringing up the subject or make an excuse when it comes up if you frequently quarrel about the same thing with the same folks. (Wafula, M., & Nyaboga, E. 2019). Condense your to-do list. Examine your obligations, schedule, and everyday responsibilities. If you have too much on your plate, decide which obligations are "musts" and which are "shoulds." Move less-important chores to the bottom of the list or do away with them entirely.

Alter the Situation

Try to change a stressful situation if you can't prevent it. Determine what you can do to make the situation different so that the issue doesn't arise again. Frequently, this entails altering how you speak and behave in everyday situations. Instead of holding your emotions inside, express them. Communicate your concerns in an honest and courteous manner if something or someone is troubling you. Resentment will grow if you don't express your feelings, and things will probably stay the same. Be open to negotiating. Be prepared to alter your own conduct when you ask someone else to. Finding a pleasant middle ground is likely if both of you are ready to budge just a little. Be more adamant. Don't let your personal life fall to the wayside. Face issues head-on and make every effort to foresee and stop them. If your chatty roommate just got home and you have an exam to study for, let them know up front that you only have five minutes to talk. Organize your time better. It can be extremely difficult to have time management issues. When you're stretched too thin and behind schedule, it's hard to stay calm and focused. However, you can change how stressed you are if you prepare ahead of time and watch out for overcommitting yourself. (Atheya, R., & Arora, R. 2014).

Adapt to the Stressor

If you can't change the stressor, change yourself. You can deal with challenging situations and regain control by changing your expectations and attitude. Reframe issues. Consider situations that are difficult from a more optimistic standpoint. Consider a traffic delay a time to pause, collect your thoughts, tune in to your favourite radio station, or just relax rather than becoming irate at it. Focus on the positive. When stress is getting to you, take a moment to reflect on all the things you love in your life, including your own positive attributes and abilities. You can maintain perspective with the aid of this straightforward technique (Bansal, R., & Minocha, K. 2017). Changing Your Mentality Your mental health can have a significant impact on your emotional and physical health. Your body responds as though it were experiencing a tense state whenever you have a negative idea about yourself. You are more likely to feel well about yourself if you think well of yourself, but the opposite is also true. Substitute words like "always," "never," "should," and "must" for others.

Accept the Things

You can't change Certain pressures simply cannot be avoided. Stressors like the death of a loved one, a life-threatening illness, or a general economic downturn are inescapable and uncontrollable. In these situations, the best way to manage stress is to accept things as they are. (Evolve. 2021, June 8). Acceptance can be difficult, but in the end, it's easier than whining about something you can't change. Do not try to control the uncontrollable. We have no control over a lot of things in life, most notably what other people do. Instead of worrying about the things you cannot control, put your attention on the things you can, such the way you decide to respond to problems. Consider the positives. What doesn't kill us makes us stronger, as the adage goes up (Bansal, R., & Saini, S. 2022). When faced with significant obstacles, strive to see them as chances for personal development. If you made bad choices that resulted in a stressful situation, reflect on them and use the chance to learn from them. Describe your feelings. (Bansal, R. 2018).

Make Time for Fun and Relaxation

In addition to taking charge and being optimistic, you may lessen stress in your life by taking care of yourself. If you routinely carve out time for enjoyment and rest, you'll be better equipped to handle life's inevitable stresses. sane techniques for unwinding and recharging Take a walk. Spend some time outside. Make a call to a trustworthy buddy. Exercise will help you sweat out your stress. (Rao, M. S. 2016). You should journal. Go for a long bath. ignite some scented candles. Enjoy a steaming cup of tea or coffee. Have fun with a pet. Do some gardening. Receive a massage. Lie down and read a good book. Play some music. Observe a comedy. Avoid becoming so stressed out by regular life that you forget to take care of your own needs.

Adopt a Healthy Lifestyle

By improving your physical health, you can better withstand stress. routine exercise Physical activity can greatly reduce and even avoid the effects of stress. Plan to work out for at least 30 minutes three times per week (Bansal, R., & Saini, S. 2022). The best approach to release accumulated stress and worry is through aerobic exercise. Eat a healthy diet. Pay attention to what you eat because properly fueled bodies can handle stress better. You may maintain high energy levels and mental clarity throughout the day by eating balanced, nutrient-rich meals. (Hannigan, B., Edwards, D., & Burnard, P. 2004). While using alcohol or drugs as self-medication may make it simple to escape stress, the calm is only temporary. Track down the cause of your stress. Along with looking outside, you also need to look inside. Talk to people about your worries.

- Talking to someone could be beneficial. Perhaps a friend, member of your family, a teacher, or a counsellor can offer you new perspective on the issue. You can seek professional assistance from a psychologist, psychiatrist, or social worker if you believe your issue is significant (Bansal, R., & Saini, S. 2022). Knowing when to seek for assistance can help you avoid later, more significant issues.
- Know your boundaries. Avoid fighting an issue if it is out of your control or cannot be changed right now. Recognize what you can't alter and learn to accept it. It will occasionally be appropriate

to act and reduce the stress. But other times, you might just have to adjust your perspective and deal with things as they are. (Kalliath, T., & Brough, P. 2008). Never waste time second-guessing a choice you've made, no matter what it may be.

- Cross off your to-do list. It can be stressful to try to handle everything at once. As a result, you might not get anything done. 4 Make a list of the chores you need to complete instead, and complete each one at a time. Don't forget to start with the most crucial chores and cross them off as you finish them. Consider assigning jobs that can be completed by others as well. Keep in mind that YOU DO NOT HAVE TO DO EVERYTHING! (Murphy, L. R. 1996).
- Resist the urge to constantly be "right." Do other people irritate you, especially when they don't do things the way you want them to?
- Instead of hostility, try cooperation. Instead of arguing and demanding your way, compromise is preferable. Everyone will feel more at ease and the strain will be reduced if both sides are willing to compromise.
- Take some time off from it. You should take a "time out" when tensions rise and you become too emotional to reason rationally or make responsible decisions. There are several ways to accomplish this, like counting to fifty, moving on to another room, or delaying the choice until later. When we step away from a problem for a while, they frequently find a way to resolve themselves. (Ladegård, G. 2011).
- Set up a calm environment. Although you might not be able to flee, you can "dream the impossible dream." You can escape the agitation of a stressful circumstance by visualizing a peaceful place in your mind. To induce calmness, try reading a nice book or listening to soothing music.
- Become more at ease — LAUGH! Even when you don't feel like smiling, there are occasions when doing so will reduce stress and help you feel much more at ease. If the smile can develop into a belly laugh, the tension will go. To not take ourselves too seriously is a key component of the secret. The second step is to adopt the mentality that "this too shall pass."

CONCLUSION

It is paradoxical that despite having large incomes, most of it is spent on illnesses brought on by stress. They must develop the ability to balance pressure and enjoyment. They need to be capable of juggling their social, professional, and personal lives. Some people spend their entire lives working. Earning money without considering the purpose of life. Sound sleep, exercise, and a healthy appetite are the final three signs of excellent health. If you take advantage of these, you'll be in good health, manage your stress, and have a fulfilling life.

REFERENCES

Asamoah-Appiah, W., & Aggrey-Fynn, I. (2017). The impact of occupational stress on employee's performance: A study at Twifo oil palm plantation limited. *African Journal of Applied Research, 3*(1), 14–25.

Asiedu-Appiah, F., Dufie-Marfo, I., & Frempong, E. (2016). *Work-life balance as a tool for stress management in selected banking institutions in Ghana*. Academic Press.

Atheya, R., & Arora, R. (2014). Stress and its brunt on employee's work-life balance (wlb): A conceptual study. *IOSR Journal of Humanities and Social Science, 19*(3), 58-61.

Bansal, R. (2018). Stress management at workplace. *International Journal of Techno-Management Research, 5*(04), 29–32.

Bansal, R., Masood, R., & Dadhich, V. (2014). Social media marketing-a tool of innovative marketing. *Journal of Organizational Management, 3*(1), 1–7.

Bansal, R., & Minocha, K. (2017). Impact of social media on Consumer Attitude Towards A Brand With Special Reference to Hospitality Industry. *International Research Journal of Management and Commerce, 4*(8), 106–120.

Bansal, R., & Pruthi, N. (2021). Developing Customer Engagement Through social media: A Review of Literature. *Marketing 5.0: Putting Up Blocks Together, 80.*

Bansal, R., & Saini, S. (2022). Leveraging role of social media influencers in corporate world-An overview. *NOLEGEIN-Journal of Global Marketing, 5*(1), 1–5.

Bansal, R., & Saini, S. (2022). Exploring the Role of social media: An Innovative Tool for Entrepreneurs. In *Applying Metalytics to Measure Customer Experience in the Metaverse* (pp. 34–43). IGI Global. doi:10.4018/978-1-6684-6133-4.ch004

Hannigan, B., Edwards, D., & Burnard, P. (2004). Stress and stress management in clinical psychology: Findings from a systematic review. *Journal of Mental Health (Abingdon, England), 13*(3), 235–245. do i:10.1080/09638230410001700871

Kalliath, T., & Brough, P. (2008). Work–life balance: A review of the meaning of the balance construct. *Journal of Management & Organization, 14*(3), 323–327. doi:10.5172/jmo.837.14.3.323

Ladegård, G. (2011). Stress management through workplace coaching: The impact of learning experiences. *International Journal of Evidence Based Coaching and Mentoring, 9*(1).

Murphy, L. R. (1996). Stress management in work settings: A critical review of the health effects. *American Journal of Health Promotion, 11*(2), 112–135. doi:10.4278/0890-1171-11.2.112 PMID:10163598

Rao, M. S. (2016). Innovative tools and techniques to manage your stress to ensure work-life balance. *Industrial and Commercial Training, 48*(6), 320–324. doi:10.1108/ICT-05-2015-0035

Stress archives. (2021, June 8). *Evolve*. Retrieved December 28, 2022, from https://evolveinc.io/mental-health/stress/

Wafula, M., & Nyaboga, E. (2019). Stress management and employee performance: Use of psychotherapy as mitigation in selected schools (School of business and economics and Health sciences) in Kisii University, Kenya. *Merit Research Journal of Business and Management, 7*(3), 19–27.

ADDITIONAL READING

Boss, P., Bryant, C. M., & Mancini, J. A. (2016). *Family stress management: A contextual approach*. Sage Publications.

Pettinger, R. (2002). *Stress management*. Capstone.

Powell, T., & Enright, S. (2015). *Anxiety and stress management*. Routledge. doi:10.4324/9781315683867

Quick, J. C., Wright, T. A., Adkins, J. A., Nelson, D. L., & Quick, J. D. (1997). *Preventive stress management in organizations*. American Psychological Association. doi:10.1037/10238-000

Schafer, W. (1996). *Stress management for wellness*. Harcourt Brace College Publishers.

Sutherland, V., & Cooper, C. (2000). *Strategic stress management: An organizational approach*. Springer. doi:10.1057/9780230509146

Van den Bergh, O. (2021). *Principles and practice of stress management*. Guilford Publications.

Yadav, R. K., & Yadav, S. S. (2014). Impact of work life balance and stress management on job satisfaction among the working women in public sector banks. *International Letters of Social and Humanistic Sciences*, *26*, 63–70. doi:10.18052/www.scipress.com/ILSHS.26.63

KEY TERMS AND DEFINITIONS

Stress: Stress is a typical bodily response to change that causes physical, emotional, and cognitive reactions.

Stress Management: The variety of methods, plans, and treatments used to assist people control their stress is known as stress management.

Work-Life Balance: A phrase that refers to the idea that you need to have time for both work and other facets of your life, such as your family and personal interests.

Work-Life Conflict: Work-life conflict is a type of inter-role conflict in which demands in the work and family spheres are contradictory, making it challenging to meet demands in both.

Chapter 15
Cultivating Compassion for Resilience and Wellbeing:
Applications for Individuals and Workplaces

Justin D. Henderson
https://orcid.org/0000-0003-4379-5045
Lewis & Clark College, USA

Alexia de León
Lewis & Clark College, USA

Jeffrey K. Christensen
Lewis & Clark College, USA

ABSTRACT

Global rates of stress and mental health distress have reached all-time highs. Given the scale of the problem, the development and dissemination of stress management strategies ought to be accessible, trainable, and low-cost. Growing evidence indicates that the utilization of compassion-based skills has positive effects on stress reduction, enhanced mental wellbeing, and emotional resilience. In this chapter, the science of compassion will be highlighted and reviewed. This chapter explores the psychological and neurobiological foundations of compassion and how those factors can be trainable motivations and behaviors. The science of compassion demonstrates that people can reduce stress in their lives by engendering the perspective taking, emotion regulation, and relational skills within compassionate behaviors. Given contemporary workplace stressors, the application of compassion to address stress and wellbeing in the workplace is explored.

INTRODUCTION

Problems with stress and mental health were pervasive prior to the COVID-19 pandemic and have only

DOI: 10.4018/978-1-6684-8565-1.ch015

grown more significant over time. In 2019, an estimated 970 million people worldwide were living with a mental disorder, accounting for about one in eight adults (WHO, 2022). Similarly, nearly 50 million American adults experienced a mental illness in 2019 (Reinert, Fritz, & Nguyen, 2021). The COVID-19 pandemic has led to significant global social and economic disruptions that have resulted in a compounding effect of stress and overwhelm.

The Global Burdens of Disease (GBD) estimates a 25-27% rise in the prevalence of depression and anxiety since the beginning of the pandemic (Santomauro et al., 2021). Additionally, workers have reported the highest stress levels on record (Gallup State of the Global Workplace Report, 2022). Thus, there is a strong need to respond to the mental health needs of adults, including how to mitigate the adverse effects of stress and crisis. When humans, individually or collectively, are activated by stress and threat, compassion is both a motivational framework and an evidence-based skill set that can enhance emotion regulation, appropriately orient problem-solving, and activate a sense of belonging (Gilbert, 2017; Kolts & Chodron, 2013).

Modern people have to contend with a chronic contextual overload. There are so many stressors– including personal, societal, and global –that people have to manage in their lives. Additionally, there are many contextual constraints placed on maintaining peoples' wellbeing including time, money, and other resource limitations. Addressing issues of stress, therefore, cannot only include expensive, high-resource strategies if they are to be applicable and distributable at scale. Modern stress management strategies need to include interventions and practices that are highly accessible, trainable, and affordable. Compassion-based interventions meet this criterion.

Since the 1970s, researchers have established a clear link between mindfulness practice and stress reduction (Kabat Zinn, 2013). Programs like Mindfulness-Based Stress Reduction (MBSR) have been shown to effectively reduce stress and enhance wellbeing (Khoury, Sharma, Rush, & Fournier,2015). While mindfulness contemplative interventions may have elements of compassion interventions within them, practices that focus primarily on developing compassion offer something unique to individuals and workplaces (Brito-Pons, Campos, & Cebolla, 2018). Over the past decade, an emergence of research has investigated the benefits of compassion practices on stress and wellbeing. Compassion cultivation is a type of mind training that translates to tangible intrapersonal and interpersonal outcomes leading to greater resilience and wellbeing (Roca et al., 2021).

The following chapter explores the function and importance of compassion in the wellbeing of individuals and groups. The authors will explore the definitions of compassion and what facets contribute toward compassionate motivations and behaviors. The chapter will explore the positive outcomes compassion practice has on stress, health, and wellbeing. The authors provide an overview of how compassion training programs are structured and implemented. Lastly, the authors discuss how compassion can be applied to workplace settings to reduce stress, burnout, and increase group cohesion.

DEFINITIONS OF COMPASSION

Compassion comes from the Latin *compati*, which means "to suffer with." In contemporary contexts, compassion is a word with a myriad of definitions of varying degrees of clarity (Gilbert, 2017). These various definitions and lack of consensus are partly due to compassion being used in various cultures and eras to describe disparate phenomena. The original Latin-derived term described processes more akin to what would be understood as sympathy or empathy (Gilbert, 2017; Goetz, Keltner, & Simon-

Thomas, 2010). To advance the understanding of the applications of compassion, it is necessary to sort out the common usages of compassion and locate a workable definition that captures the essence of the construct relevant to the application of stress management.

Locating a Working Definition of Compassion

Compassion is multifaceted and requires some explicit unpacking. Feldmen and Kuyken (2011) described compassion as an *orientation* to human suffering. The word orientation is derived from the word *orient,* which means to 'point oneself toward' something. Similar to how in sea navigation a compass orients a sailor to due north, compassion offers direction in the sea of human suffering. Compassion becomes a helpful framework given the disorienting force pain and suffering can have on people. In this way, compassion points people toward human suffering rather than avoidance.

In addition to an orientation or direction, compassion is also a *motivational force*–an evolved system that motivates human beings to engage in care-oriented behaviors. Compassion is a motivation to see the suffering in others or self be relieved and/or prevented (Gilbert & Chodron, 2014). Succinctly, the Dalai Lama (1995) offered a definition of compassion that summarizes the two parts of compassion (orientation and motivation). He defined compassion as *the sensitivity to the suffering in ourselves and others with a deep motivation and commitment to alleviate and prevent it* (Dalai Lama, 1995).

Differentiating Compassion from Other Constructs

The lack of consensus and clarity about compassion as a construct has been due, at times, to a lack of conceptual clarity in distinguishing compassion from other related phenomena. Compassion is sometimes described as sympathy, an emotion, empathy, or altruism. If compassion is to be understood as not only a psychological contract but also a skill set that can be trained, compassion must be clearly differentiated from other psychological constructs.

Sometimes compassion is likened to *pity*, a top-down approach to another's suffering where the person extending pity feels very little for the person experiencing suffering. Both pity and compassion recognize the suffering of another. However, pity assumes a relational asymmetry between the person who suffers and the person observing said suffering. This is antithetical to practices of compassion that emphasize equanimity and common humanity (Dalai Lama, & Cutler, 1998).

Compassion has been commonly described as an *emotion* or affiliative feeling (Goetz, Keltner, & Simon-Thomas, 2010). As Gilbert (2017) notes problems with conceptualizing compassion as a discrete emotion given that compassionate behavior may occur with people exhibiting a number of emotional states, including blended emotions. In other words, people do not have to feel a particular emotion, like love, to be compassionate–quite the contrary. In more advanced compassion cultivation, people learn to extend compassion to people whom they might struggle to relate to or might see as interpersonally challenging (Jinpa, 2015).

Similar to emotion, compassion is sometimes described as a form of *empathy* (Gilbert, 2009). Empathy is the capacity to feel others' feelings. Empathy is a process of emotionally connecting to another's experience because the person extending empathy has some resonating experience (Leblanc, Gingles & Byers, 2016). Compassion does require an emotional resonance on the part of the person extending compassion. However, beyond merely emotionally resonating with someone, compassion is action oriented. Neurological research has been able to differentiate between empathic activation and compassion activation in the brain in highly trained meditators, suggesting that empathy and compassion are fundamentally different brain states (Klimecki, Leibert, Ricard, & Singer, 2013).

MINDFULNESS AND COMPASSION

Mindfulness is the awareness that arises through paying attention, on purpose, in the present moment, non-judgmentally (Kabat-Zinn, 2013). The deployment of compassion-based skills requires a mindful presence. Mindfulness and compassion as constructs are separate but related. Mindfulness is an awareness of personal consciousness while compassion notes humanity's interdependence in the presence of suffering (Kolts & Chodron, 2013). In other words, it is commonly understood that compassion is a deliberate use of mindful presence with specific motivations and intention as will be described later. Compassion skills are most often taught within a curriculum that includes training in foundational mindfulness skills (e.g., Germer & Neff, 2019; Jinpa, 2015).

Components Of Compassion

Compassion is multifaceted and contains psychological, biological, and social elements. Each of these elements have important considerations both in the training of compassion and the use of compassion to mitigate the effects of stress. Compassion is an evolved capacity toward caregiving (Gilbert, 2009) that can be strengthened by training (Jinpa, 2015). In order to effectively train and enhance this capacity requires trainers and those interested in compassion to first understand the components underlying compassion.

Psychological Dimensions of Compassion

Compassion can be understood as a coping strategy that promotes wellbeing in the presence of stressors (Allen & Leary, 2010). Both training in compassion skills and deploying these skills involve two separate but equally important psychological dimensions. These two dimensions are described by Tirch, Schoendorff, & Silberstein (2014) as the *psychology of engagement* and the *psychology of alleviation*. Each of the dimensions of compassion also contains psychological qualities within them (see Figure 1).

Table 1. The Psychological dimensions of compassion

Psychological Dimensions of Compassion	
Engagement	*Alleviation*
• Awareness of suffering (cognitive) • Feeling of concern for and connection to the one who is suffering (affective)	• Desire to relieve suffering (intention) • Willingness to respond or take action (motivation)

The Psychology of Engagement

The psychology of engagement describes a process by which people intentionally draw their awareness to suffering. Gilbert and Choden (2014) describe engagement as a motivation to notice and identify suffering. Compassionate processes counteract behavioral responses aimed at distracting or numbing away from distress (Allen & Leary, 2010). Engagement also promotes a motivational awareness to recognize the suffering in self and others, sensitizing the individual to the needs of those who are the focus of compassionate response.

Within the psychology of engagement, there are cognitive processes that are critical to activating compassion–namely, a person's focus and attention. A compassionate person is paying attention to others and noticing the presence of suffering. When engaged in self-compassion, a person is attending to their own suffering non-judgmentally. Critical to engagement is also an affective component, specifically affiliative emotions. The compassionate person is affectively sensitive to the presence of suffering in another. This is the point of divergence from feeling states such as sympathy or pity that do not require affiliative emotional activation.

When applied to stress and wellbeing, the psychology of engagement appropriately encourages people to inventory and address the stress. At first, compassion may allow a person to attend mindfully, without avoidance, to the difficulties of their life (Allen & Leary, 2010; Germer, 2009). When the focus of compassion is on another person, there is an extension of tenderness and kindness for the person experiencing stress. When the focus is self-compassion, there is an intentional softening of the difficulties faced. The psychology of engagement allows a person experiencing stress to identify the nature of the pain and what they might need to address the issue (Gilbert & Choden, 2014).

The Psychology of Wise Alleviation

The psychology of alleviation contains processes aimed at preventing or extinguishing suffering (Gilbert, 2017). Within compassion is a desire for those experiencing suffering to no longer suffer. Compassion is an active process. For example, research investigating the impacts of increased self-compassion have shown that people experience a significant increase in self-improvement motivation as their self-compassion is improved (Breines & Chen, 2012).

Some have noted that the cultivation of compassion also contributes toward the development of wisdom because a compassionate motivation focuses on solutions that keep longer-term consequences in mind (Siegel & Germer, 2012). In other words, wise alleviation contrasts with seeking out momentary, short-term pleasures amid challenging contexts. Germer (2009) noted the positive impact that compassion has on bringing about happiness that is not propagated from a hedonic treadmill of surface-level pleasures.

Active compassionate behaviors, then, seek to find longer-term and deeper satisfaction to the challenges and stressors faced. Self-compassion, in particular, has been associated with constructive problem-solving motivations and behaviors (Allen & Leary, 2010). In an experimental setting, Leary et al. (2007) found that—after being inducted into self-compassion—participants took greater responsibility in addressing stressful events and experienced less negative distress. Finding wise alleviation also includes efforts to prevent future suffering, which might include building new responses and coping strategies applicable to future stress (Gilbert, 2017).

Neurobiological and Evolutionary Components of Compassion

Humanity's capacities for compassion are deeply rooted in the evolutionary history of the human species (Ricard, 2013). Archaeological evidence suggests that early humanity was characterized by a wide capacity to care for others (Spikins, 2017; Gilbert, 2022). Darwin posited that human beings' capacity toward altruistic behavior was an evolved instinct that was selected based on survival value (Wang, 2005).

Like other mammals, human parents are neurologically primed to care for offspring. This nurturance impulse is critically important given the elongated maturation of humans compared to most other animals. Human infants are helpless and remain immature for many years–requiring mature humans to tend to children's needs and protection. The neurobiological substrates of compassion have been theorized as expanded capacities of evolved caregiving capacities (Gilbert, 2022). Humans possess the unique ability to extend care and concern for others far outside of their own children and kin relationships. In compassion skills training a practitioner intentionally refines these capacities by extending compassion first to a loved one, then to a stranger, and then to those considered aversive in some manner (Jinpa, 2015). Not only does the human capacity to care for others provide greater survival prospects, it also provides a soothing environment that has direct implications for stress inoculation (Gilbert, 2009).

Evolved Systems of Affect Regulation

Stress is not only a psychological experience but a physiological process as well. Gilbert (2009) proposed a framework for understanding how compassion evolved from broader systems of affective regulation. This framework is referred to as the *Three Circles Model of Emotions* because it organizes three separate yet interrelated patterns of affect regulation. What Gilbert (2009) proposes is that human survival is dependent on balancing the survival tasks of resource-seeking and protection with affiliative care. Basic human emotions manifest in contexts where the need for seeking out resources, a human's survival is threatened, or where care and soothing are received.

First, humans possess a *threat self-protection system*, which aims to identify and respond to perceived physical or social dangers (Gilbert 2009). When activated, it primes threat-focused emotions such as fear, anxiety, or disgust and urges protection and safety-seeking behaviors. Cortisol, the stress hormone, is primarily activated when this system is primed.

Next, survival requires more than merely protecting oneself. Humans must seek resources necessary for survival (e.g., food, shelter, sexual partners). According to this model, this is referred to as the *drive system* and is responsible for incentivizing wanting, pursuing, achieving, and consuming behaviors through the emotions of excitement and pleasure. The neurotransmitter dopamine is proposed as the substance that is particularly relevant to this system activation (Gilbert, 2009).

Lastly, humans seek out connection and contentment. This system is largely affiliative and offers mechanisms for soothing distress and promoting a felt sense of safeness (Gilbert 2022). The capacity to soothe oneself is first developed through exposure to a secure base and safe haven (e.g., caregivers). The proximity of caring others provides the context whereby a child learns to regulate their drive and threat systems. As maturation progresses, people internalize this secure base and safe haven–expanding their internal capacities to self-sooth, ground, and downregulate threat activation. The *contentment/soothing system* helps regulate the central nervous system from the potential stress or distress that can result from imbalances in threat or drive activation (Gilbert, 2022).

The hormone oxytocin is associated with this soothing system (Gilbert, 2009). Oxytocin is strongly associated with social behaviors and has been shown to increase with compassion practice (Bellosta-Batalla et al., 2020). The oxytocinergic system is involved with social bonding, social conflict resolution, understanding others' feelings, and self-related and other-related processing (Colonnello, Petrocchi, & Heinrichs, 2017). This system plays a particularly important role in our ability to manage stressors and threats since oxytocin regulates aspects of the parasympathetic nervous system and modulates the vagal dorsal motor nucleus. The vagal dorsal nerve activity is linked to our capacity to regulate emotional distress (Porges, 2011). In experimental research, training in compassion has shown increases in oxytocin levels Bellosta-Batalla, et al., 2020).

Relational Components of Compassion

Compassion is also a socioemotional process that enhances people's capacities to take various perspectives (Kolts & Chodron, 2013; Strosahl, Robinson, & Gustavsson, 2015). Compassion skills training focuses on three relational modes: extending compassion toward another, toward themselves (self-compassion), or being the recipient of compassion. Employing a compassionate orientation toward another means taking on the perspective of another person and the perspective of the whole of humanity in an effort to reduce distress (Jinpa, 2015). When extending compassion to others, compassion training encourages an ever-widening zone of concern to include others beyond our immediate social environments. This process is not merely an abstraction but rather a pointed effort at gathering our affiliative capacities and extending them to strangers and even those that we find challenging in our lives. Compassion meditations like 'Just Like Me' as described in Compassion Cultivation Training, encourage people to see the suffering of others as similar to one's own suffering (Jinpa, 2015).

When a person employs self-compassion, a relational framework is still emphasized. In Neff's (2011) conceptualization of self-compassion, tapping into an appreciation of common humanity is a vital part of engaging compassion processes. To soften the propensity toward self-contempt, participants may be encouraged to relate to their own struggles with the same kindness they would extend to a close friend (Gilbert, 2009). Acknowledging humanity's common experience of suffering bridges, a felt sense of connection in the midst of struggle and distress. This can, in turn, reduce self-judgment and combat shame while facilitating a broadening and building of wider solutions (Neff, 2011). Self-compassion can help combat shame and self-attacking by improving self-relations that promote kindness and softening self-criticism (Kolts, 2019).

In the most extreme cases, compassionate individuals have demonstrated their capacity to sacrifice themselves for the wellbeing of others–sometimes without knowing who they are saving (Ricard, 2013). While outliers to the typical contexts where compassion arises, these incidents illustrate the uniquely human capacity to tend to others in unselfish ways. In more ordinary contexts, compassionate interpersonal behavior can mitigate stressful contexts and promote prosocial problem-solving. Wang (2005) notes important neurobiological differences in the activation of self-preservation versus species-preservation systems of the brain. When a threatening context is engaged through self-preservation, cortisol promotes stress arousal and fear response. Conversely, when a stressful context is organized within our species-preservation system, cortisol is associated with *engagement* and *sensitivity toward others* in addition to the activation of oxytocin (Wang, 2005). In other words, compassion helps prime a wider relational perspective of the stress people experience–thereby helping promote care taking behaviors and solving problems at a community level.

THE BENEFITS OF COMPASSION ON STRESS AND MENTAL HEALTH

In contemplative traditions, compassion emerges from a deep motivation to be free from suffering and to aspire toward humanity's grandest version of happiness (Dalai Lama, 1995; Kolts & Chodron, 2013). While compassion-based skills were not developed to target stress reduction specifically, this deep motivation of compassion certainly includes stress and other mental health-related concerns.

The emergence of compassion-based skills to address mental health concerns follows a familiar pathway that other mindfulness-based interventions have navigated. Since the 1970's, research has demonstrated the benefits of mindfulness on stress and mental health. The positive effects of mindfulness skills in reducing stress have been empirically demonstrated in the literature (Gotlink et al., 2015; Khoury et al., 2015). Programs such as Mindfulness-Based Stress Reduction (MBSR) were developed with the purpose of reducing stress through a low-cost low-entry intervention (Kabat-Zinn, 2013). While the development of compassion is implicitly a part of programs like MBSR, the question remained as to whether compassion-focused programs had any meaningful impact on stress and mental wellbeing. In their study, Roca, Vazquez, Diez, Brito-Pons, & McNally (2021) compared MBSR with Compassion Cultivation Training (CCT) and found that both programs were equally effective at reducing psychological distress (e.g., stress, anxiety) and maladaptive cognitive processes while increasing wellbeing. While the science of compassion is relatively new compared to the broader science of mindfulness, emerging research offers promising outcomes. In this section, the scientific study of compassion on stress and mental health distress will be reviewed and explored.

Compassion, Stress, and Perspective-Taking

Wellbeing is partially contingent on the capacity to cope effectively with stressful life events. The skills of compassion could be used as a direct coping strategy for stress and a growing body of research has demonstrated that training in compassion reduces stress (e.g., Allen & Leary, 2010; Irons & Heriot-Maitland, 2021; Roca, Diez, McNally, & Vazquez, 2021).

A compassionate perspective toward stress helps to reduce stress through a psychological pathway that includes people's capacity to engage in shifts to self and context perspective-taking. Self-compassion is a specific form of perspective-taking in the presence of stressful life circumstances. When people recruit a compassionate stance in this way, they have a tendency to refrain from overgeneralizing negative events to themselves (Leary et al., 2007) and espouse a greater degree of acceptance in response to life challenges (Neff, 2003). Strosahl, Robinson, & Gustavsson (2015) refer to this skill set as *softening*–which involves putting distance between stressful contexts and self-critical narratives in reaction to stress.

When adopting a compassionate self-identity in the face of distress, people are more able to skillfully work with their distress by paying greater attention to the clear causes of their issues and what wise actions need to be taken to improve their situation (Irons & Heriot-Maitland, 2021). For example, Finlay-Jones, Reese, and Kane (2015) found that self-compassion allowed for a reduction in emotion regulation difficulties which, in turn, reduced participants' levels of stress. In the study, participants with higher self-compassion could more easily accept difficult emotions and expressed greater emotional clarity of how to resolve the situation. In fact, simply engaging in the act of compassionate thinking (e.g., interpreting a stressful situation deliberately through an understandable, supportive, kind, and encouraging perspective) has been shown to quickly and significantly reduce negative emotions (Arimitsu & Hofmann, 2017).

Deploying self-compassion in stressful contexts also may help reduce dysregulation provoked by self-criticism (Gilbert, 2010). Negative self-evaluations can compound already stressful contexts and reduce capacities to engage in meaningful problem-solving (Finlay-Jones, Rees, & Kane, 2015). In other words, self-compassion reduces self-critical, judgmental factors that have a tendency to conflate or obstruct meaningful solutions to stressful situations.

In addition to a self-compassionate stance, compassion allows people to shift their perspective of stress toward the wider spectrum of the human experience (e.g., common humanity). In their study comparing MBSR to CCT, Roca et al. (2021) found that CCT's reduction in stress outcomes was uniquely mediated by socio-emotional mechanisms (e.g., skills of common humanity and empathic concern). This suggests that people can reduce the stress-inducing consequences of a difficult situation by contextualizing the issue within a wider scope of human suffering and human connection. This perceptual shift enhances a sense of relatedness and reduces a feeling of isolation and disconnection in the face of challenges (Finlay-Jones, Rees, & Kane, 2015).

Compassion and Mental Health Improvement

The application of compassion-based skills has been incorporated into therapeutic interventions that address a host of mental health concerns including depression, anxiety, trauma, and eating disorders (e.g., Germer & Siegel, 2012). Outside of these clinical contexts, there is strong evidence that compassion can improve mental health while reducing common forms of psychopathology such as depression, anxiety, and stress.

In a meta-analysis study, MacBeth and Gumley (2012) found that those with higher self-compassion demonstrated lower levels of psychopathology and greater wellbeing. Participants reported lower levels of depression and anxiety while also exhibiting an increased resiliency to stress. Conversely, people with lower levels of self-compassion are more vulnerable to psychopathology–suggesting that compassion is a protective factor for mental health (Muris & Petrocchi, 2017).

People who reported higher levels of self-compassion also had lower levels of depression, anxiety, and stress during the COVID-19 pandemic (Matos, McEwan, Kanovský et al., 2022). One of the possible explanations for this is that compassion impacts how people cognitively process events and themselves–leading to improved mental health outcomes. People who express a higher level of self-compassion show higher levels of cognitive wellbeing, which includes the capacity to recall positive memories and interpret current situations with more positive hopeful dispositions (Zessin, Dickhäuser, & Garbade, 2015). Compassion practices have also been shown to reduce psychopathological variables such as rumination and psychological distress known to impact global health negatively (Roca, Diez, McNally, & Vazquez, 2021).

Being a recipient of compassion also has meaningfully positive mental health outcomes. Receiving compassion from others has been shown to reduce depression symptomology of the receiver (Hermanto et al. 2016). Furthermore, Matos, McEwan, Kanovský et al. (2022) found, in their transcontinental international study during the COVID-19 pandemic, that those who received compassion from others expressed greater social safeness, greater sense of social connection, and lower depression symptoms regardless of their fear of COVID-19.

Resiliency and Health

Compassion may also help people be more resilient to stressors and challenges. In their longitudinal study involving university freshmen adjusting to college life, Hope, Koestner, & Milyavskaya (2014) found that participants higher in self-compassion were more resilient in the face of thwarted goals and were able to maintain motivation behind goal pursuit despite daily fluctuations in goal progress. One possible explanation as to why compassion can produce resiliency is that greater self-compassion is associated with increases in competence, autonomy, and belonging despite challenging circumstances (Gunnell et al., 2017).

Compassion appears to help people improve their psychological adjustment to challenging circumstances. For example, self-compassion aids those going through divorce to adjust better psychologically (Sbarra et al., 2012). Compassion can also help those experiencing chronic pain (Wren et al., 2012), spina bifida (Hayter & Dorstyn, 2013), and cancer (Gillanders, Sinclair, MacLean, & Jardine, 2014) to resiliently adjust to these medical conditions. Compassion practices also have shown to help people accept distressing life contexts without the need to necessarily affectively regulate distress (Jazaiere, McGonigal, Lee, et al., 2018). In an interesting finding in their study, Jazaiere, McGonigal, Lee, et al. (2018) found that participants who attended a multiweek compassion training program had two things occur. First, participants experienced a greater self-efficacy in their capacity to regulate their negative emotional distress. But secondly, the participants reported a lower need to engage in these forms of affective regulation. This outcome suggests that when people utilize compassionate practices, they are more willing to engage in acceptance processes that reduce overall distress of a given situation.

In addition to coping with distressing contexts, people who engage in frequent compassion also tend to engage in more frequent health behaviors and report better overall health as a result (Homan & Sirois, 2017). Part of what might explain this is that people who engage in compassion tend to also demonstrate action-oriented coping (Allen & Leary, 2010). Given that part of compassion involves the psychology of alleviation, it makes sense that when people are actively in a compassionate space they are more action oriented. People who engage in self-compassion also tend to have increases in self-improvement motivations (Breines & Chen, 2012).

Compassion is also associated with attenuated physiological responses to stress. Specifically, compassion has a direct relationship to the sympathetic nervous system, consistent with Gilbert's (2010) emotion regulation model that suggests the soothing system is associated with compassion. Breines et al. (2015) showed that people higher in self-compassion display lower sympathetic nervous system activation and lower inflammation response after exposure of stress. In fact, compassion-based practices have shown improvements to heart rate variability–a marker for adequate parasympathetic nervous system tone (Kirby, Doty, Petrocchi, & Gilbert, 2017).

Challenging Modern Conceptions of a Happy Life

The development and utilization of compassion skills serve people well in addressing the stressors of modern life. Compassion training also challenges cultural assumptions of happiness that might not serve long-term wellbeing.

Despite significant social and economic progress, many countries with economic affluence have not improved mental well-being and happiness (Davidson, 2012). This comparative finding is sometimes referred to as the *progress paradox* and offers insight into the nature of human happiness (Easterbrook,

2003). As mentioned previously, the drive system of emotion regulation evolved to motivate humans to pursue resources critical to survival. In the modern world, however, this system can be co-opted as a significant strategy for managing stress and wellbeing (Lembke, 2021). An example is using material consumption behaviors (e.g., shopping) as a coping strategy. While people need a minimum level of material resources to improve wellbeing, pursuing material resources has a ceiling effect on health and wellbeing (Davidson, 2012). Buddhist psychology, generally, and compassion practices, specifically, assert that human wellbeing and mental happiness cannot be fulfilled simply by acquiring pleasantries (Jinpa, 2015). Dubbed the hedonic treadmill, people who endlessly pursue material pleasures in pursuit of contentment report higher, rather than lower, stress levels and dissatisfaction (Germer, 2009). Incidentally, these same processes of flooding the reward pathway to resolve discontent are what is thought to be responsible for addiction (Lembke, 2021).

COMPASSION TRAINING AND CULTIVATION

Compassion training has traditionally been produced in contemplative traditions. Buddhist practices such as Tibetan *tonglen* (Chodron, 2001) and Vipassana *metta* (Salzberg, 2002) are explicit examples of formal compassion practices developed from these traditions. In recent years, skills of compassion have been broadened and secularized for the purpose of distributing them widely outside of any particular religious or cultural group (Jinpa, 2015). The benefit of such methods is broader generalizability; compassionate motivations and practices can be integrated within the cultural backdrop of the people being taught without a subscription to any specific religious belief or cultural viewpoint. Most of the compassion-based skills and methods described in the research literature are an amalgamation of Eastern contemplative traditions (e.g., Buddhism) and Western scientific and therapeutic methods. Compassion cultivation training, whether it be a formal training program or part of a contemplative practice, operates under the assumption that compassion is trainable. People can strengthen their compassionate capacities through both frequency and persistence of practice.

In the last two decades, a number of compassion training programs have been developed and delivered in a number of communities and medical contexts (Kirby, 2017). While the scope of this chapter does not include an in-depth analysis of each of these programs, Kirby (2017) provides a thorough overview. Most formal compassion training programs are based on a weekly group skills training model where a certified trainer leads participants through a series of didactic, experiential, and discussion-based interventions aimed at developing and practicing compassion skills (Kirby, 2017). Great care and time is used to train instructors in the methods of both compassion training and group facilitation. Increasingly these training programs have offered both online and in-person options, showing compatible results (Eriksson, Germundsjo, Astrom, & Ronnlund, 2018).

Compassion programs work to sensitize participants toward their suffering and the suffering of humanity. Rather than merely emphasizing stress management at the onset, participants are encouraged to contemplate the capacities of human suffering first. Gilbert (2009) summarizes this point well, stating, "Thinking about the pervasiveness of the human tragedy is one of the first steps on the journey into compassion; indeed, it is one of the inspirations of compassion" (p. 64). In other words, these programs emphasize the psychologies of engagement *and* alleviation.

These programs also share some teaching methodological similarities. All of the programs emphasize experiential learning and an inquiry-based form of instruction. Participants are encouraged to engage in activities, including formal meditation practices, that emphasize the topic being trained. Participants also take part in informal practices and group discussions aimed at exploring the processes that were relevant to the training. Teachers facilitate an inquiry-based discussion of practice to ensure that participants reach the contours and navigate the challenges of compassionate practice (Germer & Neff, 2019). Teachers also rely on didactic training to convey concepts, research, and technical components of the training. Exposure to the science of compassion is also commonly used.

While programs may differ in their emphasis on mindfulness meditation practice, all of the programs mentioned below focus the early part of training on developing a stable mindful awareness capacity before moving to more compassion-focused skill sets. The rationale for this is twofold: (1) a person who is attempting to employ compassion skills needs to be aware of the state of their mind prior, and (2) they need to be able to have clarity of their intentions and motivations prior to expressly engaging in compassionate behaviors. Taken together, a person engaged in compassionate behaviors responds to suffering stimuli rather than mindlessly reacting (Kolts, 2019).

Compassion Training Programs Overview

Below is an overview of prominent compassion skills training programs that have been developed and offered some research support. The programs presented below are not an exhaustive list. Instead, these programs represent both the most popular and most researched programs at present.

Mindful Self Compassion

Mindful Self Compassion (MSC) was developed to help participants enhance emotional wellbeing and resilience using a combination of mindfulness awareness training and compassion training (Germer & Neff, 2019). As the name implies, the primary focus of MSC is the development of compassion for the self. Developed in part by Neff's (2011) model of self-compassion, MSC is well suited to help people who struggle with negative self-judgments and criticism. According to the program, self-compassion comprises three components: self-kindness, a sense of common humanity, and mindfulness (Germer & Neff, 2019). These components combat the negative effects of self-judgment, isolation, and over-identification with distressing content (Neff & Germer, 2013). MSC is delivered in 8 weekly sessions, five intensive days, or ten weekly online session formats. Weekly formats also tend to offer a retreat opportunity.

Compassion Cultivation Training

Compassion Cultivation Training (CCT) was developed at Stanford University by Thupten Jinpa and colleagues. The broad goal of CCT is to cultivate deeper happiness in the participant's life (Jazaieri, Jinpa, McGonigal, et al., 2013). The CCT curriculum includes training based on Tibetan Buddhist contemplative practices and Western psychology. The program involves eight, two-hour weekly sessions. The curriculum consists of developing skills of settling the mind, extending loving-kindness to others, and compassion that can be applied to loved ones, strangers, challenging others, and to oneself. The program is well suited to help people develop capacities toward kindness toward self and more productive relationships with others.

Compassion Mind Training

Compassion mind training (CMT) is derived from the theoretical and empirical work that resulted in Compassion Focused Therapy. Based on evolutionary psychology, CMT aims to help participants cultivate a compassionate self-identity that promotes a caring motivation and to engage this motivation during daily struggles and difficulties (Irons & Heriot-Maitland, 2021). The program involves 8-two-hour sessions that cover topics related to the evolved emotion systems, the self as multiple parts, compassion as flow, compassion to self and others, and a compassionate mind toward difficulties (Irons & Heriot-Maitland, 2021). The program is a good fit for participants struggling with shame, self-criticism, depression, and negative self-evaluations.

Cultivating Emotional Balance

The Cultivating Emotional Balance (CEB) program was developed by prominent psychologist Paul Eckman and his colleagues (Eckman & Eckman, 2013). CEB aims to help people develop methods of managing emotions to build greater happiness and wellbeing (Kirby, 2017). The program combines modern psychology–particularly research on emotion–with Buddhist contemplative practices. The program consists of 8 weekly sessions with participants gaining exposure to several practices including mindfulness, loving-kindness meditation, compassion, and psychoeducation of emotion. The program is well suited to help people struggling with relationship issues, understanding others, and emotion dysregulation.

Compassion in Psychotherapy

Compassion training and skill acquisition have also increasingly become utilized within psychotherapeutic contexts aimed at addressing a number of psychological and psychiatric concerns (Kirby, 2017). Entire therapeutic modalities, like Compassion Focused Therapy, have been developed specifically for the application of compassion skills toward mental health conditions such as depression and anxiety (Gilbert, 2010). Other therapies have incorporated the use of some compassion-based skills development within their treatment programs (Germer & Siegel, 2012). These are often referred to as Compassion Infused Therapies (CIT). CFT and CITs have demonstrated meaningful clinical and empirical outcomes in treating people with depression, anxiety, and anger issues, among other mental health concerns (Kolts, 2019).

PROMOTING COMPASSION IN THE WORKPLACE

Navigating the workplace in contemporary times comes with many stressors. Since the COVID-19 pandemic, workplaces have had to navigate the personal and professional wellbeing of their workers against the onslaught of local and global challenges (Gallup State of the Global Workplace Report, 2022). Government agencies have acknowledged that the pandemic has brought a greater awareness of the relationship between work and wellbeing (Office of the Surgeon General, 2022). Increasingly there is a growing demand that workplaces address worker wellbeing in direct and intentional ways. There is evidence that shows compassion is an essential component of a healthy and productive work environment for employees, leaders, and the organization (Dutton, Workman, & Hardin, 2014).

Stress and Wellbeing at Work

Promoting compassion in the workplace requires an organization's motivation to assess and connect with the suffering of workers (Lilius, Worline, Maitlis, Kanov et al., 2008). Employee stress comes from personal and professional sources–sometimes converging in unhelpful ways that negatively impact them (Dutton, Workman, & Hardin, 2014). Stress and burnout rates are presently at staggering levels (Gallup State of the Global Workplace Report, 2022; Maslach & Leiter, 202). Worker shortages, financial strain, workplace relationship stressors, larger community stressors, and exhaustion can all play a role in workplace stress. The modern worker faces multiple crises, including a global pandemic, political unrest, ecological stressors, racial tension, and more that can impact worker engagement and productivity. Additionally, the lack of appropriate safety, inclusion, and belonging in the increasingly diverse workplaces workers inhabit can lead to additional stressors for those most disenfranchised (Shell, Teodorescu, & Williams, 2021).

Many costs are incurred when employees are burned out and unwell including increased sick time off, leave of absence due to health-related issues, and less productivity due to emotional and physical exhaustion–all of which place additional burdens on an organization (Andersson et al., 2021). For the employee, burnout and stress can result in lower job satisfaction, job insecurity, increased isolation, and threat activation, as well as elevated levels of stress and poorer overall wellness (Maslach & Leiter, 2022).

Compassion in the Workplace

Compassion is a useful framework for work because it encourages relational and cooperative frameworks. Because people are hardwired to connect and can experience emotions collectively, promoting compassion in the workplace is a well suited intervention to improve the overall wellbeing of a workplace community (Boyatzis & McKee, 2005; Dutton, Workman, & Hardin, 2014). Compassion in organizations and workplaces includes many benefits, such as decreased stress, anxiety, and emotional distress, leading to increased resilience and better conflict resolution skills for staff and employees (Hougaard & Carter, 2022; Ko, Kim, & Choi, 2021).

Implementing compassion practices, including self-compassion in the workplace, can lead to increased job satisfaction and improvement in overall wellness of employees, thus resulting in better retention rates (Hougaard & Carter, 2022). When workers intentionally support each other collectively, in a caring and compassionate manner, work related issues can be addressed productively (Fowler, & Christakis, 2010; Goetz, Keltner, & Simon-Thomas, 2010). Additionally, employees who receive compassion at work show higher affective commitment toward the organization (Lilius, Worline, Maitlis, Kanov et al., 2008). According to Chowdhury (2019) compassion in the workplace could include: more importance placed on employees' wellbeing, more positive relationships at the workplace, more open-hearted interactions, wider perspective-taking, and increased self-compassion of individual workers.

Compassion at work can also take the form of promoting deliberate and thoughtful diversity, equity, and inclusion strategies (Zheng, 2022). Increasingly many corporations have shifted their focus to include more awareness and training surrounding issues of diversity, equity, and inclusion and how these issues impact their employees and organizational culture (Tynes, 2020). When people are able to commit to viewing social injustices from a compassionate space, they show up as allies who are working toward the active disruption of such injustices (Aboul-Ela, 2017). Promoting an equitable and inclusive workplace encourages the social and psychological safety of workers (Zheng, 2022). Those with a more compassionate orientation at work are less likely to support inequitable social dominance frameworks at work and more likely to see the benefits of efforts aimed at greater inclusion (Martin, Seppala, Heineberg, Rossomando, et al. 2015).

Using compassion-based skills to improve workplace connections and conflict resolution is also important. Because navigating relationships is a crucial part of an organization, it is important to consider how compassion-focused skills may improve the overall work climate and employee relationships (Boyatzis & McKee, 2005). Workplace relationships can be challenging to navigate at times. Applying compassion as a tool for interpersonal workplace challenges allows for a more human centric method to address these concerns and promote more prosocial behaviors (Jazaieri & Rock, 2021). Compassion skills guide workers to be present for others, engage in purposeful perspective-taking, practice nonjudgmental connection, and clarify the intentions set at work (Jazaieri & Rock, 2021).

The use of compassion in the workplace also helps with a worker's overall wellbeing. Choi, Lee, No, & Kim (2016) found that compassion can increase the self-esteem and self-efficacy of workers. They also observed that those with higher levels of compassion tended to have lower levels of anxiety, burnout, and workplace deviance. Other advantages of compassion practices in the workplace include a sense of connection and belonging for employees, reduced stress and anxiety, and effective methods for addressing toxic work behaviors (Dutton, Workman, and Hardin, 2014). When people feel a sense of connectedness with one another, they are more likely to engage with one another in a positive manner and work towards common goals. At the onset of the COVID-19 pandemic, for example, it was observed that those who embodied the strongest sense of compassion for others tended to be more prosocial responsive to engaging in mitigation strategies to protect the most vulnerable in their communities (Pfattheicher, S., Nockur, L., Böhm, R., Sassenrath,2020). Conversely, when employees receive a lack of compassion from colleagues and managers, they report feelings of greater disconnection and lower organizational commitment (Lilius, Worline, Maitlis, Kanov et al., 2008).

Compassion skills are particularly potent when used by leadership. When managers utilize compassion-based skills, they are more likely to treat people with greater consideration and less likely to dehumanize workers (Frost, 2003; Hougaard & Carter, 2022). Leaders can model compassionate interpersonal behaviors by how they respond to their employees both by being sensitive to employee suffering and being action-oriented in addressing employee needs. Even in difficult contexts, leaders can model compassionate responses. Leaders are sometimes required to make difficult decisions that might negatively impact individuals in the organization. Leaders who approach these difficult contexts, like having to lay off workers, can still demonstrate a compassionate orientation to a challenging task (Hougaard & Carter, 2022).

Promoting Compassion Practices in the Workplace

Organizations strongly impact the utilization of compassion in the workplace (Boyatzis & McKee, 2005). Engaged compassion in the workplace requires motivation to identify and respond to workplace suffering in meaningful ways. Aboul-Ela (2017) offers concrete suggestions for cultivating compassion in the workplace in small, tangible ways, such as: (1) leaders in the workplace modeling compassionate behaviors that demonstrate respect and trust; (2) promoting an emotionally supportive workplace that offers authentic interactions with employees; (3) scheduling and prioritizing meetings amongst staff to investigate work-related issues leading to conflict; (4) encouraging positive attitudes toward employees from upper management and leadership; (5) recognition and positive reinforcement for employees who demonstrate compassion; and (6) attuning to empathetic listening to avoid disruptive behaviors.

In a similar viewpoint, Dutton, Workman, and Hardin (2014) encourage organizations wanting to promote workplace compassion to consider treating individuals as whole people with emotions, encouraging permeable work and life boundaries, facilitating high-quality relationships among employees, and implementing practices that support compassion including practices that notice and respond to worker distress. By centering acts of compassion and leadership consistently modeling and encouraging this, the hope is that job satisfaction and performance would increase, as well as a decrease in work-related stress and anxiety (Hougaard & Carter, 2022). Another way of engaging employees in compassion practices is offering compassion training at no additional cost to the employee, including training that aids the development of self-compassion that, in turn, has empirical support for improving health and wellbeing (Germer & Neff, 2019). Lastly, organizations should strive to infuse compassion into daily interactions and celebrate moments of gratitude in the community with each other.

Given the state of global workforce rates of stress and the crisis-prone contexts of modern work, compassion practices are vital resources to foster connection and hope for collective healing within organizations. This transformation and healing will benefit all employees, as well as the consumers and stakeholders of businesses. The authors suggest that now is an opportune time to invest in compassion-focused leadership and practices in the workplace.

CONCLUSION

The world is experiencing a host of stressors and crises that, in turn, bring myriad forms of suffering for individuals involved. Compassion is an orientation to suffering and a skillful means of action in the presence of suffering. The construct of compassion has psychological, biological, and relational domains that make it particularly well-suited to address stress-related contexts and to provide direction in the face of so much global uncertainty. Research on compassion has demonstrated meaningful outcomes including reduced stress, anxiety, and depression. Additionally, compassion research has demonstrated improved interpersonal relationships, health, wellbeing, a sense of resilience, and genuine happiness. While emerging research has demonstrated meaningful knowledge, there are many gaps that future research should address. Research could explore the dose-effect of compassion training on short-term and long-term outcomes. Exploring the effects of formal versus informal compassion practices could illuminate what people might continue to utilize on the outset of formal training. Research on the benefits of self-help/self-initiated compassion training could illuminate the viability of training modalities that don't require group training processes. Additionally, research on the application of compassion at work with a wider range of professions would be helpful in building a broader understanding of applications in the workplace.

Compassion offers a wise path through the turbulent and uncertain spaces of human suffering. The modern era benefits from the capacity to integrate ancient wisdom practices with modern scientific knowledge of human psychology, biology, and organizational behaviors.

REFERENCES

Aboul-Ela, G. M. B. E. (2017). Reflections on Workplace Compassion and Job Performance. *Journal of Human Values, 23*(3), 234–243. doi:10.1177/0971685817713285

Allen, A. B., & Leary, M. R. (2010). Self-compassion, stress, and coping. *Social and Personality Psychology Compass, 4*(2), 107–118. doi:10.1111/j.1751-9004.2009.00246.x PMID:20686629

Andersson, C., Stenfors, C. U. D., Lilliengren, P., Einhorn, S., & Osika, W. (2021). Benevolence – Associations with Stress, Mental Health, and Self-Compassion at the Workplace. *Frontiers in Psychology, 12*, 568625. doi:10.3389/fpsyg.2021.568625 PMID:34140909

Arimitu, K., & Hofman, S. G. (2017). Effects of compassionate thinking on negative emotions. *Cognition and Emotion, 31*(1), 160–167. doi:10.1080/02699931.2015.1078292 PMID:26362245

Bellosta-Batalla, M., Blanco-Gandía, M. C., Rodríguez-Arias, M., Cebolla, A., Pérez-Blasco, J., & Moya-Albiol, L. (2020). Increased Salivary Oxytocin and Empathy in Students of Clinical and Health Psychology After a Mindfulness and Compassion-Based Intervention. *Mindfulness, 11*(4), 1006–1017. doi:10.100712671-020-01316-7

Breins, J. G., & Chen, S. (2012). Self-compassion increases self-improvement motivation. *Personality and Social Psychology Bulletin, 38*(9), 1133–1143. doi:10.1177/0146167212445599 PMID:22645164

Brito-Pons, G., Campos, D., & Cebolla, A. (2018). Implicit or explicit compassion? Effects of Compassion Cultivation Training and comparison with Mindfulness-based Stress Reduction. *Mindfulness, 9*(5), 1494–1508. doi:10.100712671-018-0898-z

Chodron, P. (2001). *Tonglen: The Path of Transformation*. Shambhala.

Choi, L., Lee, S., No, S.-R., & Kim, E. I. (2016). Effects of Compassion on Employees' Self-regulation. *Social Behavior and Personality, 44*(7), 1173–1190. doi:10.2224bp.2016.44.7.1173

Chowdhury, M. R. (2019, April 30). Compassion in the workplace: 9+ examples and tips for leaders. *Positive Psychology*. https://positivepsychology.com/compassion-at-work-leadership /#comment-list

Colonnello, V., Petrocchi, N., & Heinrichs, M. (2017). The psychobiological foundation of prosocial relationships: The role of oxytocin in daily social exchanges. In P. Gilbert (Ed.), *Compassion: Concepts, research, and applications*. Routledge. doi:10.4324/9781315564296-6

Dalai Lama. (1995). *The power of compassion.* HarperCollins.

Dutton, J., Workman, K., & Hardin, A. (2014). Compassion at work. *Annual Review of Organizational Psychology and Organizational Behavior, 1*(1), 277–304. doi:10.1146/annurev-orgpsych-031413-091221

Ekman, E., & Ekman, P. (2013). Cultivating emotional balance: structure, research, and implementation. In T. Singer & M. Boz (Eds.), *Compassion: Bridging practice and science* (pp. 398–414). Max Planck Society.

Eriksson, T., Germundsjo, L., Astrom, E., & Ronnlund, M. (2018). Mindful self-compassion training reduces stress and burnout symptoms mong practicing psychologists: A randomized controlled trial of a brief web-based intervention. *Frontiers in Psychology*, *9*, 2340. Advance online publication. doi:10.3389/fpsyg.2018.02340 PMID:30538656

Feldmen, C., & Kuyken, W. (2011). Compassion in the landscape of suffering. *Contemporary Buddhism*, *12*(1), 143–155. doi:10.1080/14639947.2011.564831

Finlay-Jones, A. L., Rees, C. S., & Kane, R. T. (2015). Self-compassion, emotion regulation and stress among Australian psychologists: Testing an emotion regulation model of self-compassion using structural equation modeling. *PLoS One*, *10*(7), e0133481. doi:10.1371/journal.pone.0133481 PMID:26207900

Fowler, J. H., & Christakis, N. A. (2010). Cooperative behavior cascades in human social networks. *Proceedings of the National Academy of Sciences of the United States of America*, *107*(12), 5334–5338. doi:10.1073/pnas.0913149107 PMID:20212120

Gallop. (2022). *State of the global workplace: 2022 report.* Gallop Press.

Germer, C., & Neff, K. (2019). *Teaching the mindful self-compassion program: A guide for professionals*. Guilford.

Germer, C. K. (2009). *The mindful path to self-compassion.* Guilford.

Gilbert, P. (2009). *The Compassionate Mind: A New Approach to Life's Challenges*. New Harbinger.

Gilbert, P., & Choden. (2014). *Mindful compassion: How the science of compassion can help you understand your emotions, live in the present, and connect deeply with others*. New Harbinger.

Gilbert, P. (2017). Compassion: Definitions and controversies. In P. Gilbert (Ed.), *Compassion: Concepts, research, and applications*. Routledge. doi:10.4324/9781315564296-1

Gilbert, P. (2022). The evolved functions of caring connections as a basis for compassion. In P. Gilbert (Ed.), *Compassion focused therapy: Clinical practice and applications*. Routledge. doi:10.4324/9781003035879-4

Gilbert. (2010). *Compassion focused therapy: Distinctive features*. Routledge.

Gillanders, D. T., Sinclair, A. K., MacLean, M., & Jardine, K. (2015). Illness cognitions, cognitive fusion, avoidance, and self-compassion as predictors of distress and quality of life in a heterogeneous sample of adults, after cancer. *Journal of Contextual Behavioral Science*, *4*(4), 300–311. doi:10.1016/j.jcbs.2015.07.003

Global Burden of Diseases. (2020). *Injuries and Risk Factors Study*. Author.

Goetz, J. L., Keltner, D., & Simon-Thomas, E. (2010). Compassion: An evolutionary analysis and empirical review. *Psychological Bulletin*, *136*(3), 351–374. doi:10.1037/a0018807 PMID:20438142

Gotlink, R. A., Chu, P., Busschbach, J. J. V., Benson, H., Friccione, G. L., & Hunink, M. G. M. (2015). Standardised mindfulness-based interventions in healthcare: An overview of systematic reviews and meta-analyses of RCTs. *PLoS One*, *10*(4), e0124344. doi:10.1371/journal.pone.0124344 PMID:25881019

Gunnell, K. E., Mosewich, A. D., McEwen, C. E., Eklund, R. C., & Crocker, P. R. E. (2017). Don't be so hard on yourself! Changes in self-compassion during the first year of university are associated with changes in well-being. *Personality and Individual Differences, 107*, 43–48. doi:10.1016/j.paid.2016.11.032

Hayter, M. R., & Dorstyn, D. S. (2013). Resilience, self-esteem, and self-compassion in adults with spina bifida. *Spinal Cord, 52*(2), 167–171. doi:10.1038c.2013.152 PMID:24322213

Homan, & Sirois, F. M. (2017). Self-compassion and physical health: Exploring the roles of perceived stress and health-promoting behaviors. *Health Psychology Open, 4*(2). doi:10.1177/2055102917729542

Hope, N., Koestner, R., & Milyavskaya, M. (2014). The Role of Self-Compassion in Goal Pursuit and Well-Being Among University Freshmen. *Self and Identity, 13*(5), 579–593. doi:10.1080/15298868.2014.889032

Hougaard, R., & Carter, J. (2022). *Compassionate leadership: How to do hard things in a human way*. Harvard Business Review Press.

Irons & Heriot-Maitland, C. (2021). Compassionate Mind Training: An 8-week group for the public. *Psychology and Psychotherapy, 94*(3), 443–463. doi:10.1111/papt.12320

Jazaieri, H., Jinpa, G. T., McGonigal, K., Rosenberg, E. L., Finkelstein, J., Simon-Thomas, E., Cullen, M., Doty, J. R., Gross, J. J., & Goldin, P. R. (2013). Enhancing compassion: A randomized controlled trial of a compassion cultivation training program. *Journal of Happiness Studies, 14*(4), 1113–1126. doi:10.100710902-012-9373-z

Jazaieri, H., McGonigal, K., Lee, I. A., Jinpa, T., Doty, J. R., Gross, J. J., & Goldin, P. R. (2018). Altering the Trajectory of Affect and Affect Regulation: The Impact of Compassion Training. *Mindfulness, 9*(1), 283–293. doi:10.100712671-017-0773-3

Jazaieri, H., & Rock, M. (2021). Putting compassion to work: Compassion as a tool for navigating challenging workplace relationships. *Mindfulness, 12*(10), 2552–2558. doi:10.100712671-021-01695-5

Jinpa, T. (2015). *A fearless heart: How the courage to be compassionate can transform our lives*. Avery.

Kabat-Zinn, J. (2013). *Full catastrophe living*. Bantam Dell Publishing Group.

Khoury, B., Sharma, M., Rush, S. E., & Fournier, C. (2015). Mindfulness-based stress reduction for healthy individuals: A meta-analysis. *Journal of Psychosomatic Research, 78*(6), 519–528. doi:10.1016/j.jpsychores.2015.03.009 PMID:25818837

Kirby, J. N. (2017). Compassion interventions: The programs, the evidence, and implications for research and practice. *Psychology and Psychotherapy: Research and Practice, 90*(3), 432–455. doi:10.1111/papt.12104 PMID:27664071

Kirby, J. N., Doty, J. R., Petrocchi, N., & Gilbert, P. (2017). The current and future role of heart rate variability for assessing and training compassion. *Frontiers in Public Health, 5*. Advance online publication. doi:10.3389/fpubh.2017.00040 PMID:28337432

Klimecki, O. M., Leiberg, S., Ricard, M., & Singer, T. (2013). Differential pattern of functional brain plasticity after compassion and empathy training. *Social Cognitive and Affective Neuroscience*. Advance online publication. doi:10.1093can/nst060 PMID:23576808

Ko, S.-H., Kim, J., & Choi, Y. (2021). Compassion and workplace incivility: Implications for open innovation. *Journal of Open Innovation*, *7*(1), 95. doi:10.3390/joitmc7010095

Kolts, R., & Chodron, T. (2015). *An open-hearted life: Transformative methods for compassionate living from a clinical psychologist and a Buddhist nun*. Shambhala.

Kolts, R. L. (2019). *CFT Made Simple: Competency-Based Training for Mindfulness-Based Therapies*. New Harbinger Publications.

Dalai Lama & Cutler, H. C. (1998). *The art of happiness*. Riverhead Books.

Leary, M. R., Tate, E. B., Adams, C. E., Batts Allen, A., & Hancock, J. (2007). Self-compassion and reactions to unpleasant self-relevant events: The implications of treating oneself kindly. *Journal of Personality and Social Psychology*, *92*(5), 887–904. doi:10.1037/0022-3514.92.5.887 PMID:17484611

Lembke, A. (2021). *Dopamine nation: Finding balance in the age of indulgence*. Dutton.

MacBeth, A., & Gumley, A. (2012). Exploring compassion: A meta-analysis of the association between self-compassion and psychopathology. *Clinical Psychology Review*, *32*(6), 545–552. doi:10.1016/j.cpr.2012.06.003 PMID:22796446

Martin, S., Seppala, E., Heineberg, Y., Rossomando, T., Doty, J., Zimbardo, P., Shiue, T.-T., Berger, R., & Zhou, Y. Y. (2015). Multiple Facets of Compassion: The Impact of Social Dominance Orientation and Economic Systems Justification. *Journal of Business Ethics*, *129*(1), 237–249. doi:10.100710551-014-2157-0

Maslach, C., & Leiter, M. P. (2022). *The burnout challenges*. Harvard Press.

Matos, M., McEwan, K., Kanovský, M., Halamová, J., Steindl, S. R., Ferreira, N., Linharelhos, M., Rijo, D., Asano, K., Márquez, M. G., Gregório, S., Vilas, S. P., Brito-Pons, G., Lucena-Santos, P., da Silva Oliveira, M., de Souza, E. L., Llobenes, L., Gumiy, N., Costa, M. I., ... Gilbert, P. (2022). Compassion Protects Mental Health and Social Safeness During the COVID-19 Pandemic Across 21 Countries. *Mindfulness*, *13*(4), 863–880. doi:10.100712671-021-01822-2 PMID:35003380

Muris & Petrocchi, N. (2017). Protection or Vulnerability? A Meta-Analysis of the Relations Between the Positive and Negative Components of Self-Compassion and Psychopathology: Self-compassion: Protection or vulnerability? *Clinical Psychology and Psychotherapy*, *24*(2), 373–383. doi:10.1002/cpp.2005

Neff, K. D. (2011). *Self-compassion: Stop beating yourself up and leave insecurity behind*. William Morrow.

Neff, K. D., & Germer, C. K. (2013). A Pilot Study and Randomized Controlled Trial of the Mindful Self-Compassion Program. *Journal of Clinical Psychology*, *69*(1), 28–44. doi:10.1002/jclp.21923 PMID:23070875

Office of the Surgeon General. (2022). *The U.S. Surgeon General's Framework for Workplace Mental Health & Well-Being*. Department of Health and Human Services.

Pfattheicher, S., Nockur, L., Böhm, R., Sassenrath, C., & Petersen, M. B. (2020). The Emotional Path to Action: Empathy Promotes Physical Distancing and Wearing of Face Masks During the COVID-19 Pandemic. *Psychological Science, 31*(11), 1363–1373. doi:10.1177/0956797620964422 PMID:32993455

Porges, S. W. (2011). *The polyvagal theory: Neurophysiological foundations of emotions, attachment, communication, and self-regulation*. W W Norton & Co.

Ricard, M. (2013). *Altruism: The power of compassion to change yourself and the world*. Bay Back Books.

Roca, P., Diez, G., McNally, R. J., & Vazques, C. (2021). The impact of compassion meditation training on psychological variables: A network perspective. *Mindfulness, 12*(4), 873–888. doi:10.100712671-020-01552-x

Roca, V., Vazquez, C., Diez, G., Brito-Pons, G., & McNally, R. J. (2021). Not all types of meditation are the same: Mediators of change in mindfulness and compassion meditation interventions. *Journal of Affective Disorders, 283*, 354–362. doi:10.1016/j.jad.2021.01.070 PMID:33578349

Salzberg, S. (2002). *Lovingkindness: The Revolutionary Art of Happiness*. Shambhala.

Santomauro, D. F., Mantilla Herrera, A. M., Shadid, J., Zheng, P., Ashbaugh, C., Pigott, D. M., Abbafati, C., Adolph, C., Amlag, J. O., Aravkin, A. Y., Bang-Jensen, B. L., Bertolacci, G. J., Bloom, S. S., Castellano, R., Castro, E., Chakrabarti, S., Chattopadhyay, J., Cogen, R. M., Collins, J. K., ... Ferrari, A. J. (2021). Global prevalence and burden of depressive and anxiety disorders in 204 countries and territories in 2020 due to COVID-19 pandemic. *Lancet, 398*(10312), 1700–1712. doi:10.1016/S0140-6736(21)02143-7 PMID:34634250

Sbarra, D. A., Smith, H. L., & Mehl, M. R. (2012). When leaving your ex, love yourself: Observational rating of self-compassion predict the course of emotional recovery following marital separation. *Psychological Science, 23*(3), 261–269. doi:10.1177/0956797611429466 PMID:22282874

Shell, E. M., Teodorescu, D., & Williams, L. D. (2021). Investigating Race-related Stress, Burnout, and Secondary Traumatic Stress for Black Mental Health Therapists. *The Journal of Black Psychology, 47*(8), 669–694. doi:10.1177/00957984211033963

Siegel, R. D., & Germer, C. K. (2012). Wisdom and compassion: Two wings of a bird. In C. K. Germer & R. D. Siegel (Eds.), *Wisdom and compassion in psychotherapy: Deepening mindfulness in clinical practice*. Guilford.

Spikins, P. (2017). Prehistoric origins: The compassion of far distant strangers. In P. Gilbert (Ed.), *Compassion: Concepts, research, and applications*. Routledge. doi:10.4324/9781315564296-2

Stellar, J. E., Cohen, A., Oveis, C., & Keltner, D. (2015). Affective and physiological responses to the suffering of others: Compassion and vagal activity. *Journal of Personality and Social Psychology, 108*(4), 572–585. doi:10.1037/pspi0000010

Strosahl, K. D., Robinson, P. J., & Gustavsson, T. (2015). *Inside this moment: A clinician's guide to promoting radical change using acceptance and commitment therapy*. Context Press.

Tirch, D., Schoendorff, B., & Silberstein, L. R. (2014). *The ACT practitioner's guide to the science of compassion*. New Harbinger.

Tynes, B. (2020, March). The Importance of Diversity and Inclusion for Today's Companies. *Forbes Magazine*.

Wang, S. (2005). A conceptual framework for integrating research related to the physiology of compassion and the wisdom of Buddhist teachings. In P. Gilbert (Ed.), *Compassion: Conceptualisations, research and use in psychotherapy*. Routledge.

Wren, S., Somers, T. J., Wright, M. A., Goetz, M. C., Leary, M. R., Fras, A. M., Huh, B. K., Rogers, L. L., & Keefe, F. J. (2012). Self-Compassion in Patients with Persistent Musculoskeletal Pain: Relationship of Self-Compassion to Adjustment to Persistent Pain. *Journal of Pain and Symptom Management, 43*(4), 759–770. doi:10.1016/j.jpainsymman.2011.04.014 PMID:22071165

Zessin, U., Dickhäuser, O., & Garbade, S. (2015). The relationship between self-compassion and well-being: A meta-analysis. *Applied Psychology, 7,* 340–364. doi:10.1111/aphw.12051

Zheng, L. (2022). *DEI deconstructed: Your no-nonsense guide to doing the work and doing it right.* Berrett-Hoehler.

Chapter 16
Does Voluntary Simplicity Lifestyle Support Psychological Resilience During Crises?
Evidence From the COVID-19 Pandemic

Hediye Yürüyen Kılıç
Gebze Technical University, Turkey

Inci Dursun
https://orcid.org/0000-0002-9856-3914
Gebze Technical University, Turkey

Ebru Tumer Kabadayi
https://orcid.org/0000-0002-0673-6866
Gebze Technical University, Turkey

ABSTRACT

This study aims to investigate the contribution of voluntary simplicity to psychological resilience during the Covid-19 pandemic. Distinctively, the study investigates (1) how a voluntary simplicity lifestyle (VSL) supports psychological well-being in terms of the valuation of life, mental health, and boredom experienced during the pandemic crisis and (2) whether pandemic-induced psychological states encourage the intention for a future VSL. Data were collected in Turkey through an online survey of 541 participants in the Covid-19 period. Analysis results revealed that not all but certain VSL aspects supported psychological resilience by promoting the valuation of life, mental health, and alleviating boredom during the pandemic. Material independency appeared as the most prominent VSL value contributing to psychological resilience. Findings revealed that a high valuation of life and high mental stress during the pandemic motivates individuals for future simple lives. The present study enhances the current knowledge about voluntary simplicity during highly stressful periods.

DOI: 10.4018/978-1-6684-8565-1.ch016

INTRODUCTION

The Covid-19 pandemic is considered the most severe global health crisis of the century, with more than 6.37 million deaths and 562.672.324 confirmed cases worldwide (WHO, 2022). In the two and a half years of the pandemic, Covid-19 is spreading worldwide, with new variants signaling the pandemic is far from being completely over. In addition to the vast human loss, the pandemic has destructed economic, social, and psychological well-being worldwide. Substantial research investigated the impacts of Covid-19, which is an unexpected, hard to control, and still unpredictable crisis, and revealed negative consequences on psychological well-being (Morgul et al., 2021; Casagrande et al., 2020; Wang et al., 2020; Odriozola-Gonzáleza et al., 2020). Varying degrees of anxiety, depression, stress, poorer sleep quality, loneliness, and boredom were experienced during the pandemic (Droit-Volet et al., 2020; Tutzer, 2021; Mazza et al., 2020). Although limited in number, some research on the correlates of severity of pandemic-induced psychological strain reveals that some individuals are more vulnerable to the destructive effects of this crisis while others appear to be psychologically more resilient. Particularly, young, single, low-income people and women experience psychological distress, loneliness, boredom (Tutzer, 2021), and depression more intensively than other individuals (Ustun, 2021). In addition to those demographic factors, some personality traits such as self-security and conscientiousness (Hampshire et al., 2021), self-compassion, gratitude (Nguyen & Le, 2021), mindfulness (Conversano et al., 2020); activities for personal care (Adamson et al., 2020), leisure activities and connection with family/friends (Ryerson, 2020) were found to support psychological resilience during the pandemic.

However, previous studies have not yet dealt with the role of pre-pandemic lifestyles in psychological responses to the pandemic. This is surprising since the pandemic-induced psychological strain is mainly attributed to the destruction of well-established lifestyles because of confinement and multiple restrictive measures (Brooks et al., 2020; Picó-Pérez et al., 2021; Znazen et al., 2021). Social distancing and varying levels of quarantine precautions changed individuals' working, studying, socializing, shopping, traveling, cleaning, eating, praying routines, and leisure time activities for a significant period. Besides, many individuals suffered financially on various scales because of job or income losses due to the negative economic impact of Covid-19 (Adams-Prassl et al., 2020; Acs & Karpman, 2020). This financial stress and future economic uncertainty led to a remarkable change in consumption patterns (Sheth, 2020) and disrupted contemporary consumerist lifestyles in many ways. This sudden and unwilling change in preferred lifestyle, isolation from loved ones, the loss of freedom, and uncertainty over disease are argued to have dramatic effects on psychological states (Brooks et al., 2020). However, the empirical evidence regarding the psychological well-being of individuals during the pandemic with different lifestyles is hardly scarce. In this research, to fill the gap to some extent, we focus on voluntary simplicity as a pre-pandemic lifestyle and investigate its role in psychological responses to the ongoing Covid-19 crisis.

Voluntary simplicity lifestyle (VSL), both a belief system and a practice, stemmed in the 1960s as a response to the consumption culture (Tosun & Sezgin, 2021). It refers to "choice out of free will to limit expenditures on consumer goods and services, and to cultivate non-materialistic sources of satisfaction and meaning" (Etzioni, 1998, pp. 620). Although VSL was mainly studied in the pro-environmental consumption context, it comprises a group of practices and motivations beyond sustainability concerns (Rebouças & Soares, 2021). Accordingly, voluntary simplicity is not only a reduction of material consumption but also a way of life where people choose freely to live a simple life, search for internal growth and well-being, personal fulfillment and control, self-sufficiency, and include values such as environmentalism, social consciousness, spirituality, self-determination, self-development, and humanism (Zavestoski, 2002; Craig-Lees & Hill, 2002; Rebouças & Soares, 2021). In their literature review, Hook et al. (2021) summarize the empirical evidence of a consistent positive relationship between voluntary simplicity and well-being built primarily due to restraint of consumption desires, replacement of materialistic values, and psychological need satisfaction. One crucial question here is whether a VSL may also support psychological well-being through crisis periods such as the Covid-19 pandemic? To provide theoretical and empirical evidence on the subject, this study investigates the interaction between voluntary simplicity and psychological resilience in terms of the positive and negative valuation of life, positive and negative mental health, and boredom experienced during the pandemic.

Furthermore, we also investigate if pandemic-induced psychological states encourage the intention to engage in a voluntary simplicity lifestyle in the future. Although there is much research on drivers and motivations for having a VSL, this is the first research that suggests "crisis-resilience" as a VSL engagement motivator and crisis-induced psychological states as a driver of intention for voluntary simplicity, to the best of our knowledge. This research also expands the current state of knowledge on the psychological impacts of the Covid-19 pandemic and its correlates.

LITERATURE REVIEW

Voluntary Simplicity Lifestyle

A growing body of research on VSL provides particular but conceptually related definitions of voluntary simplicity, emphasizing certain motivations, values, and behaviors. The concept of voluntary simplicity was first defined by Gregg (1936, pp. 4) as avoiding items that are not related to one's main purpose in life and embodying sincerity, honesty, and a unique purpose that help to secure a greater abundance of life in relatively more important directions (cited in Shama, 1985, pp. 57). Leonard-Barton (1981) defined voluntary simplicity as a lifestyle aimed at maximizing the control of the individual in his/her daily life and minimizing his/her dependency and consumption. For Shama (1985), it is a lifestyle of self-sufficiency, low consumption, and ecological responsibility. Iwata (1997) states that the concept refers to a low-consumption lifestyle with low material dependency. Craig-Lees and Hill (2002, pp. 191) states that voluntary simplicity is a way of life where people choose freely to live a simple life, reduce material consumption, have personal fulfillment and control, and include values such as environmentalism, spirituality, self-determination, self-development, and humanism. According to this philosophy of living; self-development of the individual or social progress does not occur with the evidence of status and wealth, but with the development of relationships in daily life, with increases in the qualitative richness of life such as social, aesthetic, and intellectual resources (Alexander, 2007, pp. 1).

Elgin and Mitchell (1977), Etzioni (1998), and Shama (1985) are among the pioneering scholars in the literature on voluntary simplicity who propose dimensions of voluntary simplicity values. According to Shama (1985, pp. 57-58), voluntary simplicity has six core values: material simplicity, human scale value, appropriate technology, self-determination, ecological awareness, and personal growth. Similarly, Elgin and Mitchell (1977) examined voluntary simplicity in five dimensions: material simplicity, human scale value, self-determination, ecological awareness, and personal growth. Material simplicity is the simplifying or uncluttering of an individual's life as a consumer (Shama, 1985, pp. 57-58); appropriate technology, rather than the automatic use of high technology, is the use of appropriate technology that will provide functionality, efficiency, and energy savings in the product (Shama, 1985, pp. 57-58). The other value expressed as self-determination is having more control over one's destiny (Elgin & Mitchell, 1977). Ecological awareness identifies sustainable consumption tendency in which a person acts with the awareness of the interdependence of resources and makes witting choices to use natural resources less (Elgin & Mitchell, 1977). Voluntary simplicity does not only mean reducing consumption. With this lifestyle, individuals tie better human relations and improve themselves psychologically. In this context, the humane scale value, which has an essential place in the set of values of voluntary simplicity, means humanizing the living and working environment of the individual and making it non-mechanical. It also includes making human relations more emotional and marvelous in the working environment (Elgin & Mitchell, 1977; Shama, 1985, pp. 57-58). Also, personal growth is becoming less dependent on the outside to heal oneself and create spiritual and psychological space. It refers to the concern for self-realization by developing practical, creative, or intellectual skills to discover and develop oneself in one's inner journey. Values such as material simplicity, human scale, self-determination, appropriate technology, and ecological awareness sweep away impediments to personal growth (Elgin & Mitchell, 1977; Shama, 1985, pp. 57-58).

Voluntary Simplicity and Individual Well Being

Does voluntary simplicity promote individual well-being beyond contributing to environmental well-being? The literature provides empirical evidence regarding the encouraging impact of VSL on satisfaction with life (Boujbel & d'Astous, 2012; Rich, Hanna & Wright, 2017; Ezell, 2019; Kuanr et al., 2020) and happiness (Alexander & Ussher 2012; Monopolis, 2010; Balderjahn et al., 2020; 2021).

Some other studies help to understand how and by which way VSL improves life satisfaction and happiness. Accordingly, VSL can promote life satisfaction and well-being by restraining consumption desires, replacing materialistic values, and satisfying psychological needs (Hook et al., 2021). Through voluntary simplicity, individuals depend on internal factors that will meet their psychological needs rather than external factors such as saving their wealth to be happy (Hook et al., 2021). For example, those who choose this lifestyle due to stress, dissatisfaction, and too much work, which are common in capitalist consumption societies, aim to have meaningful and, at the same time, happy lives, to find the inner focus of life and regain the sense of autonomy lost with overconsumption (Rodriquez, 2018; Ugla, 2019; Hausen, 2019). In addition, those who voluntarily simplify their lives achieve goals such as working less and earning less money, spending more time with their friends and family and contributing to their personal development (Etzioni, 1998; Huneke, 2005). Furthermore, voluntary simplicity was also found to be positively related to increased relationship quality (Beecher, 2007), personal fulfillment (Beecher, 2007; McGouran & Prothero, 2016), and communal/personal well-being (Chowdhury, 2018). VSL, in turn, leads to longer-term happiness, life satisfaction or satisfaction, and lower stress levels (Etzioni, 1998; Carter & Gilovich, 2010; Tatzel, 2002).

Ambrose (2011) found that the benefits of voluntary simplicity included experiencing a sense of personal control, happiness, feeling healthy, well-being, and peace of mind. The study of Kang, Martinez, and Johnson (2021) on minimalism show that people with this lifestyle tend to have more satisfaction and respect, and at the same time, they are less likely to experience depression. According to Connelly (2020), voluntary simplicity is endowed with psychological benefits such as decreasing stress and anxiety, improving relationships with people, independence, and mindfulness. In addition, it has been observed that people with this lifestyle are healthier, more peaceful, and calm (Ezell, 2019).

The Contributions of Pre-pandemic VSL to Psychological Resilience during Covid-19 Pandemic

Following the results above, it is safe to conclude that VSL promotes individual well-being in normal life rutin. What about highly stressful crisis periods, such as the Covid-19 pandemic? Does VSL support psychological resilience during crises? To provide an answer to the issue, the recent research focuses on the impact of pre-pandemic VSL adoption on psychological well-being indicators, including (1) valuation of life, (2) mental health, and (3) boredom during the pandemic.

Valuation of life, which is an aspect of psychological well-being, refers to the subjectively experienced worth of a person's life and is reflected as an attachment to the present life (Lawton et al., 2001; Lawton et al., 1999). The concept comprises positive and negative valuation of life influenced by personal background characteristics and external and internal aspects of quality of life (Lawton et al., 1999). For this reason, it is safe to suggest a reduced positive and an increased negative value of life due to the Covid-19 pandemic since the well-established life routines were altered and quality of life decreased during this period (Colucci et al., 2022; Ferreira et al., 2021; Suryavanshi et al., 2020). However, we posit that VSL should contribute to the valuation of life during the pandemic. Particularly, we expect voluntary simplifiers to value their lives during the pandemic relatively more due to the values on which their lives are built. This is partly because the positive value of life was promoted, and the negative value of life was alleviated by certain well-being indicators such as personal growth, positive relationships, and environmental mastery (Lawton et al., 2001). Here, personal growth refers a continued personal development, realizing the personal potential and improvement in self, while positive relationships indicate trusting relationships with others, and environmental mastery describes an ability to choose or create contexts suitable to personal needs and values (Ryff, 1989). These are the aspects in which voluntary simplifiers predominate their counterparts due to their lifestyle orientation. Through their commitment to the non-material aspects of life (Zavestoski, 2002), voluntary simplifiers reduce their consumption and working hours, focus on personal development, spend quality time with their friends and family, and live a satisfying, happy and meaningful life (Etzioni, 1998; Huneke, 2005; Hausen, 2019) which should support the valuation of their life during crisis periods. Thus we propose:

H1. Adoption of VSL before the Covid-19 pandemic has a positive impact on the valuation of life during Covid-19 pandemic.

One other psychological well-being indicator is mental health, referring "a state of well-being in which the individual realizes his or her own abilities, can cope with the normal stresses of life, can work productively and fruitfully, and is able to make a contribution to his or her community" (WHO, 2004, pp. 10). Following this definition and prior research (Lau et al., 2006) negative and positive mental health conditions in Covid-19 pandemic are examined in this research. Positive mental health refers to individuals' ability to successfully cope with the pandemic's stresses and focus on enhancing their personal, psychological and physical well-being. In contrast, negative mental health defines extended Covid-related stress, anxiety, and feelings of helplessness. A well-accepted finding of a two-year literature review is that the Covid-19 pandemic negatively impacts individuals' mental health. The higher levels of distress (Casagrande et al., 2020; Yu et al., 2021), anxiety (Casagrande et al., 2020; Wang et al., 2020; Evanoff et al., 2020; Odriozola-Gonzáleza et al., 2020), depression (Wang et al., 2020; Odriozola-Gonzáleza et al., 2020; Mazza et al., 2020), post-traumatic stress disorder (Brooks et al., 2020; Wang et al., 2020), lower sleep quality (Casagrande et al., 2020; Bartoszek et al., 2020), higher levels of loneliness (Bartoszek et al., 2020; González-Sanguino et al., 2020) and have less positive emotions (Losda-Baltar et al., 2020)

and general mental distress was reported to be related with quarantine and isolation precautions (Schnell & Krampe, 2020; Pierce et al., 2020). It appears that the fear of losing family members, contracting an infection, the economic destruction, risk of unemployment, and disrupted contemporary consumerist lifestyle poss a significant threat to the physical and mental health of individuals (Asmundson et al., 2020; Hetkamp et al., 2020; Humphrey & Vari, 2021).

We suggest that during highly stressful periods such as Covid-19, people who previously had a VSL should be more resilient to negative mental impacts. This is partly because they are expected to adopt quarantine and confinement situations which are addressed as mental health hindering factors, more easily (Schnell & Krampe, 2020). Thanks to their relatively higher control over life, slowness, balance, and activities contributing to becoming more mindful and accepting (Osikominu & Bocken, 2020), they are likely to maintain positive mental health and experience less stress and anxiety during quarantine and confinement periods. Besides, voluntary simplifiers are likely to be more resilient to stress rooted in job insecurity and financial loss stemming from economic disruption in the Covid-19 era (Zhang et al., 2020; Probst et al., 2020). Indeed, VSL adoption is often triggered by personal economic problems such as bankruptcy (Osikominu & Bocken, 2020) or macro events such as stagflation (Shama, 1981) and results in the adoption of values of "material simplicity", "function over style" and "small is beautiful". Thanks to these values, voluntary simplifiers avoid overconsumption and obtain financial well-being, which will eliminate financial stress during the pandemic and help to maintain positive mental health. Contrary, a materialistic lifestyle is known to cause anxiety and depression, lower happiness and life satisfaction, some personality disorders, and physical problems such as headaches (Kasser, 2002). Lloyd and Pennington (2020) revealed that the clutter and complexity of individuals' lives make them feel more stressed, overwhelmed, and anxious, which may be a more severe case during the pandemic. Thus:

H2. Adoption of VSL before the Covid-19 pandemic has a positive impact on mental health during the Covid-19 pandemic.

The final psychological state investigated in the current research is boredom, defining "an aversive experience of wanting but failing to engage in satisfying activity" (Eastwood et al., 2012, pp. 482). It is experienced as being disengaged from the world and stuck in a seemingly endless and dissatisfying present (Fahlman et al., 2013). During the pandemic, people whose working, studying, socializing, shopping, and traveling routines changed and stayed at home with their thoughts due to confinement and multiple restrictive precautions are likely to experience boredom (Wolff et al., 2020). It is evident that individuals perceive time passing slower, especially in lock-down periods, and this perception promotes boredom (Droit-Volet et al., 2020). Boredom was found to be a risk factor for stress, depression, anxiety (Chao et al., 2020), fear (Bösselmann et al., 2021), anger (Droit-Volet et al., 2020), and adversely related to life satisfaction (Waterschoot et al., 2021) and happiness (Droit-Volet et al., 2020). The literature identifies some antecedents of boredom that help to understand its association with VSL. It was found that people with high self-control have less boredom during the pandemic (Wolff et al., 2020). Besides, mindful individuals, who are aware, attentive, and open to the present experiences, are less likely to feel boredom during the pandemic (Waterschoot et al., 2021). Boredom is especially the case for people who are less aware of the potential resources to satisfy their inner needs (Weissinger et al., 1992). With voluntary simplicity, individuals can achieve goals such as focusing more on their inner world and having more life satisfaction. Shama (1985) states that personal growth, or the desire to improve oneself psychologically and spiritually, is a core value of voluntary simplifiers. More spare time should encourage their purpose rather than the feeling of boredom. Thus:

H3. Adoption of VSL before the Covid-19 Pandemic has a positive impact on boredom during the Covid-19 pandemic.

Determinants of Intention for Engaging in VSL in the Post-Pandemic Period

The VSL focuses on the idea that personal satisfaction and happiness stem from a commitment to the non-material aspects of life (Zavestoski, 2002). This approach involves meeting material needs as simply and directly as possible, minimizing consumption of consumer goods and services (Alexander, 2011). While people minimize their consumption with a more minimalist lifestyle, they also aim to maximize their personal development. There are specific motivations for living simply, such as being healthier, saving money, environmental concern, more time for community involvement, more time for oneself, more time with family, decluttering life/minimalism, self-reliance/self-sufficiency, humanitarian or social justice concerns, to live more spiritually or mindfully (Huneke, 2005; Alexander & Ussher, 2012). Zavestoski (2002) states that the motivation of people who learn to adopt a VSL can be both positive, such as increasing life satisfaction, and negative, such as getting tired of consumption pressure and environmental concerns. Besides, in the study of Kraleva (2017), the participants expressed the reasons for choosing a simpler life as spirituality, the desire to save the self from institutional hegemony, the effect of the individual on nature, the inconsistency with the values of modern society, dissatisfaction with individual's own life and the desire for inner growth. With these motivations, it is predicted that people who had a simple lifestyle before the Covid-19 period intend to continue this lifestyle after the pandemic. Based on all these, the following hypothesis is provided:

H4. Adoption of VSL before the Covid-19 Pandemic has a positive impact on the intention for adapting VSL after Covid-19 Pandemic.

In addition to the pre-pandemic VSL adoption's direct impact on the lifestyle's future intention, we also expect it to increase the intention indirectly through its positive role on Covid-19 induced psychological states. We propose that positive or negative psychological states during the pandemic, which are expected to be related to the pre-pandemic VSL adoption, may help to increase the intention to live a simple life after the pandemic. Broaden and Build Theory (Fredrickson, 2001) can constitute a basis for this proposition. According to the Theory in which Fredrickson (2001) draws attention to the benefits of positive and negative emotions in individual functioning, emotions such as satisfaction, interest, love, joy, and pride in the individual can expand the actions and thoughts that the individual wants to do, and it can provide the necessary resources for lead a better life. Fredrickson (2001) argued that individuals who experience such emotions tend to have more social, psychological, and cognitive resources than those in negative moods. Another form of positive emotions mentioned in Broaden and Build Theory can be indicated as the fact that individuals overcome such a stressful pandemic era more efficiently with a VSL and experience fewer pandemic-induced psychological strains than others. Therefore, it is predicted that the psychological states that are positively affected by the pre-pandemic VSL will enhance the intentions for a post-pandemic simple life.

Additionally, the Upward Spiral Theory of Lifestyle Change (Fredrickson, 2013) may explain the indirect impact of pre-pandemic VSL on future intention through its impact on individuals' psychological strain. The theory predicts that as long as a positive effect is experienced in exhibiting behavior and it is supported by certain personal resources, cognitive, social, psychological, and biological, the behavior is maintained. The positive effects experienced in these lifestyle changes provide unconscious motivations for behavior, and it is argued that this increases the possibility of continuing the behavior in the future

(Fredrickson, 2013; Rice & Fredrickson, 2017). In support of this; Kang, Martinez and Johnson (2021) stated that if behaviors representing a minimalist lifestyle are associated with positive emotions, these positive emotions strengthen the logic of engaging in minimalism, as these positive emotions provide an impetus to help motivate, encourage and maintain the behavior.

Besides, the negative emotional states proposed to be experienced more intensively by individuals during this period may lead individuals who did not lead a voluntarily simple life pre-pandemic to a post-pandemic simple life. Individuals in a negative mood state engage in behaviors that can reduce or eliminate the effect of the negative mood state (Clark & Isen, 1982). Clark and Isen (1982) stated that when individuals are in a negative mood, they may turn to more pessimistic thinking and demoralizing behaviors with automatic cognitive processes; instead, controlled cognitive processes can improve their negative mood and at least prevent it from getting worse. VSL can be considered as a coping strategy to improve negative emotional states. Because with this lifestyle, individuals establish a better work and life balance, spend more time with family and friends, or achieve goals such as establishing more meaningful and harmonious relationships with nature and the environment (Bekin, et al., 2005). Based on all these, the following hypothesis is provided:

H5. Psychological states during the Covid-19 Pandemic have positive impacts on the intention for adapting VSL after Covid-19 Pandemic.

Control Variables

In previous studies on psychological states during the pandemic, demographic factors such as age (Pierce et al., 2020; Casagrande et al., 2020), gender (Pierce et al., 2020; Casagrande et al., 2020; Bartoszek et al., 2020), education (Morgul et al., 2021; Tutzer et al., 2021), income (Pierce et al., 2020; Morgul et al., 2021), marital status (De Pedraza et al., 2020; Alirezaei et al., 2022), household size (Morgul et al., 2021) and Covid-19 induced health issues (Wang, 2020; Mazza, 2020) and Covid-19 related income reduction (De Pedraza et al., 2020) have been found to impact on psychological states during the Covid-19 outbreak. Besides, in previous studies, demographic factors such as age, gender, education, income, and marital status have been found to impact the intention to adapt VSL (Leonard-Barton, 1981; Özgül, 2011; Chang, 2021; Çınar, 2021). Thus, these variables were considered as control variables in the research. Figure 1 represents the research model considered in the context of Covid-19.

METHOD

Instruments

Data was collected through an online survey conducted in Turkey between March and August 2020. In this process, Turkey was one of the countries most affected by the Covid-19 pandemic. During this period, many precautions were taken in Turkey regarding education, entertainment, home confinement, and traveling (MoI, 2022; MoH-TR, 2022). For this reason, it is safe to state that evaluating pandemic-induced psychological states at the time of the study is appropriate.

The questionnaire included multi-item scales for measuring participants' pre-pandemic VSL, intention for adapting VSL after the Covid-19 pandemic, boredom, valuation of life, and mental health. Voluntary simplicity lifestyle was measured by Iwata's (2006) scale comprising five sub-dimensions, including

Figure 1. Research model

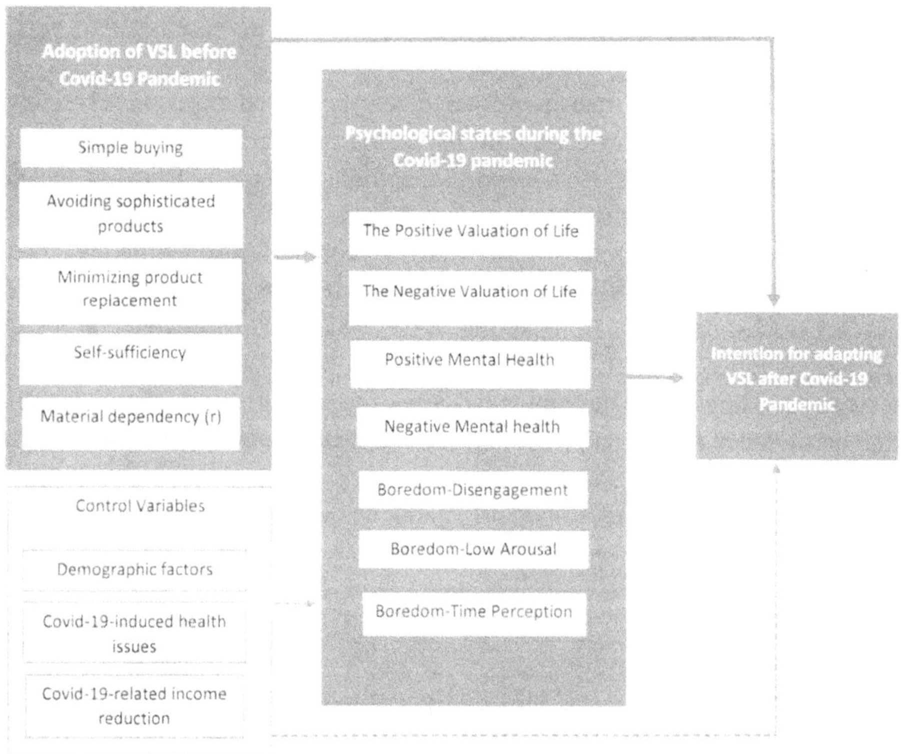

simple buying, avoiding sophisticated products, minimizing product replacement, self-sufficiency, and material independency. Intention for adapting VSL after the Covid-19 pandemic was measured using five items from Iwata (1997). The boredom scale consisting of 12 items was modified from Fahlman et al. (2013), comprising three dimensions: disengagement, low arousal, and time perception. The positive and negative valuation of life was measured using 14 items from Lawton et al. (2001), and the positive and negative mental health was measured using 11 items from Lau et al. (2006). The original items were tailored to the Covid-19 context and asked in the form of a 5-point Likert scale (1 = Strongly disagree, 5 = Strongly agree). In the last part of the questionnaire, demographic questions about the participants' age, gender, education level, income status, marital status, and household size were included. In this section, questions were also asked to indicate whether they experienced any health problems during the Covid-19 period and whether there was a decrease in their income during the pandemic period.

Clarity of wording and ease of responding was ensured through a pilot test of the online questionnaire. Then, an invitation link was sent to participants, who were drawn by convenience sampling, through e-mail, instant messaging applications (e.g., Telegram, WhatsApp), and social media platforms (e.g., Instagram, Facebook). A total of 554 valid questionnaires were obtained. Respondents were on average 28,09 years old (standard deviation = 6,97). Of the respondents, approximately 73,4% were female, and 69,1% were single. Regarding educational attainment, 1,7% held a primary and secondary school education, 18,9% had graduated from high school, 56,2% held undergraduate degrees, and 23,1% held graduate degrees. Lastly, 35,5% of the respondents had a monthly income of more than 5.000₺.

ANALYSES

Evaluation of Measurement Validity and Reliability

To evaluate the construct validity of the scales, an exploratory factor analysis (EFA) was conducted on 65 items using principal component analysis and varimax rotation. 13 factors were obtained that had eigenvalues greater than one and cumulatively explained 67% of the total variance. However, seven items were problematic due to low factor loadings and were eliminated in an iterative process. Final EFA resulted in a 13-factor solution which explained 70% of the total variance in the data set. As presented in Table 2, each scale item was loaded to their relevant factors with satisfactory factor loadings revealing the construct validity of scales. Table 2 also provides Cronbach's alpha coefficients which were estimated to evaluate the reliability of the scales. Satisfactory alpha coefficients ranging from 0,61 to 0,93 confirmed the scales' reliability (Nunnaly, 1978).

Following the validation of scales, composite scores were derived for each scale by estimating the arithmetic means of the relevant items. Besides, an overall score of a simple lifestyle was calculated through the arithmetic mean of the five sub-dimensions. When the kurtosis and skewness values of the variables were examined, it was seen that all the variables had a normal distribution. Table 3 provides descriptive statistics of the variables, while Table 4 displays correlations across variables.

A series of multiple linear regression analyses were performed with relevant dependent variables to test the research hypotheses. In the first regression model, the positive valuation of life was regressed on control variables (age, gender, education, income, marital status, household size) and five sub-dimensions of VSL (i.e., simple buying, avoiding sophisticated products, minimizing product replacement, self-sufficiency, material independence). As displayed in Table 5, the regression model was found to explain 12% of the observed variance in the positive valuation of life, which is significantly greater than zero (F=6,639; p<0,01). After controlling for the impacts of control factors, VSL-Avoiding sophisticated products (b=0,135, p<0,01) and VSL-Self-sufficiency (b=0,118, p<0,01) have significant positive impacts on the positive valuation of life. In contrast, other dimensions of the VSL were found to have no significant impact on the positive valuation of life. Based on standardized beta coefficients, VSL-Self-sufficiency was the strongest predictor of positive valuation of life. A further examination of the results found that the control variables such as age (b=-0.082, p<0,05), education (b=0.107, p<0,05), marital status (b=0.093, p<0,05), Covid-19 induced health issues (b=-0.115, p<0,01), Covid-19 related income reduction (b=-0.089, p<0,05) had significant impact on positive valuation of life.

In the second regression analysis, the negative valuation of life was regressed on control variables and five sub-dimensions of VSL. The regression model was found to explain 10,3% of the observed variance in the negative valuation of life, which was significantly greater than zero (F=5,749; p<0,01). After controlling for the impacts of control factors, VSL-Material independency (b=-0,135, p<0,01) significantly impacted the negative valuation of life. In contrast, other dimensions of the VSL were found to have no significant impact. A further evaluation of the results found that the control variables such as education (b=-0.163, p<0,01), marital status (b=-0.171, p<0,01), household size (b=-0.089, p<0,05), Covid-19 related income reduction (b=0.083, p<0,05) had significant impact on negative valuation of life. In line with these data, the H1 hypothesis was partially supported.

In the following regression model, the positive mental health was regressed on control variables and five sub-dimensions of VSL. Consistent with the test results, the regression model explained 4,6% of the observed variance in positive mental health, which was found to be significant (F=3,023; p<0,01).

Table 1. Factor loadings and reliability coefficients for dimensions

Items/Factors	Factor loadings
VSL dimension - Simple buying before Covid-19 pandemic α=,79	
VSL1	,734
VSL2	,810
VSL3	,762
VSL6	,524
VSL dimension - Avoiding sophisticated products α=,61	
VSL9	,641
VSL8	,622
VSL10	,724
VSL dimension - Minimizing product replacement α=,76	
VSL14	,699
VSL15	,851
VSL16	,683
VSL dimension - Self-sufficiency α=,77	
VSL11	,705
VSL12	,779
VSL13	,813
VSL dimension -Material independency α=,71	
VSL17 (r)	,759
VSL18 (r)	,782
VSL21 (r)	,726
Positive valuation of life α=,92	
POS-VOL1	,594
POS-VOL2	,612
POS-VOL3	,632
POS-VOL4	,807
POS-VOL5	,826
POS-VOL6	,780
POS-VOL7	,743
POS-VOL8	,655
Positive mental health α=,86	
POS-MH1	,609
POS-MH2	,847
POS-MH3	,862
POS-MH4	,764
POS-MH5	,648
Boredom-Disengagement (DIS) α=,90	
DIS-BOR1	,668
DIS-BOR2	,783
DIS-BOR3	,624
DIS-BOR4	,712
DIS-BOR5	,628
DIS-BOR6	,590
Boredom-Low Arousal (LA) α=,88	
LA-BOR1	,676
LA-BOR4	,553
LA-BOR5	,740
Boredom-Time Perception (TP) α=,93	
TP-BOR1	,824
TP-BOR2	,778
TP-BOR3	,826
Negative mental health α=,91	
NEG-MH1	,637
NEG-MH2	,751
NEG-MH3	,737
NEG-MH4	,771
NEG-MH5	,793
NEG-MH6	,702
Negative valuation of life α=,86	
NEG-VOL1	,649
NEG-VOL2	,773
NEG-VOL3	,683
NEG-VOL4	,781
NEG-VOL5	,455
NEG-VOL6	,527
Intention for a simple lifestyle after Covid-19 pandemic α=,87	
Intention1	,825
Intention2	,791
Intention3	,767
Intention4	,674
Intention5	,733

Avoiding the sophisticated products aspect of VSL (b=0,122, p<0,05) significantly promoted positive mental health. A further evaluation of the results revealed that the age (b=-0.136, p<0,01) variable among the control variables significantly impacts positive mental health. Any other control variables had no significant relation to positive mental health.

In the next regression analysis, negative mental health was the dependent variable, while control variables and five sub-dimensions of VSL were held as independent variables. The regression model was found to be significant (F=6,424; p<0,01), and the model was found to explain 11,5% of the observed variance. VSL-Material independency (b=-0,099, p<0,05) was found to alleviate negative mental

Table 2. Descriptive statistics of the variables

N= 541	Mean	Std. Deviation	Skewness		Kurtosis	
			Statistic	Std. Error	Statistic	Std. Error
VSL before the Covid-19 pandemic						
Simple buying	3.8253	.82845	-.735	.105	.315	.210
Avoiding sophisticated products	3.5539	.81512	-.340	.105	-.023	.210
Minimizing product replacement	4.1466	.69230	-.698	.105	.305	.210
Self-sufficiency	3.6753	.92626	-.524	.105	-.305	.210
Material independency	2.2964	.93727	-.764	.105	.380	.210
Overall VSL	3.7810	.54361	-.331	.105	.265	.210
Positive valuation of life	3.2077	.94512	-.406	.105	-.379	.210
Negative valuation of life	3.2733	.98608	-.200	.105	-.629	.210
Positive mental health	3.5305	.87731	-.449	.105	-.050	.210
Negative mental health	3.5832	1.06195	-.447	.105	-.581	.210
Boredom-Disengagement (DIS)	3.6377	1.02649	-.632	.105	-.315	.210
Boredom-Low Arousal (LA)	3.1319	1.22015	-.067	.105	-1.059	.210
Boredom-Time Perception (TP)	3.1707	1.31462	-.100	.105	-1.219	.210
Intention for adapting VSL after Covid-19 Pandemic	3.8680	.82081	-.576	.105	.189	.210

health significantly. As seen in the table, control variables such as income (b=-0,111, p<0,05), marital status (b=-0,172, p<0,01), Covid-19 induced health issues (b=0,102, p<0,05), Covid-19 related income

Table 3. Correlation coefficients

		1	2	3	4	5	6	7	8	9	10	11	12	13	14
1	VSL-Simple buying	1													
2	VSL-Avoiding sophisticated products	.439**	1												
3	VSL-Minimizing product replacement	.459**	.258**	1											
4	VSL-Self-sufficiency	.374**	.348**	.329**	1										
5	VSL-Material independency (r)	.245**	.104*	.174**	.071	1									
6	Overall VSL adoption before the Covid-19 pandemic	.765**	.654**	.644**	.668**	-.519**	1								
7	Positive valuation of life	.201**	.218**	.134**	.199**	-.003	.228**	1							
8	Negative valuation of life	-.040	.020	-.035	-.018	-.174**	-.081	-.483**	1						
9	Positive mental health	.144**	.166**	.131**	.119**	.069	.191**	.531**	-.265**	1					
10	Negative mental health	-.067	-.061	.036	.009	-.143**	-.076	-.483**	.596**	-.318**	1				
11	Boredom-Disengagement (DIS)	-.078	-.019	-.010	-.014	-.171**	-.096*	-.511**	.655**	-.354**	.681**	1			
12	Boredom-Low Arousal (LA)	-.097*	-.032	-.018	-.016	-.165**	-.106*	-.505**	.571**	-.318**	.608**	.687**	1		
13	Boredom-Time Perception (TP)	-.061	.007	-.033	.027	-.240**	-.098*	-.363**	.517**	-.185**	.522**	.594**	.528**	1	
14	Intention for adapting VSL after Covid-19 Pandemic	.437**	.418**	.403**	.407**	.215**	.574**	.215**	.019	.189**	.059	.003	-.022	.008	1

** Correlation is significant at the 0.01 level (2-tailed) * Correlation is significant at the 0.05 level (2-tailed)

Table 4. Multiple linear regression analyses of variables

	Dependent Variables											
	The positive valuation of life			**The negative valuation of life**			**Positive mental health**			**Negative mental health**		
	Std. Beta	t	Sig.	Std. Beta	t	Sig.	Std. Beta	t	Sig.	Std. Beta	t	Sig.
(Constant)		1,808	,071		8,503	,000		4,807	,000		7,254	,000
Age	**-,082**	**-2,006**	**,045**	,076	1,834	,067	**-,136**	**-3,180**	**,002**	,044	1,075	,283
Gender	,004	,093	,926	,063	1,481	,139	-,019	-,422	,673	-,032	-,744	,457
Education	**,107**	**2,474**	**,014**	**-,163**	**-3,716**	**,000**	,083	1,837	,067	-,058	-1,344	,179
Income	,083	1,705	,089	-,075	-1,511	,131	,029	,569	,569	**-,111**	**-2,267**	**,024**
Marital status	**,093**	**1,995**	**,047**	**-,171**	**-3,629**	**,000**	,003	,064	,949	**-,172**	**-3,683**	**,000**
Household size	,031	,711	,477	**-,089**	**-2,017**	**,044**	-,043	-,952	,342	-,022	-,506	,613
Covid-19-induced health issues	**-,115**	**-2,798**	**,005**	,079	1,898	,058	-,046	-1,077	,282	**,102**	**2,478**	**,014**
Covid-19-related income reduction	**-,089**	**-2,132**	**,033**	**,083**	**1,975**	**,049**	,035	,802	,423	**,159**	**3,787**	**,000**
VSL-Simple buying	,092	1,801	,072	-,007	-,139	,890	,043	,797	,426	-,045	-,881	,379
VSL-Avoiding sophisticated products	**,135**	**2,887**	**,004**	,061	1,294	,196	**,122**	**2,513**	**,012**	-,052	-1,108	,268
VSL-Minimizing product replacement	,042	,888	,375	-,020	-,420	,674	,072	1,477	,140	,074	1,571	,117
VSL-Self-sufficiency	**,118**	**2,590**	**,010**	-,024	-,520	,603	,037	,778	,437	,018	,388	,698
VSL-Material independency	-,076	-1,764	,078	**-,135**	**-3,123**	**,002**	,038	,844	,399	**-,099**	**-2,291**	**,022**
Adjusted R2		,120			,103			,046			,115	
F		6,639			5,749			3,023			6,424	
Significance		,001			,001			,001			,001	

reduction (b=0,159, p<0,01) had a significant impact on negative mental health. Based on all of these, the H2 hypothesis was partially supported.

Table 5. Multiple linear regression analyses of variables (cont.)

	Dependent Variables								
	Boredom-Disengagement			**Boredom-Low Arousal**			**Boredom-Time Perception**		
	Std. Beta	**t**	**Sig.**	**Std. Beta**	**t**	**Sig.**	**Std. Beta**	**t**	**Sig.**
(Constant)		8,745	,000		5,886	,000		3,600	,000
Age	,088	2,128	,034	,015	,363	,717	-,050	-1,191	,234
Gender	,053	1,234	,218	,053	1,207	,228	,075	1,743	,082
Education	**-,112**	**-2,575**	**,010**	-,043	-,973	,331	-,018	-,414	,679
Income	-,075	-1,528	,127	-,053	-1,050	,294	-,061	-1,216	,225
Marital status	**-,223**	**-4,754**	**,000**	**-,197**	**-4,119**	**,000**	**-,125**	**-2,627**	**,009**
Household size	-,073	-1,667	,096	-,055	-1,221	,223	,036	,816	,415
Covid-19-induced health issues	**,101**	**2,436**	**,015**	,038	,895	,371	,048	1,141	,254
Covid-19-related income reduction	,063	1,493	,136	**,089**	**2,061**	**,040**	,074	1,736	,083
VSL-Simple buying	-,061	-1,184	,237	-,085	-1,621	,106	-,032	-,615	,539
VSL-Avoiding sophisticated products	,027	,583	,560	,021	,429	,668	,028	,594	,553
VSL-Minimizing product replacement	,028	,600	,549	,037	,759	,448	,004	,094	,925
VSL-Self-sufficiency	-,003	-,057	,955	,003	,064	,949	,030	,648	,517
VSL-Material independency	**-,120**	**-2,770**	**,006**	**-,105**	**-2,384**	**,017**	**-,192**	**-4,394**	**,000**
Adjusted R2		,108			,071			,088	
F		6,041			4,186			4,989	
Significance		,001			,001			,001	

In the next stage, three distinct regression analyses were conducted where three sub-dimensions of boredom were regressed on control variables and dimensions of VSL. All regression models were found to be significant. The regression model, which included the disengagement dimension of boredom as the dependent variable, was significant (F=6,041; p<0,01) and explains 10,8% of the observed variance. Results revealed that VSL-Material independency (b=-0,120, p<0,01) was the unique VSL dimension

Table 6. Multiple linear regression analyses of variables (cont.)

	Dependent Variable		
	Intention for adapting VSL after Covid-19 Pandemic		
	Std. Beta	t	Sig.
(Constant)		,700	,484
Age	,041	1,160	,247
Gender	,018	,495	,621
Education	-,012	-,322	,748
Income	**-,081**	**-1,963**	**,050**
Marital status	**,118**	**2,926**	**,004**
Household size	-,035	-,929	,353
Covid-19-induced health issues	**-,086**	**-2,449**	**,015**
Covid-19-related income reduction	,060	1,663	,097
VSL-Simple buying	**,127**	**2,910**	**,004**
VSL-Avoiding sophisticated products	**,190**	**4,702**	**,000**
VSL-Minimizing product replacement	**,176**	**4,411**	**,000**
VSL-Self-sufficiency	**,180**	**4,603**	**,000**
VSL-Material independency	**,143**	**3,780**	**,000**
Positive valuation of life	**,158**	**3,192**	**,001**
Negative valuation of life	,040	,814	,416
Positive mental health	069	1,661	,097
Negative mental health	**,140**	**2,694**	**,007**
Boredom-Disengagement (DIS)	,029	,496	,620
Boredom-Low Arousal (LA)	-,001	-,026	,979
Boredom-Time Perception (TP)	,021	,467	,641
Adjusted R2		0,374	
F		17,158	
Significance		,001	

that significantly impacted the boredom-disengagement. Besides, control variables including education (b=-0,112, p<0,05), marital status (b=-0,223, p<0,01), Covid-19 induced health issues (b=0,101, p<0,05) were significantly related with disengagement.

Then, the boredom-low arousal dimension was regressed on control variables and five sub-dimensions of VSL. The results showed that the observed variance explained in the boredom-low arousal variable was 7,1%. VSL-Material independency had a significant mitigating impact (b=-0,105, p<0,05) on the low arousal. As seen in the table, marital status (b=-0,197, p<0,01) and Covid-19 related income reduction (b=0,089, p<0,05) were found to significantly explain boredom-low arousal variable.

The final regression model with the boredom dimension, namely time perception, as a dependent variable, was found to be significant (F=4,989; p<0,01). Results showed again that VSL-Material independency had a significant impact (b=-0,192, p<0,01) while other VSL dimensions had no significant impact. Besides marital status (b=-0,125, p<0,01), one of the control variables, had a significant impact. The regression model explained 8,8% of the total variance in boredom-time perception. In line with these findings, the H3 hypothesis was partially supported.

At the final step of the analysis process, the intention for adapting VSL after the Covid-19 pandemic was regressed on control variables, five subdimensions of VSL, and psychological states during the Covid-19 pandemic. The regression model was found to explain 3,7% of the observed variance in the intention, which was significantly greater than zero (F=17,158; p<0,01). All sub-dimensions of pre-pandemic VSL were found to significantly encourage the intention of adapting VSL after the Covid-19 pandemic. So H4 hypothesis was supported.

Findings also showed that positive valuation of life during pandemic ($b=0,158$, $p<0,01$) and negative mental health during pandemic levels ($b=0,140$, $p<0,01$) were statistically significant predictors of the intention for adapting VSL after Covid-19 pandemic variable. In line with these data, the H5 hypothesis was partially supported. It was seen that psychological states, especially positive valuation of life and negative mental health during the Covid-19 pandemic, positively impacted intention for adapting VSL after the Covid-19 pandemic. A further evaluation of the results revealed that the control variables such as income ($b=-0,081$, $p<0,05$), marital status ($b=0,118$, $p<0,01$) Covid-19 induced health issues ($b=-0,086$, $p<0,05$) had significant impact on the intention for adapting VSL after Covid-19 pandemic.

DISCUSSION

It is a well-documented fact now that the Covid-19 pandemic hindered the psychological well-being of individuals directly or indirectly. Some researchers revealed that specific individuals are more vulnerable to this crisis's destructive effects, while others appear to be psychologically more resilient (e.g., Tutzer, 2021; Ustun, 2021; Hampshire et al., 2021). This study focused on the contribution of voluntary simplicity as a pre-pandemic lifestyle to psychological resilience during the Covid-19 crisis. Particularly the study investigates the impact of having a VSL on the valuation of life, mental health, and boredom in times of crisis such as the Covid-19 pandemic. It was also investigated whether pandemic-induced psychological states would motivate engaging in VSL in the future. Depending on the research findings, we can generally conclude that pre-pandemic VSL partially contributed to psychological resilience during the stressful Covid-19 pandemic period. Since VSL and psychological well-being are both broad concepts, detailed information regarding the dynamics of the relationship between the two concepts is needed for complete comprehension.

Relatively Higher Valuation of Life

Results revealed that not all but some VSL aspects, including avoiding sophisticated products, self-sufficiency, and material independency, contributed to the valuation of life during the pandemic. Accordingly, people who want to prefer products with simple functions to those with complex functions, be less dependent on businesses that sell goods and provide services, grow their own fruits and vegetables, and do their own repairs before the pandemic, feel more hopeful and think that their lives have a purpose during the Covid-19 period. Besides, it can be said that people who buy something new shortly after it comes out, even if they have a similar product, and who think that a simple life is an indicator of poverty and misery, have an even more negative valuation of life during the pandemic period. Here, it is seen that voluntary simplifiers value their lives during the pandemic relatively more due to the values their lives are built on. Previous researchers confirmed these findings (Etzioni, 1998; Huneke, 2005; Hausen, 2019). This study tested the effect of voluntary simplicity on the valuation of life in the context of Covid-19, and empirical support was provided for the relevant holistic effect.

Relatively Better Mental Health

Results showed that pre-pandemic VSL also promoted mental health to some extent. A specific aspect, avoiding sophisticated products, was found to encourage positive mental health. Besides, material independency, another aspect of VSL, contributed to well-being by alleviating negative mental health. Accordingly, a simple and uncluttered life contributes to mental health. On the other hand, it can be said that materialistic people were more likely to feel stressed, anxious, and nervous during the pandemic. Simplifiers appear to be more resilient to mental health problems caused by quarantine and other precautions during the pandemic. This finding is consistent with previous findings on VSL and mental health relation (Kasser, 2002; Lloyd & Pennington, 2020; Zhang et al., 2020; Probst et al., 2020). This study provided unique empirical evidence showing that VSL supports mental health in the context of the pandemic process.

Relatively Lower Level of Boredom

Material independency, as a specific aspect of the VSL, was found to reduce boredom during the pandemic period. People with a higher level of material dependency were found to experience all forms of boredom more intensively. Individuals with a consumerist lifestyle are relatively more prone to feel isolated and stuck in a situation in which time passes too slowly, and everything is repetitive, meaningless, and irritating during the pandemic period. Destruction of a well-established, shopping-oriented lifestyle because of confinement and multiple restrictive measures appear to make them feel bored, low aroused, and aimless (Brooks et al., 2020; Picó-Pérez et al., 2021; Znazen et al., 2021). On the other side, simplifiers are more resilient to boredom because it has been determined that people who live in a simple way are less bored during the pandemic due to high self-control and awareness (Wolff et al., 2020; Waterschoot et al., 2021).

Relatively Higher Intention for Engaging VLS in the Post-Pandemic Period

The research also investigated the determinants of intention for adopting VSL after the pandemic. As expected, people who had a simple lifestyle before the Covid-19 period were found to have a stronger intention for VSL after the pandemic. Accordingly, people who have experienced VSL before are more motivated to continue this lifestyle after the pandemic. However, findings revealed that VSL adopting intention for the post-Covid-19 period is not merely an extension of a typical VSL but also encouraged by certain pandemic-induced psychological states. According to the results, two psychological states, one positive and one negative, promote the intention for a future simple life.

First, results revealed that a positive valuation of life during the pandemic promotes the future intention for engaging in VSL. This finding provides partial empirical evidence for Broaden and Build Theory and Upward Spiral Theory of Lifestyle Change since positive valuation of life is increased by the VSL aspects to some extent. It can be stated that voluntary simplifiers who are hopeful for the future, purposeful, and have high energy for living during the pandemic with the help of their simple lifestyle are likely to have a stronger motivation for pursuing VSL in the future. In other words, when the individuals realize that they overcome such a stressful period more efficiently with a positive valuation of life thanks to their lifestyle, this encourages them to maintain the lifestyle after the pandemic. This finding is consistent with Kang, Martinez, and Johnson (2021) argument that if behaviors representing a minimalist lifestyle are associated with positive emotions, these positive emotions strengthen the logic of engaging in minimalism.

However, not only hopeful individuals but also those with an intensive psychological strain reported higher intention for a post-pandemic VSL since negative mental health was found to promote people's intention to live a more simple life after the pandemic. It appears that Covid-19-related stress, anxiety, and feeling of helplessness lead individuals to think over their previous lifestyle and provide motivation for a better quality of life with higher personal, social, and environmental benefits. Here the financial benefits of the VSL may be a prominent factor for a higher intention for simple life since individuals countered the risk of losing income or employment during the pandemic, which was a significant stress trigger. This stress may make individuals aware of their previous excessive, dysfunctional purchases in the past and, in turn, promote the intention for a simple life.

CONCLUSIONS AND LIMITATIONS

The current research contributes to knowledge of VSL by providing information about the role of voluntary simplicity in psychological well-being during an unexpected and unpredictable crisis. In addition to its well-accepted environmental benefits, VLS appeared as a lifestyle that partially supports psychological resilience in a highly stressful crisis era. Through its various aspects, VSL supports certain positive psychological states and alleviates negative states during the pandemic. Here the role of material independency aspect of the VSL appeared as the most prominent value contributing to psychological resilience. Furthermore, the research uncovered if pandemic-induced psychological states encourage the intention for future simple life. In addition to the dominant influence of pre-pandemic consistent lifestyle, certain crisis-induced psychological states appeared to trigger the intention for voluntary simplicity. Two adverse psychological states, including a positive valuation of life and negative mental health status, motivated a future VSL through different routes. In sum, the results of the present study enhance the current knowledge about voluntary simple lifestyle by explaining how it influences and is influenced by the psychological states during an unpredictable, highly stressful period.

In addition to its contributions, the study also has some limitations. First of all, the data was collected only in Turkey. Because pandemic conditions and precautions may differ in other countries, the psychological states of this period and the level of people living in these countries to adopt a voluntary simplicity may differ. For this reason, the study can be extended to other countries. Another limitation is that we included certain psychological states in the study. Future studies may focus on more diverse psychological states. In addition, the study's findings can be expanded based on different lifestyles at the point of sustainable consumption and contribute to the literature on the presented relationships.

REFERENCES

Acs, G., & Karpman, M. (2020). Employment, income, and unemployment insurance during the Covid-19 Pandemic. Urban Institute, 1-11.

Adams-Prassl, A., Boneva, T., Golin, M., & Rauh, C. (2020). Inequality in the impact of the coronavirus shock: Evidence from real time surveys. *Journal of Public Economics*, *189*, 104245. doi:10.1016/j.jpubeco.2020.104245

Adamson, M. M., Phillips, A., Seenivasan, S., Martinez, J., Grewal, H., Kang, X., Coetzee, J., Luttenbacher, I., Jester, A., Harris, O. A., & Spiegel, D. (2020). International prevalence and correlates of psychological stress during the global COVID-19 pandemic. *International Journal of Environmental Research and Public Health*, *17*(24), 9248. doi:10.3390/ijerph17249248 PMID:33321950

Alexander, S. (2007). Voluntary simplicity movement. The Blackwell Encyclopedia of Sociology, 1-2. doi:10.1002/9781405165518.wbeos0693

Alexander, S. (2011). God's away on business: The spiritual significance of voluntary simplicity. *EarthSong Journal: Perspectives in Ecology, Spirituality and Education, 2*(2), 7-9. https://search.informit.org/doi/10.3316/informit.676595747751645

Alexander, S., & Ussher, S. (2012). The voluntary simplicity movement: A multi-national survey analysis in theoretical context. *Journal of Consumer Culture*, *12*(1), 66–86. doi:10.1177/1469540512444019

Alirezaei, M., Eskandarieh, S., Sahraian, M. A., & Naser Moghadasi, A. (2022). Depression, anxiety, and fear of COVID-19 in patients with multiple sclerosis in pandemic era: A cross-sectional study. *Neurological Sciences*, *43*(1), 59–66. doi:10.100710072-021-05612-5 PMID:34554334

Ambrose, M. S. (2011). Voluntary simplicity as an urban lifestyle: resisting a consumer economy/by Michelle Ambrose. Library and Archives Canada=Bibliothèque et Archives Canada.

Asmundson, G. J., Paluszek, M. M., Landry, C. A., Rachor, G. S., McKay, D., & Taylor, S. (2020). Do pre-existing anxiety-related and mood disorders differentially impact COVID-19 stress responses and coping? *Journal of Anxiety Disorders*, *74*, 102271. doi:10.1016/j.janxdis.2020.102271 PMID:32673930

Balderjahn, I., Lee, M. S., Seegebarth, B., & Peyer, M. (2020). A sustainable pathway to consumer well-being. The role of anticonsumption and consumer empowerment. *The Journal of Consumer Affairs*, *54*(2), 456–488. doi:10.1111/joca.12278

Balderjahn, I., Seegebarth, B., & Lee, M. S. (2021). Less is more! The rationale behind the decision-making style of voluntary simplifiers. *Journal of Cleaner Production*, *284*, 124802. doi:10.1016/j.jclepro.2020.124802

Bartoszek, A., Walkowiak, D., Bartoszek, A., & Kardas, G. (2020). Mental well-being (Depression, loneliness, insomnia, daily life fatigue) during COVID-19 related home-confinement—A study from Poland. *International Journal of Environmental Research and Public Health*, *17*(20), 7417. doi:10.3390/ijerph17207417 PMID:33053787

Beecher, T. S. (2007). *Questioning the consumer culture: A qualitative study on voluntary simplicity [PhD]*. University of North Dakota.

Bekin, C., Carrigan, M., & Szmigin, I. (2005). Defying marketing sovereignty: Voluntary simplicity at new consumption communities. *Qualitative Market Research*, *8*(4), 413–429. doi:10.1108/13522750510619779

Bösselmann, V., Amatriain-Fernández, S., Gronwald, T., Murillo-Rodríguez, E., Machado, S., & Budde, H. (2021). Physical activity, boredom and fear of COVID-19 among adolescents in Germany. *Frontiers in Psychology, 12*, 624206. Advance online publication. doi:10.3389/fpsyg.2021.624206 PMID:34012413

Boujbel, L., & d'Astous, A. (2012). Voluntary simplicity and life satisfaction: Exploring the mediating role of consumption desires. *Journal of Consumer Behaviour, 11*(6), 487–494. doi:10.1002/cb.1399

Brooks, S. K., Webster, R. K., Smith, L. E., Woodland, L., Wessely, S., Greenberg, N., & Rubin, G. J. (2020). The psychological impact of quarantine and how to reduce it: Rapid review of the evidence. *Lancet, 395*(10227), 912–920. doi:10.1016/S0140-6736(20)30460-8 PMID:32112714

Carter, T., & Gilovich, T. (2010). The relative relativity of material and experiential purchases. *Journal of Personality and Social Psychology, 98*(1), 146–159. doi:10.1037/a0017145 PMID:20053039

Casagrande, M., Favieri, F., Tambelli, R., & Forte, G. (2020). The enemy who sealed the world: Effects quarantine due to the COVID-19 on sleep quality, anxiety, and psychological distress in the Italian population. *Sleep Medicine, 75*, 12–20. doi:10.1016/j.sleep.2020.05.011 PMID:32853913

Chang, H. H. (2021). Exploring consumer behavioral predispositions toward voluntary simplicity. *Current Psychology (New Brunswick, N.J.), 40*(2), 731–743. doi:10.100712144-018-9994-4

Chao, M., Chen, X., Liu, T., Yang, H., & Hall, B. J. (2020). Psychological distress and state boredom during the COVID-19 outbreak in China: The role of meaning in life and media use. *European Journal of Psychotraumatology, 11*(1), 1769379. doi:10.1080/20008198.2020.1769379 PMID:33029315

Çınar, D. (2021). A research on the evaluation of consumers' voluntary simplicity lifestyle tendency in the Covid-19 period. *International Journal of Social Sciences and Education Research, 7*(1), 12–23. doi:10.24289/ijsser.832065

Clark, M. S., & Isen, A. M. (1982). Toward understanding the relationship between feeling states and social behavior. In A. Hastorf & A. M. Isen (Eds.), *Cognitive socialpsychology* (pp. 73–108). Elsevier.

Colucci, E., Nadeau, S., Higgins, J., Kehayia, E., Poldma, T., Saj, A., & de Guise, E. (2022). COVID-19 lock-downs' effects on the quality of life, perceived health and well-being of healthy elderly individuals: A longitudinal comparison of pre-lockdown and lock-down states of well-being. *Archives of Gerontology and Geriatrics, 99*, 104606. doi:10.1016/j.archger.2021.104606 PMID:34896795

Connelly, J. (2020). *The experience of voluntary simplicity: A consensual qualitative research study* [Unpublished doctoral dissertation]. Marquette University.

Conversano, C., Di Giuseppe, M., Miccoli, M., Ciacchini, R., Gemignani, A., & Orrù, G. (2020). Mindfulness, age and gender as protective factors against psychological distress during COVID-19 pandemic. *Frontiers in Psychology, 11*, 1900. doi:10.3389/fpsyg.2020.01900 PMID:33013503

Craig-Lees, M., & Hill, C. (2002). Understanding voluntary simplifiers. *Psychology and Marketing, 19*(2), 187–210. doi:10.1002/mar.10009

De Pedraza, P., Guzi, M., & Tijdens, K. (2020). *Life Dissatisfaction and Anxiety in COVID-19 pandemic* (No. 2020-03). MUNI ECON Working Paper.

Droit-Volet, S., Gil, S., Martinelli, N., Andant, N., Clinchamps, M., Parreira, L., Rouffiac, K., Dambrun, M., Huguet, P., Dubuis, B., Pereira, B., Bouillon, J.-B., & Dutheil, F. (2020). Time and Covid-19 stress in the lock-down situation: Time free,«Dying» of boredom and sadness. *PLoS One*, *15*(8), e0236465. doi:10.1371/journal.pone.0236465 PMID:32776990

Eastwood, J. D., Frischen, A., Fenske, M. J., & Smilek, D. (2012). The unengaged mind: Defining boredom in terms of attention. *Perspectives on Psychological Science*, *7*(5), 482–495. doi:10.1177/1745691612456044 PMID:26168505

Elgin, D., & Mitchell, A. (1977). Voluntary simplicity. *Planning Review*, *5*(6), 13–15. doi:10.1108/eb053820

Etzioni, A. (1998). Voluntary simplicity: Characterization, select psychological implications, and societal consequences. In *Essays in Socio-Economics* (pp. 1–26). Springer.

Evanoff, B. A., Strickland, J. R., Dale, A. M., Hayibor, L., Page, E., Duncan, J. G., Kannampallil, T., & Gray, D. L. (2020). Work-related and personal factors associated with mental well-being during the COVID-19 response: Survey of health care and other workers. *Journal of Medical Internet Research*, *22*(8), e21366. doi:10.2196/21366 PMID:32763891

Ezell, D. (2019). *Consumer well-being: A typology and examination of voluntary simplicity [PhD]*. University of Mississippi.

Fahlman, S. A., Mercer-Lynn, K. B., Flora, D. B., & Eastwood, J. D. (2013). Development and validation of the multidimensional state boredom scale. *Assessment*, *20*(1), 68–85. doi:10.1177/1073191111421303 PMID:21903683

Ferreira, L. N., Pereira, L. N., da Fé Brás, M., & Ilchuk, K. (2021). Quality of life under the COVID-19 quarantine. *Quality of Life Research: An International Journal of Quality of Life Aspects of Treatment, Care and Rehabilitation*, *30*(5), 1389–1405. doi:10.100711136-020-02724-x PMID:33389523

Fredrickson, B. L. (2001). The role of positive emotions in positive psychology: The broadenand-build Theory of positive emotions. *The American Psychologist*, *56*(3), 218–226. doi:10.1037/0003-066X.56.3.218 PMID:11315248

Fredrickson, B. L. (2013). Positive emotions broaden and build. *Advances in Experimental Social Psychology*, *47*, 1–53. doi:10.1016/B978-0-12-407236-7.00001-2

González-Sanguino, C., Ausín, B., Castellanos, M. Á., Saiz, J., López-Gómez, A., Ugidos, C., & Muñoz, M. (2020). Mental health consequences during the initial stage of the 2020 Coronavirus pandemic (COVID-19) in Spain. *Brain, Behavior, and Immunity*, *87*, 172–176. doi:10.1016/j.bbi.2020.05.040 PMID:32405150

Gregg, R. B. (1936). *The Voluntary Simplicity*. Pendle Hill Publications.

Hampshire, A., Hellyer, P. J., Soreq, E., Mehta, M. A., Ioannidis, K., Trender, W., Grant, J. E., & Chamberlain, S. R. (2021). Associations between dimensions of behaviour, personality traits, and mental-health during the COVID-19 pandemic in the United Kingdom. *Nature Communications*, *12*(1), 1–15. doi:10.103841467-021-24365-5 PMID:33397941

Hausen, J. E. (2019). Minimalist life orientations as a dialogical tool for happiness. *British Journal of Guidance & Counselling*, *47*(2), 168–179. doi:10.1080/03069885.2018.1523364

Hetkamp, M., Schweda, A., Bäuerle, A., Weismüller, B., Kohler, H., Musche, V., Dörrie, N., Schöbel, C., Teufel, M., & Skoda, E. M. (2020). Sleep disturbances, fear, and generalized anxiety during the COVID-19 shut down phase in Germany: Relation to infection rates, deaths, and German stock index DAX. *Sleep Medicine*, *75*, 350–353. doi:10.1016/j.sleep.2020.08.033 PMID:32950879

Hook, J. N., Hodge, A. S., Zhang, H., Van Tongeren, D. R., & Davis, D. E. (2021). Minimalism, voluntary simplicity, and well-being: A systematic review of the empirical literature. *The Journal of Positive Psychology*, 1–12. doi:10.1080/17439760.2021.1991450

Humphrey, A., & Vari, O. (2021). Meaning matters: Self-perceived meaning in life, Its predictors and psychological stressors associated with the COVID-19 pandemic. *Behavioral Sciences (Basel, Switzerland)*, *11*(4), 50. doi:10.3390/bs11040050 PMID:33924422

Huneke, M. E. (2005). The face of the un-consumer: An empirical examination of the practice of voluntary simplicity in the United States. *Psychology and Marketing*, *22*(7), 527–550. doi:10.1002/mar.20072

Iwata, O. (1997). Attitudinal and behavioral correlates of voluntary simplicity lifestyles. *Social Behavior and Personality*, *25*(3), 233–240. doi:10.2224bp.1997.25.3.233

Iwata, O. (2006). An evaluation of consumerism and lifestyle as correlates of a voluntary simplicity lifestyle. *Social Behavior and Personality*, *34*(5), 557–568. doi:10.2224bp.2006.34.5.557

Kang, J., Martinez, C. M. J., & Johnson, C. (2021). Minimalism as a sustainable lifestyle: Its behavioral representations and contributions to emotional well-being. *Sustainable Production and Consumption*, *27*, 802–813. doi:10.1016/j.spc.2021.02.001

Kasser, T. (2002). *The high price of materialism*. A Bradford Book, The MIT Press.

Kraleva, V. (2017). Understanding voluntary simplifiers in Bulgaria. *Marketing and Business Development Journal*, *3*(1). Advance online publication. doi:10.2139srn.2987904

Kuanr, A., Pradhan, D., & Chaudhuri, H. R. (2020). I (do not) consume; therefore, I am: Investigating materialism and voluntary simplicity through a moderated mediation model. *Psychology and Marketing*, *37*(2), 260–277. doi:10.1002/mar.21305

Lau, J. T., Yang, X., Tsui, H. Y., Pang, E., & Wing, Y. K. (2006). Positive mental health-related impacts of the SARS epidemic on the general public in Hong Kong and their associations with other negative impacts. *The Journal of Infection*, *53*(2), 114–124. doi:10.1016/j.jinf.2005.10.019 PMID:16343636

Lawton, M. P., Moss, M., Hoffman, C., Grant, R., Have, T. T., & Kleban, M. H. (1999). Health, valuation of life, and the wish to live. *The Gerontologist*, *39*(4), 406–416. doi:10.1093/geront/39.4.406 PMID:10495578

Lawton, M. P., Moss, M., Hoffman, C., Kleban, M. H., Ruckdeschel, K., & Winter, L. (2001). Valuation of life: A concept and a scale. *Journal of Aging and Health*, *13*(1), 3–31. doi:10.1177/089826430101300101 PMID:11503845

Leonard-Barton, D. (1981). Voluntary simplicity lifestyles and energy conservation. *The Journal of Consumer Research*, *8*(3), 243–252. doi:10.1086/208861

Lloyd, K., & Pennington, W. (2020). Towards a theory of minimalism and well-being. *International Journal of Applied Positive Psychology*, 1-16. doi:10.1007/s41042-020-00030-y

Losda-Baltar, A., Jiménez-Gonzalo, L., Gallego-Alberto, L., Pedroso-Chaparro, M. D. S., Fernandes-Pires, J., & Márquez-González, M. (2020). "We're Staying at Home". Association of Self-Perceptions of Aging, Personal and Family Resources and Loneliness With Psychological Distress During the Lock-Down Period of COVID-19. *The Journals of Gerontology: Series B*, *76*(2), e10–e16. doi:10.1093/geronb/gbaa048

Mazza, C., Ricci, E., Biondi, S., Colasanti, M., Ferracuti, S., Napoli, C., & Roma, P. (2020). A nation-wide survey of psychological distress among Italian people during the COVID-19 pandemic: Immediate psychological responses and associated factors. *International Journal of Environmental Research and Public Health*, *17*(9), 3165. doi:10.3390/ijerph17093165 PMID:32370116

McGouran, C., & Prothero, A. (2016). Enacted voluntary simplicity–Exploring the consequences of requesting consumers to intentionally consume less. *European Journal of Marketing*, *50*(1/2), 189–212. doi:10.1108/EJM-09-2013-0521

MoH-TR. (2022). *Ministry of Health, Republic of Turkey*. Available at https://covid19.saglik.gov.tr/TR-66935/genel-koronavirus-tablosu.html

MoI. (2022). *Ministry of Interior (Turkey)*. Available at https://www.icisleri.gov.tr/koronavirus-salgini-yeni-tedbirler

Monopolis, A. N. (2010). *Voluntary simplicity, authentic happiness, and ecological sustainability [PhD]. University of California.*

Morgul, E., Bener, A., Atak, M., Akyel, S., Aktaş, S., Bhugra, D., Ventriglio, A., & Jordan, T. R. (2021). COVID-19 pandemic and psychological fatigue in Turkey. *The International Journal of Social Psychiatry*, *67*(2), 128–135. doi:10.1177/0020764020941889 PMID:32650681

Nguyen, T. M., & Le, G. N. H. (2021). The influence of COVID-19 stress on psychological well-being among Vietnamese adults: The role of self-compassion and gratitude. *Traumatology*, *27*(1), 86–97. doi:10.1037/trm0000295

Nunnally, J. C. (1978). *Psychomtietrictheory*. McGraw-Hill.

Odriozola-González, P., Planchuelo-Gómez, Á., Irurtia, M. J., & de Luis-García, R. (2020). Psychological effects of the COVID-19 outbreak and lock-down among students and workers of a Spanish university. *Psychiatry Research*, *290*, 113108. doi:10.1016/j.psychres.2020.113108 PMID:32450409

Osikominu, J., & Bocken, N. (2020). A voluntary simplicity lifestyle: Values, adoption, practices and effects. *Sustainability*, *12*(5), 1903. doi:10.3390u12051903

Özgül, E. (2011). Tüketicilerin sosyo-demografik özelliklerinin hedonik tüketim ve gönüllü sade yaşam tarzları açısından değerlendirilmesi. *Ege Akademik Bakış*, *11*(1), 25–38. doi:10.21121/eab.2011119578

Picó-Pérez, M., Ferreira, S., Couto, B., Raposo-Lima, C., Machado-Sousa, M., & Morgado, P. (2021). Sociodemographic and lifestyle predictors of mental health adaptability during COVID-19 compulsory confinement: A longitudinal study in the Portuguese population. *Journal of Affective Disorders*, *295*, 797–803. doi:10.1016/j.jad.2021.08.150 PMID:34517254

Pierce, M., Hope, H., Ford, T., Hatch, S., Hotopf, M., John, A., Kontopantelis, E., Webb, R., Wessely, S., McManus, S., & Abel, K. M. (2020). Mental health before and during the COVID-19 pandemic: A longitudinal probability sample survey of the UK population. *The Lancet. Psychiatry*, *7*(10), 883–892. doi:10.1016/S2215-0366(20)30308-4 PMID:32707037

Probst, T. M., Lee, H. J., & Bazzoli, A. (2020). Economic stressors and the enactment of CDC-recommended COVID-19 prevention behaviors: The impact of state-level context. *The Journal of Applied Psychology*, *105*(12), 1397–1407. doi:10.1037/apl0000797 PMID:33271028

Rebouças, R., & Soares, A. M. (2021). Voluntary simplicity: A literature review and research agenda. *International Journal of Consumer Studies*, *45*(3), 303–319. doi:10.1111/ijcs.12621

Rice, E. L., & Fredrickson, B. L. (2017). Do positive spontaneous thoughts function as incentive salience? *Emotion (Washington, D.C.)*, *17*(5), 840–855. doi:10.1037/emo0000284 PMID:28206793

Rich, S. A., Hanna, S., & Wright, B. J. (2017). Simply satisfied: The role of psychological need satisfaction in the life satisfaction of voluntary simplifiers. *Journal of Happiness Studies*, *18*(1), 89–105. doi:10.100710902-016-9718-0

Rodriquez, J. (2018). The US minimalist movement: Radical political practice? *The Review of Radical Political Economics*, *50*(2), 286–296. doi:10.1177/0486613416665832

Ryerson, N. C. (2020). Behavioral and psychological correlates of well-being during COVID-19. *Psychological Reports*, *125*(1), 200–217. doi:10.1177/0033294120978160 PMID:33302799

Ryff, C. D. (1989). Happiness is everything, or is it? Explorations on the meaning of psychological well-being. *Journal of Personality and Social Psychology*, *57*(6), 1069–1081. doi:10.1037/0022-3514.57.6.1069

Schnell, T., & Krampe, H. (2020). Meaning in life and self-control buffer stress in times of COVID-19: Moderating and mediating effects with regard to mental distress. *Frontiers in Psychiatry*, *11*, 983. doi:10.3389/fpsyt.2020.582352 PMID:33173525

Shama, A. (1981). Coping with staglation: Voluntary simplicity. *Journal of Marketing*, *45*(3), 120–134. doi:10.1177/002224298104500310

Shama, A. (1985). The voluntary simplicity consumer. *Journal of Consumer Marketing*, *2*(4), 57–63. doi:10.1108/eb008146

Sheth, J. (2020). Impact of Covid-19 on consumer behavior: Will the old habits return or die? *Journal of Business Research*, *117*, 280–283. doi:10.1016/j.jbusres.2020.05.059 PMID:32536735

Suryavanshi, N., Kadam, A., Dhumal, G., Nimkar, S., Mave, V., Gupta, A., Cox, S. R., & Gupte, N. (2020). Mental health and quality of life among healthcare professionals during the COVID-19 pandemic in India. *Brain and Behavior*, *10*(11), e01837. doi:10.1002/brb3.1837 PMID:32918403

Tatzel, M. (2002). 'Money worlds' and well-being: An integration of money dispositions, materialism and price-related behavior. *Journal of Economic Psychology*, *23*(1), 103–126. doi:10.1016/S0167-4870(01)00069-1

Tosun, P., & Sezgin, S. (2021). Voluntary simplicity: A content analysis of consumer comments. *Journal of Consumer Marketing*, *38*(5), 484–494. doi:10.1108/JCM-04-2020-3749

Tutzer, F., Frajo-Apor, B., Pardeller, S., Plattner, B., Chernova, A., Haring, C., Holzner, B., Kemmler, G., Marksteiner, J., Miller, C., Schmidt, M., Sperner-Unterweger, B., & Hofer, A. (2021). Psychological Distress, Loneliness, and Boredom Among the General Population of Tyrol, Austria During the COVID-19 Pandemic. *Frontiers in Psychiatry*, *12*, 921. doi:10.3389/fpsyt.2021.691896 PMID:34177672

Uggla, Y. (2019). Taking back control: Minimalism as a reaction to high speed and overload in contemporary society. *Sociologisk Forskning*, *56*(3–4), 233–252. doi:10.37062f.56.18811

Ustun, G. (2021). Determining depression and related factors in a society affected by COVID-19 pandemic. *The International Journal of Social Psychiatry*, *67*(1), 54–63. doi:10.1177/0020764020938807 PMID:32605422

Wang, C., Pan, R., Wan, X., Tan, Y., Xu, L., Ho, C. S., & Ho, R. C. (2020). Immediate psychological responses and associated factors during the initial stage of the 2019 coronavirus disease (COVID-19) epidemic among the general population in China. *International Journal of Environmental Research and Public Health*, *17*(5), 1729. doi:10.3390/ijerph17051729 PMID:32155789

Waterschoot, J., Van der Kaap-Deeder, J., Morbée, S., Soenens, B., & Vansteenkiste, M. (2021). "How to unlock myself from boredom?" The role of mindfulness and a dual awareness-and action-oriented pathway during the COVID-19 lock-down. *Personality and Individual Differences*, *175*, 110729. doi:10.1016/j.paid.2021.110729 PMID:36540053

Weissinger, E., Caldwell, L. L., & Bandalos, D. L. (1992). Relation between intrinsic motivation and boredom in leisure time. *Leisure Sciences*, *14*(4), 317–325. doi:10.1080/01490409209513177

Wolff, W., Martarelli, C. S., Schüler, J., & Bieleke, M. (2020). High boredom proneness and low trait self-control impair adherence to social distancing guidelines during the COVID-19 pandemic. *International Journal of Environmental Research and Public Health*, *17*(15), 5420. doi:10.3390/ijerph17155420 PMID:32731369

World Health Organization. (2004). *Promoting mental health: Concepts, emerging evidence, practice: Summary report*. World Health Organization.

Yu, Y., She, R., Luo, S., Xin, M., Li, L., Wang, S., Ma, L., Tao, F., Zhang, J., Zhao, J., Li, L., Hu, D., Zhang, G., Gu, J., Lin, D., Wang, H., Cai, Y., Wang, Z., You, H., ... Lau, J. T. F. (2021). Factors influencing depression and mental distress related to COVID-19 among university students in China: Online cross-sectional mediation study. *JMIR Mental Health*, *8*(2), e22705. doi:10.2196/22705 PMID:33616541

Zavestoski, S. (2002). The social–psychological bases of anticonsumption attitudes. *Psychology and Marketing*, *19*(2), 149–165. doi:10.1002/mar.10007

Zhang, S. X., Wang, Y., Rauch, A., & Wei, F. (2020). Unprecedented disruption of lives and work: Health, distress and life satisfaction of working adults in China one month into the COVID-19 outbreak. *Psychiatry Research*, *288*, 112958. doi:10.1016/j.psychres.2020.112958 PMID:32283450

Znazen, H., Slimani, M., Bragazzi, N. L., & Tod, D. (2021). The Relationship between Cognitive Function, Lifestyle Behaviours and Perception of Stress during the COVID-19 Induced Confinement: Insights from Correlational and Mediation Analyses. *International Journal of Environmental Research and Public Health*, *18*(6), 3194. doi:10.3390/ijerph18063194 PMID:33808777

KEY TERMS AND DEFINITIONS

Boredom: A the state of being stuck in an endless and dissatisfying time, in which the person perceives that time passes more slowly.

Ecological Awareness: The awareness that resources are limited and that there is a need to protect resources and that pollution should be reduced.

Human Scale Value: Humanizing the living and working environment of the individual and removing it from being mechanical.

Material Simplicity: Emphasizing the joy of life and the beauties of life by reducing the ostentatiousness and luxury of life.

Mental Health: A state of well-being in which individual can cope with stress in the daily routine of life, work productively, realize his or her own abilities and be successful.

Personal Growth: The individual's moral and spiritual development of individual's inner world by making himself/herself independent from the external world.

Self-Determination: The individual's desire to decide for himself or herself the ample time required for self-improvement and the formation of creativity.

Valuation of Life: The positive and negative evaluation of individual's life, which is affected by individual's own personal characteristics and quality of life, and the subjectively experienced value of individual's life.

Voluntary Simplicity Lifestyle: A practice and belief system in which a person limits her spending on consumer goods and services and aims to increase a person's internal growth, personal fulfillment, control, and self-sufficiency by choosing a simple life.

Chapter 17
A Conceptual Framework to Guide Psychological Resilience Knowledge and Practice Regarding COVID-19:
Towards Maintaining Psychological Wellbeing in Pandemic Situations

Karen T. Odhiambo
University of Nairobi, Kenya

ABSTRACT

Resilience is perceived within the context of perceived risk, fear, and vulnerability. The purpose of the theme chosen is to help contribute and help reduce suffering and to improve overall psychological wellbeing while strengthening resilience within guiding resilience principles of practice. COVID-19 continues to ravage the world and so there is a need for interventions that will help in managing the vulnerabilities that arise. The author hopes to contribute to this important topic and to come up with a conceptual framework and to instigate dialogue and guide even as it ensures management of vulnerability through resilience, resolve, and optimization.

BACKGROUND

It is important to understand different levels of engagement in preventive behaviors for current global COVID-19 pandemic. It is also important to know levels of fear, perceived risk and vulnerability and those affected most and how to reduce these levels and effects. Further, it is helpful to know perceived risk and vulnerabilities as well as how these can be significantly linked to preventive behaviours as well as the extent to which these do predict these behaviors over and above the demography variables. The chapter arises from the fact that covid-19 pandemic having had a major effect on the human population

DOI: 10.4018/978-1-6684-8565-1.ch017

globally, since 2020 and still does, it has led to a global experience of increased levels of distress and anxiety due to social isolations consequences and other tragedies. The result as stated by the call is vulnerabilities, behavior related, with the human race being overwhelmed while causing strong emotions on the human race. Learning to cope with these stressors is healthy and does make one become more resilient. Thus, the decision to address psychological wellness regarding RESILIENCE at such a time as this, that which is covid-19 related, comes at an opportune time. This writer will look into resilience as the adversary and risk factor based on social distance and isolation consequences all within the frame of psychological wellbeing.

The given concepts of risk, protection and resilience have emerged as concepts for conceptualizing and managing social and health problems arising from on-going covid-19. However, according to Fraser, M.W., Galinsky, M.J., & Richman, J.M. (1999), these terms are elusive. The author takes up the task of writing the chapter while being well aware of this elusive nature of resilience and the fact that even it's conceptualization is not in harmony. Regarding the psychological perspectives of behavior response to the pandemic, there has been a shift from deficits of individuals to focusing on ones strengths. Thus a construct such as resilience, the essence of stress perspective becomes a positive construct. Being the ability to bounce back, resilient becomes a suitable aspect of the chapter, for bouncing back is relevant in the current situation of pandemic. As stated the situation prevails and it is not known how and when covid-19 will come end.

The risk of stress and negative life events arising from covid-19, more so regarding isolation and constant hand washing is new to the world as there is yet to be such a pandemic on such global scale. Concern is more on the role of potential *mediators* in the link between *resilience* and *wellbeing*. Research on resilience has however evolved over the years but is not complete and continues to develop. The intent here is for psychology researchers to better understand even as they create new knowledge on the subject and greater realization of the complexities arising from what the world faces in the present, past, in real time and in future. The given concepts of risk, protection and resilience have emerged as concepts for conceptualizing social and health problems such as the world is now facing. Psychological resilience should allow one to cope successfully with adversities occurring during stressful periods, which may otherwise trigger mental illness. Recent models suggest that inhibitory control (IC), the executive control function (ECF) which supports our *goal-directed behavior* and regulates our *emotional response*, may underlie *resilience*. However, the ways in which this is manifested during stressful situations in real life is still unclear. The construct resilience derives from the Latin verb resilient which means to rebound or "leap back." It is a term used in many fields originally coming from ecology. This brings to bear new thinking thus the aspect of "positive psychology." The term resilience connotes a psychological meaning.

As a result of the paradigm shift the interest regarding this write up is on *positive aspects of "human functioning"* more so how these can assist individual's resolve and optimize their psychological functioning during a pandemic. There is need for knowledge to provoke forethought between practitioners and persons in the society towards a better conceptualization of the construct resilience while in a crisis from a global point of view, as a localized phenomenon even as resilience becomes a personal characteristics as well as a perspective on stress and wellness management. The author is cognizance of the fact that even although the concept of resilience has been studied for decades there remains a lack of consensus on the definition, conceptualization, and measurement of resilience. These issues are even more evident in relation to resilience in the context of perceived risk, fear, and vulnerability. Even though there is no agreed definition of resilience, all definitions of resilience are fundamentally comprising a reference to both *adversity and positive outcomes*. Debate continues over conceptualization of resilience. It is in this state of conceptualization to operationalize that this author writes this chapter. The hope is to factor in these challenges and still come up with some harmony on conceptualization of resilience into a framework that comprise adversity and positive outcomes, that which leads to better understanding and operationalization to best guide resilience practice in crisis with the goal to reduce negative behavior effects.

The Basis of the Undertaking

The chapter write up is knowledge oriented, practice oriented even as it is a guide to practitioners. It is hoped it will provide an avenue to help reduce suffering, and to improve overall psychological wellbeing and strengthen resilience of the thematic perspective, that is, "Covid-19 pandemic regarding social isolation consequences. Secondly to come up with a common frame as a reference point for understanding and determining practice of resilience in risk situations of pandemics globally. Demographic variables will not be considered. Resilience will be the positive effect with mediators and wellbeing. Mediator in this case is "social distancing and isolation," while wellness is based on "psychological wellbeing." The model is *Risk-Protection-Resilience-Goal Directed Behavior* with the manifestation being evidenced and demonstrated wellness or positive behavior prospective of human functioning. The goal is for a conceptual frame of thought that which will result in resolve and optimization of psychological functioning within the context of perceived risk, fear and vulnerability. The end result is a model that will lead to regulating behavior that underlie psychological resilience arising from a compromise between adversity and positive outcome.

The hope is to provide knowledge for understanding, a framework to guide practice, to motivate dialogue and debates since the field is still emerging more so covid-19 adversity and behavior implications. Basically the chapter is also to contribute towards providing an avenue to help reduce suffering, and to improve overall psychological wellbeing and strengthen resilience within guiding resilience principles of practice. The author researcher will explain and present content within the given goal moving across the literature towards a theoretical justification supported by a growing body of empirical research and to conclude with a "*framework for resilience based on psychological purpose and practice.*" The intention is also to provide and create a narrative of sorts, that leads to a dialogue that is knowledge based even as it provides an avenue for critique.

The approach taken is to equip one with tools towards overcoming the adversity and those that lead to improving mental health and in turn outcomes of psychological functioning. It will be presented in a handy table that with summarize "what works" while supporting people's resiliency. The author will provide summarized set of ideas and practices that promote resilience. The ideas have been split into headings, compartments, components, elements. It will be in a manner that one can navigate across the table to determine more. The summary table generally looks simple but it is based on a lot of background activity of literature review, research evaluation and critique.

The chapter constitutes the following sub-headings:

- Background
- Conceptualizing Resilience
- Resilience and Covid-19 Pandemic
- Psychological Wellbeing
- The Conceptual Framework Intended

Table 1. Defining resilience

The Term Resilience	Author
The *capacity for* or the result of successful adaptation regarding the adversity	Masten
A *dynamic process* which results in positive adaption within a context of severe adversity.	Later, Luthar and Zigler [5
A reflection of a diverse set of processes that alter ones(children's) transactions within adverse life conditions to reduce negative effects and promote mastery normalcy	Wyman et al.
Develops thanks to an *intrinsic or extrinsic driving force* that emerges from the processes of overcoming trauma. Based on this theoretical model	Richardson et al
A set of *personal qualities* that enables one to prosper in situations of adversity	Connor and Davidson
to restore from stressful events or *maintain equilibrium* under significant threats	(Wagnild & Young, 1993; Ryff & Singer, 2003
To bounce back from adversities *adopting positive coping strategies*	Smith et al., 2008
A *process adaptive response* to different adversities, ranging from ongoing daily hassles to major life events, or on the side as the results deriving from the interactive influence of psychological characteristics within the context of the stress process.	Fletcher and Sarkar, 2013

CONCEPTUALISING RESILIENCE

The Concept of Resilience

As an attribute that encompasses positive adaptation within a context of adversity, resilience is a dynamic process with two critical conditions. These according to Roisaman et. al. (2002) are exposure to significant threat or severe adversity and the achievement of positive adaptation despite major assaults on the developmental process. It was given even more prominence when the world was impacted with covid-19_ and still is. Masten describes resilience as positive adaptation to adversity despite serious threats to adaptation or development. The literature states that the term resilience as used was coined by Roisman, Padrón and colleagues in 2002. Resilience is an emergent property of a hierarchically organized set of protective systems that cumulatively buffer the effects of adversity and can therefore rarely, if ever, be regarded as an intrinsic property of individuals (Roisman et al., 2002). Basically, resilience has to do with bouncing back as well as beating the odds. It is how well one copes with adversity that they face that determines resiliency for one to be declares as resilient, thus demonstrating resiliency.

Much as resilience is an object of concern in many disciplines, there is however, no single definition of the term that has been agreed upon by the scientific community. According to Blandina (2016), he states that almost all definitions are built around two key aspects, that is, significant exposure to risk and positive adaptation. Thus, resilience becomes a process of adapting well in the face of adversity, trauma, tragedy, threats, or significant sources (American Psychological Association). The result is a number of definitions as reflected in the table below. What they agree on is that in the definitions one can see a sense of human-centered perspective and that it involves resistance to or a positive and effective way of desire to cope with situations of risk and adversity. Resistance resilience is viewed as a process, the capacity for, a result of successful adaptation, a dynamic process within a context of severe adversity.

Different writers have referenced resilience depending on the focus they want to maintain. Definitions are important as it enables professionals write in harmony. According to (Fletcher & Sarkar, 2013; Kolar, 2011) resilience has been referred to in many forms such as intrinsic to the individual, others as a more holistic sense, still others as competencies or capacities of people, while others positive functioning in the face of adversity. Thus, this write up is developed with these considerations in mind. The authors do agree however, that resilience has roots in the theme adversity and how these can impact upon people harmfully (or not). This is generally referred to as a breakdown in wellness, a term that has dominated clinical sciences and the field of behavior science. The studies around this area of resilience have looked at risks while demonstrating that vulnerability contributes to outcomes while in a diverse situation or later after the adverse situation. They also realized that the aftereffects are not universal in the sense that some do dip but some do not while others came out of it and others don't come out of it easily.

Outcome here refers to "A stable trajectory of healthy functioning after a highly adverse event," so states Bonanno (2014). Those who adapt are known to have a stable trajectory of healthy functioning after the effect and achieve positive and unexpected resilience related outcomes. This is referred to as state of being resilient which is the outcome of what is termed '*construction*' of resilience. There is a distinction between those with better outcome and those without. This is what the origins of health or psychosocial functioning is. This means that there are other processes that mediate the adversity and the negative outcomes.

There are also definitions which view resilience as a process. In this sense these authors distinguished three main aspects to this construct: adversity, positive adaptation, and the emotional, cognitive and sociocultural mechanisms. In other words, the individual is exposed to a high-intensity risk and yet, at the same time, deploys a series of adaptive behaviors despite the impact of possible threats to their resiliency. Resilience has also been understood as the individual capacity or ability to survive and regain one's balance after experiencing certain traumatic events. Yet in others, resilience has been defined as a synonym of vulnerability reduction, the ability to tolerate experiences of change and adversity, the ability to adapt to adversity, effective coping, a complex behavioral repertoire and personal stability or recovery.

The Basis of Resilience Theory

Behavior and rallying around adversity regarding risks is the reason for *Resilient Theory*. In this case the resilient theory is Why some succeed in bouncing back and some don't is the reason why and the power to change about understanding biology, psychology, and social aspects behind what enables people to bounce back from adversity experiences what is referred to as being resilient and having resilience. It is agreed that with the events such as covid-19 to which solutions are yet to be fully determined, work on possible solutions is what the world needs, that which psychologists should play a role within the frame of behavior science approach such as psychological wellness. The need for more resilient people has brought about the intent of this write up what would be referred to as on-going work. Thus, in this section the idea is to collate what is in the literature and present the current view of resilient theory.

What resilience means has been presented. The term resilience originates from the Latin word RESILIENS which refers to pliant or elastic quality of a substance. Resilience theory wasn't really developed by one person only. Dr. Norman Garmezy was one of the first to use the word resilience in the 1900s in his pioneering work on stress, competence, and individual development. And a few years before him, developmental psychologist Erik Erikson laid some of the groundwork for the ideas of resilience in his work on psychosocial development. Since then, there have been countless great researchers that have carried on the work regarding covid-19 and resilience. Regarding covid-19 and resilience, the context is that of perceived risk, fear, and vulnerability. This compromises adversity, positive outcomes. Two aspects are considered, that of exposure and positive adaptation. The model arising is that which contains the adversary or covid-19 pandemic, positive adaptability, behaviors repertoire, cognition or persistent thinking and social demographics as mechanisms that influence mitigative effects.

RESILIENCE AND COVID-19 PANDEMIC

Psychological Perspectives and Correlates of Covid-19 and Resilience Factor

The issue in this write up is help in constructing ones resilience as well as understanding and linking the constructs that arise so as to avoid preventing harmful behavior resulting from ***covid-19 within a social distancing strategy for managing the pandemic. This is*** to help reduce risks arising from covid-19 adversity, risks that arise and the vulnerabilities that are associated with the individual. These are not universal. It depends on the mediating factors such as human centeredness, capacities and skills, potential, and personal agency drivers. These could be physical and social ecologically.

The dictionary description gives the following regarding the risk factor of social distancing and isolation:

- Physical distance maintained between individuals in order to avoid catching or transmitting an infectious disease. Regarding covid-19, attention was to public health messages on social distance, hand washing, and face covering.
- The perceived or desired degree of *remoteness* between a member of one social group and the members of another, as evidenced in the level of *intimacy tolerated* between them. Generally, this definition states that "*material differences*" provided members with a constant stimulus for social distance"
- Limiting physical *closeness* and contact with other people, especially in order to avoid catching or *transmitting* an infectious disease. This is very true of covid-19. Thus beyond social distancing is the wearing of the mask.

In the case of covid-19, the belief is that limiting contact with people does slow down virus transmission and flatten the epidemic curve so that the number of cases occurring at the peak of the epidemic can reduce and social distance will be lifted and the adversity risk reduced. Psychological distance theory, which describes how far away an object, event, or person is from someone's perception of reality, can help explain these differences. If distance is high, people are less likely to alter their behavior than when distance is low. The psychologically factors that arise are: the nature of relationships, the experience of ease of stress in the social environment and the experience of trauma. The effects of social distancing on mental health range from increased attention to effects and the virus' death toll to poor understanding and decreased decision-making abilities, which may hinder control of the epidemic. Then there is psychophysical whereby, exhaustion, anxiety, fear and pain, anguish, trauma, and anger arise. These emotions alternate, mix, and grow in intensity to the point of overwhelming, leading to clinically significant psychological disorders, such as "reactive depression."

Put into theoretical and psychological perspective it becomes a construct to the extent to which people experience isolation as a result of a number of things depending on the nature and context of the adversity and possible risks one is exposed to. This is related to a sense of familiarity (nearness and intimacy) or unfamiliarity (farness and difference) between themselves and people belonging to different social, ethnic, occupational, and religious groups from their own. Sociologists recognize three key types of social distance or affective, normative and interactive. These have a bearing on psychological distance also explained below.

- ***Affective:*** The degree to which a person from one group feels sympathy or empathy for persons from other groups. The pandemic resulted in more of the north suffering than the south
- ***Normative***: The kind of difference perceived between oneself and members of groups and others who are not members
- ***Interactive***: The focus is on the frequency and intensity of interactions claiming that the more the members interact, the closer they are socially. With covid-19 lock downs, this was not possible (Coleman, 2006)

The interest is in psychological aspect of the write up. The four dimensions of psychological distance arising are:

- ***Temporal distance***: The extent to which imagined future events or recalled past events deviate from the present in time (Bar-Anan et al., 2006). A measure of physical change of _ the ability to time the past, the present and the future
- ***Spatial distance:*** The extent to which imagined future events or recalled past events deviate from the present in time (Bar-Anan et al., 2006). mental representations and processes evolved in living organisms to cope with the physical dimension of space, be it the space immediately experienced through a sensory modality (visual space, auditory space, etc.) or the whole environment in which behavior is occurring
- ***Social distance***: physical distance maintained between individuals in order to avoid catching or transmitting an infectious disease. This permeates all aspects of intractable conflict. While history, perceptions and identity are inherently present in the escalation of conflict. They are also intrinsic to managing conflict and contributing to a sustainable peace.
- ***Hypothetically:*** by making an assumption for the sake of discussion or argument: in a hypothetical way. Speaking hypothetically this is a conjectured entity, process, or event that is not observed directly but is assumed to explain an observable phenomenon (Coleman, 2006)

What arises are attributes that affect social and psychological functioning and so wellbeing a sense of psychological adjusted Ness. These are related to mental conditions and power play regarding Power and social distancing.

Mental Conditions

Thus things like cognitive distance arise or viewing your own thoughts (or beliefs) as constructions of "*reality*" rather than as "*reality itself.* Emotional distancing, or emotional detachment as the inability of an individual to completely engage with their own feelings, or the feelings of others. The result of the above can lead to severe emotional distancing that can start interfering with a person's social, emotional, psychological, as well as physical development. One can use the above social and psychological dimensions to build distance and gain back control of one's life one of which is through resilience, the construct in this write up. Each dimension is related to the other (Fiedler et al., 2012). Social isolation and loneliness has been linked to higher risks for a variety of physical and mental conditions lifestyle related such as high blood pressure, heart disease, obesity, a weakened immune system, anxiety, depression and cognitive decline and even death. The result is symptoms of social isolation that relate to many behaviors from mere dysfunctions of stress and anxiety to schizophrenia. These begin as aspects of ddepression and anxiety because of one's social isolation and results in behaviors such as aggression, lethargy, insomnia, even memory loss and poor self-care among others.

Power Relations in Social Distancing

Joe C. Magee & Pamela K. Smith has addressed an important component of social distancing. They proposes that asymmetric dependence between individuals, or what we call power in social distance produces asymmetric social distance, with high-power individuals feeling more distant than low-power individuals. From this they articulated how power relations affects. These are in terms of social comparison, susceptibility to influence, mental state inference and responsiveness, and emotions. It is believed this leads to greater experienced social distance that leads to engagement in more abstract mental representation. This mediating process of construal level generates predictions about how power affects. This has a direct bearing on what results in resiliency in a person as to whether one would retain and not. As a mechanism it does have limitations. The authors have illuminated the following as those things that would affect psychological functioning as drivers of behavior in an adversity in regards to power relations from a social distance perspective:

- Goal selection and pursuit
- Attention to desirability and feasibility concerns
- Subjective certainty
- Value-behavior correspondence
- Self-control, and,
- Person perception

Joe C. Magee & Pamela K. Smith

Below are aspects of psychological perspectives of Covid-19 related behaviors that have a bearing on covid-19 pandemic, that is, dysfunctional thought process and cognitive distortions.

Dysfunctional Thought Process

This has to do with persistent thinking that has a bearing on mental health and psychological functioning. There have been many studies that have looked into this and states that the outbreak of covid-19 pandemic has had an impact on the daily function of individuals. According to Skalski et. al. (2022), this has effects on moods, sense of well-being and overall mental health. There have been studies showing consequences of PTSD_ post-traumatic stress disorders, chronic psychologic dysfunctions such as stress, anxiety and depression, social anxiety. The result is a situation known as dysfunctional thought processes of persistent thinking thus an event that is devastating to mental health and wellbeing. He goes on to state that this kind of thinking in regards to covid-19 pandemic may have manifested into dissipation of epidemic threats in the form of a number of things such as: intrusive personal memories, tormenting dreams with epidemic-related content, repetitive dissociative reactions associated with a sense of the unreality of the threat, and, a persistent sense of hurt and suffering as psychological effects.

He goes on to state that these serve as psychopathologic symptoms that imply recurring thoughts, ideas, or impulses that are known to impede daily functioning. This causes buildup of emotional tension of worry and fear. It can at times lead to intrusive activities of compulsive behavior that occur with obsessions. These are the symptoms that are typical of obsessive-compulsive disorder. The result in obsessions that occur against ones will (ego dystonic), that disrupts thinking leading to emotional tension of anxiety, worry and fear. This can further lead to intrusive activities or compulsions. These usually occur with obsession or obsessive-compulsive disorder. The author cautions that not all compulsive behavior arises from pandemic situations.

Cognitive Distortions

The given dysfunctions give rise to cognitive distortions. According to Beck et. Al. in Skalti et. al. (2022), the basis of persistent thinking. These generally distort negatively the way we see the world, ourselves and others as well as events that surround one as they go through the pandemic phase. Regarding the threat and coping with it, these distortions causes one to absorb the threat and underestimate the ability to cope with it, which ultimately leads to pathological anxiety. This extends this issue to mind and behavior, an aspect that will not be explored in this write up. However, at this level, one has to have the capacity of behavior response mechanism or the knowledge as well as the will and drive to evaluate, name, and with understanding the problem act, thus ***resilience power.*** This is what will determine and lead to one becoming aware of their situation that then lead to restructuring the mental representation of emotional arousal. The way in which one deals with their situation even as a community determines the quality of response and the intensity as well as persistence with which they generate their specific behavior responses.

Resilience Practice and Processes Psychological Harm Reduction and Health Promotion

Resilience practice is geared towards persons undergoing risks of pandemics in this case as to the way they develop capacity to face the ongoing crisis activities. The objective is to enable one's ability to tackle life's challenges arising from the adversity. Psychologists who give services begin by framing positive goals. They then assess one's strengths and weaknesses and strategies aimed at reducing risks while ensuring adaptive systems. They do this even as they determine the level of risk, symptoms, vulnerabilities, and disorders. Also emphasized is *social and emotional well-being*. Generally, the practice is to align the philosophical with the harm reduction and health promotion movements. The persons who need to be more resilient are enabled so as to increase control and to manage their well-being thus making changes in their behavior. In this case, the issue is preventing harmful behavior resulting from ***covid-19 social distancing with the view*** to reducing risks arising from covid-19. What is to be improved is psychological wellbeing and to strengthen resilience. Generally, there is increased levels of distress and anxiety leading to depression due to these social isolation consequences. To rebound one needs to be resilient in which case resilient is looked at as perceived risk, fear and vulnerability. The frame of thought and guide desired is towards a better understanding and operationalization as well as guide to resilience practice.

However, much as overcoming adversity is important, it is believed resilience is more than that. Hart, et. Al. (2016) states that it is actually "beating *the odds whilst also changing the odds*." However, the odds can arise due to people's circumstances. Consider various disadvantages arising from many reasons. It could be geographical, gender, poverty among others. Thus, resilience is also about challenges arising from inequalities.

Perceptions of Risk and Vulnerability in Covid-19 Pandemic Situations

There are many ways to conceptualize and measure perceptions of risk and vulnerability. One can go ahead and examine the content of individual risk and vulnerability beliefs—identifying those things that worry or concern them, as well as the degree of anxiety generated by these concerns. The other was is to observe whether people recognize the risks inherent in a given situation, or we can look at how accurately someone judges a specific risk. Risk judgments may focus on situations and their potential outcomes such as the chance that they will violate social distancing. Personal risk can be viewed in absolute terms how one's behavior on response to social distancing compares with others. There is also the element to how one ranks the risk as to the important of various risks that arise. The perception on these risks can also be measured to form a comprehensive whole towards response to the pandemic and so potential of one's resilience.

The magnitude assessment of risk is also important and so risk judgement. This focuses only on the outcome behaviors. Focusing on outcome only is considered non-conditional. There is also there is also situational or conditional risk judgement. When assessment of risk does not include magnitude, we use the term risk identification. Thus, the issue is what would happen if you fail to socially isolate. There are legal, health and social issues that leads to even financial implications and loneliness. Identification is the best possible way to tap assessment in social isolation, however, individual affective responses can also be informative. When assessment focuses on degree of psychological dysfunction occur on the dysfunctions such as anxiety, stress, or outcomes of fear and worry then these become feelings or perception of vulnerability.

There are also the cognitive aspects of risk perception which can be conditional or unconditional. For example, in asking one to state what concerns them. Consider health, lacking resources, that one's condition can further aggregate the vulnerability. Also individual differences such as generalized anxiety or pessimism may influence the degree to which the or outcomes are identified, judged or experienced as risk.

PSYCHOLOGICAL WELLBEING: THE STATE OF PSYCHOLOGICAL FUNCTIONING

An element of wellbeing or happiness is affected by a number of psychological factors including RESILIENCE. That, resilience is positively associated with satisfaction with life. It is further it is negatively associated with negative affect and positively associated with positive affect. It is argued that resilient people who strive to attain their goals have higher levels of positive affect and satisfaction with life. This means that, those who cope with and adapt better to stressful situations and adversity feel better about themselves and are happier than their non-resilient counterparts. In terms of resilience, this reflects a situation of Selman's 3Ps' Model.

Well-being does provide a measure of how well one is coping and feeling good about themselves in their adverse circumstance. In broad terms, subjective well-being provides a measure of how good we feel about ourselves and how happy we are. Although we are dealing here with a concept that is difficult to delimit, most authors agree that the following elements should, at least, be taken into account: its subjective nature, which is rooted in each individual's own experience; its global dimension, since it encompasses an assessment or judgment about all aspects of life; and the need to include positive measures, since its nature goes beyond the mere absence of negative factors. It is therefore important to consider the effect of resilience on two major dimensions: the cognitive and the emotional or affective dimension, that is, personalization, pervasiveness and permanence. These attributes helps one understand how ones thoughts, mindset, and beliefs affects ones experiences by recognizing their role in our ability to adapt positively. Then one can start becoming more resilient and learn to bounce back from life's challenges.

Well-being does provide a measure of how well one is coping and feeling good about themselves in their adverse circumstance. The elements that should be included which is agreed by most authors has to do with its subjective nature, it's global dimension by the fact that it encompasses assessment or judgement on all aspects of life. There is also the need to include positive measures since its nature is more than just negative in essence. Thus, the need to consider the effect of resilience on two major dimensions, that is, cognitive and the emotional or affective dimension.

Thus, one of the psychological traits that foster satisfaction with life is the individual capacity to overcome adversity and grow despite it. It seems that those who adapt better to stressful situations and more easily to adversity are also those who feel most satisfied with their lives, unlike their non-resilient counterparts. There is also a strong link between psychological resilience and positive emotional states whereby those with resilience profile experience more positive emotions in stressful situations than less resilient subjects, even though they experience similar levels of negative emotions. Being positively resilient means having greater capacity to overcome the adversity. Thus, these people are enthusiastic with energetic attitude as well as curiosity and openness to new experiences. They also deploy positive emotions in order to cope including humor, relaxation and optimistic thought. That including positivity to events, having problem centered coping style are useful. In this sense, resilience facilitates positive effects and alleviates negative affect.

At the most basic level, psychological wellbeing (PWB) is quite similar to other terms that refer to positive mental states, such as happiness or satisfaction, and in many ways, it is not necessary, or helpful to worry about fine distinctions between such terms. If I say that I'm happy, or very satisfied with my life you can be pretty sure that my psychological wellbeing is quite high! Psychological wellbeing has two important facets. The first of these refers to the extent to which people experience positive emotions and feelings of happiness. Sometimes this aspect of psychological wellbeing is referred to as subjective wellbeing (*Diener, 2000*). Subjective wellbeing is a necessary part of overall psychological wellbeing but on its own it is not enough.

For a person to achieve high levels of subjective well-being, they need to feel satisfied with life, have a predominantly positive affectivity and a low level of negative affect. Thus, psychological well-being is purely evaluative and subjective, the most important element being how everyone assesses his or her own life even as they react and respond to their life. There is significant correlate thus making these two attributes independent. The most recent study found corroborates this, since satisfaction with life was observed to correlate significantly with both positive and negative affect, with all correlations being moderately strong, while positive and negative affect were not found to be significantly correlated with each other, thus indicating that they are independent constructs.

Main Orientations of Wellbeing

Subjective Wellbeing

Subjective well-being (SWB), also known as self-reported well-being, refers to how people experience and evaluate different aspects of their lives. It is often used to measure mental health and happiness, and it can be an important predictor of individual health, wellness, and longevity, Kendra Chryy (2022). affective and cognitive _ It has become a useful measure of societal health. In addition to providing psychologists a way to assess how people feel about their lives, it also offers insights that can be used to guide public health, economic, and social policies. Policymakers utilize assessments of subjective well-being to gauge the health of societies and measure the impact of social policies.

Social Wellbeing

Social well-being can be defined as the sharing, developing, and sustaining of *meaningful relationships* with others. This allows you to feel authentic and valued, and provides a sense of connectedness and belonging. Without awareness, development, and maintenance of our social well-being, we run the risk of becoming socially isolated. This is different from choosing to have some time alone to enjoy solitude. Social isolation isn't really a choice. Withdrawal from human relationships becomes a self-reinforcing spiral, as isolation leads to negative feelings of fear and threat that lead to more isolating behaviors. Social isolation leads to loneliness, which can be incredibly damaging, Jenna Sinclaire (2021). Focus is on optimal functioning of individual in social life with the five dimensions, that is social perspective that includes the following acceptance, actualization, coherence and integration (Keyyes, 1998). Psychological well-being can be further divided into three basic components. These are related to:

Satisfaction with Life

This is a cognitive component of subjective well-being that arises from an individual's global judgment of their life. This becomes a result of the comparisons made by the adversity they are facing in this case covid-19 pandemic with social distances as a strategy. Satisfaction with life becomes a variable that assesses the self-perception of global satisfaction.

Positive Affect/ Negative Affect

As regards positive/negative affect, a person's position on the psychological well-being scale is a result of their position in two independent dimensions: positive affect and negative affect. Thus, an individual will have a high level of psychological well-being to the extent to which positive affect predominates over the negative affect. These two dimensions are independent from each other, making it impossible to predict a subject's score in the negative dimension on the basis of their score in the positive affect one and vice versa.

The Psychological Functioning_Covid-19 Social Isolated behavior Related Perspective

A person is resilient to the extent that they evident sound functioning outcomes during the life of the adversity or that the resilience of the person is supportive and so attainment of positive effects. If then adversity is on-going and resilience are at work, then, adversity has passed, and the system is recovering. This is the state that is desirable for management of stressful situation during and after an ongoing pandemic. Below is an attempt to harmonize information, a situation that usually leads to behaviors being crafted as psychological dysfunctions of anxiety, stress and depression without a basic theoretical basis of the adversary and the risk factors clearly defined and demonstrated and behavior repertoires clearly spelt out. Many times, these are generalized across different perspectives. The psychological functions have been derived from the given foundation that is equated with adversity of covid-19 within am social distant and isolation perspective as the risk factor. It is this that will be used as a background to guide the conceptual model intended.

The model is on resilience which is within the context of adversity, risks, and positive factors of behaviors. Thus, the model perceived is within the basis of:

- The adversity_ Covid-19
- Adaptation_ Positive factors, coping, and adaptive processes
- Behavior repertoire
- Cognitive construction of realities
- Social mechanisms_ context specific of physical, social and daily occurrences

THE CONCEPTUAL FRAMEWORK: THE RESILIENCE FRAME OF THOUGHT AND DETERMINANTS OF RESILIENCE AND WELLBEING

Foundational Basis and Thinking of the Conceptual Framework Intended

This is the conceptual framework for establishing the thinking behind and the determinants of psychological adjustment as derived from the background literature in the write up and the background on *Summary Table* given in the first table below. The concern is towards potential mediators and their link between the risk or social distancing and wellbeing or psychological functioning. This is a theoretical model for resilience development that allows one to understand the role of potential mediators and how these link the identified risks and wellbeing. The frame of thought provides potential users as a guide and frame of thought.

The table is a handy table that summarizes "*what works*" supporting resilience according to the *"basis for intention"* to find a link between social distancing and wellbeing. The nature of the logic is a summary of a set of attributes and constructs of the domain, processes and practices that promote resiliency. The table will be presented in a summary table where ideas have been split into headings and compartments. One has to navigate through the table to find out more. The table looks simply but it requires a lot of work to arrive at. It is hoped that anyone using the framework will be able to understand, conceptualize what resilience is, it's operations in terms of practice and process(therapy) and to be led towards practice and process that will reduce suffering, improve psycho-social wellbeing and strengthen resilience and ability to be resilient.

Basically, the purpose as stated is how to reduce these levels, to prevent behaviors not desirable and how these can predict preventive behaviors over and above the demographic variable regarding covid-19. The assumption made is that there is generally increased levels of distress and anxiety due to social isolations consequences. That a person's resilience is significantly related to mental health outcomes and that resilience obtains good measures of good psychological functioning. The hope is to factor in all these attributes and still have an efficient and effective conceptual framework that will lead one t design yet another based on their context and context depending on the risk one that would lead to ensuring resilient psychological support intervention. The frame of thought of resilience should allow one to understand the role of potential mediators in the link between social distancing and isolation and wellbeing even as it provides foundations for establishing determinants of psychological adjustment.

The frame is divided into-3:

- ***The conceptualization phase***: Perceived risk, fear and vulnerability arising from the adversity of covid-19 pandemic within a social distancing and isolation risk factor
- ***Operationalization phase:*** Synergies created between risk, mediators and wellbeing perspective as psychological functioning strategies with the view to provide knowledge and guide the development of resiliency to resolve situation and optimize response thus reducing vulnerabilities
- ***Psychological Wellness phase:*** or outcome. A state of psychological human functioning that evidence coping and adaptiveness to wellness

Background Summary of Theoretical Basis of the Conceptual Framework

The background information was thought important to summarize and inform on the thinking that resulted in the *'conceptual framework'* for practice and process regarding resilience. Table 3 below is guided by this summary information. Focus is on the adversity and the risks affiliated with the vulnerabilities that affect psychological functioning.

The table 3 below is a logic that arise and is to conceptualize, operationalize and outcome arising as a result of resiliency within the context of perceived risk arising from adversity of covid-19. The hope is for a successful model that will ensure resolve and optimize psychological functioning towards psychological wellness.

CONCLUSION

To provide an avenue to help reduce suffering, and to improve overall psychological wellbeing and strengthen resilience within guiding resilience principles of practice., the writer sort to provide literature on concept of resilience and to devise a frame of thought, a theoretical basis. As stated, the framework is both knowledge based, practice oriented and a guide towards common frame of thought on "perspective on stress and wellness management in times of crisis, in this case, COVID-19, with resilience as the intervention. Covid-19 has brought to bear new realities of life in real time as it is still on-going. Adapting to these lifestyle changes and managing the fear of contracting the virus are challenging globally and individuals in homes and personally. One word that comes up from a psychological point

Table 2. Summary background for conceptual framework on resilience

	Covid-19 Pandemic and Resilience Background for Building a Conceptual Frame of Knowledge and Practice [Behavior Repertoire] ::::	
	Attribute	**Description**
	Key constructs	Covid-19 and resilience factor a) Adversary: Covid-19 Pandemic b) Risk factor: Social distancing and isolation c) Adaptivity: Resilience d) Wellness: Psychological functioning Types of Resilience: i. Physical ii. Social iii. Psychological iv. Community based
a)	Resilient Model	Within the context of perceived • Risk_ Psychological responses • Fear _ State of being • Vulnerability _ Reductive basis
b)	Goal	To resolve and optimize positive psychological functioning
c)	Aspects of Covid-19	Comprises adversity and positive outcomes; 2 aspects: • exposure to risk_ isolation, and, • positive adaptation_ resiliency
d)	Processes of risk management	• Positive coping strategies • Process of adaptive response • Construction processes
c)	Vulnerabilities	• Has to do with abilities to: • Tolerate experiences of change and adversity • Effective coping strategies and skills • Personality stability of recovery
f)	Isolation and Psychological Factors	• Nature of relationships • Experience and ease arising from the risk factor • The nature of social environment • Experience of the trauma
g)	Effects of Social Distance(Mental Health Related)	• Increased attention and knowledge to effects • Virus death toll perspective • The disadvantaged • Lack of understanding and conceptualization • Media influence • Decreased decision making ability • Others hindrances to pandemic control and management
h)	Psychological Behavior Repertoire	• As Related to: Exhaustion, anxiety, fear, pain, anguish, trauma, anger arising, • When overwhelmed: Psychological disorders and reactive depression
Dr. Karen T. Odhiambo _ 2023		

of view in pandemic challenging times is RESILIENCE, a process of adapting in the face of tragedy, trauma, threats and stress. There is need for a better understanding of resilience practice and process in global pandemics more so covid-19. The framework developed is to ensure positive perspective of human functioning towards resolving and optimizing psychological functioning to manage risk factors of pandemics of global level.

Table 3. Perceived conceptual framework on covid-19 and wellbeing

CONCEPTUAL FRAMEWORK **A GUIDE TO PSYCHOLOGICAL RESILIENCE, KNOWLEDGE AND PRACTICE COVID-19 and PSYCHOLOGICAL WELLBEING**		
Conceptualization _ [Perceived risk, fear and vulnerability from covid-19 pandemic]	**Operationalization _ [Synergies between risk and wellbeing to develop resilience _Resolve and Optimization]**	**Outcome: Psychological Wellbeing _ [Psychological Human Functioning_ Evidence of coping and adaptiveness to recovery]**
Thematic Perspective: Resilience and covid-19 adversity within the risk of social distancing and isolation consequences	*To alter the trajectory from risk situations through development of resilience in covid-19 situations_ process and Practice*	*Outcome related to psychological functioning from a behavior science perspective*
Resilience: To rebound, to be resilient Adversity: Covid-19 as the pandemic Perceived risk: Focus_ Preventing behavior from social distancing and isolation in covid-19 pandemic with Psychological determinants of Vulnerabilities_ anxiety, stress, depression, fear as social isolation consequences Framework: _Wellbeing pillars_ internal and external capacities, perceived vulnerabilities, risks to be mitigated, resources to be strengthened _Resilience Capacities _Socio-Ecological approaches Practice principles: Is based on_ strength, human relations, catalyst for development of resilience, prevailing societal norms, interaction and available opportunity that is the pandemic of covid-19 Predictors of preventive behaviours: age, gender, education level, culture and association between these	Resiliency enabled: ensuring mediators that create a link between adversity risks and wellbeing. Potential mediators_ linking resilience and well being Resilience Models: Compensatory, Protective Challenge Resilience strategies_ building confidence, self efficacy, copying style Psychological assessment: for Knowledge needed such as vulnerabilities levels of fear, perceived risk, vulnerabilities Goal Directed Behaviour: Resilience _Psychological resilience and wellbeing: inhibitory control(IC) and Executive control function(ICF) Towards effectiveness: Better understanding, Operationalisation, Guiding practice towards mitigating factors, to prevent and predict preventive behavior over and above demographic variables Predictors of preventive behaviours: to determine whether these have a bearing on preventing behaviours	Evidence of resiliency_ there is resolve and optimization of psychological. functioning Processes: ability to develop ones resiliency Capacity: For successful adaptation, a dynamic process linking risk, adversity and wellbeing Products: reduction of negative effects, promotion of mastery of normative development task, intrinsic and extrinsic driving force Resilient characteristics, and Capabilities: Resilience skills_ development of self awareness, self regulation, coping, increased optimism, connected, knowing strength. , problem solving skills Psychological Resilience: Ability to cope and adapt, emotionally stable, ability to adapt, ability of groups to response Positive Relationship: Potential: In social skills, supportive response, understanding people, willing to engage, capacity _ physical-social-ecological, exercising personal agency Self-care: Management of self-care vs mismanagement
Dr. Karen T. odhiambo _ 2023		

REFERENCES

Bonanno, G. A., & Diminish, E. D. (2012). *Annual Research Review: Positive adjustment to adversity—trajectories of minimal-impact resilience and emergent resilience.* Advance online publication. doi:10.1111/jcpp.12021 PMID:23215790

Brooker, R. W., Kikvidze, Z., Kunstler, G., Liancourt, P., & Seifan, M. (2013). The concept and measurement of importance: A comment on Rees et al. 2012. *Journal of Ecology*, *101*(6), 1369–1378. Advance online publication. doi:10.1111/1365-2745.12164

Diener, E. (2000). Subjective well-being: The science of happiness and a proposal for a national index. *The American Psychologist*, *55*(1), 34–43. doi:10.1037/0003-066X.55.1.34 PMID:11392863

Eur, J. P. (2014). Resilience: Revisiting the Concept and its Utility for Social Research. *International Journal of Mental Health and Addiction*, *9*(4), 421–433.

Fraser, M. W., GalInsky, M. J., & RIchman, J. M. (1999). Risk, Protection, and Resilience: Toward a Conceptual Framework for Social Work Practice. *Social Work Research, 23*, 131-143. http://dx.doI.org/10.1093/swr/23.3.131

Glenn, L. R. (2002). Earned-Secure Attachment Status in Retrospect and Prospect. *Child Development*, *73*(4), 1204–1219. doi:10.1111/1467-8624.00467 PMID:12146743

Keyes, C. L. M. (1998). Social Well-Being. *Social Psychology Quarterly*, *61*(2), 121–140. doi:10.2307/2787065

Klaus, F., Florian, K., & Joachim, K. (2012). The Long Way From -Error Control to Validity Proper: Problems with a Short-Sighted False-Positive Debate. *Perspectives on Psychological Science*, *7*(6), 661–669. doi:10.1177/1745691612462587 PMID:26168128

Robert J. H. & Emmanuel C. & Amanah A., (2016). *Scientific Reports Supplementary Info*. License. CC BY 4.0.

Skalski S. B. (2022). Resilience and Mental Well-Being During the COVID-19 Pandemic: Serial Mediation by Persistent Thinking and Anxiety About Coronavirus. *Front. Psychiatry, Sec. Public Mental Health, 12*. doi:10.3389/fpsyt.2021.810274

Steven M. S. (2014). *Resilience definitions, theory, and challenges: interdisciplinary perspectives.* doi:10.3402/ejpt.v5.25338

Ungar, M. (Ed.). (2012). The social ecology of resilience: A handbook of theory and practice. Springer Science + Business Media. doi:10.1007/978-1-4614-0586-3

Yoav, B. (2006). The Association Between Psychological Distance and Construal Level: Evidence From an Implicit Association Test. *Journal of Experimental Psychology. General*, *135*(4), 609–622. doi:10.1037/0096-3445.135.4.609 PMID:17087576

KEY TERMS AND DEFINITIONS

Adaptation: At its most basic, adaptation that refers to a process or action that changes a living thing so that it is better able to survive in a new environment.

Adversity: Is harsh conditions that falls into two categories of chronic that is distal and proximal-onset and acute has a definite starting point unlike chronic and has a brief duration and limited impact. These define different resilient pathways (Bonnanno & Diminich, 2013).

Coping: Coping is defined as the thoughts and behaviors mobilized to manage internal and external stressful situations

Mediators: Resilience as a Mediator Between Interpersonal Risk Factors and Hopelessness in Depression.

Psychological Functioning: Is an outcome arising from an adversity from given points of vulnerability and is further divided into maladaptive and adaptive, negative, and positive related.

Resilience Competence: Resilience is the ability to face and adapt to challenges to overcome them. A person with strong resilience skills can handle disappointments because they don't let setbacks keep them from progressing.

Resilience Practice: It describes the strategies and processes put in place that leads to building capacities or ability that leads one to anticipate and cope with shocks, and to recover from their impacts in a timely and efficient manner.

Resilience Processes: Is development in that one can help develop resilience as a process and is categorized as individually related even as it is personally spirited as optimism, social such as family and friends and the environment such as disasters to foster positive relationships.

Risk Factor: That which arises from the effects of the adversity in this case social distancing and its behavior rapporteur.

Vulnerability: This is the quality or state of being exposed to the possibility of being attacked or harmed, either physically or emotionally, and is on a reduction basis.

Chapter 18
Worry Control in Education for People With Special Needs:
The Case of Enko Cameroon in the Times of COVID-19

Helen Chwienui Ghogomu Gayelle
https://orcid.org/0000-0002-9612-8871
University of the People, Pasadena, USA

ABSTRACT

This study captures a precise moment in controlling worry derived from the COVID-19 pandemic in the context of Cameroon as implemented by Enko Education. It shows how people with disability undergo double exclusion in times of general crisis. The chapter draws inspiration from pertinent concepts by Paulo Freire, Thierry Anderson, and Margaret Wehrenberg insofar as they relate to pedagogy and crisis management. The study documents and suggests methods to manage worries from future crisis or pandemic. One substantial contribution of the study is to highlight the continuation's necessity of more pertinent and innovative research for a more inclusive and fairer human society. The chapter will certainly help teachers, educational stakeholders, parents, and students easily identify what worry derived from crisis refers to.

INTRODUCTION

The sudden eruption of COVID-19 in Wuhan/China, has imposed a multidimensional stream of concern worldwide. Due to COVID-19, academia, NGOs, governments, nations, and many other significant stakeholders unanimously became concerned by the issue. Considerable amounts of economic, socio-political, and sanitary reports do now exist that address consequences of the pandemic and that suggest adequate behaviors for the future.

In education, challenges of COVID-19 and their rapid dilation turns out to be a very productive motive. This situation raises the management of these wide-ranging challenges to the substantial challenge of the

DOI: 10.4018/978-1-6684-8565-1.ch018

pandemic in education. This paper thus sets out to address and document methods put in place by Enko Education in Cameroon for their pertinence and exemplarity. Consequences of COVID-19 in education made the transition from traditional face-to-face to homeschooling format a necessity. Contrary to the Cameroonian national education where the majority of stakeholders were not prepared to such innovations, online schooling was already applicable within Enko Education before the outbreak of COVID-19.

In fact, the transnational nature of Enko Education and its ambitions make it unimaginable without online schooling as it seeks to "unlock potentials across Africa[1]" by "offering international programs and degrees recognized around the world" (Enko Education Homepage, 2023). In the times of COVID-19, this specific condition made the transition from face-to-face class to home schooling very ordinary in Cameroon Enko Education. As far as home schooling is concerned, the typical situation of Enko Education enables an easier discernment and clearer identification of measures put in place to exclusively manage worry in times of crises. Consequently, the study displaces and documents methods of controlling worry from COVID-19 as deployed at Cameroon Enko Education which could help address future pandemics or crises.

The place chosen for the study is an international school site that offers both the International Baccalaureate (IB) and Cambridge Assessment International Education (CAIE) curricula. As such, online schooling appears to be its alter ego in so far as Enko Education translates the dematerialization and deterritorialization of education. As compare to Cameroon government schools and contrary to prejudices, Enko Education faced the challenges of COVID-19 more severely because of the diverse and foreign origins of its students and workers in times of massive migration's restriction. In fact, with COVID-19, migration became a true sanitary thread irrespective of any meaningful reason as to why people migrate. The complex condition of Enko Education (favorable on one side and disadvantageous on the other) makes it acquire a paradigmatical status from which adequate and sustainable policies against crisis are made.

The following research questions guide the study: What reactions did Enko Education have to COVID-19 which were not represented in other Cameroonian educational institutions? What online methods in controlling worry are available as didactic targets are achieved? What significant problems of online learning overpower the strengths of homeschooling? How does worry control affect people with disability based on Enko Education experience?

The study shows how people with disability undergo double exclusion in times of general crisis. It also suggests to pedagogues and to decision makers on education and specifically in times of crisis, to consider the disparities highlighted in relation to people with disability if a more inclusive and fairer human society is to be achieved. The study itself is informed by data collected from the field, and their qualitative interpretation. It also draws inspiration from pertinent concepts as elaborated by scholars such as Paulo Freire (Freire, 1970), Thierry Anderson (Anderson, 2016) and Margaret Wehrenberg (Wehrenberg, 2005) whose works focus predominantly on pedagogy and crisis management. The study will help teachers, educational stakeholders, parents, and students identify what worry, or stress derived from crisis refer to. It will finally help them with different methods to manage worries derived from crises or from any future pandemic.

LITERATURE REVIEW

E-Learning and the 21st Century

Arkorful (2015) reviews the use of E-learning and technologies to access teaching and learning materials online in higher education. Thus, the importance of e-learning, which takes place through the use of the internet in 21st-century education, is undeniable, especially for "digital natives" (Bennett et al., 2008, Prensky 2001a). Prensky & Amory (2010b) suggest that e-learning makes course contents available online through technological evolution. This evolution enables students to freely access courses at their place irrespective of the challenges resulting from such as the COVID pandemic outbreak of 2019.

Nevertheless, some studies argue that no matter the advancement of technology, face-to-face learning is irreplaceable. It is the cornerstone of every learning institution, even if the current discourse and technological revolution demand the use of e-learning (Liu & Long, 2014; Nikoubakht & Kiamanesh, 2019). These studies demonstrate a conundrum between face-to-face and e-learning. Nonetheless, scholars like Anderson (2016) and Bates (2018), argue that a combination of the two is the best way to give students a variety of ways to access curriculum content following their diverse learning styles. However, compelling conditions like the outbreak of COVID-19 can make solid advocates for the need and relevance of e-learning.

Online Education in Cameroon

Yufek's (2021) report entitled "Holiday Classes: MINESEC Boss Visits Schools in Yaoundé" is the legal documents about how teachers in public schools misunderstand the concept of online studies. According to the minister:

If schools decide to create a platform for distance learning, it should not be just about putting lessons on a board and asking students to copy. It is all about distance teaching in which the teacher and students effectively interact during the process. (Yufek, 2021, para. 4)

The statement made by the minister of secondary education, in Cameroon, Nalova Lyonga displays the wrong implementation of online education by Cameroonian teachers in the public sector. Nalova regrets that instead of teachers promoting interaction between students and them, they use various online platforms as Nearpod, prodigy and Moodle on which notes are posted for students. This shocking admission by the main authority in charge of secondary education highlights better than any other statistics the level of misunderstanding of online education effectivity in the public education which is contrary to what takes place in the private sector.

Despite the misconception of online studies in the public sector, some private schools like Enko La Gaieté had long been using online studies before the outbreak of COVID-19. In line with this, the admin of the Enko blog attests on July 31st 2021 that:

Ultimately, emergency distance learning measures or not, thanks to the IB's pedagogy system, our students already have experience in self-regulatory learning methodology using technology. As such we are confident in their academic success in these exceptional times (Enko Blog Admin, 2020, para. 9)

They even go as far as providing the example of Florent Dusengue an Enko La Gaieté alumnus from Cameroon, who was able to skip some of his University Classes at the University of British Columbia, thanks to classes he had taken during his 2 years of IBDP[2] (Enko Blog Admin, 2020, para. 8). The long experience of Enko La Gaieté justifies why the setting is appropriate for the current work alongside with their internet connection. However, Macdonald highlights in "Obstacles Facing Cameroon's E-learning Drive" that Cameroon faces unstable internet connection due to poor infrastructure and the higher costs associated with it (Macdonald, 2020). As a consequence, many students and parents are unable to meet up with online schooling due to network.

Online Education and Memory

UNESCO is one of the institutions interested in archiving pandemics that affect humanity amongst which is COVID-19. Since the pandemic outbreak, the UNESCO updated its website in order to include a variety of initiatives against COVID-19. These initiatives are regularly stored and advertised on UNESCO homepage. The objective being that future generations could find instrumental statistics or methods in the archives on how today's generations control worry arisen from the COVID-19 pandemic in their time. The website is a repertoire of initiatives about worry control in COVID-19 time. Some initiatives to be mentioned as they relate to the current study are:

Creatives Against COVID-19 the Photography Edition

As part of Creatives against COVID-19 initiative, the Africa Digital Media Foundation (Kenya) launched webinar series to explore the ways in which Kenyan artists overcame the COVID-19 crisis. The initiative aimed at initiating a vibrant discussion on how photographers managed the COVID-19 crises in Kenya, and how they could come out stronger. Lock downs and social distancing measures strongly affected Kenya artists economically. They were for instance unable to organise festivals and expositions. The webinar series is an initiative created against their economic crises. In so doing, they were able to continue advertising their activity using photography and being paid. UNESCO taught this initiative was of interest to the future generations because photography keeps artist creative during confinement. One can learn more about the UNESCO COVID-19 initiatives by visiting the UNESCO home website.

However, though promoting creativity like the current study does, the initiative focuses exclusively on Kenyan artists financial interests. Photography being viewed by many as a controversial activity as it relates to arts, the possibility that this controversy curbs the reception of this creative initiative is very high. In order to avoid the waste of time, it is maybe advisable to diversify perspectives and actors, which the current study does.

A Film About Teenagers Surviving COVID-19 in Different Countries

The project is about a film which was produced in 2020 in Aglaia in France. The film displays teenagers who talk about their experiences during COVID-19 crises. They are from France, Russia, Finland, Singapore, USA, Italy and Spain. They do not just express the challenges they face but also about strategies they invented in other to overcome the consequences. One strength of this initiative is that youth speak to youth. It wise to sensitized the youth that way because young people belief each other and easily trust one another. This is one reason why UNESCO supported the initiative because, according to the organization, if one teenager says, act responsibly, wear a mask, wash your hands, other teenagers are likely to listen and put it in practice (UNESCO, 2020). The film is tagged online as "Teens in Confinement: COVID-19 story" with the title Quarantine project Covid-19.

However, the film perspectives on youth makes it at the same time bias. In fact, not only teenagers face consequences of COVID-19. alone cannot make a society. Thus, the current study which takes into account the perspective of young people, teenagers and adults. In fact, the current study postulates education as a melting pot between young people and adult deconstructing indeed the sense of essentialism inherent in Quarantine project Covid-19.

IMPORTANCE OF THE WORRY CONTROL CONCEPT

Everyone has worries. Worry is a daily burden to the human beings (Tallis, Davey & Capuzzo, 1994) and its magnitude varies depending on the behavioral and cognitive dispositions. Economically difficulties, uncertainty of the future, terrible sickness, political repression, exile, repression due to sexual orientation, etc. are few conditions that nurture worry. It is however very important to differentiate between "practical" and "hypothetical" worry (Thewellnesssociety, 2020, p. 5). "Practical" worry is one on which one can act on (Chellingsworth & al., 2013, p. 5). An instance is when someone worries about the little time, they have to complete their assignment. Hypothetical worry is one that something might happen when it rarely ever comes true (Shandel Group, 2017). In relation to Coronavirus, a good example of hypothetical worry is when someone knows they follow all the guidelines to avoid Corona but still ask themselves what if they catch the virus (Thewellnesssociety, 2020).

In this relation, home schooling appears like sort of capturing and addressing hypothetical worry. Following Margaret Wehrenberg, the concept of worry control specifically refers in this study to home schooling as a consensual method and tool for managing practical and hypothetical worries (Wehrenberg, 2005) from COVID-19 pandemic.

DYNAMISM OF WORRY CONCEPT

Human psychology being essentially fluid, the concept of worry control which tries to contain some aspects of it does not always succeed as evidenced by a variety of terms fighting over their legitimacy. A clear representation of this diversity is provided by terms such as anxiety management (Wehrenberg, 2005) worry deal (Chellingsworth, et al., 2020), worry management (Smith & Boxal, 2020). It is noteworthy to observe that, based on the literature consulted (worry management, worry deal, anxiety management) have in common the facts of being conceived as packages of regular activities, steps, methods provided to patients by a psychotherapist in order to heal their various worries. One of the preliminary steps being the "classification of worries into practical and hypothetical anxiety (Chellingsworth, et al., 2020, p. 7).

Worry control though integrative of the content of the other terms have the advantage of going beyond them because it incorporates a proactive dimension. The proactive dimension refers to fighting against eventual worry manifestation through the documentation for instance as the current study attempts to do.

OPERATIONALIZATION OF WORRY CONTROL

In this study worry merges both the worry due to the Corona pandemic and, worry arose from the transition to online schooling. Worry control then refers to methods used to control all these worries and to remain pro-active against similar situations in the future. The following figure systematized the perspective about worry control in this study whereby worry C symbolizes the worry being managed in this study.

Figure 1. Illustration of the worry being addressed in the study

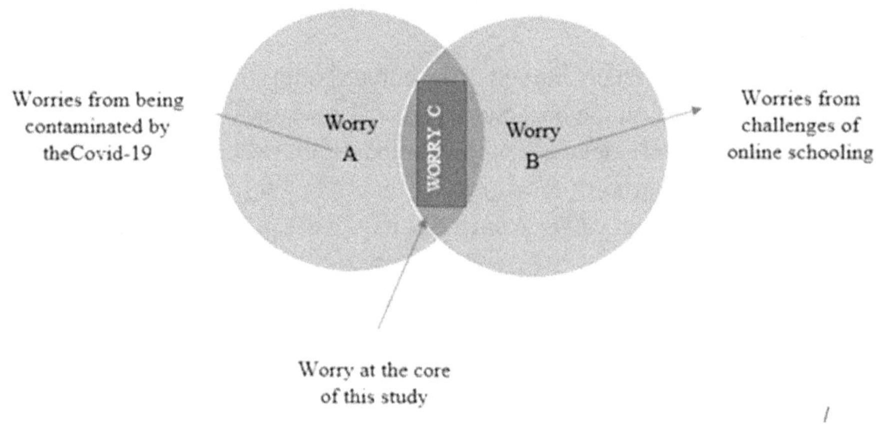

CONCLUSION

This research document methods in controlling worry arisen from the COVID-19, through a didactic approach which is different from previous studies. This study is significant because many researchers have distinguished various perspectives of controlling worries arisen from the COVID-19 pandemic or focus on online learning as a method to control the worry. The current study attempts to document worries arisen from the intersection between worries caused by the COVID-19 pandemic and the worry caused by online studies. This inquiry field is critical as its centre on the effectivity of online class amongst stake holders in the school milieu due to the worries created during the Coronavirus pandemic. Though much research has been conducted and archives documented, more study and investigation are required to understand the worries arisen from the link between COVID-19 and online class.

METHODOLOGY

Purpose of the Study

The purpose of this study is to document methods in controlling worry arisen from COVID-19 threat and discuss them as they apply in an international school context. More specifically, the current work will address the relevance and accuracy of online method to control anxieties derive from COVID -19 both at institutional (school system) and individual (teacher, student) levels. The study also takes into account the situation of people with disabilities. It does not segregate the society into two considering only "healthy" people.

Research Questions

1- What reactions did Enko La Gaieté have to COVID-19 which were represented in other educational institutions?
2- What online methods in controlling worry are available as didactic targets are achieved?
3- What significant problems of online learning overpower the strengths of homeschooling?
4- How does worry control affect people with disability at Enko La Gaieté?

Study Population

The study was carried out at the International School Complex La Gaieté. The reason that guided the choice is good internet capacities, so far as online class involves the internet. Evidence of their good internet band wit is provided from past teaching experience in that complex. As of date, the school has close to a thousand students. The work is exclusively focused on students enrolled for International Baccalaureate at Enko La Gaieté and their teachers. Print copy questionnaires were used to answer questions. Participants were from diverse gender, social and economic backgrounds.

Population Justification

The current work deals with worry control in times of COVID-19 in an international school context with International Baccalaureate students that essentially form Enko La Gaieté. The International Baccalaureate program which these students follow and the certificate they acquire is valued as it contributes in "increasing students access to the world's best universities for learners across Africa" (Home - La Gaieté International School, 2022, para. 1). The choice is a balanced one in the sense that, participants are made up of 10 girls and 15 boys.

INTERVENTION

Some of the strategies and processes that were put in place to collect data were sensitization of the population about the benefits and risks of their participation. I expected by so doing to gain participants' confidence so that they provide me with authentic data.

In case some participants were to condition their participation by requiring tips from the researcher, I was to think about a better offer that would not have compromised a good research policy. I for instance thought of providing them with past questions papers.

Intervention Plan

Week One: preparation of strategies for the Intervention like Searching for past questions paper. In case participants ask for incentives. The aim is to collect Data without corrupting participants (students)

Week Two: Research online what risk and benefits can be in participation. The purpose is to diversify my arguments, to be convincing and appealing to the students.

Week Three: Sensitization about the risks and benefits of participating using PowerPoint presentation. In the case where any participant asks for incentives, the researcher will print the numbers of past question papers equivalent to the number in class and give to all the learners. Give them a few days to reflect on my proposal.

Week four: distribution of a questionnaire to participants and guiding them where to put the filled questionnaire.

Week Five: collection of the filled questionnaire and data analyses.

SOURCES OF DATA

The main source of data for this research was the questionnaire. Two different questionnaires were conceived, one for teachers and one for students. The questions were simple and orientated to provide the best data. One of the questions is "how will you grade your satisfaction about online classes as a measure toward worry control?" The instruction was valid for all the 20 questions minimum. Tick what matches your feeling. All the questions were followed by grading criteria ranging from (1-6).

Instrumentation

The questionnaire consisted of 20 questions. One of the questions, as highlighted in the previous section, is for instance "how will you grade your satisfaction about online class as a measure toward worry control"? The question aimed at measuring the level of satisfaction of the participants with online classes. This level of participation is important for this research so far as it helps find suitable answers to the last question of my research. Which is (Why is the online method problematic despite its strengths?). The dissatisfaction of the participants enables the study looks for reasons why online classroom is problematic. The choice of 20 questions is justified by the first 5 questions which guide in providing pertinent answers to the first research question, the next 5, the second research question, the next 5, the third research question and the last 5, the last research question.

RESEARCH PROCEDURE

The procedure for acquiring research permission consists of the following steps:

The researcher searched the contact of the school online, in newspapers and on the city map.

Establishing Contact

The researcher emailed, phoned the schools individually, and when necessary, appeared on the spot to book appointments and establish connections with the school.

Direct Contact with School Authorities

After appointments were granted, the researcher introduced herself to the school authority, briefed the school authority about the content, objective of the study, and the use of data she was collect. She then handed the consent forms to the school authorities until permission to collect data was granted

Soliciting Participants

Enrolment of participants occurred following the subsequent steps:

Determining Participants

Based on the topic, the researcher needed to identify participants that best represent the target population and study requirement (Hulley et al.2013). The researcher also considered what age, and what level matches best with the research. The researcher had to finally consider a diverse range of participants (Mishna et al. 2012) from different socio-economic and gender backgrounds for equity reasons.

Appropriate Questionnaire

Questionnaires are series of prints or written questions with choices of answers conceive by the researcher to gather information from the informants. The researcher will conceive the questions in such a way that the minimum of questions require reflects the preoccupations of the topic such as to enable them to acquire the best data for the research. Johnson (2008) sustains this argument by stating that questionnaires permit a teacher-researcher to gather a lot of, as well as a variety of information relatively quickly. Questionnaires are simple and compose of open-ended questions where informants are given choices to provide their responses.

Sensitization About the Process of the Project of Collecting Data

The researcher went to the classroom with sample questionnaires, read the questions, and showed to the participants how to fill them. The researcher let participants fill the questionnaires on their own and minors could seek explanation from their parents at home. Though, only what they thought and not what their parent's thought was needed, copies were given out as well as explanations about where to deliver the filled questionnaires.

Informed Consent

Having had the supervisors' consent to research Enko La Gaieté, a meeting was scheduled on the school campus with the potential participation for approximately 10-15 minutes. During this session, participants were fully informed regarding the objectives of the study. The researcher also explained to them what the risks and benefits of their participation in the research is. The researcher insisted on the acquisition of practical skills about applied research as one of the benefits in case the young participants decide to carry out such research in the future. They were reassured that their answers were to be treated with confidentiality and strictly to the benefit of this academic research.

The participants were equally assured that at the end of the research a copy of the work will be available in their school library for them to be able to verify in case there was a bridge of contract. Participants were informed about the rights to decline their participation and were given time (two days) to reflect before taking part in the study.

Distribution of Informed Concern Forms

Those who were under 18 took to their parent/guardians, brought them back to school the following day acknowledging their consent for the child to participate in the study. The signed consent letter aimed at re-assuring the participants that their participation in the research is voluntary. Participants were either to return the document to the researcher while on campus or deposit in the box placed in their class.

Data Collection Procedures

The data collection method used is a qualitative one. Since it provides a standard format for collecting information, it has helped reduced bias in answering the research questions. Though each group of participants (teachers/students) required a specific set of questionnaires.

Conception of a Clear, Appropriate and Simple Questionnaire

Based on the variety of participants the researcher has conceived two different sets of questionnaires: one for teachers, one for students. Both questionnaires complied with the linguistic level of the participants.

Sensitization of Participants

The researcher met the potential participants in other to facilitate the filling of the questionnaire. That phase was important because it enables the researcher to get pertinent data. For example, Rubrics designed are on a scale of 1 - 6 where 1 is the descriptor for "excellent" 2 for "very good", 3 for "average", 4 for "bad", 5 for "very bad" and 6 for "not matching". The instruction was "tick" what matches your feelings.

Distribution of the Questionnaires

The researcher spread and explained where the filled questionnaires were to be deposited.

Some sample questions that were included in the questionnaires are:

Question 1: How will you grade your satisfaction with the online class as a measure toward worry control?

Question 2: I am not satisfied with the online class because it is…?

Question 3: I am satisfied with the online class because it is…?

ETHICAL CONSIDERATIONS

Ethical Research Practices are important in applied research because applied research involves many stakeholders (society, researcher, informants, values, regulations for good research practice, and regulations) in society. The more the researcher respects the ethical research practices the better and more valuable the quality of the research is. The ethical research practices that are deemed adequate for the current study are consent forms and questionnaires. The consent form has two parts (a) an information sheet describing the research and nature of participants involving in it and (b) participants consent.

Consent Form

The consent form is discussed by some scholars as guidelines about ethical research practices (Bhattacharya & Preissle, 2003). In this study, the consent form is an authorization given by Enko La Gaieté School Complex authorities for the researcher to research on their campus. As an ethical practice, the consent form protects both the researcher and the informant. It protects the researcher from participants' refusal to take part or provide the researcher with the data needed. When the collaborators realized the document has been signed, they will willingly take part. It also protects the researcher from time wasting and useless expenditure without which the researcher could not complete the work thus, showing the importance of ethical rules. It also protects the informant in case that the researcher gives wrong information, which can lead to character defamation, the informant has the right to take the researcher to court in order to face judiciary issues.

Questionnaire

World Health Organization, (2001) defines a questionnaire as a sample list of mimeographed or printed questions that is completed by a respondent. In this study questionnaire is a psychometric collection of 15 questions whereby the informant has to rate the question from 1-6) using ("good", "average", "bad", "too bad", "not applicable", "excellent", "very bad"). Each series of five questions enables the researcher to adequately address the three research questions introduced previously. This study considers questionnaire appropriate as ethical research practice because it complies with one of the ethical principles called anonymity. However, the questionnaire for the current research was conceived for two different informants (a) students (b) teachers.

Considerations During Intervention

Intervention in this research consists of sets of possible situations which the researcher has to foresee when carrying out research. Some of them could be potential informants who could ask for tips or incentives, and researcher can be involved in an accident. Some of them are briefly discussed in the subsequent lines.

- Some informants could have conditioned their taking part in the research process by asking for money

Some scholars are of the opinion that offering compensation demonstrates respect, for the time and contribution made by participants (Grady, 2001). Considering that justice is one of the basic ethical principles in applied research (See Belmont Report, 1979, for more) and the data collection procedure must be fair, the researcher will bring past question papers to share with the whole class. Past question paper is the fairest means as money cannot be considered an adequate means for "fairness" (Belmont Report, 1979, p. 7). The ethics of offering incentives to participants limits the exploration in qualitative research (Head, 2009). Paying participants will have implications and have consequences in terms of data collection (Head, 2009).

Money symbolizes injustice as it makes some people rich and others poor. though, most

people value money based on their social conviction. To stingy people money has a great value. Giving informants money means they will be tempted to give the researcher information based on the amount given and the researcher will have insufficient authentic data due to retention. Money cannot therefore be considered a fair means because it is an "improper reward meant to obtain compliance" (Belmont Report, 1979, p. 11). Money can therefore not be considered a symbol of justice which is one of the ethical principles of applied research.

- The researcher could have been involved in a car accident.

In the case where the researcher's leg is broken, it will impact the data collection procedure as the researcher will need immediate medical attention. This explains why it is necessary for the researcher to have a good relationship with the school administrations. The researcher would call the school and tell them where to keep the filled questionnaire.

Considerations During Data Collection

The process of gathering qualitative information, aiming at evaluating the outcome is known as data collection. In this research, data collection is conceived of as a process that involves sets of activities like planning, implementation, and selection of adequate methods.

Planning

During this process, the researcher considered the type of data to be collected, in relation to the cost and time allocation. The researcher equally determined the kind of data that would be appropriate for the research, where the data would be collected from, and determine the amount of data sufficient for the study. According to COPE, good research should be well adjusted, well-planned, appropriately designed, and ethically approved (COPE, 2005).

Method and Adequate Implementation

What could be the appropriate method for data collection? When the researcher knows which method to use, and what procedure to follow during the survey, for instance, it helps them determine what types of survey to use. In this study, the method used is a questionnaire. To collect data, the researcher administered two different kinds of surveys to the two different groups of participants made up of 15 questions each. Participants have been trained on how to answer the survey.

Considerations of Researcher Bias

Research is generally considered bias when it does not include participants that are representative of the society. For instance, gender, religion socio-political, and ideologically. Research is a bias when it does not promote inclusion. On this basis, the researcher planned not only to get male informants but, also females so as to have a balanced rate of participation. The same thing applied to social classes. Another important point is that the researcher ensured not to get bias data in the sense of misunderstanding the question. That is why the researcher spent enough time in explaining what each question meant to the participants.

CONCLUSION

From the above, there is no doubt that the methodology chooses for this research complies with ethical research principles.

Data Analysis and Results

The data collection process started with the identification of a problem. The problem being identified as previously indicated; the researcher split the problem into four research questions as already stated. In order to balance the results, the researcher decided to attribute to each research question, five questions which finally generated two types of questionnaires, each made up of twenty questions. The first questionnaire is meant for the teachers and the second for students. This division was necessary because students being teenagers in their majority the researcher alleged that their reaction to the questionnaire could be superficial.

In fact, research on youth has proven that teenagers are very much distracted, joyful, playful, carelessly, and inconsistent. That is the reason why the data collected from them works in the study as support to the ones collected from the teachers who, contrary to teenagers, are alleged as reasonable, thoughtful, and rational. It was also necessary to divide the questionnaire in that way in order to meet the language level of the informants. The second reason of dividing the questionnaire is that the concentration level in filling the questionnaire by informants could be the same.

The questionnaire being conceived, it was time for the researcher to meet up with all the administrative procedures before going to the field to collect data. A regular parent's concern form was conceived and validated by both parts: researcher and the school. It is then that the researcher went to the field, Enko La Gaieté, to collect data from the informants. The data collected are being analyzed in the following section.

Data Analysis Procedure

Data analysis aims at answering the research questions based on the data provided by the informants. The proper analysis of data collected in relation to the topic at stake consists of three various steps. The first step consists in the description of facts about what the data collected exactly reflect. In other words, this first step is all about observing and uttering factually what the data collected say. Secondly, a close examination is given to the data collected as they provide a pertinent answer to the research questions or not. Methodologies for the said close examination vary from comparisons, contrasts, transpositions of the issue at stake or artifacts to different contexts and paradigms. The last step in the data analysis procedure consists in evaluating the answer obtained from the data collected. In the case where answers achieved are not satisfactory, suggestions or perspectives are raised which can lead to further fundamental or applied research in the times ahead.

Data Analysis

The questionnaires used for data collection respected the ethical consideration as they were anonymous, and informants participated willingly in the data collection. First of all, the filled questionnaires were classified according to whether they were filled by learners or teachers. Then, questions in the questionnaires were considered in relation to the four research questions. Five of each question in the questionnaire aimed at providing satisfactory answer to each research question. Operationally, rankings in terms of how many participants reacted to the questionnaires in general and how many did effectively provide an answer, were used in order to draw satisfactorily answer to each research question. Reasons why some informants did react or not to this or that question from the questionnaires were attempted to be provided based on parallel artifacts and the researcher's own rationality or intuition.

Validity and Reliability

Under this section, results refer to both the data collected and the answers to the research questions obtained from the data analysis. It therefore goes without saying how important the data in this study are. This is because the reliability of the results exclusively depends on the reliability of the data collected. How then did the researcher ensure that the results in this study are going to be both valid and reliable at all?

To ensure that the data collected are valid and reliable, the researcher generated two types of questionnaires for the sake of data collection. The first questionnaire was meant for the teachers and the second for students. This division was necessary, useful and even strategical because students being teenagers in their majority the researcher alleged that their reaction to the questionnaire could be superficial. In fact, research on youth has proven that teenagers are very much distracted, joyful, playful, careless and inconsistent. That is the reason why the data collected from them, works in the study as support to the ones collected from the teachers who, contrary to teenagers, are alleged to be more reasonable, thoughtful, and rational. It was also necessary to divide the questionnaire that way in order to meet the language level of the informants. The said questionnaires are provided in the appendix of the final document.

Also, to ensure the reliability and validity of results the researcher though it useful to diversify the data collection methods. Therefore, other artifacts like articles, book chapters, interviews, newspapers, videos, diagrams, etc. are used either to support, contrasts or even challenge the data collected.

Moreover, the principles of anonymity and ethics were rigorously observed as no name of any participant is mentioned in the data collection and analysis and no bribe was undertaken during data collection. These two principles grant the data collected their authenticity and therefore their reliability at least in the context of the study.

Last but not the least, reliability formula by Miles and Huberman (1994) is used to sustain the reliability of the findings in the study. Miles and Huberman formula reads as follows:

Reliability = Consensus/(Agreement+Dissagreement) x 100

As applied to the data collected, the above formula takes the following form:

Reliability = 36/(36+15) x 100 = 70.5%.

Seventy-point five percent, is above the average of a hundred. Miles and Huberman would have had no other term to qualify the data collected for this study than reliable.

RESULTS

To present the results, the perspective adopted is a combination of apposite explanations with diagrams and figures which account of statistics about informants' reactions to research questions. Also, consultation of concurrent artifacts is made in other to high light with more insight the pertinence or values of the results obtained. The results are presented below from the framework of four complementary chapters, each chapter's heading being a derivation of the respective research questions.

Descriptive Findings

Out of 22 informants under (teachers) expected 14 effectively took part in the Data collection. Though 14 could appear small as compared to the 22 expected, it must be stressed that, the 14 informants were neither forced nor corrupted by any other means to take part in the data collection. The 14 informants amongst the teachers willingly filled out the questionnaires. 14 is therefore representative for, it grants the data collected their qualitative value so far as it enables comparisons, contrasts, and complementarity with other artifacts. The same observations apply with students though out of the 29 informants expected, 22 effectively took part in the data collection.

To the research question about the reaction of Enko La Gaieté towards COVID-19, the questionnaire enables the researcher to witness various perspectives. For example, 14 informants out of 24 were not aware that homeschooling started at Enko La Gaieté before the COVID-19 outbreak. Whereas all the informants amongst teachers were fully aware that homeschooling was not implemented at Enko La Gaieté due to COVD-19 outbreak. This situation enabled the researcher to view the reaction of Enko La Gaieté toward COVID-19 as more of reinforcing the internet provision and reorganizing homeschooling regulation as evidenced by the report of the minister of secondary education, in Cameroon, Nalova Lyonga, (Yufek, 2021).

The table one below shows the rationale between the number of expected participants to the field work and the effective number of participants (both students and teachers) to the research question number 1.

Now that it is clear what Enko La Gaieté 's reaction toward COVID-19 is, the question one could ask is whether the re-enforcement of internet connection effectively worked. This question is pertinent because during the period of COVID-19 countries experimented a boom in the internet demand and Cameroon being classified by the International Monetary Fund (IMF) as a poor country, one is not wrong to doubt the quality of internet provision under such circumstances.

In relation to the research question about what significant problems of online learning overpower the strengths, the question to know how satisfactorily, informants felt about homeschooling was raised. The data collected provided four categories of answers. While 4 informants out of 24 amongst students were not at all satisfied with homeschooling, 3 informants out of 14 teachers were equally not at all satisfied. While none of the informants amongst the 14 teachers ticked extremely satisfied, two informants out of the 24 students thought that they were extremely satisfied with homeschooling. While 1 informant out of 14 teachers were very satisfied, none of the informants out of 24 amongst students were very satisfied. 18 informants amongst the 24 students ticked moderately satisfied meanwhile 10 teachers out of 14 were of the same opinion.

The table two below shows the rationale between the total number of participants (students and teachers) satisfied with online class to those not satisfied with it. The rationale helps in answering the research question number 2.

Figure 2. Statistics on participation to RQ1

Figure 3. Statistics on dissatisfaction with distance schooling (RQ2)

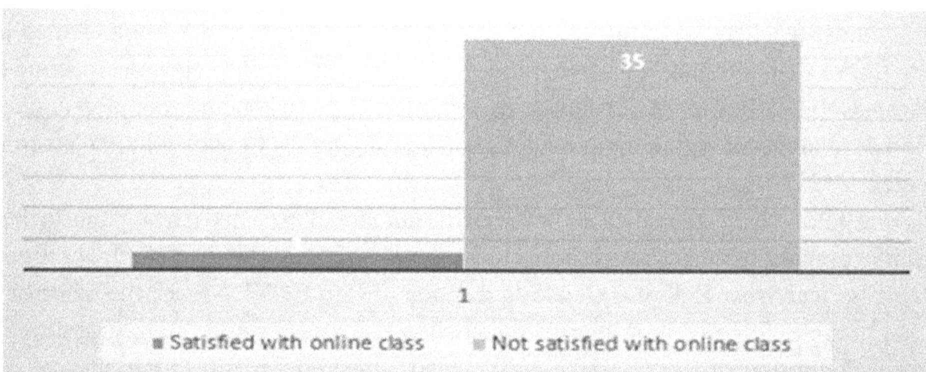

The results presented as such, though not clear about what problems overpower the strengths of homeschooling, show that majority of informants are not satisfied with homeschooling. This situation suggests somehow the effectiveness of a problem somewhere. Is the problem not maybe related to the discomfort of informants to deal with technological tools? Is the problem also not maybe due to electricity shortages very common in the Cameroonian contexts? It is clear based on each of these two questions raised and based on the interdependency of schools and educational processes, that shortage or discomfort with technological tools effectively affect quality education. The problem becomes more crucial when related to the situation of people with disability as the next paragraph attempts to show.

As far as people with disability are concerned, questions were asked to the informants whether people with disability had the same chances in homeschooling as "normal" people? Based on the informant's experiences, the data collected highlight a general unanimity. For, they all believe that people with disability did not have the same chances as others. It is noteworthy observing that for the reliability of data collected in relation to people with disability, a question was asked to make sure whether the informants knew what it meant to be a person with disability. The data collected provided a general satisfaction. All the 38 informants were very much aware of what it meant to be a person with disability.

The table three below shows the rationale between the total number of participants (students and teachers) who believe that online class is very challenging to people with disability. The rationale helps in answering the research question number 3. \

Figure 4. Statistics on distance schooling as challenging for people with disability (RQ3)

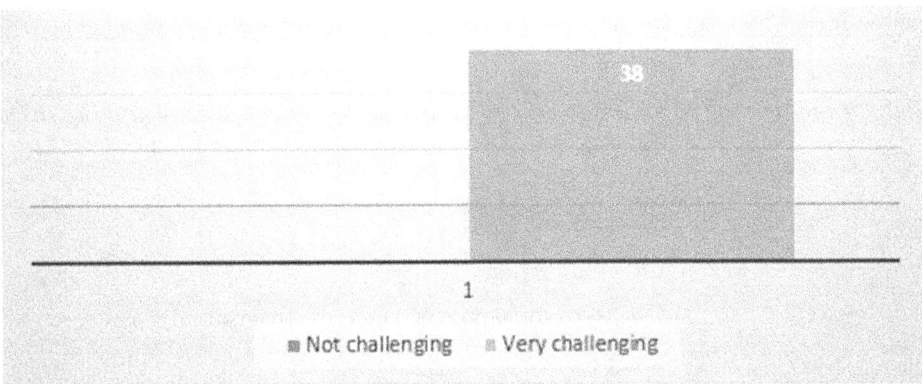

What problems then do people with disability face with homeschooling? The data collected are silent on that question inviting for consideration of other artifacts. People with disability in Cameroon faced multiple challenges during the COVID-19 pandemic as the journalist Moki Edwin Kindzeka reports in *Voice of Africa* (Kindzeka, 2020). The journalist reports that hundreds of people with disability fanned out across Cameroon's capital, protesting the neglect they suffered during the COVID-19 pandemic. As evident in the report by Kindzeka, which he backed up with interviews from representatives of people with disability from Cameroon, disable people found themselves abandoned and excluded from the society. In fact, COVID-19 is felt by people with disabilities as a situation which worsened the social exclusion which people with disability has always been undergoing. One therefore can easily guess the situation with people with disability in schools as disable artists and workers demonstrated in the street to complaint about their abandonment.

The above examples that capture the conditions of people with disability in Cameroon show that people with disability in general, learners at Enko La Gaieté in particular suffered double. They suffered double because the control of COVID-19 worries promoting social exclusion appeared as re-enforcement of the previous exclusion they were facing. This explains why in the suddenness of the COVID-19 outbreak, preliminary training for teachers on behalf of people with disability were neglected if they were not even strongly forgotten.

The last research question which was raised is to know what online methods in controlling worry are available as didactic targets are achieved? One didactic target was drilling students to discipline, informants were asked to judge whether online class assured discipline. Results from the data collection brought out 3 categories of answers. One informant out of the 24 students was of the opinion that online class matches the requirement of discipline in the classroom. On the teacher's side, only one informant out of the 14 informants was also of the same opinion. Out of the 24 informants amongst the students 6 were of the opinion that it is challenging for teachers to get students' attention during homeschooling. On the other side, out of the 14 informants for teachers, 6 were of the opinion that getting students' attention during online class is challenging. Amongst the 24 informants for students 18 reacted by stressing how very challenging it was for homeschooling to assure discipline. Out of the 14 informants for teachers, 5 were of the opinion that homeschooling was very challenging to get students' attention.

The table below shows the rationale between the total number of participants (students and teachers) who believe that online class fails to achieve discipline in education. The orange portion represents the percentage of the informants who responded positively and the blue portion the percentage of those who were against the idea. The rationale helps in answering the research question number 4.

Figure 5. Statistics in relation to failure to discipline learners during online schooling (RQ4)

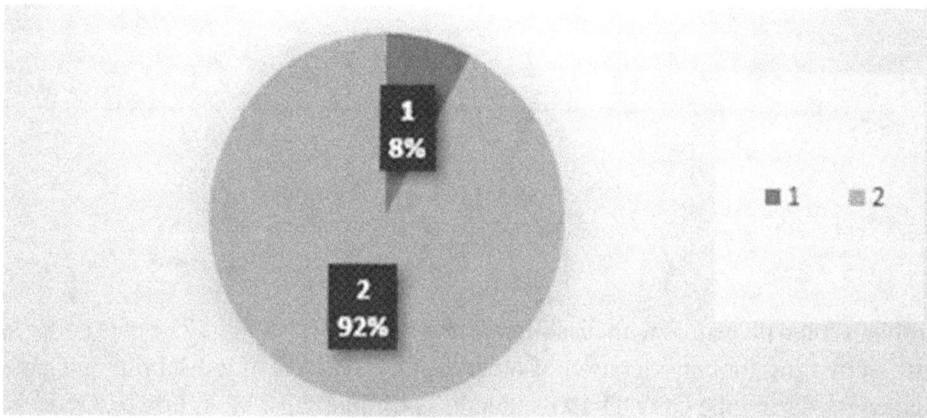

All in all, and given that "very challenging" is almost the same as "challenging", it is to be said that 35 informants in total out of the 38 informants say homeschooling to be a disciplinary loss, failure, or even crisis. This situation unveils a significant weakness of online classes as related to education. Future generations are, therefore. Invited to start searching or carrying on research on methods to achieve optimal discipline in homeschooling.

Outcome Analysis/Discussion

Finding description is referred in this section as one step in outcome (findings) analysis. Therefore, the researcher thought it wise to merged finding description alongside with analysis of findings as evident in the following paragraphs.

Reaction of Enko La Gaieté Toward COVID-19

The analysis of the data collected enabled the study to evidence the reaction of Enko La Gaieté toward COVID-19 as being one of reinforcement of its internet provision and reorganization of homeschooling-regulation. The study validated this specific reaction of Enko La Gaieté toward COVID-19 as it considered a different artifact, the Cameroon government daily magazine, *Cameroon Tribune,* Nr. 12320/8519.

Significant Problems of Online Learning Overpowering the Strengths

The data collected and their analysis highlighted the dissatisfaction of the informants with homeschooling, suggesting therefore the existence of a problem with online class. It is not by chance that not only students but also teachers are not satisfied with online schooling. Their dissatisfaction in the proportions as evidenced by the statistics in the data analysis says more about this significant problem. For, human beings are a combination of reasoning, behavior, practicing and moods.

Homeschooling as Marginalization of People with Disability

The data collected and their analysis proved that at Enko La Gaieté, people with disability did not have the same chances as others. In fact, due to the suddenness and unpredictability of COVID-19, teachers, educators could not have time to attain professional development classes which could have helped them teach students with disability using IT-tools.

Online Methods in Controlling Worry and Achievement of Didactic Targets

One relevant didactic target being to drill students to discipline, the data collected and their analysis emphasized the failure of online schooling in doing so. In fact, though online schooling upholds autonomy and freedom on the side of learners, it does not allow direct control by the supervisor about what learners are doing at the same time they are being taught. Online schooling therefore fails to discipline the learners proportionately like face-to-face class. The younger the learners are, the more awful the idea of the situation appears.

Learning Themes

This applied research attempt has been a necessary and useful journey. It has enabled the researcher measure the challenges of dealing with people characterized by their unpredictability. One lesson from it is that each person builds a whole world in its own. Therefore, dealing with people calls on values such as patience, tolerance, humility, prudence and lucidity on the side of the researcher. This research left the researcher with few points of thoughts which are listed and discussed under learning themes as follows:

Disaffection as a Challenge to Education

The problem raised under this theme is whether it is possible to permanently lead people to a destination they do not like? Education aiming at achieving democracy (Kom, 1985) this condition appears as unreliable if educational values are to be hand over to the next generations. Therefore, it becomes a requirement from educators to always ensure whether the needs and the satisfaction of the learners are met if not at least taken into account. It is on this condition that the banking system by Paulo Freire will be challenge for ever in education.

Double Exclusion of People with Disability in Times of COVID-19

The lesson one can draw from the current COVID-19 pandemic is that like other sudden crisis, societies never have enough time to prepare themselves on how to deal with consequences of those crises. People with disability from this study have the merit because they suffered double exclusion I times of COVID-19 has the merit strongly to highlight the necessity for society to start making pro activity their habit. In fact, what people with disability teach the community is that community should not wait until the crisis is there before they start looking for means how to challenge them. For, the consequences of waiting are heavier than the consequences of anticipating.

If one were to restart a study from these premises, one could have focused on the message uttered by disable people in times of crisis. It could have been the occasion to question the wait-and-see-attitude of people and its consequences not only on education but also in the whole society at large. It could also have been the occasion to take into account to make profit of the few weaknesses observed during this applied research.

CONCLUSION

At the eve of this study, it is necessary to recall what it was all about and what its ambition was. The study attempted to meet the requirements of an applied research on didactics survey about worry management in the times of COVID-19 at an international school from Cameroon. Enko La Gaieté has been selected as the adequate place to carry on the study because of its specificity, which has been repeatedly highlighted in the study as far as homeschooling is involved. The study finally ought to capture a moment in the management of worry as displayed at Enko La Gaieté from a didactics point of view.

The main motivation which led to the study was the concern whether homeschooling which, all of a sudden, became the consensual method of managing didactic worries from the COVID-19 pandemic, could satisfactorily replace traditional school format. The necessity to split this main preoccupation in to a complementary preoccupation occurred as the researcher was exposed to disability studies in both the course of the study and the Master Program as a whole. Thus, the subsequent main preoccupation which was whether the management of COVID-19 through homeschooling did consider the needs of people with disability.

To answer these questions, the study relied predominantly, but not exclusively, on two types of questionnaires filled by learners and teachers from Enko La Gaieté. Ethical principles, rigor and impartiality were strictly observed during data collection and data analysis. The study made it clear that, though it works efficiently in managing worries due to COVID-19 in conventional education, homeschooling does not satisfactorily replace traditional education. It fails for instance to achieve discipline in the same proportion as face-to-face class. Homeschooling does not fully achieve the disciplinary mission which is one relevant purpose of education. The study also made it clear that disable people underwent double exclusion, as the sudden outbreak of COVID-19 did not give educators enough time to update their teaching methods such as to meet the needs of people with disability.

Researchers from all fields in general, those on education in particular, are put on trial by the weakness of homeschooling underlined in this study. It is maybe the responsibility of future researches to closely address this weakness of homeschooling which, if not given the necessary attention, threatens harmony and ethics in human society severely. Though one can deplore insufficiency of theoretical approach in the study, the study has tried to remain modest, rigorous, and empirical.

REFERENCES

American psychiatric Association. (2000). *Diagnostic and statistics: Manual of mental.* APA.

Amory, A. (2010). Education technology and hidden ideological contradictions. *Journal of Educational Technology & Society, 13*(1), 69–79.

Anderson, T. (2016). Theories for Learning with Emerging Technologies. *Emerging Technologies in Distance Education, 7*(1), 7-23.

Arkorful, V. (2015). The role of e-learning, advantages and disadvantages of its adoption in higher education. *Int J Instruct Technol Distance Learn, 12*(1), 29–42.

Bates, A. (2018). *Teaching in a digital age: Guidelines for designing teaching and learning for a digital age*. Tony Bates Associates Ltd.

Bennett, S., Maton, K., & Kervin, L. (2008). The 'digital natives' debate: A critical review of the evidence. *British Journal of Educational Technology, 39*(5), 775–786. doi:10.1111/j.1467-8535.2007.00793.x

Bhattacharya, K., & Preissle, J. (2003). *Ethics and Research Interviewing*. Paper presented at the American Educational Studies Association, Mexico City, Mexico.

Cameroon COVID-19 situation report. (2021). World Health Organization Publication in UNOCHA.

Chellingsworth, M., Farrand, P., & Rayson, K. (2013). *Dealing with worry. CEDAR*. University of Exeter.

Copeland, M. E. (1998). *The worry control workbook*. New Harbinger Pubns Inc.

Dana Di Pardo, L.-H. (2021). *What is the difference between didactics and pedagogy in reflective teaching. Disorders*.

Enko Blog Admin. (2020, March 26). Why are Enko Students more prepared for distance learning? *Enko Blog*.

Freire, P. (1970). *"Banking" concept of Education. In Ways of Reading*. St. Martin's.

Grady, C. (2005). Payment of clinical research subjects. *The Journal of Clinical Investigation, 115*(7), 1681–1687. doi:10.1172/JCI25694 PMID:16007244

Head, E. (2009). The ethics and implications of paying participants in qualitative research. *International Journal of Social Research Methodology, 12*(4), 335–344. doi:10.1080/13645570802246724

Hulley, S. B., Cummings, S., Browner, W., Grady, D.G., & Newman, T. B. (2013). Designing Clinical Research. An epidemiological approach (2nd ed.). Lippincott Williams & Wilkins.

International Council of Archives. (2020). *The Role-of-achieves-in-the COVID-19 crisis*. Author.

Johnson, D. H. (2008). In defense of indices: The case of bird surveys. *The Journal of Wildlife Management, 72*(4), 857–868. doi:10.2193/2007-294

Kom, A. (1996). *Éducation et démocratie en Afrique. Le temps des illusions.* l'Harmattan.

Liu, C., & Long, F. (2014). The discussion of traditional teaching and multimedia teaching approach in college English teaching. *2014 International Conference on Management, Education and Social Science (ICMESS 2014).* 10.2991/icmess-14.2014.9

Long Beach. (n.d.). *Data collection strategies II: Qualitative research.* California State University.

Macdonald, A. (2020, September 30). *Obstacles Facing Cameroon's E-learning Drive. E-Learning in Cameroon.* iafrikan.com

Mishna, F., Muskat, B., & Cook, C. (2012). Anticipating Challenges: School-Based social work intervention research. *Children & Schools, 34*(3), 135–144. doi:10.1093/cs/cds002

Munir, S., Gondal, A. Z., &Takov, V. (2019). *Generalized Anxiety Disorder.* Academic Press.

National Commission for the Protection of Human Subjects of Biomedical and Behavioral Research. (1979). *The Belmont Report: Ethical Principles and Guidelines for the protection of Human Subjects of Research.* Author.

Nikoubakht, A., & Kiamanesh, A. (2019). The comparison of the effectiveness of computer-based education and traditional education on the numerical memory in students with mathematics disorder. *J. Psychol Sci, 18*(73), 55–65.

Prensky,M.(2001a).DigitalNativesDigitalImmigrants.*Horizon*,*9*(5),1–6.doi:10.1108/10748120110424816

Shandel Group. (2017). *Worry-is-a-false-sense-of-control.* Group Leadership Blog.

Smith, M. & Boxall, R. (2020). *Managing Worry Group Handbook.* Academic Press.

Tallis, F., Davey, G. C. L., & Capuzzi, N. (1994). *The phenomenology of non-pathological worry: A preliminary investigation. In Worrying: Perspectives on theory, assessment, and treatment.* Wiley.

Thewellnesssociety. (2020). *Coronavirus anxiety workbook.* Author.

UNESCO. (2020). *COVID-19 Educational disruptions and response, 2020.* UNESCO.

UNESCO. (2020). *Turning the threat of COVID-19 into an opportunity for greater support to document heritage.* UNESCO.

UNESCO COVID-19 Initiatives. (2020). *A film about teenagers surviving COVID in different countries.* UNESCO.

UNESCO COVID-19 Initiatives. (2020). *Creatives against COVID-19: The photography edition.* UNESCO.

Wehrenberg, M. (2005). *10 Best-Ever Anxiety-Management Techniques.* Academic Press.

WHO. (2020). *WHO Director-General's opening remarks at the media briefing on COVID-19.* WHO.

World Health Organizations Regional Office for the Western Pacific. (2001). *Health research methodology: A guide for training in research methods* (2nd ed). WHO regional Office of the Western Pacific.

Yufek, B. (2021). *Holiday classes: MINESEC boss visits schools in Yaoundé*. Academic Press.

ENDNOTES

1. Enko Education has representations in Botswana, Burkina Faso, Cameroon, Ivory Coast, Mali, Mozambique, Senegal, South Africa, and Zambia.
2. International Baccalaureate Diploma Programme.

Compilation of References

Abdullah, D. N. M. A., & Lee, O. Y. (2012). Effects of wellness programs on job satisfaction, stress and absenteeism between two groups of employees (attended and not attended). *Procedia: Social and Behavioral Sciences*, *65*, 479–484. doi:10.1016/j.sbspro.2012.11.152

Aboul-Ela, G. M. B. E. (2017). Reflections on Workplace Compassion and Job Performance. *Journal of Human Values*, *23*(3), 234–243. doi:10.1177/0971685817713285

Acs, G., & Karpman, M. (2020). Employment, income, and unemployment insurance during the Covid-19 Pandemic. Urban Institute, 1-11.

Adamson, M. M., Phillips, A., Seenivasan, S., Martinez, J., Grewal, H., Kang, X., Coetzee, J., Luttenbacher, I., Jester, A., Harris, O. A., & Spiegel, D. (2020). International prevalence and correlates of psychological stress during the global COVID-19 pandemic. *International Journal of Environmental Research and Public Health*, *17*(24), 9248. doi:10.3390/ijerph17249248 PMID:33321950

Adams-Prassl, A., Boneva, T., Golin, M., & Rauh, C. (2020). Inequality in the impact of the coronavirus shock: Evidence from real time surveys. *Journal of Public Economics*, *189*, 104245. doi:10.1016/j.jpubeco.2020.104245

Adderholdt-Elliott, M., & Eler, S. H. (1989). Counseling students who are gifted through bibliotherapy. *Teaching Exceptional Children*, *22*(1), 26–31. doi:10.1177/004005998902200106

Adelmann, P. K. (1994). Multiple roles and psychological well-being in a national sample of older adults. *The Journals of Gerontology. Series B, Psychological Sciences and Social Sciences*, *49*(6), S277–S285. PMID:7963284

Afolayan, J. A. (1992). Documentary perspective of bibliotherapy in education. *Reading Horizons*, *33*(2).

Agai–Demjaha, T., Karadzinska Bislimovska, J., & Mijakoski, D. (2015). Level of Work-Related Stress among Teachers in Elementary Schools. *OA Maced J Med Sci.*, *3*, 484-488. doi:10.3889/oamjms.2015.076

Agrawal, S. (2019). Anasakti and Adjustment. *Journal of Indian Council of Philosophical Research*, *36*(1), 39–51. doi:10.100740961-018-0155-9

Aguilar Yuste, M. (2021). Leadership and Emotional Intelligence during a Crisis. Revista de Relaciones Internacionales. *Estrategia y Seguridad*, *16*(2), 47–60.

Ahmad, M. B., Ali, H. F., Malik, M. S., Humayun, A. A., & Ahmad, S. (2019). Factors affecting impulsive buying behavior with mediating role of positive mood: An empirical study. *European Online Journal of Natural and Social Sciences*, *8*(1), 17.

Ahmed, R. R., Streimikiene, D., Rolle, J.-A., & Duc, P. A. (2020). The COVID-19 pandemic and the antecedents for the impulse buying behavior of US citizens. *Journal of Competitiveness*, *12*(3), 5–27. doi:10.7441/joc.2020.03.01

Ahrens, C. J. C., & Ryff, C. D. (2006). Multiple roles and well-being: Socio-demographic and psychological moderators. *Sex Roles*, *55*(11-12), 801–815. doi:10.100711199-006-9134-8

AjayiS. (2018). Effect of stress on employee performance and job satisfaction: A case study of Nigerian banking industry. *Available at* SSRN 3160620. doi:10.2139/ssrn.3160620

Akellaa, D., & Lewis, V. (2019). The Modern Face of Workplace Incivility. *Organization Management Journal*, 1-7. do i:10.1080/15416518.2019.1604202

Al Lily, A. E., Ismail, A. F., Abunasser, F. M., & Alhajhoj, R. H. (2020). Distance education as a response to pandemics: Coronavirusand Arab culture. *Technology in Society*, *63*, 101317. doi:10.1016/j.techsoc.2020.101317 PMID:32836570

Albers, B., & Pattuwage, L. (2017). Implementation in education: Findings from a scoping review. Evidence for Learning, 10.

Albrecht, S. L., & Marty, A. (2020). Personality, self-efficacy and job resources and their associations with employee engagement, affective commitment, and turnover intentions. *International Journal of Human Resource Management*, *31*(5), 657–681. doi:10.1080/09585192.2017.1362660

Alexander, S. (2007). Voluntary simplicity movement. The Blackwell Encyclopedia of Sociology, 1-2. doi:10.1002/9781405165518.wbeos0693

Alexander, S. (2011). God's away on business: The spiritual significance of voluntary simplicity. *EarthSong Journal: Perspectives in Ecology, Spirituality and Education*, *2*(2), 7-9. https://search.informit.org/doi/10.3316/informit.676595747751645

Alexander, S., & Ussher, S. (2012). The voluntary simplicity movement: A multi-national survey analysis in theoretical context. *Journal of Consumer Culture*, *12*(1), 66–86. doi:10.1177/1469540512444019

Alirezaei, M., Eskandarieh, S., Sahraian, M. A., & Naser Moghadasi, A. (2022). Depression, anxiety, and fear of COVID-19 in patients with multiple sclerosis in pandemic era: A cross-sectional study. *Neurological Sciences*, *43*(1), 59–66. doi:10.100710072-021-05612-5 PMID:34554334

Allen, A. B., & Leary, M. R. (2010). Self-compassion, stress, and coping. *Social and Personality Psychology Compass*, *4*(2), 107–118. doi:10.1111/j.1751-9004.2009.00246.x PMID:20686629

Allen, T. (2013). The work-family interface: a synthesis of research from industrial and organizational psychology. In I. Weiner (Ed.), Handbook of psychology (2nd ed., Vol. 12, pp. 698–718). Wiley.

Allen, T. D., & Kiburz, K. M. (2012). Trait mindfulness and work–family balance among working parents: The mediating effects of vitality and sleep quality. *Journal of Vocational Behavior*, *80*(2), 372–379. doi:10.1016/j.jvb.2011.09.002

Almhdawi, K. A. (2022). Influencing Medical Students' Knowledge and Attitudes Related to Disability: A Randomized Controlled Trial. *American Journal of Physical Medicine & Rehabilitation*, *101*(2), 113–118. doi:10.1097/PHM.0000000000001740 PMID:33657029

Almojali, A. I., Almalki, S. A., Alothman, A. S., Masuadi, E. M., & Alaqeel, M. K. (2017). The prevalence and association of stress with sleep quality among medical students. *Journal of Epidemiology and Global Health*, *7*(3), 169–174. doi:10.1016/j.jegh.2017.04.005 PMID:28756825

Alola, U. V., Avcı, T., & Öztüren, A. (2021). The nexus of workplace incivility and emotional exhaustion in hotel industry. *Journal of Public Affairs*, *21*(3), e2236. doi:10.1002/pa.2236

Alonazi, W. B. (2020). The impact of emotional intelligence on job performance during COVID-19 crisis: A cross-sectional analysis. *Psychology Research and Behavior Management*, *13*, 749–757. doi:10.2147/PRBM.S263656 PMID:33061691

Altamirano, M. A., & Collazo, C. E. R. (2020). Leading with emotional intelligence: How leaders of a diverse-based urban college in New York successfully respond to the COVID-19 crisis of 2020. *Communication is Robust when Nations Come Together: The Importance of Collaboration during a Global Crisis*.

Amatea, E. S., Cross, E. G., Clarke, J. E., & Bobby, C. L. (1986). Assessing the work and family role expectations of career-oriented men and women: The Life Role Salience Scales. *Journal of Marriage and Family*, *48*(4), 831–838. doi:10.2307/352576

Ambrose, M. S. (2011). Voluntary simplicity as an urban lifestyle: resisting a consumer economy/by Michelle Ambrose. Library and Archives Canada=Bibliothèque et Archives Canada.

American psychiatric Association. (2000). *Diagnostic and statistics: Manual of mental.* APA.

American Psychological Association (APA). (2020, May 30). *Stress in the time of COVID 19*. APA.

Amory, A. (2010). Education technology and hidden ideological contradictions. *Journal of Educational Technology & Society*, *13*(1), 69–79.

Ancona, D., Malone, T. W., Orlikowski, W. J., & Senge, P. M. (2007). In praise of the incomplete leader. *Harvard Business Review*, *85*(2). PMID:17345683

Anderson, T. (2016). Theories for Learning with Emerging Technologies. *Emerging Technologies in Distance Education, 7*(1), 7-23.

Anderson, C. M., & MacCurdy, M. M. (2000). *Writing and healing: Toward an informed practice*. National Council of Teachers of English.

Andersson, C., Stenfors, C. U. D., Lilliengren, P., Einhorn, S., & Osika, W. (2021). Benevolence – Associations with Stress, Mental Health, and Self-Compassion at the Workplace. *Frontiers in Psychology*, *12*, 568625. doi:10.3389/fpsyg.2021.568625 PMID:34140909

Andersson, L., & Pearson, C. (1999). Tit for tat? The spiralling effect of incivility in the workplace. *Academy of Management Review*, *24*(3), 452–471. doi:10.2307/259136

Anitha, J. (2014). Determinants of employee engagement and their impact on employee performance. *International Journal of Productivity and Performance Management*, *63*(3), 308–323. doi:10.1108/IJPPM-01-2013-0008

Antonakis, J. (2012). Transformational and charismatic leadership. *The Nature of Leadership*, 256-288.

Arias Gallegos, W. L., Huamani Cahua, J. C., & Ceballos Canaza, K. D. (2019). Burnout Syndrome in School Teachers and University Professors: A Psychometrical and Comparative Analysis from Arequipa City. *Journal of Educational Psychology-Propositos y Representaciones*, *7*(3), 92–113.

Arimitu, K., & Hofman, S. G. (2017). Effects of compassionate thinking on negative emotions. *Cognition and Emotion*, *31*(1), 160–167. doi:10.1080/02699931.2015.1078292 PMID:26362245

Arkorful, V. (2015). The role of e-learning, advantages and disadvantages of its adoption in higher education. *Int J Instruct Technol Distance Learn*, *12*(1), 29–42.

Armstrong, M. (2006). A handbook of human resource management practice (10th ed.). Kogan Page.

Arslan, G., Yıldırım, M., Karataş, Z., Kabasakal, Z., & Kılınç, M. (2020). Meaningful living to promote complete mental health among university students in the context of the COVID-19 pandemic. *International Journal of Mental Health and Addiction*, 1–13. doi:10.100711469-020-00416-8 PMID:33169074

Arvanitis, S. (2005). Modes of labour flexibility at firm level: Are there any implications for performance and innovation? Evidence for the Swiss economy. *Industrial and Corporate Change*, *14*(6).

Arvidsdotter, T., Marklund, B., Kylén, S., Taft, C., & Ekman, I. (2016). Understanding persons with psychological distress in primary health care. *Scandinavian Journal of Caring Sciences*, *30*(4), 687–694. doi:10.1111cs.12289 PMID:26463897

Aryee, S., Srinivas, E. S., & Tan, H. H. (2005). Rhythms of life: Antecedents and outcomes of work–family balance in employed parents. *The Journal of Applied Psychology*, *90*(1), 132–146. doi:10.1037/0021-9010.90.1.132 PMID:15641894

Asamoah-Appiah, W., & Aggrey-Fynn, I. (2017). The impact of occupational stress on employee's performance: A study at Twifo oil palm plantation limited. *African Journal of Applied Research*, *3*(1), 14–25.

Asiedu-Appiah, F., Dufie-Marfo, I., & Frempong, E. (2016). *Work-life balance as a tool for stress management in selected banking institutions in Ghana*. Academic Press.

Asmundson, G. J., Paluszek, M. M., Landry, C. A., Rachor, G. S., McKay, D., & Taylor, S. (2020). Do pre-existing anxiety-related and mood disorders differentially impact COVID-19 stress responses and coping? *Journal of Anxiety Disorders*, *74*, 102271. doi:10.1016/j.janxdis.2020.102271 PMID:32673930

Atheya, R., & Arora, R. (2014). Stress and its brunt on employee's work-life balance (wlb): A conceptual study. *IOSR Journal of Humanities and Social Science, 19*(3), 58-61.

Atulkar, S., & Kesari, B. (2018). Role of consumer traits and situational factors on impulse buying: Does gender matter? *International Journal of Retail & Distribution Management*, *46*(4), 386–405. Advance online publication. doi:10.1108/IJRDM-12-2016-0239

Aunión, J. A., & Romero, J. M. (2020). *Educación: cómoreparar los destrozos*. Madrid: El País. Available online at: https://elpais. com/ideas/2020-09-05/educacion-como-reparar-los-destrozos. html

Avolio, B. J., Walumbwa, F. O., & Weber, T. J. (2009). Leadership: Current theories, research, and future directions. *Annual Review of Psychology*, *60*(1), 421–449. doi:10.1146/annurev.psych.60.110707.163621 PMID:18651820

Azorín, C. (2020). Beyond COVID-19 supernova. Is another education coming? *Journal of Professional Capital and Community*, *5*(3), 381–390. doi:10.1108/JPCC-05-2020-0019

Baba, M. M. (2020). Navigating COVID-19 with emotional intelligence. *The International Journal of Social Psychiatry*, *66*(8), 810–820. doi:10.1177/0020764020934519 PMID:32583710

Babicka-Wirkus, A., Wirkus, L., Stasiak, K., & Kozłowski, P. (2021). University students' strategies of coping with stress during the coronavirus pandemic: Data from Poland. *PLoS One*, *16*(7), e0255041. doi:10.1371/journal.pone.0255041 PMID:34310649

Bacchus, D. N. (2008). Coping with work-related stress: A study of the use of coping resources among professional *Black women. Journal of Ethnic & Cultural Diversity in Social Work*, *17*(1), 60–81. doi:10.1080/15313200801906443

Badgaiyan, A. J., & Verma, A. (2015). Does urge to buy impulsively differ from impulsive buying behaviour? Assessing the impact of situational factors. *Journal of Retailing and Consumer Services*, *22*, 145–157. doi:10.1016/j.jretconser.2014.10.002

Baesu, C. (2019). Leadership based on emotional intelligence in modern organizations. *The USV Annals of Economics and Public Administration*, *18*(28), 73-78.

Bagozzi, R. P., Gopinath, M., & Nyer, P. U. (1999). The role of emotions in marketing. *Journal of the Academy of Marketing Science*, *27*(2), 184–206. doi:10.1177/0092070399272005

Bagozzi, R. P., & Yi, Y. (1988). On the evaluation of structural equation models. *Journal of the Academy of Marketing Science*, *16*(1), 74–94. doi:10.1007/BF02723327

Bakırtaş, H. (2013). SOR paradigması temelinde mağaza atmosferi ve duyguların pazarlamadaki önemi: bir literatür incelemesi. *Karamanoğlu Mehmetbey Üniversitesi Sosyal ve Ekonomik Araştırmalar Dergisi, 2013*(2), 47-55. https://dergipark.org.tr/en/pub/kmusekad/issue/10211/125472

Balderjahn, I., Lee, M. S., Seegebarth, B., & Peyer, M. (2020). A sustainable pathway to consumer well-being. The role of anticonsumption and consumer empowerment. *The Journal of Consumer Affairs*, *54*(2), 456–488. doi:10.1111/joca.12278

Balderjahn, I., Seegebarth, B., & Lee, M. S. (2021). Less is more! The rationale behind the decision-making style of voluntary simplifiers. *Journal of Cleaner Production*, *284*, 124802. doi:10.1016/j.jclepro.2020.124802

Bandura, A. (1990). Perceived self-efficacy in the exercise of control over AIDS infection. *Evaluation and Program Planning*, *13*(1), 9–17. doi:10.1016/0149-7189(90)90004-G

Banerjee, D., & Rai, M. (2020). Social isolation in COVID-19: The impact of loneliness. *The International Journal of Social Psychiatry*, *66*(6), 525–527. doi:10.1177/0020764020922269 PMID:32349580

Banjanirat. (2022). Stress and burnout during crisis. *Journal of Higher Education*, *97*(8), 1603-1609.

Bansal, R., & Pruthi, N. (2021). Developing Customer Engagement Through social media: A Review of Literature. *Marketing 5.0: Putting Up Blocks Together, 80.*

Bansal, R., Shuklaa, G., & Pruthi, N. (n.d.). *Higher education sector in India: Disruptions by COVID-19 and post covid trends*. Academic Press.

Bansal, R. (2017). Challenges and future trends in commerce education in India. *International Journal of Techno-Management Research*, *5*(3), 25–35.

Bansal, R. (2018). Stress management at workplace. *International Journal of Techno-Management Research*, *5*(04), 29–32.

Bansal, R., Gupta, A., Singh, R., & Nassa, V. K. (2021, July). Role and impact of digital technologies in E-learning amidst COVID-19 pandemic. In *2021 Fourth International Conference on Computational Intelligence and Communication Technologies (CCICT)* (pp. 194-202). IEEE. 10.1109/CCICT53244.2021.00046

Bansal, R., Masood, R., & Dadhich, V. (2014). Social media marketing-a tool of innovative marketing. *Journal of Organizational Management*, *3*(1), 1–7.

Bansal, R., & Minocha, K. (2017). Impact of social media on Consumer Attitude Towards A Brand With Special Reference to Hospitality Industry. *International Research Journal of Management and Commerce*, *4*(8), 106–120.

Bansal, R., & Saini, S. (2022). Exploring the Role of social media: An Innovative Tool for Entrepreneurs. In *Applying Metalytics to Measure Customer Experience in the Metaverse* (pp. 34–43). IGI Global. doi:10.4018/978-1-6684-6133-4.ch004

Bansal, R., & Saini, S. (2022). Leveraging role of social media influencers in corporate world-An overview. *NOLEGEIN-Journal of Global Marketing*, *5*(1), 1–5.

Banth, S., & Talwar, C. (2012). Anasakti, the Hindu ideal, and its relationship to well-being and orientations to happiness. *Journal of Religion and Health*, *51*(3), 934–946. doi:10.100710943-010-9402-3 PMID:20953711

Barakat, M. A. (2019). A proposed model for factors affecting consumers' impulsive buying tendency in shopping malls. *Journal of Marketing Management*, *7*(1), 120–134. doi:10.15640/jmm.v7n1a10

Barkley, J. E., Lepp, A., Glickman, E., Farnell, G., Beiting, J., Wiet, R., & Dowdell, B. (2020). The acute effects of the COVID-19 pandemic on physical activity and sedentary behavior in university students and employees. *International Journal of Exercise Science*, *13*(5), 1326. PMID:33042377

Barlow, D. H. (1988). *Anxiety and Its Disorders*. The Guilford Press.

Barnett, R. C., & Hyde, J. S. (2001). Women, men, work, and family. *The American Psychologist*, *56*(10), 781–796. doi:10.1037/0003-066X.56.10.781 PMID:11675985

Baron, R., & Neuman, J. (1996). Workplace violence and workplace aggression: Evidence on their relative frequency and potential causes. *Aggressive Behavior*, *221*(3), 161–173. doi:10.1002/(SICI)1098-2337(1996)22:3<161::AID-AB1>3.0.CO;2-Q

Bartoszek, A., Walkowiak, D., Bartoszek, A., & Kardas, G. (2020). Mental well-being (depression, loneliness, insomnia, daily life fatigue) during COVID-19 related home-confinement—A study from Poland. *International Journal of Environmental Research and Public Health*, *17*(20), 7417. doi:10.3390/ijerph17207417 PMID:33053787

Bashar, A., Ahmad, I., & Wasiq, M. (2013). A study of influence of demographic factors on consumer impulse buying behavior. *Journal of Management Research*, *13*(3).

Bates, A. (2018). *Teaching in a digital age: Guidelines for designing teaching and learning for a digital age*. Tony Bates Associates Ltd.

Batista, E. C., Matos, L. A. L., & Nascimento, A. B. (2017). A entrevista como técnica de investigação na pesquisa qualitativa. *Revista Interdisciplinar Científica Aplicada*, *11*(3), 23–38.

Baumeister, R. F. (2002). Yielding to temptation: Self-control failure, impulsive purchasing, and consumer behavior. *The Journal of Consumer Research*, *28*(4), 670–676. doi:10.1086/338209

Bayram, N., & Bilgel, N. (2008). The prevalence and socio-demographic correlations of depression, anxiety and stress among a group of university students. *Social Psychiatry and Psychiatric Epidemiology*, *43*(8), 667–672. doi:10.100700127-008-0345-x PMID:18398558

Bean-Mellinger, B. (2017). *Six leadership styles*. Academic Press.

Beddoes-Jones, F., & Swailes, S. (2015). Authentic leadership: Development of a new three pillar model. *Strategic HR Review*, *14*(3), 94–99. doi:10.1108/SHR-04-2015-0032

Beecher, T. S. (2007). *Questioning the consumer culture: A qualitative study on voluntary simplicity [PhD]*. University of North Dakota.

Bekin, C., Carrigan, M., & Szmigin, I. (2005). Defying marketing sovereignty: Voluntary simplicity at new consumption communities. *Qualitative Market Research*, *8*(4), 413–429. doi:10.1108/13522750510619779

Bellosta-Batalla, M., Blanco-Gandía, M. C., Rodríguez-Arias, M., Cebolla, A., Pérez-Blasco, J., & Moya-Albiol, L. (2020). Increased Salivary Oxytocin and Empathy in Students of Clinical and Health Psychology After a Mindfulness and Compassion-Based Intervention. *Mindfulness, 11*(4), 1006–1017. doi:10.100712671-020-01316-7

Bennett, S., Maton, K., & Kervin, L. (2008). The 'digital natives' debate: A critical review of the evidence. *British Journal of Educational Technology, 39*(5), 775–786. doi:10.1111/j.1467-8535.2007.00793.x

Bergner, S. (2021). The role of the European Union in global health: The EU's self-perception (s) within the COVID-19 pandemic. *Health Policy (Amsterdam).* PMID:34802748

Berkman, L. F., & Syme, S. L. (1979). Social network, host resistance, and mortality: A nine-year follow-up of study of Alamed county residents. *American Journal of Epidemiology, 109*(2), 186–204. doi:10.1093/oxfordjournals.aje.a112674 PMID:425958

Berry, S. (2020). *An Assessment of Acne, Stress, and Psychological Symptoms in College Students: A Daily Diary Study.* Academic Press.

BerryL.MirabitoA. M.BaunW. B. (2020). What's the hard return on employee wellness programs? SSRN.

Besser, A., Lotem, S., & Zeigler-Hill, V. (2020). Psychological stress and vocal symptoms among university professors in Israel: Implications of the shift to online synchronous teaching during the COVID-19 pandemic. *Journal of Voice.* PMID:32600872

Bhandari, K., & Soni, H. (2015). Impact of Gender, Age and Work Experience on Satisfaction towards Work Life Balance (with special reference to Bank of Baroda, Udaipur). *IOSR Journal of Business and Managemen, 17*(3). doi:10.9790/487X-17324853

Bharathi, K., & Sudha, S. (2017). Store ambiance influence on consumer impulsive buying behavior towards apparel: SOR model. *Indian Journal of Public Health Research & Development, 8*(4), 4140. doi:10.5958/0976-5506.2017.00329.1

Bhatia, A., & Mohsin, F. (2020). Determinants of college teachers' hapinness- A comprehensive review. *J.Crit. Rev., 7*(9), 9–17.

Bhattacharya, K., & Preissle, J. (2003). *Ethics and Research Interviewing.* Paper presented at the American Educational Studies Association, Mexico City, Mexico.

Bhumika. (2020). Challenges for work-life balance during COVID-19 induced nationwide lockdown: exploring gender difference in emotional exhaustion in the Indian setting. *Gender in Management, 35*(7-8), 705-718.

Bibliotherapy. (n.d.). *Good Therapy.* www.goodtherapy.org/learn-about-therapy/types/bibliotherapy

Bigham, E., McDannel, L., Luciano, I., & Salgado-Lopez, G. (2014). Effect of a Brief Guided Imagery on Stress. *Biofeedback, 42*(1), 28–35. doi:10.5298/1081-5937-42.1.07

Blau, G., & Andersson, L. (2005). Testing a measure of instigated incivility. *Journal of Occupational and Organizational Psychology, 78*(4), 595–614. doi:10.1348/096317905X26822

Blau, P. M. (1964). *Exchange and power in social life.* John Wiley and Sons.

Boermans, S., Delahaij, R., Korteling, H., & Euwema, M. (2012). Training Resilience for High-risk Environments: Towards a Strength-based Approach within the Military. In International Handbook of Workplace Trauma Support (pp. 313–330). John Wiley & Sons, Ltd. doi:10.1002/9781119943242.ch20

Bokde, V., Kharbikar, H. L., Roy, M. L., Joshi, P., & Ga, A. (2020). Possible impacts of COVID-19 pandemic and lockdown on education sector in India. *Food and Scientific Reports, 1*(Special Issue), 30–33.

Bolden, R., Gosling, J., Marturano, A., & Dennison, P. (2003). *A review of leadership theory and Competency frameworks*. Centre for leadership studies, University of Exeter. Retrieved on January 21, 2023 from http//: centers.exeter.ac.uk/cls/documents/mgmt.sandardspdf

Bonanno, G. A., & Diminish, E. D. (2012). *Annual Research Review: Positive adjustment to adversity—trajectories of minimal-impact resilience and emergent resilience*. Advance online publication. doi:10.1111/jcpp.12021 PMID:23215790

Bono, J., Glomb, T., Shen, W., Kim, E., & Koch, A. (2013). Building positive resources: Effects of positive events and positive reflection on work stress and health. *Academy of Management Journal*, *56*(6), 1601–1627. doi:10.5465/amj.2011.0272

Bosma, A. R., Boot, C. R. L., De Maaker, M., Boeije, H. R., Schoonmade, L. J., Anema, J. R., & Schaafsma, F. G. (2019). Exploring self-control of workers with a chronic condition: A qualitative synthesis. *European Journal of Work and Organizational Psychology*, *28*(5), 653–668. doi:10.1080/1359432X.2019.1631801

Bösselmann, V., Amatriain-Fernández, S., Gronwald, T., Murillo-Rodríguez, E., Machado, S., & Budde, H. (2021). Physical activity, boredom and fear of COVID-19 among adolescents in Germany. *Frontiers in Psychology*, *12*, 624206. Advance online publication. doi:10.3389/fpsyg.2021.624206 PMID:34012413

Boujbel, L., & d'Astous, A. (2012). Voluntary simplicity and life satisfaction: Exploring the mediating role of consumption desires. *Journal of Consumer Behaviour*, *11*(6), 487–494. doi:10.1002/cb.1399

Bower, G. H. (1981). Mood and memory. *The American Psychologist*, *36*(2), 129–148. doi:10.1037/0003-066X.36.2.129 PMID:7224324

Boyatzis, R., Boyatzis, R. E., & McKee, A. (2005). *Resonant leadership: Renewing yourself and connecting with others through mindfulness, hope, and compassion*. Harvard Business Press.

Bradberry. (2016). *Why The Best Leaders Have Conviction*. https://www.forbes.com/sites/travisbradberry/2016/06/28/why-the-best-leaders-have-conviction/?sh=231474001c8d

Brailovskaia, J., Cosci, F., Mansueto, G., Miragall, M., Herrero, R., Baños, R. M., Krasavtseva, Y., Kochetkov, Y., & Margraf, J. (2021). The association between depression symptoms, psychological burden caused by Covid-19 and physical activity: An investigation in Germany, Italy, Russia, and Spain. *Psychiatry Research*, *295*, 113596. doi:10.1016/j.psychres.2020.113596 PMID:33261924

Branco, F., & Farçadas, M. (2012). O Serviço Social nos cuidados de saúde primários: contexto, perspetivas e desafios. In M. I. Carvalho (Ed.), *Serviço Social na Saúde* (pp. 1–24). Pactor.

Braun, S.S., Schonert-Reichl, K.A., & Roeser, R.W. (2020). Effects of teachers' emotion regulation, burnout, and satisfaction with life on student well-being. *J. Appl. Dev Psychol. 69*, 1–13.

Braun, V., & Clarke, V. (2006). Using thematic analysis in psychology. *Qualitative Research in Psychology*, *3*(2), 77–101. doi:10.1191/1478088706qp063oa

Breins, J. G., & Chen, S. (2012). Self-compassion increases self-improvement motivation. *Personality and Social Psychology Bulletin*, *38*(9), 1133–1143. doi:10.1177/0146167212445599 PMID:22645164

Brief, A. (1998). *Attitudes in and Around Organizations*. Thousand Oaks ed. CA. *Sage (Atlanta, Ga.)*.

Brito-Pons, G., Campos, D., & Cebolla, A. (2018). Implicit or explicit compassion? Effects of Compassion Cultivation Training and comparison with Mindfulness-based Stress Reduction. *Mindfulness*, *9*(5), 1494–1508. doi:10.100712671-018-0898-z

Brooker, R. W., Kikvidze, Z., Kunstler, G., Liancourt, P., & Seifan, M. (2013). The concept and measurement of importance: A comment on Rees et al. 2012. *Journal of Ecology, 101*(6), 1369–1378. Advance online publication. doi:10.1111/1365-2745.12164

Brooks, S. K., Webster, R. K., Smith, L. E., Woodland, L., Wessely, S., Greenberg, N., & Rubin, G. J. (2020). The psychological impact of quarantine and how to reduce it: Rapid review of the evidence. *Lancet, 395*(10227), 912–920. doi:10.1016/S0140-6736(20)30460-8 PMID:32112714

Brough, P., & O'Driscoll, M. (2005). Work-family conflict and stress. In A. Antoniou & C. Cooper (Eds.), *Research companion to organizational Health Psychology* (pp. 346–365). Edward Elgar Publisher. doi:10.4337/9781845423308.00032

Brough, P., O'Driscoll, M. P., & Kalliath, T. J. (2007). Work-family conflict and facilitation: achieving workfamily balance. In A. I. Glendon, B. M. Thompson, & B. Myors (Eds.), *Advances in organisational psychology* (pp. 73–92). Australian Academic Press.

Buffer. (2020). *The 2020 state of remote work.* Retrieved from https://lp.buffer.com/state-of-remote-work-2020

Bunk, J. A., & Magley, V. J. (2013). The role of appraisals and emotions in understanding experiences of workplace incivility. *Journal of Occupational Health Psychology, 18*(1), 87–105. doi:10.1037/a0030987 PMID:23339748

Burke, R. J., & Richardsen, A. M. (2014). Corporate wellness programs: An overview. In Corporate wellness programs: Linking employee and organizational health. Edward Elgar Publishing.

Burke, R. J., Moodie, S., Dolan, S. L., & Fiksenbaum, L. (2012). *Job demands, social support, work satisfaction and psychological well-being among nurses in Spain.* ESADE Business School Research Paper, (233).

Burrows, V. (2015). *The medicalization of stress: Hans Selye and the transformation of the postwar medical marketplace.* City University of New York.

Byron, K. (2008). Carrying too heavy a load? The communication and miscommunication of emotion by email. *Academy of Management Review, 33*(2), 309–327. doi:10.5465/amr.2008.31193163

Cachón-Zagalaz, J., Sánchez-Zafra, M., Sanabrias-Moreno, D., González-Valero, G., Lara-Sánchez, A. J., & Zagalaz-Sánchez, M. L. (2020). Systematic review of the literature about the effects of the COVID-19 pandemic on the lives of school children. *Frontiers in Psychology, 11*, 2457. doi:10.3389/fpsyg.2020.569348 PMID:33162910

Cacioppo, J. T., Hawkley, L. C., Berntson, G. G., Ernst, J. M., Gibbs, A. C., Stickgold, R., & Hobson, J. A. (2002). Do lonely days invade the nights? Potential social modulation of sleep efficiency. *Psychological Science, 13*(4), 384–387. doi:10.1111/1467-9280.00469 PMID:12137144

Caldwell, C. (2009). Identity, self-awareness, and self-deception: Ethical implications for leaders and organizations. *Journal of Business Ethics, 90*(S3), 393–406. doi:10.100710551-010-0424-2

Callahan, K., Christman, G., & Maltby, L. (2018). Battling burnout: Strategies for promoting physician wellness. *Advances in Pediatrics, 65*(1), 1–17. doi:10.1016/j.yapd.2018.03.001 PMID:30053918

Cameroon COVID-19 situation report. (2021). World Health Organization Publication in UNOCHA.

Caraballo, V., & Gates, D. (2011). *Innovation Among Latinos: Exploring Differences Across Genders.* Universidad y Empresa, Universidad del Rosario.

Cardoso, J., Vilar, D., & Casquilho-Martins, I. (2020). Desafios ao Serviço Social no contexto da COVID-19. *Intervenção Social, 55/56*, 9–87. doi:10.34628/9y57-1x20

Carlson, D. S., Kacmar, K. M., Wayne, J. H., & Grzywacz, J. G. (2006). Measuring the positive side of the workfamily interface: Development and validation of a work-family enrichment scale. *Journal of Vocational Behavior*, *68*(1), 131–164. doi:10.1016/j.jvb.2005.02.002

Carnevale, J. B., & Hatak, I. (2020). Employee adjustment and well-being in the era of COVID-19: Implications for human resource management. *Journal of Business Research*, *116*, 183–187. doi:10.1016/j.jbusres.2020.05.037 PMID:32501303

Carney, T., & Stanford, J. (2018). *The dimensions of insecure work: A factbook*. Retrieved from Canberra: https://www.tai.org.au/sites/default/files/Insecure_Work_Factbook.pdf

Carrera, J. F. G. F. (2011). *Stress e Burnout: um estudo de caso de assistentes sociais que trabalham com idosos em IPSS's* [Master's Thesis, Instituto Superior de Ciências Sociais e Políticas]. http://hdl.handle.net/10400.5/3097

Carrillo-Gonzalez, A., Camargo-Mendoza, M., & Cantor-Cutiva, L. C. (2021). Relationship between sleep quality and stress with voice functioning among college professors: A systematic review and meta-analysis. *Journal of Voice*, *35*(3), 499–e13. doi:10.1016/j.jvoice.2019.11.001 PMID:31866075

Carter, T., & Gilovich, T. (2010). The relative relativity of material and experiential purchases. *Journal of Personality and Social Psychology*, *98*(1), 146–159. doi:10.1037/a0017145 PMID:20053039

Cartmill, C. (2020). New survey shows 87% of staff wish to work from home in post lockdown world. *Belfast Newsletter, 28.*

Carvalho, M. I. (Ed.). (2012). *Serviço Social na Saúde*. Pactor.

Carver, C. S. (1997). You want to measure coping but your protocol'too long: Consider the brief cope. *International Journal of Behavioral Medicine*, *4*(1), 92–100. doi:10.120715327558ijbm0401_6 PMID:16250744

Casagrande, M., Favieri, F., Tambelli, R., & Forte, G. (2020). The enemy who sealed the world: Effects quarantine due to the COVID-19 on sleep quality, anxiety, and psychological distress in the Italian population. *Sleep Medicine*, *75*, 12–20. doi:10.1016/j.sleep.2020.05.011 PMID:32853913

Casquilho-Martins, I. (2022). Consequences of COVID-19: Limitations to the Quality of Palliative Care and Social Work Intervention. *Journal of Social Work in End-of-Life & Palliative Care*, *18*(3), 195–198. doi:10.1080/15524256.2022.2050338 PMID:35333687

Casquilho-Martins, I., & Ferreira, S. (2022). Migrants' Health Policies and Access to Health Care in Portugal within the European Framework. *Societies (Basel, Switzerland)*, *12*(2), 55. doi:10.3390oc12020055

Chaaya, C., Devi Thambi, V., Sabuncu, Ö., Abedi, R., Osman Ahmed Osman, A., Uwishema, O., & Onyeaka, H. (2022). Ukraine – Russia crisis and its impacts on the mental health of Ukrainian young people during the COVID-19 pandemic. *Annals of Medicine and Surgery (London)*, *79*, 104033. doi:10.1016/j.amsu.2022.104033 PMID:35765517

Chakravorty, A., & Singh, P. (2020). Work/family interference and burnout among primary school teachers: The moderating role of emotional intelligence. *Decision (Washington, D.C.)*, *47*(3), 251–264.

Chang, H. H. (2021). Exploring consumer behavioral predispositions toward voluntary simplicity. *Current Psychology (New Brunswick, N.J.)*, *40*(2), 731–743. doi:10.100712144-018-9994-4

Chang, H. H., Tsai, Y. C., Chen, S. H., Huang, G. H., & Tseng, Y. H. (2015). Building long-term partnerships by certificate implementation: A social exchange theory perspective. *Journal of Business and Industrial Marketing*, *30*(7), 867–879. doi:10.1108/JBIM-08-2013-0190

Chang, H. J., Eckman, M., & Yan, R. N. (2011). Application of the Stimulus-Organism-Response model to the retail environment: The role of hedonic motivation in impulse buying behavior. *International Review of Retail, Distribution and Consumer Research*, *21*(3), 233–249. doi:10.1080/09593969.2011.578798

Chang, W.-H. (2020). Understanding the COVID-19 pandemic from a gender perspective. *Taiwanese Journal of Obstetrics & Gynecology*, *59*(6), 801–807. doi:10.1016/j.tjog.2020.09.004 PMID:33218392

Chan, X. W., Kalliath, T., Brough, P., Siu, O. L., O'Driscoll, M. P., & Timms, C. (2016). Work–family enrichment and satisfaction: The mediating role of self-efficacy and work–life balance. *International Journal of Human Resource Management*, *27*(15), 1755–1776. doi:10.1080/09585192.2015.1075574

Chao, M., Chen, X., Liu, T., Yang, H., & Hall, B. J. (2020). Psychological distress and state boredom during the COVID-19 outbreak in China: The role of meaning in life and media use. *European Journal of Psychotraumatology*, *11*(1), 1769379. doi:10.1080/20008198.2020.1769379 PMID:33029315

Chauhan, S., Banerjee, R., & Dagar, V. (2021). Analysis of impulse buying behaviour of consumer during COVID-19: An empirical study. *Millennial Asia*. Advance online publication. doi:10.1177/09763996211041215

Chellingsworth, M., Farrand, P., & Rayson, K. (2013). *Dealing with worry. CEDAR*. University of Exeter.

Chen, C. C., & Yao, J. Y. (2018). What drives impulse buying behaviors in a mobile auction? The perspective of the Stimulus-Organism-Response model. *Telematics and Informatics*, *35*(5), 1249–1262. doi:10.1016/j.tele.2018.02.007

Chin, S. T. S., Anantharaman, R. N., & Tong, D. Y. K. (2011). The roles of emotional intelligence and spiritual intelligence at the workplace. *Journal of Human Resources Management Research*, *2011*, 1–9. doi:10.5171/2011.582992

Chodron, P. (2001). *Tonglen: The Path of Transformation*. Shambhala.

Choi, H. M., Mohammad, A. A., & Kim, W. G. (2019). Understanding hotel frontline employees' emotional intelligence, emotional labor, job stress, coping strategies and burnout. *International Journal of Hospitality Management*, *82*, 199–208. doi:10.1016/j.ijhm.2019.05.002

Choi, L., Lee, S., No, S.-R., & Kim, E. I. (2016). Effects of Compassion on Employees' Self-regulation. *Social Behavior and Personality*, *44*(7), 1173–1190. doi:10.2224bp.2016.44.7.1173

Chowdhury, M. R. (2019, April 30). Compassion in the workplace: 9+ examples and tips for leaders. *Positive Psychology*. https://positivepsychology.com/compassion-at-work-leadership/#comment-list

Chung, H., Quan, W., Koo, B., Ariza-Montes, A., Vega-Muñoz, A., Giorgi, G., & Han, H. (2021). A Threat of Customer Incivility and Job Stress to Hotel Employee Retention: Do Supervisor and Co-Worker Supports Reduce Turnover Rates? *International Journal of Environmental Research and Public Health*, *18*(12), 6616. doi:10.3390/ijerph18126616 PMID:34205422

Çınar, D. (2021). A research on the evaluation of consumers' voluntary simplicity lifestyle tendency in the Covid-19 period. *International Journal of Social Sciences and Education Research*, *7*(1), 12–23. doi:10.24289/ijsser.832065

Cladellas-Pros, R., Castelló-Tarrida, A., & Parrado-Romero, E. (2018). Satisfaction, health, and work-related stress of the university professorship according to their contractual status. *Revista de Salud Publica (Bogota, Colombia)*, *20*(1), 53–59. PMID:30183885

Clark, S., McGrane, A., Boyle, N., Joksimovic, N., Burke, L., Rock, N., & O' Sullivan, K. (2021). You're a teacher you're a mother, you're a worker. In Gender Inequality during COVID-19 in Ireland. Academic Press.

Clark. (2020). *8 Ways to Manage Your Team While Social Distancing*. https://hbr.org/2020/03/8-ways-to-manage-your-team-while-social-distancing

Clarke, V., Braun, V., & Hayfield, N. (2015). Thematic analysis. *Qualitative Psychology: A Practical Guide to Research Methods, 3*, 222-248.

Clark, M. S., & Isen, A. M. (1982). Toward understanding the relationship between feeling states and social behavior. In A. Hastorf & A. M. Isen (Eds.), *Cognitive socialpsychology* (pp. 73–108). Elsevier.

Clark, S. C. (2000). Work/family border theory: A new theory of work/family balance. *Human Relations, 53*(6), 747–770. doi:10.1177/0018726700536001

Colonnello, V., Petrocchi, N., & Heinrichs, M. (2017). The psychobiological foundation of prosocial relationships: The role of oxytocin in daily social exchanges. In P. Gilbert (Ed.), *Compassion: Concepts, research, and applications*. Routledge. doi:10.4324/9781315564296-6

Colucci, E., Nadeau, S., Higgins, J., Kehayia, E., Poldma, T., Saj, A., & de Guise, E. (2022). COVID-19 lock-downs' effects on the quality of life, perceived health and well-being of healthy elderly individuals: A longitudinal comparison of pre-lockdown and lock-down states of well-being. *Archives of Gerontology and Geriatrics, 99*, 104606. doi:10.1016/j.archger.2021.104606 PMID:34896795

Comissão Nacional de Cuidados Paliativos. (2021). *Plano Estratégico para o Desenvolvimento dos Cuidados Paliativos 2021–2022*. http://www.acss.min-saude.pt/wp-content/uploads/2017/01/PEDCP-2021_2022.pdf

Connelly, J. (2020). *The experience of voluntary simplicity: A consensual qualitative research study* [Unpublished doctoral dissertation]. Marquette University.

Conselho Nacional de Saúde. (2020). *Portugal e a resposta à covid-19 a posição do Conselho Nacional de Saúde e o contributo das entidades que o constituem*. https://www.cns.min-saude.pt/wp-content/uploads/2020/10/CNS_Reflexao-Conselho-Nacional-Saude-resposta-COVID-19.pdf

Consolo, K., Fusner, S., & Staib, S. (2008). Effects of diaphragmatic breathing on stress levels of nursing students. *Teaching and Learning in Nursing, 3*(2), 67–71. doi:10.1016/j.teln.2007.10.003

Conversano, C., Di Giuseppe, M., Miccoli, M., Ciacchini, R., Gemignani, A., & Orrù, G. (2020). Mindfulness, age and gender as protective factors against psychological distress during COVID-19 pandemic. *Frontiers in Psychology, 11*, 1900. doi:10.3389/fpsyg.2020.01900 PMID:33013503

Cooper, C. L., & Marshall, J. (1976). Occupational sources of stress: A review of the literature relating to coronary heart disease and mental ill health. *Journal of Occupational Psychology, 49*(1), 11–28. doi:10.1111/j.2044-8325.1976.tb00325.x

Copeland, M. E. (1998). *The worry control workbook*. New Harbinger Pubns Inc.

Corbin, C. B., & Pangrazi, R. P. (2001). Toward a uniform definition of wellness: A commentary. *President's council on physical fitness and sports research digest*.

Cornelius, J. (2017). *Five minute meditation used to impact workplace meetings* [Doctoral dissertation]. Pepperdine University.

Cortina, L., Magley, V., Williams, J., & Langhout, R. (2001). Incivility in the workplace: Incidence and impact. *Journal of Occupational Health Psychology, 6*(1), 64–80. doi:10.1037/1076-8998.6.1.64 PMID:11199258

Courtois, C. A. (2019). *Understanding Complex Trauma, Complex Reactions, and Treatment Approaches*. aaets.org.

Craig-Lees, M., & Hill, C. (2002). Understanding voluntary simplifiers. *Psychology and Marketing*, *19*(2), 187–210. doi:10.1002/mar.10009

Crayne, M. P., & Medeiros, K. E. (2021). Making sense of crisis: Charismatic, ideological, and pragmatic leadership in response to COVID-19. *The American Psychologist*, *76*(3), 462–474. doi:10.1037/amp0000715 PMID:32772539

Cresswell, J. W. (2003). *Research design: Qualitative, quantitative, and mixed methods approach* (2nd ed.). Sage Publications.

Creswell, J. W. (2014). *Research Design: Qualitative*. Quantitative and Mixed Methods.

Creswell, J. W., & Poth, C. N. (2016). *Qualitative inquiry and research design: Choosing among five approaches*. Sage publications.

Cropanzano, R., & Wright, T. A. (2001). When a" happy" worker is really a" productive" worker: A review and further refinement of the happy-productive worker thesis. *Consulting Psychology Journal: Practice and Research*, *53*(3), 182-199.

Cropanzano, R., & Mitchell, M. S. (2005). Social exchange theory: An interdisciplinary review. *Journal of Management*, *31*(6), 874–900. doi:10.1177/0149206305279602

Cropanzano, R., & Wright, T. A. (1999). A 5-year study of change in the relationship between well-being and job performance. *Consulting Psychology Journal*, *51*(4), 252–265. doi:10.1037/1061-4087.51.4.252

Csikszentmihalyi, M., & Csikszentmihalyi, I. S. (2006). *A Life Worth Living: Contributions to Positive Psychology*. Oxford University Press.

Cuervo, T. C., Orviz, N. M., Arce, S. G., & Fernández, I. S. (2018). Technostressin Communication and Technology Society: Scoping Literature Review from the Web of Science. *Archivos de Prevencion de Riesgos Laborales*, 18–25. doi:10.12961 / aprl.2018.21.1.04

Currie, C., Molcho, M., Boyce, W., Holstein, B., Torsheim, T., & Richter, M. (2008). Researching health inequalities in adolescents: The development of the Health Behaviour in School-Aged Children (HBSC) family affluence scale. *Social Science & Medicine*, *66*(6), 1429–1436. doi:10.1016/j.socscimed.2007.11.024 PMID:18179852

D'ambra, A. M., & Andrews, D. R. (2014). Incivility, retention and new graduate nurses: An integrated review of the literature. *Journal of Nursing Management*, *22*(6), 735–742. doi:10.1111/jonm.12060 PMID:23927565

D'Auria, G., & De Smet, A. (2020). Leadership in a crisis: Responding to the coronavirus outbreak and future challenges. *Psychology (Irvine, Calif.)*, *22*(2), 273–287.

D'Cruz, P., & Rayner, C. (2014). The incidence of interpersonal workplace bullying in India"s ITES-BPO sector. *Indian Journal of Labour Economics*, *57*(2), 221–242.

Dagli, R. (2020). Fear and anxiety-coping strategies during COVID-19 pandemic in lockdown. *Journal of International Oral Health: JIOH*, *12*(3), 187–188. doi:10.4103/JIOH.JIOH_133_20

Dalai Lama & Cutler, H. C. (1998). *The art of happiness*. Riverhead Books.

Dalai Lama. (1995). *The power of compassion*. HarperCollins.

Dana Di Pardo, L.-H. (2021). *What is the difference between didactics and pedagogy in reflective teaching. Disorders*.

Dangi, R. R., & George, M. (2020). Psychological perception of students during COVID-19 outbreak in India. *High Technology Letters*, *26*(6), 142–144.

Dash, S. P. (2022). Post Pandemic: The New Advanced Society. *The New Advanced Society: Artificial Intelligence and Industrial Internet of Things Paradigm,* 1-14.

Das, S. S., & Mishra, S. A. (2016). A Study on Work Life Balance of Women Working in IT Sectors of Mumbai City. *International Journal of Humanities and Social Science Invention*, *5*(9), 43–47. www.ijhssi.org

Day, D. V. (2011). Leadership development. The SAGE Handbook of Leadership, 22, 37-50.

De Clercq, D., Haq, I. U., & Azeem, M. U. (2019). Time-related work stress and counterproductive work behavior: Invigorating roles of deviant personality traits. *Personnel Review*, *48*(7), 1756–1781. doi:10.1108/PR-07-2018-0241

de la Fucntc, J. (2017). Theory of self- vs. externally-regulated learning: Fundamentals, evidence, and applicability. *Frontiers in Psychology*, *8*, 1675. doi:10.3389/fpsyg.2017.01675 PMID:29033872

de la Fuente, J., Amate, J., González-Torres, M. C., Artuch, R., García-Torrecillas, J. M., & Fadda, S. (2020a). Effects of levels of self-regulation and regulatory teaching on strategies for coping with academic stress in undergraduate students. *Frontiers in Psychology*, *11*, 22. doi:10.3389/fpsyg.2020.00022 PMID:32082213

de la Fuente, J., Pachón-Basallo, M., Santos, F. H., González-Torres, M. C., Artuch Garde, R., Peralta-Sánchez, F. J., ... Gaeta, M. L. (2021). How has the COVID-19 crisis affected the academic stress of university students? The role of teachers and students. *Frontiers in Psychology*, *12*, 1554. doi:10.3389/fpsyg.2021.626340 PMID:34140911

de la Fuente, J., Peralta-Sánchez, F. J., Martínez-Vicente, J. M., Sander, P., Garzón-Umerenkova, A., & Zapata, L. (2020c). Effects of Self-Regulation vs. External Regulation on the Factors and Symptoms of Academic Stress in Undergraduate Students. *Frontiers in Psychology*, *11*, 1773. doi:10.3389/fpsyg.2020.01773 PMID:32982819

De Pedraza, P., Guzi, M., & Tijdens, K. (2020). *Life Dissatisfaction and Anxiety in COVID-19 pandemic* (No. 2020-03). MUNI ECON Working Paper.

De Vaus, D. (2001). Research design in social research. *Sage (Atlanta, Ga.).*

Değirmenci, B., Durmaz, Y., Fidanoğlu, A., & Değirmenci, S. (2023). Psychological effects of COVID-19 phobia on industrial consumers: A case study in Turkey. *Journal of Business and Industrial Marketing*, *38*(1), 170–187. doi:10.1108/JBIM-04-2021-0221

Deguchi, Y., Iwasaki, S., Konishi, A., Ishimoto, H., Ogawa, K., Fukuda, Y., Nitta, T., & Inoue, K. (2016). The Usefulness of Assessing and Identifying Workers' Temperaments and Their Effects on Occupational Stress in the Workplace. *PLoS One*, *11*(5), e0156339. doi:10.1371/journal.pone.0156339 PMID:27227771

Delahaij, R., Gaillard, A. W., & van Dam, K. (2010). Hardiness and the response to stressful situations: Investigating mediating processes. *Personality and Individual Differences*, *49*(5), 386–390. doi:10.1016/j.paid.2010.04.002

DeSarbo, W. S., & Edwards, E. A. (1996). Typologies of compulsive buying behavior: A constrained clusterwise regression approach. *Journal of Consumer Psychology*, *5*(3), 231–262. doi:10.120715327663jcp0503_02

Dever, C., & Justice, G. (2020). *Coming together in crisis times.* Retrieved from https://www.insidehighered.com/advice/2020/03/27/during-pandemic-crisis-faculty-and-administrators-must-move-beyond-thei r

Dhobale, R. S. (2009). Stress Management Training: A Boon to Employee Wellness! *The IUP Journal of Soft Skills*, *3*(1), 39–44.

Di Blasi, M., Gullo, S., Mancinelli, E., Freda, M. F., Esposito, G., Gelo, O. C. G., ... Coco, G. L. (2021). Psychological distress associated with the COVID-19 lockdown: A two-wave network analysis. *Journal of Affective Disorders*, *284*, 18–26. doi:10.1016/j.jad.2021.02.016 PMID:33582428

Diener, E. (2000). Subjective well-being: The science of happiness and a proposal for a national index. *The American Psychologist*, *55*(1), 34–43. doi:10.1037/0003-066X.55.1.34 PMID:11392863

Dirani, K. M., Abadi, M., Alizadeh, A., Barhate, B., Garza, R. C., Gunasekara, N., Ibrahim, G., & Majzun, Z. (2020). Leadership competencies and the essential role of human resource development in times of crisis: A response to Covid-19 pandemic. *Human Resource Development International*, *23*(4), 380–394. doi:10.1080/13678868.2020.1780078

Dovey, C. (n.d.). Can Reading Make You Happier? *The New Yorker*. www.newyorker.com/culture/cultural-comment/can-reading-make-you-happier

Drigas, A., & Papoutsi, C. (2019). Emotional Intelligence as an Important Asset for HR in Organizations: Leaders and Employees. *International Journal of Advanced Corporate Learning*, *12*(1), 58. doi:10.3991/ijac.v12i1.9637

Droit-Volet, S., Gil, S., Martinelli, N., Andant, N., Clinchamps, M., Parreira, L., Rouffiac, K., Dambrun, M., Huguet, P., Dubuis, B., Pereira, B., Bouillon, J.-B., & Dutheil, F. (2020). Time and COVID-19 stress in the lockdown situation: Time free,«Dying» of boredom and sadness. *PLoS One*, *15*(8), e0236465. doi:10.1371/journal.pone.0236465 PMID:32776990

Drvaric, L., Gerritsen, C., Rashid, T., Bagby, R. M., & Mizrahi, R. (2015). High stress, low resilience in people at clinical high risk for psychosis: Should we consider a strengths-based approach? *Canadian Psychology*, *56*(3), 332–347. doi:10.1037/cap0000035

Dumulescu, D., & Muţiu, A. I. (2021). Academic leadership in the time of COVID-19—Experiences and perspectives. *Frontiers in Psychology*, *12*, 648344. doi:10.3389/fpsyg.2021.648344 PMID:33959076

Dursun, İ., Gökmen Köksal, C., & Tümer Kabadayı, E. (2022). COVID-19 salgını döneminde sürdürülebilir tüketim davranışlarında yaşanan değişim. *Journal of Management and Economics Research*, *20*(3), 302–324.

Dutot, V. (2020). A social identity perspective of social media's impact on satisfaction with life. *Psychology and Marketing*, *37*(6), 759–772. doi:10.1002/mar.21333

Dutton, J., Workman, K., & Hardin, A. (2014). Compassion at work. *Annual Review of Organizational Psychology and Organizational Behavior*, *1*(1), 277–304. doi:10.1146/annurev-orgpsych-031413-091221

Duxbury, L., & Higgins, C. (2001). *Work–life balance in the new millennium: Where are we? Where do we need to go?* CPRN.

Eastwood, J. D., Frischen, A., Fenske, M. J., & Smilek, D. (2012). The unengaged mind: Defining boredom in terms of attention. *Perspectives on Psychological Science*, *7*(5), 482–495. doi:10.1177/1745691612456044 PMID:26168505

Efron, B. (1979). Bootstrap methods. Another look at jackknife. *Annals of Statistics*, *7*(1), 1–26. doi:10.1214/aos/1176344552

Eisenberg, D., Gollust, S. E., Golberstein, E., & Hefner, J. L. (2007). Prevalence and correlates of depression, anxiety, and suicidality among university students. *The American Journal of Orthopsychiatry*, *77*(4), 534–542. doi:10.1037/0002-9432.77.4.534 PMID:18194033

Eka, N. G., & Chambers, D. (2019). Incivility in nursing education: A systematic literature review. *Nurse Education in Practice*, *39*, 45–54. doi:10.1016/j.nepr.2019.06.004 PMID:31382114

Ekman, E., & Ekman, P. (2013). Cultivating emotional balance: structure, research, and implementation. In T. Singer & M. Boz (Eds.), *Compassion: Bridging practice and science* (pp. 398–414). Max Planck Society.

Elgin, D., & Mitchell, A. (1977). Voluntary simplicity. *Planning Review*, *5*(6), 13–15. doi:10.1108/eb053820

Elliott, R. (1994). Addictive consumption: Function and fragmentation in postmodernity. *Journal of Consumer Policy*, *17*(2), 159–179. doi:10.1007/BF01016361

Embse, V., Sandilos, N., Pendergast, L., & Mankin, A. (2016). Teacher stress, teaching-efficacy, and job satisfaction in response to test-based educational accountability policies. *Learning and Individual Differences*, *50*, 308–317. doi:10.1016/j.lindif.2016.08.001

Enko Blog Admin. (2020, March 26). Why are Enko Students more prepared for distance learning? *Enko Blog*.

Erdogan, B., Bauer, T. N., Truxillo, D. M., & Mansfield, L. R. (2012). Whistle while you work: A review of the satisfaction with life literature. *Journal of Management*, *38*(4), 1038–1083. doi:10.1177/0149206311429379

Eriksson, T., Germundsjo, L., Astrom, E., & Ronnlund, M. (2018). Mindful self-compassion training reduces stress and burnout symptoms mong practicing psychologists: A randomized controlled trial of a brief web-based intervention. *Frontiers in Psychology*, *9*, 2340. Advance online publication. doi:10.3389/fpsyg.2018.02340 PMID:30538656

Esteban, R. E. C., Mamani-Benito, O., Chaparro, J. E. T., Lingan-Huaman, S. K., & Pajares, A. E. (2021). Psychological distress and workload as predictors of satisfaction with life in Peruvian female university professors with a family burden. *Heliyon*, *8*, 2022. PMID:35071805

Etzioni, A. (1998). Voluntary simplicity: Characterization, select psychological implications, and societal consequences. In *Essays in Socio-Economics* (pp. 1–26). Springer.

Eurich. (2018). *What Self-Awareness Really Is (and How to Cultivate It)*. https://hbr.org/2018/01/what-self-awareness-really-is-and-how-to-cultivate-it

Eurich, T. (2018). What self-awareness really is (and how to cultivate it). *Harvard Business Review*, 1–9.

Eur, J. P. (2014). Resilience: Revisiting the Concept and its Utility for Social Research. *International Journal of Mental Health and Addiction*, *9*(4), 421–433.

Eurofound, I. L. O. (2017). Working anytime, anywhere: The effects on the world of work. Author.

Evanoff, B. A., Strickland, J. R., Dale, A. M., Hayibor, L., Page, E., Duncan, J. G., Kannampallil, T., & Gray, D. L. (2020). Work-related and personal factors associated with mental well-being during the COVID-19 response: Survey of health care and other workers. *Journal of Medical Internet Research*, *22*(8), e21366. doi:10.2196/21366 PMID:32763891

Ezell, D. (2019). *Consumer well-being: A typology and examination of voluntary simplicity [PhD]*. University of Mississippi.

Faber, R. J., & O'Guinn, T. C. (1992). A clinical screener for compulsive buying. *The Journal of Consumer Research*, *19*(3), 459–469. doi:10.1086/209315

Fahlman, S. A., Mercer-Lynn, K. B., Flora, D. B., & Eastwood, J. D. (2013). Development and validation of the multidimensional state boredom scale. *Assessment*, *20*(1), 68–85. doi:10.1177/1073191111421303 PMID:21903683

Fanner & Urquhart. (2008). Bibliotherapy for mental health service users Part 1: A systematic review. *Health Information & Libraries Journal, 25*(4). doi:. doi:10.1111/j.1471-1842.2008.00821.x

Fässberg, M. M., Orden, K. A. V., Duberstein, P., Erlangsen, A., Lapierre, S., Bodner, E., Canetto, S. S., Leo, D. D., Szanto, K., & Waern, M. (2012). A systematic review of social factors and suicidal behavior in older adulthood. *International Journal of Environmental Research and Public Health, 9*(3), 722–745. doi:10.3390/ijerph9030722 PMID:22690159

Feldmen, C., & Kuyken, W. (2011). Compassion in the landscape of suffering. *Contemporary Buddhism, 12*(1), 143–155. doi:10.1080/14639947.2011.564831

Fenton-O'Creevy, M., Dibb, S., & Furnham, A. (2018). Antecedents and consequences of chronic impulsive buying: Can impulsive buying be understood as dysfunctional self-regulation? *Psychology and Marketing, 35*(3), 175–188. doi:10.1002/mar.21078

Ferguson, M., Carlson, D., Zivnuska, S., & Whitten, D. (2012). Support at work and home: The path to satisfaction through balance. *Journal of Vocational Behavior, 80*(2), 299–307. doi:10.1016/j.jvb.2012.01.001

Fernandez, A. A., & Shaw, G. P. (2020). Academic leadership in a time of crisis: The Coronavirus and COVID-19. *The Journal of Leadership Studies, 14*(1), 39–45. doi:10.1002/jls.21684

Fernandez, A., & Shaw, G. (2020). Leadership in higher education in an era of new adaptive challenges. In *INTED2020 Proceedings* (pp. 61-65). IATED. 10.21125/inted.2020.0037

Ferreira, L. N., Pereira, L. N., da Fé Brás, M., & Ilchuk, K. (2021). Quality of life under the COVID-19 quarantine. *Quality of Life Research: An International Journal of Quality of Life Aspects of Treatment, Care and Rehabilitation, 30*(5), 1389–1405. doi:10.100711136-020-02724-x PMID:33389523

Field, K. (n.d.). Lessons from campuses that closed after natural disasters. *The Chronicle of Higher Education.*

Fight or Flight Response. (2022). *Psychology Tools.* Retrieved December 16, 2022, from https://www.psychologytools.com/resource/fight-or-flight-response/

Fink, G. (2010). Stress: definition and history. *Stress Science: Neuroendocrinology, 3*(9), 319-328.

Finlay-Jones, A. L., Rees, C. S., & Kane, R. T. (2015). Self-compassion, emotion regulation and stress among Australian psychologists: Testing an emotion regulation model of self-compassion using structural equation modeling. *PLoS One, 10*(7), e0133481. doi:10.1371/journal.pone.0133481 PMID:26207900

Fisher, C. D. (2010). Happiness at work. *International Journal of Management Reviews, 12*(4), 384–412. doi:10.1111/j.1468-2370.2009.00270.x

Fitzgerald, L. (2017). Still the last great open secret: Sexual harassment as systemic trauma. *Journal of Trauma & Dissociation, 18*(4), 483–489. doi:10.1080/15299732.2017.1309143 PMID:28375711

Flick, U. (2005). Métodos Qualitativos na Investigação Científica. *Monitor (Charlottetown).*

Flook, L., Goldberg, S. B., Pinger, L., Bonus, K., & Davidson, R. J. (2013). Mindfulness for teachers: A pilot study to assess effects on stress, burnout, and teaching efficacy. *Mind, Brain and Education, 7*(3), 182–195. doi:10.1111/mbe.12026 PMID:24324528

Fluharty, M., & Fancourt, D. (2021). How have people been coping during the COVID-19 pandemic? Patterns and predictors of coping strategies amongst 26,016 UK adults. *BMC Psychology, 9*(1), 1–12. . doi:10.118640359-021-00603-9 PMID:34266498

Ford, M. T., Cerasoli, C. P., Higgins, J. A., & Decesare, A. L. (2011). Relationships between psychological, physical, and behavioural health and work performance: A review and meta-analysis. *Work and Stress*, *25*(3), 185–204. doi:10.1080/02678373.2011.609035

Forsey. (2018). *The True Meaning of Self-Awareness (& How to Tell If You're Actually Self-Aware).* https://blog.hubspot.com/marketing/self-awareness

Fowler, J. H., & Christakis, N. A. (2010). Cooperative behavior cascades in human social networks. *Proceedings of the National Academy of Sciences of the United States of America*, *107*(12), 5334–5338. doi:10.1073/pnas.0913149107 PMID:20212120

Franklin, N. (2010). The rise and fall of the 8 hour day: part one. In Hindsight. Australian Broadcasting Commission.

Fraser, M. W., GalInsky, M. J., & RIchman, J. M. (1999). Risk, Protection, and Resilience: Toward a Conceptual Framework for Social Work Practice. *Social Work Research, 23*, 131-143. http://dx.doI.org/10.1093/swr/23.3.131

Fredrickson, B. L. (2001). The role of positive emotions in positive psychology: The broadenand-build Theory of positive emotions. *The American Psychologist*, *56*(3), 218–226. doi:10.1037/0003-066X.56.3.218 PMID:11315248

Fredrickson, B. L. (2013). Positive emotions broaden and build. *Advances in Experimental Social Psychology*, *47*, 1–53. doi:10.1016/B978-0-12-407236-7.00001-2

Freire, P. (1970). *"Banking" concept of Education. In Ways of Reading.* St. Martin's.

Freitas, A. R. R., Napimoga, M., & Donalisio, M. R. (2020). Assessing the severity of COVID-19. *Epidemiologia e Serviços de Saúde: Revista do Sistema Unico de Saúde do Brasil*, *29*, e2020119. PMID:32267300

French, S. E., Lenton, R., Walters, V., & Eyles, J. (2000). An Empirical Evaluation of an Expanded Nursing Stress Scale. *Journal of Nursing Measurement*, *8*(2), 161–178. doi:10.1891/1061-3749.8.2.161 PMID:11227582

Freyd, J. J. (1999, June). *Blind to Betrayal: New Perspectives on Memory for Trauma.* Retrieved from https://dynamic.uoregon.edu/jjf/articles/freyd99.pdf

Freyd, J. J. (2021). What is a Betrayal Trauma? What is Betrayal Trauma Theory? *Definition of Betrayal Trauma Theory.* Retrieved from https://dynamic.uoregon.edu/jjf/defineBT.html

Frone, M. R., Russell, M., & Cooper, M. (1992). Antecedents and outcomes of work-family conflict: Testing a model of work-family interface. *The Journal of Applied Psychology*, *77*(1), 65–78. doi:10.1037/0021-9010.77.1.65 PMID:1556042

Fusch, P. I., & Ness, L. R. (2015). Are we there yet? Data saturation in qualitative research. *Qualitative Report*, *20*(9), 1408. doi:10.46743/2160-3715/2015.2281

Future Talent Learning. (2021). *What are the top 5 characteristics of emotional intelligence in good leadership?* https://www.futuretalentlearning.com/en/future-talent-learning-blog/what-are-the-top-5-characteristics-of-emotional-intelligence-in-good-leadership

Gallop. (2022). *State of the global workplace: 2022 report.* Gallop Press.

Gálvez, A., Tirado, F., & Martínez, M. J. (2020). Work–life balance, organizations, and social sustainability: Analyzing female telework in Spain. *Sustainability*, *12*(9), 3567. doi:10.3390u12093567

Gandolfi, F., & Stone, S. (2016). Clarifying leadership: High-impact leaders in a time of leadership crisis. *Revista de Management Comparat International*, *17*(3), 212.

Gandolfi, F., & Stone, S. (2018). Leadership, leadership styles, and servant leadership. *Journal of Management Research, 18*(4), 261–269.

Gao, G., & Sai, L. (2020). Towards a 'virtual' world: Social isolation and struggles during the COVID-19 pandemic as single women living alone. *Gender, Work and Organization, 27*(5), 754–762. doi:10.1111/gwao.12468 PMID:32837008

Garcia, H. F. (2006). Effective leadership response to crisis. *Strategy and Leadership, 34*(1), 4–10. doi:10.1108/10878570610637849

Gardner, M. P., & Rook, D. W. (1988). *Effects of impulse purchases on consumers' affective states.* ACR North American Advances.

Gardner, W. L., Avolio, B. J., Luthans, F., May, D. R., & Walumbwa, F. (2005). "Can you see the real me?" A self-based model of authentic leader and follower development. *The Leadership Quarterly, 16*(3), 343–372. doi:10.1016/j.leaqua.2005.03.003

Gardner, W. L., Cogliser, C. C., Davis, K. M., & Dickens, M. P. (2011). Authentic leadership: A review of the literature and research agenda. *The Leadership Quarterly, 22*(6), 1120–1145. doi:10.1016/j.leaqua.2011.09.007

Gates, D. (2003). Learning to play the game: An exploratory study of how African American women and men interact with others in organizations. *Electronic Journal of Communication, 12*(2-3).

Gates, D. (2008). Business communication: identifying strategies employed by Latino/a or Hispanic Americans within superior-subordinate relationships. *Business Research Yearbook, 15*(2).

Gates, D. (2009). The managerial communication process: Organizational socialization model. In S. Zhang, D. Gates, C. Nealy, & J. Stark (Eds.), *Managerial communication: Theory and application* (pp. 26–58). The Publishing House of South-China University of Technology.

Gates, D. (2010). Polarity management: Balancing stress and tranquility polarities during a recession. *Business Research Yearbook, 17*(2), 704–711.

Gates, D. (2019). *Superior-subordinate dialogue: Mastering communication with bosses / Examining communication within and across races and genders.* Lambert Publishing House.

Gates, D. (2020). *Next level learning: Mastering Organizational Socialization.* Lambert Publishing House.

Gates, D. (2021). Exploring Superior-Subordinate Communication from the Perspectives of African American and Latino American Subordinates. In R. D. Johnson (Ed.), *Handbook of Research on Multidisciplinary Perspectives on Managerial and Leadership Psychology* (pp. 148–166). IGI Global. doi:10.4018/978-1-7998-3811-1.ch008

Gates, D. (2021). Mastering Diversity and Gaining a Competitive Advantage on University Campuses. In R. D. Johnson (Ed.), *Handbook of Research on Multidisciplinary Perspectives on Managerial and Leadership Psychology* (pp. 558–570). IGI Global. doi:10.4018/978-1-7998-3811-1.ch028

Gaxiola-Villa, E. (2014). Bienestar psicol_ogico y desgaste profesional [DP] en amas de casa docentes universitarias. *J. Behav. Health Soc., 6*(1), 79–88.

George, B. (2007). *True north: Discover your authentic leadership.* Jossey-Bass.

George, B. P., & Vaoyuneyong, G. (2010). Impulsive buying and cognitive dissonance: A study conducted among the spring break student shoppers. *Young Customers, 11*(4), 291–306. doi:10.1108/17473611011093925

George, B., Sims, P., McLean, A. N., & Mayer, D. (2007). Discovering your authentic leadership. *Harvard Business Review, 85*(2), 129. PMID:17345686

Germer, C. K. (2009). *The mindful path to self-compassion*. Guilford.

Germer, C., & Neff, K. (2019). *Teaching the mindful self-compassion program: A guide for professionals*. Guilford.

Giallonardo, L. M., Wong, C. A., & Iwasiw, C. L. (2010). Authentic leadership of preceptors: Predictor of new graduate nurses' work engagement and job satisfaction. *Journal of Nursing Management*, *18*(8), 993–1003. doi:10.1111/j.1365-2834.2010.01126.x PMID:21073571

Gilbert, P., & Choden. (2014). *Mindful compassion: How the science of compassion can help you understand your emotions, live in the present, and connect deeply with others*. New Harbinger.

Gilbert. (2010). *Compassion focused therapy: Distinctive features*. Routledge.

Gilbert, P. (2009). *The Compassionate Mind: A New Approach to Life's Challenges*. New Harbinger.

Gilbert, P. (2017). Compassion: Definitions and controversies. In P. Gilbert (Ed.), *Compassion: Concepts, research, and applications*. Routledge. doi:10.4324/9781315564296-1

Gilbert, P. (2022). The evolved functions of caring connections as a basis for compassion. In P. Gilbert (Ed.), *Compassion focused therapy: Clinical practice and applications*. Routledge. doi:10.4324/9781003035879-4

Gillanders, D. T., Sinclair, A. K., MacLean, M., & Jardine, K. (2015). Illness cognitions, cognitive fusion, avoidance, and self-compassion as predictors of distress and quality of life in a heterogeneous sample of adults, after cancer. *Journal of Contextual Behavioral Science*, *4*(4), 300–311. doi:10.1016/j.jcbs.2015.07.003

Giorgi, G., Perminiene, M., Montani, F., Fiz-Perez, J., Mucci, N., & Arcangeli, G. (2016). Detrimental effects of workplace bullying: Impediment of self-management competence via psychological distress. *Frontiers in Psychology*, *7*. Advance online publication. doi:10.3389/fpsyg.2016.00060 PMID:26913013

Gismero-González, E., Bermejo-Toro, L., Cagigal, V., Roldán, A., Martínez-Beltrán, M. J., & Halty, L. (2020). Emotional impact of COVID-19 lockdown among the Spanish population. *Frontiers in Psychology*, *11*, 616978. doi:10.3389/fpsyg.2020.616978 PMID:33391136

Giumetti, G. W., Hatfield, A. L., Scisco, J. L., Schroeder, A. N., Muth, E. R., & Kowalski, R. M. (2013). What a rude e-mail! Examining the differential effects of incivility versus support on mood, energy, engagement, and performance in an online context. *Journal of Occupational Health Psychology*, *18*(3), 297–309. doi:10.1037/a0032851 PMID:23834445

Giumetti, G., McKibben, E., Hatfield, A., Schroeder, A., & Kowalski, R. (2012). Cyber incivility @ work: The new age of interpersonal deviance. *Cyberpsychology, Behavior, and Social Networking*, *15*(3), 148–154. doi:10.1089/cyber.2011.0336 PMID:22304404

Giumetti, G., Saunders, L., Brunette, J., Di Francesco, F., & Graham, P. (2016). Linking Cyber Incivility with Job Performance Through Job Satisfaction: The Buffering Role of Positive Affect. *Psi Chi Journal of Psychological Research*, *21*(4), 230–240. doi:10.24839/2164-8204.JN21.4.230

Gladding, S. T., & Gladding, C. (1991). The ABCs of bibliotherapy for school counselors. *The School Counselor*, *39*(1).

Glenn, L. R. (2002). Earned-Secure Attachment Status in Retrospect and Prospect. *Child Development*, *73*(4), 1204–1219. doi:10.1111/1467-8624.00467 PMID:12146743

Global Burden of Diseases. (2020). *Injuries and Risk Factors Study*. Author.

Glotzbecker, M. P. (2022). Crisis Leadership: Lessons Learned From the COVID Pandemic. *Journal of Pediatric Orthopedics*, *42*(Suppl 1), S56–S59. doi:10.1097/BPO.0000000000002068 PMID:35405706

Goetz, J. L., Keltner, D., & Simon-Thomas, E. (2010). Compassion: An evolutionary analysis and empirical review. *Psychological Bulletin, 136*(3), 351–374. doi:10.1037/a0018807 PMID:20438142

Goldstein, D. S., & Kopin, I. J. (2007). Evolution of concepts of stress. *Stress (Amsterdam, Netherlands), 10*(2), 109–120. doi:10.1080/10253890701288935 PMID:17514579

Goleman. (2013). *The Focused Leader - How effective executives direct their own and their organizations' attention*. https://hbr.org/2013/12/the-focused-leader

Goleman, D. (1995). *Emotional Intelligence: Why it can matter more than IQ*. Bloomsbury.

Gomes, A. R., & Cruz, J. F. (2004). A experiência de stresse e "burnout" em psicólogos portugueses: Um estudo sobre as diferenças de género. *Psicologia: Teoria, Investigação e Prática, 9*(2), 193–212.

González-Sanguino, C., Ausín, B., Castellanos, M. Á., Saiz, J., López-Gómez, A., Ugidos, C., & Muñoz, M. (2020). Mental health consequences during the initial stage of the 2020 Coronavirus pandemic (COVID-19) in Spain. *Brain, Behavior, and Immunity, 87*, 172–176. doi:10.1016/j.bbi.2020.05.040 PMID:32405150

Goode, W. J. (1960). A theory of role strain. *American Sociological Review, 25*(4), 483–496. doi:10.2307/2092933

Goodlet, K. J., Raney, E., Buckley, K., Afolabi, T., Davis, L., Fettkether, R. M., Jones, M., Larson, S., & Tennant, S. (2022). Impact of the COVID-19 Pandemic on the Emotional Intelligence of Student Pharmacist Leaders. *American Journal of Pharmaceutical Education, 86*(1), 8519. doi:10.5688/ajpe8519 PMID:34301541

Görgens-Ekermans, G., & Roux, C. (2021). Revisiting the emotional intelligence and transformational leadership debate:(How) does emotional intelligence matter to effective leadership? *SA Journal of Human Resource Management, 19*, 1279. doi:10.4102ajhrm.v19i0.1279

Gotlink, R. A., Chu, P., Busschbach, J. J. V., Benson, H., Friccione, G. L., & Hunink, M. G. M. (2015). Standardised mindfulness-based interventions in healthcare: An overview of systematic reviews and meta-analyses of RCTs. *PLoS One, 10*(4), e0124344. doi:10.1371/journal.pone.0124344 PMID:25881019

Goulão, M. P. de L. M. S. (2017). *Efeitos do clima de comunicação organizacional no "stress", "work" "engagement" e comportamentos extra-papel* [Doctoral Thesis, Iscte – Instituto Universitário de Lisboa]. http://hdl.handle.net/10071/15427

Grady, C. (2005). Payment of clinical research subjects. *The Journal of Clinical Investigation, 115*(7), 1681–1687. doi:10.1172/JCI25694 PMID:16007244

Grant, A. (2019, Feb 15). *No, you can't ignore email. It's rude*. Retrieved from The New York Times: https://www.nytimes.com/2019/02/15/opinion/sunday/email-etiquette.html

Greenberg, N., Docherty, M., Gnanapragasam, S., & Wessely, S. (2020). Managing mental health challenges faced by healthcare workers during covid-19 pandemic. BMJ, 368, 2-4.

Greenhaus, J. H., & Allen, T. D. (2011). Work-family balance: A review and extension of the literature. In J. C. Quick & L. E. Tetrick (Eds.), Handbook of occupational health psychology (2nd ed.). Washington, DC: American Psychological Association.

Greenhaus, J. H., & Beutell, N. (1985). Sources of conflict between work and family roles. *Academy of Management Review, 10*(1), 76–88. doi:10.2307/258214

Greenhaus, J. H., Collins, K. M., & Shaw, J. D. (2003). The relation between work–family balance and quality of life. *Journal of Vocational Behavior, 63*(3), 510–531. doi:10.1016/S0001-8791(02)00042-8

Greenleaf, R. K. (2002). *Servant leadership: A journey into the nature of legitimate power and greatness*. Paulist Press.

Gregg, R. B. (1936). *The Voluntary Simplicity*. Pendle Hill Publications.

Grossman, P., Niemann, L., Schmidt, S., & Walach, H. (2004). Mindfulness-based stress reduction and health benefits: A meta-analysis. *Journal of Psychosomatic Research*, *57*(1), 35–43. doi:10.1016/S0022-3999(03)00573-7 PMID:15256293

Groysberg, B., Abrahams, R. A., & Baden, K. C. (2021). *The pandemic conversations that leaders need to have now*. Harvard Business Working Paper.

Guerra, I. C. (2006). *Pesquisa qualitativa e análise de conteúdo. Sentido e formas de uso*. Principia Editora.

Guillaume, Y. R., Van Knippenberg, D., & Brodbeck, F. C. (2014). Nothing succeeds like moderation: A social self-regulation perspective on cultural dissimilarity and performance. *Academy of Management Journal*, *57*(5), 1284–1308. doi:10.5465/amj.2013.0046

Gunnell, K. E., Mosewich, A. D., McEwen, C. E., Eklund, R. C., & Crocker, P. R. E. (2017). Don't be so hard on yourself! Changes in self-compassion during the first year of university are associated with changes in well-being. *Personality and Individual Differences*, *107*, 43–48. doi:10.1016/j.paid.2016.11.032

Guo, J., Qiu, Y., & Gan, Y. (2022). Workplace incivility and work engagement: The mediating role of job insecurity and the moderating role of self-perceived employability. *Managerial and Decision Economics*, *43*(1), 192–205. doi:10.1002/mde.3377

Gupta, R., Nair, K., & Radhakrishnan, L. (2021). Impact of COVID-19 crisis on stocking and impulse buying behaviour of consumers. *International Journal of Social Economics*, *48*(12), 1794–1809. Advance online publication. doi:10.1108/IJSE-03-2021-0163

Guy, T (2022). *Betrayal Trauma & CPTSD*. CPTSDfoundation.org

Hair, J., Black, W. C., Babin, B. J., & Anderson, R. E. (2013). *Multivariate Data Analysis*. Pearson Education Limited.

Halbesleben, J. R., Neveu, J. P., Paustian-Underdahl, S. C., & Westman, M. (2014). Getting to the "COR" understanding the role of resources in conservation of resources theory. *Journal of Management*, *40*(5), 1334–1364. doi:10.1177/0149206314527130

Halkos, G., & Bousinakis, D. (2010). The effect of stress and satisfaction on productivity. *International Journal of Productivity and Performance Management*, *59*(5), 415–431. doi:10.1108/17410401011052869

Hall, J. C., Everett, J. E., & Hamilton-Mason, J. (2012). Black women talk about workplace stress and how they cope. *Journal of Black Studies*, *43*(2), 207–226. doi:10.1177/0021934711413272 PMID:22457894

Hama, Y. (2001). Shopping as a coping behavior for stress. *The Japanese Psychological Research*, *43*(4), 218–224. doi:10.1111/1468-5884.00179

Hampshire, A., Hellyer, P. J., Soreq, E., Mehta, M. A., Ioannidis, K., Trender, W., Grant, J. E., & Chamberlain, S. R. (2021). Associations between dimensions of behaviour, personality traits, and mental-health during the COVID-19 pandemic in the United Kingdom. *Nature Communications*, *12*(1), 1–15. doi:10.103841467-021-24365-5 PMID:33397941

Hanks, L., & Mattila, A. S. (2014). The impact of gender and pre-purchase mood on consumer guilt after a travel purchase. *Journal of Travel Research*, *53*(5), 625–637. doi:10.1177/0047287513506296

Hannigan, B., Edwards, D., & Burnard, P. (2004). Stress and stress management in clinical psychology: Findings from a systematic review. *Journal of Mental Health (Abingdon, England)*, *13*(3), 235–245. doi:10.1080/09638230410001700871

Haque, M. R., Hafiz, R., Azad, A. A., & Adnan, Y. (2021). Crime Detection and Criminal Recognition to Intervene in Interpersonal Violence Using Deep Convolutional Neural Network with Transfer Learning. *International Journal of Ambient Computing and Intelligence*, *12*(4), 14. doi:10.4018/IJACI.20211001.oa1

Harms, P. D., Credé, M., Tynan, M., Leon, M., & Jeung, W. (2017). Leadership and stress: A meta-analytic review. *The Leadership Quarterly*, *28*(1), 178–194. doi:10.1016/j.leaqua.2016.10.006

Harris, A. (2010). Distributed leadership: Evidence and implications. *The principles of educational leadership and management*, 55-69.

Harris, P. (2007). Flexible work policies-means business. *T+D Journal*, 32-36.

Hartmann, N. N., & Lussier, B. (2020). Managing the sales force through the unexpected exogenous COVID-19 crisis. *Industrial Marketing Management*, *88*, 101–111. doi:10.1016/j.indmarman.2020.05.005

Hasan, A. H., Sultana, S., Hossain, S., Hasan, M., Ahmed, H. U., & Sikder, T. (2020). The impact of COVID-19 pandemic on mental health & wellbeing among home-quarantined Bangladeshi students: A cross-sectional pilot study. *Journal of Affective Disorders*, *277*, 121–128. doi:10.1016/j.jad.2020.07.135 PMID:32818775

Hausen, J. E. (2019). Minimalist life orientations as a dialogical tool for happiness. *British Journal of Guidance & Counselling*, *47*(2), 168–179. doi:10.1080/03069885.2018.1523364

Hausman, A. (2000). A multi-method investigation of consumer motivations in impulse buying behavior. *Journal of Consumer Marketing*, *17*(5), 403–426. doi:10.1108/07363760010341045

Hayter, M. R., & Dorstyn, D. S. (2013). Resilience, self-esteem, and self-compassion in adults with spina bifida. *Spinal Cord*, *52*(2), 167–171. doi:10.1038c.2013.152 PMID:24322213

Head, E. (2009). The ethics and implications of paying participants in qualitative research. *International Journal of Social Research Methodology*, *12*(4), 335–344. doi:10.1080/13645570802246724

Heath, C., Sommerfield, A., & von Ungern-Sternberg, B. S. (2020). Resilience strategies to manage psychological distress among healthcare workers during the COVID-19 pandemic: A narrative review. *Anaesthesia*, *75*(10), 1364–1371. doi:10.1111/anae.15180 PMID:32534465

Hebert, T. P., & Kent, R. (2000). Nurturing social and emotional development in gifted teenagers through young adult literature. *Roeper Review*, *22*(3).

Heifetz, R. A. (2000). *Leadership without easy answers*. Harvard University Press.

Heifetz, R. A., Heifetz, R., Grashow, A., & Linsky, M. (2009). *The practice of adaptive leadership: Tools and tactics for changing your organization and the world*. Harvard Business Press.

Heifetz, R. A., & Laurie, D. L. (2001). The work of leadership. *Harvard Business Review*, *79*(11). PMID:10174450

Heischman, R. (2017). *Face to Face and Cyber Incivility*. Academic Press.

Helliker, K. (2007, July 31). *Bibliotherapy: Reading your way to mental health*. Academic Press.

Herbsleb, J. (2007). Global software engineering: The future of sociotechnical coordination. In *Proceedings of the Future of Software Engineering Conference* (pp. 188–198). IEEE.

Hetkamp, M., Schweda, A., Bäuerle, A., Weismüller, B., Kohler, H., Musche, V., Dörrie, N., Schöbel, C., Teufel, M., & Skoda, E. M. (2020). Sleep disturbances, fear, and generalized anxiety during the COVID-19 shut down phase in Germany: Relation to infection rates, deaths, and German stock index DAX. *Sleep Medicine*, *75*, 350–353. doi:10.1016/j.sleep.2020.08.033 PMID:32950879

Hill, B. (2020). Coronavirus: Origins, signs, prevention, and management of patients. *British Journal of Nursing (Mark Allen Publishing)*, *29*(7), 399–402. doi:10.12968/bjon.2020.29.7.399 PMID:32279552

Hill, E. J., Hawkins, A. J., Ferris, M., & Weitzman, M. (2001). Finding an extra day a week: The positive influence of perceived job flexibility on work and family life balance. *Family Relations*, *50*(1), 49–58. doi:10.1111/j.1741-3729.2001.00049.x

Hills, P., & Argyle, M. (2001). Emotional stability as a major dimension of happiness. *Personality and Individual Differences*, *31*(8), 1357–1364. doi:10.1016/S0191-8869(00)00229-4

Hobfoll, S. (1989). Conservation of resources: A new attempt at conceptualizing stress. *The American Psychologist*, *44*(3), 513–524. doi:10.1037/0003-066X.44.3.513 PMID:2648906

Hoch, S. J., & Loewenstein, G. F. (1991). Time-inconsistent preferences and consumer self-control. *The Journal of Consumer Research*, *17*(4), 492–507. doi:10.1086/208573

Hoert, J., Herd, A. M., & Hambrick, M. (2018). The role of leadership support for health promotion in employee wellness program participation, perceived job stress, and health behaviors. *American Journal of Health Promotion*, *32*(4), 1054–1061. doi:10.1177/0890117116677798 PMID:27920214

Hoffart, A., Johnson, S. U., & Ebrahimi, O. V. (2020). Loneliness and social distancing during the COVID-19 pandemic: Risk factors and associations with psychopathology. *Frontiers in Psychiatry*, *11*, 1297. doi:10.3389/fpsyt.2020.589127 PMID:33329136

Holguín, E. C. (2021). Implicaciones de la pandemia por COVID-19 en la salud docente. Revisión sistemática. *Temas sociológicos*, (28), 113-142.

Homan, & Sirois, F. M. (2017). Self-compassion and physical health: Exploring the roles of perceived stress and health-promoting behaviors. *Health Psychology Open, 4*(2). doi:10.1177/2055102917729542

Homans, G. C. (1958). Social behavior as exchange. *American Journal of Sociology*, *63*(6), 597–606. doi:10.1086/222355

Hook, J. N., Hodge, A. S., Zhang, H., Van Tongeren, D. R., & Davis, D. E. (2021). Minimalism, voluntary simplicity, and well-being: A systematic review of the empirical literature. *The Journal of Positive Psychology*, 1–12. doi:10.1080/17439760.2021.1991450

Hope, N., Koestner, R., & Milyavskaya, M. (2014). The Role of Self-Compassion in Goal Pursuit and Well-Being Among University Freshmen. *Self and Identity*, *13*(5), 579–593. doi:10.1080/15298868.2014.889032

Hosie, P. J., & Sevastos, P. (2009). Does the "happy-productive worker" thesis apply to managers? *International Journal of Workplace Health Management, 2*(2), 131-160.

Hougaard, R., & Carter, J. (2022). *Compassionate leadership: How to do hard things in a human way*. Harvard Business Review Press.

Huang, E. (2012). Online experiences and virtual goods purchase intention. *Internet Research*, *22*(3), 252–274. doi:10.1108/10662241211235644

Hulin, C., & Judge, T. (2003). Job attitudes. In Handbook of Psychology: Industrial and Organizational Psychology. Wiley. doi:10.1002/0471264385.wei1211

Hulley, S. B., Cummings, S., Browner, W., Grady, D.G., & Newman, T. B. (2013). Designing Clinical Research. An epidemiological approach (2nd ed.). Lippincott Williams & Wilkins.

Humphrey, A., & Vari, O. (2021). Meaning matters: Self-perceived meaning in life, Its predictors and psychological stressors associated with the COVID-19 pandemic. *Behavioral Sciences (Basel, Switzerland)*, *11*(4), 50. doi:10.3390/bs11040050 PMID:33924422

Huneke, M. E. (2005). The face of the un-consumer: An empirical examination of the practice of voluntary simplicity in the United States. *Psychology and Marketing*, *22*(7), 527–550. doi:10.1002/mar.20072

Hunsley, J., Elliott, K., & Therrien, Z. (2014). The efficacy and effectiveness of psychological treatments for mood, anxiety, and related disorders. *Canadian Psychology*, *55*(3), 161–176. doi:10.1037/a0036933

Hunter, D., McCallum, J., & Howes, D. (2019). Defining exploratory-descriptive qualitative (EDQ) research and considering its application to healthcare. *Journal of Nursing and Health Care*, *4*(1).

Hunt, P., & Greaves, I. (2017). *Oxford manual of major incident management*. Oxford University Press. doi:10.1093/med/9780199238088.001.0001

Hwang, T. J., Rabheru, K., Peisah, C., Reichman, W., & Ikeda, M. (2020). Loneliness and social isolation during the COVID-19 pandemic. *International Psychogeriatrics*, *32*(10), 1217–1220. doi:10.1017/S1041610220000988 PMID:32450943

Iaquinta, A., & Hipsky, S. (2006, July). *Bibliotherapy for the inclusive classroom*. Academic Press.

İlhan, M. N., Tüzün, H., Kiliç, R., & Yildirim, N. (2021). Nonpharmaceutical interventions in Turkey and worldwide during COVID-19 pandemic. *Turkish Journal of Medical Sciences*, *51*(SI-1), 3207–3214. doi:10.3906ag-2106-210 PMID:34590802

Ilies, R., Morgeson, F. P., & Nahrgang, J. D. (2005). Authentic leadership and eudaemonic well-being: Understanding leader–follower outcomes. *The Leadership Quarterly*, *16*(3), 373–394. doi:10.1016/j.leaqua.2005.03.002

Ilies, R., Nahrgang, J. D., & Morgeson, F. P. (2007). Leader-member exchange and citizenship behaviours: A meta-analysis. *The Journal of Applied Psychology*, *92*(1), 269–277. doi:10.1037/0021-9010.92.1.269 PMID:17227168

Imam, F. (2013). Gender differences in impulsive buying behavior and post purchasing dissonance under incentive conditions. *The Journal of Business Strategy*, *7*(1), 23.

Imran, M. K., Fatima, T., Sarwar, A., & Iqbal, S. M. J. (2021). Will I speak up or remain silent? Workplace ostracism and employee performance based on self-control perspective. *The Journal of Social Psychology*, 1–19. PMID:34498546

Insights, I. C. A. E. W. (2021). *The 5 Elements of Emotional Intelligence*. https://www.icaew.com/insights/student-insights/the-5-elements-of-emotional-intelligence

International Council of Archives. (2020). *The Role-of-achieves-in-the COVID-19 crisis*. Author.

Irons & Heriot-Maitland, C. (2021). Compassionate Mind Training: An 8-week group for the public. *Psychology and Psychotherapy*, *94*(3), 443–463. doi:10.1111/papt.12320

Iskamto, D. (2021). Stress and its impact on employee performance. *International Journal of Social and Management Studies*, *2*(3), 142–148.

Iwata, O. (1997). Attitudinal and behavioral correlates of voluntary simplicity lifestyles. *Social Behavior and Personality*, *25*(3), 233–240. doi:10.2224bp.1997.25.3.233

Iwata, O. (2006). An evaluation of consumerism and lifestyle as correlates of a voluntary simplicity lifestyle. *Social Behavior and Personality*, *34*(5), 557–568. doi:10.2224bp.2006.34.5.557

Jablin, F. (2001). *Organizational entry, assimilation, and disengagement/exit*. SAGE Publications, Inc. doi:10.4135/9781412986243.n19

Jacoby, J. (2002). Stimulus-organism-response reconsidered: An evolutionary step in modeling (consumer) behavior. *Journal of Consumer Psychology*, *12*(1), 51–57. doi:10.1207/S15327663JCP1201_05

Jakubowski, T. D., & Sitko-Dominik, M. M. (2021). Teachers' mental health during the first two waves of the COVID-19 pandemic in Poland. *PLoS One*, *16*(9), e0257252. doi:10.1371/journal.pone.0257252 PMID:34555049

Jazaieri, H., Jinpa, G. T., McGonigal, K., Rosenberg, E. L., Finkelstein, J., Simon-Thomas, E., Cullen, M., Doty, J. R., Gross, J. J., & Goldin, P. R. (2013). Enhancing compassion: A randomized controlled trial of a compassion cultivation training program. *Journal of Happiness Studies*, *14*(4), 1113–1126. doi:10.100710902-012-9373-z

Jazaieri, H., McGonigal, K., Lee, I. A., Jinpa, T., Doty, J. R., Gross, J. J., & Goldin, P. R. (2018). Altering the Trajectory of Affect and Affect Regulation: The Impact of Compassion Training. *Mindfulness*, *9*(1), 283–293. doi:10.100712671-017-0773-3

Jazaieri, H., & Rock, M. (2021). Putting compassion to work: Compassion as a tool for navigating challenging workplace relationships. *Mindfulness*, *12*(10), 2552–2558. doi:10.100712671-021-01695-5

Jena, P. K. (2020). Impact of Covid-19 on higher education in India. *International Journal of Advanced Education and Research*, *5*(3), 77–81.

Jennings, M. L. (2009). Medical student burnout: Interdisciplinary exploration and analysis. *The Journal of Medical Humanities*, *30*(4), 253–269. doi:10.100710912-009-9093-5 PMID:19865808

Jin, P. (2012). Stress and Learning. In N. M. Seel (Ed.), *Encyclopedia of the Sciences of Learning* (pp. 3202–3205). Springer US. doi:10.1007/978-1-4419-1428-6_203

Jinpa, T. (2015). *A fearless heart: How the courage to be compassionate can transform our lives*. Avery.

Johari, J., Yean Tan, F., & Tjik Zulkarnain, Z. I. (2018). Autonomy, workload, work-life balance and job performance among teachers. *International Journal of Educational Management*, *32*(1), 107–120. doi:10.1108/IJEM-10-2016-0226

Johnson, D. H. (2008). In defense of indices: The case of bird surveys. *The Journal of Wildlife Management*, *72*(4), 857–868. doi:10.2193/2007-294

Johnson, P., & Indvik, J. (2001). Rudeness at work: Impulse over restraint. *Public Personnel Management*, *30*(4), 457–465. doi:10.1177/009102600103000403

Jun, W. H., Yang, J., & Lee, E. J. (2018). The mediating effects of social support and a grateful disposition on the relationship between life stress and anger in Korean nursing students. *Asian Nursing Research*, *12*(3), 197–202. doi:10.1016/j.anr.2018.08.002 PMID:30130592

Kabat-Zinn, J. (2013). *Full catastrophe living*. Bantam Dell Publishing Group.

Kahai, S. S., & Cooper, R. B. (2003). Exploring the core concepts of media richness theory: The impact of cue multiplicity and feedback immediacy in decision quality. *Journal of Management Information Systems*, *20*(1), 263–299. doi:10.1080/07421222.2003.11045754

Kalla, S. M., & Arora, A. P. (2011). Impulse buying: A literature review. *Global Business Review*, *12*(1), 145–157. doi:10.1177/097215091001200109

Kalliath, T., & Brough, P. (2008a). Work–life balance: A review of the meaning of the balance construct. *Journal of Management & Organization*, *14*(3), 323–327. doi:10.5172/jmo.837.14.3.323

Kalliath, T., & Brough, P. (2008b). Achieving work-life balance. *Journal of Management & Organization*, *14*(3), 224–226. doi:10.5172/jmo.837.14.3.224

Kalu, F. A., & Bwalya, J. C. (2017). What makes qualitative research good research? An exploratory analysis of critical elements. *International Journal of Social Science Research*, *5*(2), 43–56. doi:10.5296/ijssr.v5i2.10711

Kamboj, S., Sarmah, B., Gupta, S., & Dwivedi, Y. (2018). Examining branding co-creation in brand communities on social media: Applying the paradigm of Stimulus-Organism-Response. *International Journal of Information Management*, *39*, 169–185. doi:10.1016/j.ijinfomgt.2017.12.001

Kang, J., Martinez, C. M. J., & Johnson, C. (2021). Minimalism as a sustainable lifestyle: Its behavioral representations and contributions to emotional well-being. *Sustainable Production and Consumption*, *27*, 802–813. doi:10.1016/j.spc.2021.02.001

Kanter, R. M. (1977). *Work and family in the United States: a critical review and agenda for research and policy*. Russell Sage Foundation.

Karimi, L., Leggat, S. G., Bartram, T., & Rada, J. (2020). The effects of emotional intelligence training on the job performance of Australian aged care workers. *Health Care Management Review*, *45*(1), 41–51. doi:10.1097/HMR.0000000000000200 PMID:29742522

Kasser, T. (2002). *The high price of materialism*. A Bradford Book, The MIT Press.

Kauffeld, S., Jonas, E., & Frey, D. (2004). Effect of a flexible work-time design on employee-and company – related aims. *European Journal of Work and Organizational Psychology*, *13*(1), 79–100. doi:10.1080/13594320444000001

Kaur, S., Kremer, M., & Mullainathan, S. (2010). Self-control and the development of work arrangements. *The American Economic Review*, *100*(2), 624–628. doi:10.1257/aer.100.2.624

Kawakami, N., & Tsutsumi, A. (2016). The stress check program: A new national policy for monitoring and screening psychosocial stress in the workplace in Japan. *Journal of Occupational Health*, *58*(1), 1–6. doi:10.1539/joh.15-0001-ER PMID:26607455

Kecojevic, A., Basch, C. H., Sullivan, M., & Davi, N. K. (2020). The impact of the COVID-19 epidemic on mental health of undergraduate students in New Jersey, cross-sectional study. *PLoS One*, *15*(9), e0239696. doi:10.1371/journal.pone.0239696 PMID:32997683

Kellaway, L. (2016, March 13). *Email: The weapon wielded by the passive aggressive colleague*. Retrieved from Financial Times, https://www.ft.com/content/dee75f5e-e635-11e5-a09b-1f8b0d268c39

Kelly, E. L., Kossek, E. E., Hammer, L. B., Durham, M., Bray, J., Charmack, K., Murphy, L. A., & Kaskubar, D. (2008). Getting there from here: Research on the effects of work-family initiatives on work-family conflict and business outcomes. *The Academy of Management Annals*, *2*(1), 305–349. doi:10.5465/19416520802211610 PMID:20589229

Kerrissey, M. J., & Edmondson, A. C. (2020). What good leadership looks like during this pandemic. *Harvard Business Review*, *13*(1).

Keyes, C. L. M. (1998). Social Well-Being. *Social Psychology Quarterly*, *61*(2), 121–140. doi:10.2307/2787065

Kezar, A., Fries-Britt, S., Kurban, E., McGuire, D., & Wheaton, M. M. (2018). *Speaking truth and acting with integrity*. American Council on Education. https://www.acenet.edu/Documents/Speaking-Truth-and-Acting-with-Integrity.pdfnoe

Kezar, A. J., & Holcombe, E. M. (2017). *Shared leadership in higher education*. American Council on Education.

Khan, H., Abbas, J., Kumari, K., & Najam, H. (2022). Corporate level politics from managers and employees perspective and its impact on employees' job stress and job performance. *Journal of Economic and Administrative Sciences*.

Khan, M. R., & Wajidi, A. (2019). Role of leadership and team building in employee motivation at workplace. *GMJACS*, *9*(1), 11–11.

Khoshbakht, F., Mohammadi, M., Naseri, R., Mirghafari, F., Safari, M., Roosta, F., & .... (2021). Evaluating the Health-Oriented Attitude of Parents of Elementary School Students towards the Reopening of Schools in the Corona Crisis. *The Journal of Educational Research*, *8*(42), 33–48.

Khoury, B., Sharma, M., Rush, S. E., & Fournier, C. (2015). Mindfulness-based stress reduction for healthy individuals: A meta-analysis. *Journal of Psychosomatic Research*, *78*(6), 519–528. doi:10.1016/j.jpsychores.2015.03.009 PMID:25818837

Kihara, L. N., & Mugambi, H. (2018). Effect of stress management strategies on employees' performance in the public service. *The Strategic Journal of Business & Change Management*, *5*(2), 2382–2405.

Kim, M. G., & Mattila, A. S. (2010). The impact of mood states and surprise cues on satisfaction. *International Journal of Hospitality Management*, *29*(3), 432–436. doi:10.1016/j.ijhm.2009.10.022

Kirby, J. N. (2017). Compassion interventions: The programs, the evidence, and implications for research and practice. *Psychology and Psychotherapy: Research and Practice*, *90*(3), 432–455. doi:10.1111/papt.12104 PMID:27664071

Kirby, J. N., Doty, J. R., Petrocchi, N., & Gilbert, P. (2017). The current and future role of heart rate variability for assessing and training compassion. *Frontiers in Public Health*, *5*. Advance online publication. doi:10.3389/fpubh.2017.00040 PMID:28337432

Kirchmeyer, C. (2000). Work–life initiatives: greed or benevolence regarding workers' time. In C. L. Cooper & D. M. Rousseau (Eds.), *Trends in Organisational Behaviour* (pp. 79–93). John Wiley and Sons.

Kirchmeyer, C. (2000). Work–life initiatives: greed or benevolence regarding workers' time? In C. L. Cooper & D. M. Rousseau (Eds.), *Trends in organizational behavior: time in organizational behavior* (Vol. 7, pp. 79–94). Wiley.

Klaus, F., Florian, K., & Joachim, K. (2012). The Long Way From -Error Control to Validity Proper: Problems with a Short-Sighted False-Positive Debate. *Perspectives on Psychological Science*, *7*(6), 661–669. doi:10.1177/1745691612462587 PMID:26168128

Klimecki, O. M., Leiberg, S., Ricard, M., & Singer, T. (2013). Differential pattern of functional brain plasticity after compassion and empathy training. *Social Cognitive and Affective Neuroscience*. Advance online publication. doi:10.1093can/nst060 PMID:23576808

Knight. (2020a). *How to Manage a Hybrid Team*. https://hbr.org/2020/10/how-to-manage-a-hybrid-team

Knight. (2020b). *How to Talk to Your Team When the Future Is Uncertain*. https://hbr.org/2020/04/how-to-talk-to-your-team-when-the-future-is-uncertain

Kobasa, S. C. (1979). Stressful life events, personality, and health: An inquiry into hardiness. *Journal of Personality and Social Psychology*, *37*(1), 1–11. doi:10.1037/0022-3514.37.1.1 PMID:458548

Koçak, O. (2021). Does emotional intelligence increase satisfaction with life during COVID-19? The mediating role of depression. Healthcare, 9(11), 1529.

Kollat, D. T., & Willett, R. P. (1967). Customer impulse purchasing behavior. *JMR, Journal of Marketing Research*, *4*(1), 21–31. doi:10.1177/002224376700400102

Kolts, R. L. (2019). *CFT Made Simple: Competency-Based Training for Mindfulness-Based Therapies*. New Harbinger Publications.

Kolts, R., & Chodron, T. (2015). *An open-hearted life: Transformative methods for compassionate living from a clinical psychologist and a Buddhist nun*. Shambhala.

Kom, A. (1996). *Éducation et démocratie en Afrique. Le temps des illusions*. l'Harmattan.

Konig, J., Jager-Biela, D. J., & Glutsch, N. (2020). Adapting to online teaching during COVID-19 school closure: Teacher education and teacher competence effects among early career teachers in Germany. *European Journal of Teacher Education*, *43*(4), 608–622. doi:10.1080/02619768.2020.1809650

Konstam, V., Moser, D. K., & De Jong, M. J. (2005). Depression and anxiety in heart failure. *Journal of Cardiac Failure*, *11*(6), 455–463. doi:10.1016/j.cardfail.2005.03.006 PMID:16105637

Koopmans, L., Bernaards, C. M., Hildebrandt, V. H., Schaufeli, W. B., De Vet, H. C., & Van Der Beek, A. J. (2011). Conceptual frameworks of individual work performance: A systematic review. *Journal of Occupational and Environmental Medicine*, *53*(8), 856–866. doi:10.1097/JOM.0b013e318226a763 PMID:21775896

Koopmans, L., Bernaards, C., Hildebrandt, V., van Buuren, S., van der Beek, A. J., & de Vet, H. C. (2012). Development of an individual work performance questionnaire. *International Journal of Productivity and Performance Management*, *62*(1), 6–28. doi:10.1108/17410401311285273

Korpa, V. (2012). *DarbaungimenesdzīvesSaskaņošanaPrivātāSektoraOrganizācijās* [ReconciliationofWorkandFamilyLifein Private Sector Organizations] [Ph.D thesis]. Available online at: https://www.szf.lu.lv/fileadmin/user_upload/szf_faili/Petnieciba/promocijas_darbi/Viola_Korpa_2012.pdf

Ko, S.-H., Kim, J., & Choi, Y. (2021). Compassion and workplace incivility: Implications for open innovation. *Journal of Open Innovation*, *7*(1), 95. doi:10.3390/joitmc7010095

Kowalski, R. M., & Robbins, C. E. (2021). *The Meaning, Prevalence, and Outcomes of Cyberbullying in the Workplace. In Handbook of Research on Cyberbullying and Online Harassment in the Workplace*. IGI Global.

Kraag, G., Zeegers, M. P., Kok, G., Hosman, C., & Abu-Saad, H. H. (2006). School programs targeting stress management in children and adolescents: A meta-analysis. *Journal of School Psychology*, *44*(6), 449–472. doi:10.1016/j.jsp.2006.07.001

Kraleva, V. (2017). Understanding voluntary simplifiers in Bulgaria. *Marketing and Business Development Journal*, *3*(1). Advance online publication. doi:10.2139srn.2987904

Kruger, J., Epley, N., Parker, J., & Ng, Z. (2005). Egocentrism over e-mail: Can we communicate as well as we think? *Journal of Personality and Social Psychology*, *89*(6), 925–936. doi:10.1037/0022-3514.89.6.925 PMID:16393025

Kuanr, A., Pradhan, D., & Chaudhuri, H. R. (2020). I (do not) consume; therefore, I am: Investigating materialism and voluntary simplicity through a moderated mediation model. *Psychology and Marketing*, *37*(2), 260–277. doi:10.1002/mar.21305

Kuhn, U., Klaas, H.S., Antal, E., Dasoki, N., Lebert, F., Lipps, O., Voorpostel, M. (2021). Who is most affected by the Corona crisis? An analysis of changes in stress and wellbeing in Switzerland. *Eur. Soc., 23*(sup1), S942–S956.

Kumar, A., De Bruyn, A. J., & Bushney, M. J. (2020). The employee wellness and employee engagement relationship in a parastatal. *Journal of Contemporary Management, 17*(1), 1–15. doi:10.35683/jcm19094.53

Kumar, S., McCalla, M., & Lybeck, E. (2009). Operational impact of employee wellness programs: A business case study. *International Journal of Productivity and Performance Management, 58*(6), 581–597. doi:10.1108/17410400910977109

Kwon, J., & Ahn, J. (2021). The effects of cruise attributes on impulse buying behavior: The mediating role of impulsive buying tendency. *International Journal of Quality and Service Sciences, 13*(3), 456–470. doi:10.1108/IJQSS-09-2020-0141

La Vanguardia. (2020). *USOC y UGT advierten de despidos de profesoresen lasescuelasconcertadas.* Barcelona: La Vanguardia. Available onlineat: https://www.lavanguardia.com/vida/20200408/48387012784/usoc-y-ugtadvierten-de-despidos-de-profesores-en-las-escuelas-concertadas.html

Laato, S., Islam, A. N., Farooq, A., & Dhir, A. (2020). Unusual purchasing behavior during the early stages of the COVID-19 pandemic: The stimulus-organism-response approach. *Journal of Retailing and Consumer Services, 57*, 102224. doi:10.1016/j.jretconser.2020.102224

Ladegård, G. (2011). Stress management through workplace coaching: The impact of learning experiences. *International Journal of Evidence Based Coaching and Mentoring, 9*(1).

Lappegard, T., Goldscheider, F., & Bernhardt, E. (2017). Introduction to the special collection on finding work-life balance: History, determinants, and consequences of new breadwinning models of the industrialized world. *Demographic Research, 37*(26), 853–865. doi:10.4054/DemRes.2017.37.26

LaSala, K. B., Wilson, V., & Sprunk, E. (2016, May-June). Nursing Academic Administrators' Lived Experiences with Incivility and Bullying From Faculty: Consequences and Outcomes Demanding Action. *Nurse Educator, 41*(3), 120–124. doi:10.1097/NNE.0000000000000234 PMID:26673315

Laschinger, H., Cummings, G., Wong, C., & Grau, A. (2014). Resonant leadership and workplace empowerment: The value of positive organizational cultures in reducing workplace incivility. *Nursing Economics, 32*(1), 5–44. doi:10.1111/j.1365-28 PMID:24689153

Laschinger, H., Leiter, M., Day, A., & Gilin, D. (2009). Workplace empowerment, incivility, and burnout: Impact on staff nurse recruitment and retention outcomes. *Journal of Nursing Management, 17*(3), 302–311. doi:10.1111/j.1365-2834.2009.00999.x PMID:19426367

Lau, J. T., Yang, X., Tsui, H. Y., Pang, E., & Wing, Y. K. (2006). Positive mental health-related impacts of the SARS epidemic on the general public in Hong Kong and their associations with other negative impacts. *The Journal of Infection, 53*(2), 114–124. doi:10.1016/j.jinf.2005.10.019 PMID:16343636

Lawton, M. P., Moss, M., Hoffman, C., Grant, R., Have, T. T., & Kleban, M. H. (1999). Health, valuation of life, and the wish to live. *The Gerontologist, 39*(4), 406–416. doi:10.1093/geront/39.4.406 PMID:10495578

Lawton, M. P., Moss, M., Hoffman, C., Kleban, M. H., Ruckdeschel, K., & Winter, L. (2001). Valuation of life: A concept and a scale. *Journal of Aging and Health, 13*(1), 3–31. doi:10.1177/089826430101300101 PMID:11503845

Lazarus, R. S. (2003). Does the Positive Psychology Movement Have Legs? *Psychological Inquiry, 14*(2), 93–109. doi:10.1207/S15327965PLI1402_02

Lazarus, R. S., & Folkman, S. (1984). *Stress, appraisal, and coping*. Springer.

Leary, M. R., Tate, E. B., Adams, C. E., Batts Allen, A., & Hancock, J. (2007). Self-compassion and reactions to unpleasant self-relevant events: The implications of treating oneself kindly. *Journal of Personality and Social Psychology, 92*(5), 887–904. doi:10.1037/0022-3514.92.5.887 PMID:17484611

Lee, E. E., Depp, C., Palmer, B. W., Glorioso, D., Daly, R., Liu, J., Tu, X. M., Kim, H.-C., Tarr, P., Yamada, Y., & Jeste, D. V. (2019). High prevalence and adverse health effects of loneliness in community-dwelling adults across the lifespan: Role of wisdom as a protective factor. *International Psychogeriatrics, 31*(10), 1447–1462. doi:10.1017/S1041610218002120 PMID:30560747

Lee, S. H., & Cotte, J. (2009). Post-Purchase Consumer Regret: Conceptualization and Development of the PPCR Scale. In A. L. McGill & S. Shavitt (Eds.), *NA - Advances in Consumer Research* (Vol. 36, pp. 456–462). Association for Consumer Research.

Lembke, A. (2021). *Dopamine nation: Finding balance in the age of indulgence*. Dutton.

Lenkowsky, R. S. (1987). Bibliotherapy: A review and analysis of the literature. *The Journal of Special Education, 2*(2).

Leonard-Barton, D. (1981). Voluntary simplicity lifestyles and energy conservation. *The Journal of Consumer Research, 8*(3), 243–252. doi:10.1086/208861

Lewis, J., & Webster, A. (2021). *Sort your brain out: boost your performance, manage stress and achieve more*. John Wiley & Sons.

Liao, H., Liang, R., He, H., Huang, Y., & Liu, M. (2022). Work stress, burnout, occupational commitment, and social support among Chinese pediatric nurses: A moderated mediation model. *Journal of Pediatric Nursing, 67*, e16–e23. doi:10.1016/j.pedn.2022.10.009 PMID:36307294

Liao, L. F. (2008). Knowledge-sharing in R&D departments: A social power and social exchange theory perspective. *International Journal of Human Resource Management, 19*(10), 1881–1895. doi:10.1080/09585190802324072

Li, B., Hu, M., Chen, X., & Lei, Y. (2021). The Moderating Role of Anticipated Regret and Product Involvement on Online Impulsive Buying Behavior. *Frontiers in Psychology, 12*, 732459–732459. doi:10.3389/fpsyg.2021.732459 PMID:34975621

Liljander, V., & Strandvik, T. (1997). Emotions in service satisfaction. *International Journal of Service Industry Management, 8*(2), 148–169. doi:10.1108/09564239710166272

Lim, J., Jeon, S., Shin, H. Y., Kim, M. J., Seong, Y. M., Lee, W. J., ... Park, S. J. (2020). Case of the index patient who caused tertiary transmission of COVID-19 infection in Korea: The application of lopinavir/ritonavir for the treatment of COVID-19 infected pneumonia monitored by quantitative RT-PCR. *Journal of Korean Medical Science, 35*(6), e79. doi:10.3346/jkms.2020.35.e79 PMID:32056407

Lim, S., & Cortina, L. (2005). Interpersonal mistreatment in the workplace: The interface and impact of general incivility and sexual harassment. *The Journal of Applied Psychology, 90*(3), 483–496. doi:10.1037/0021-9010.90.3.483 PMID:15910144

Lim, V., & Teo, T. (2009). Mind your E-manners: Impact of cyber incivility on employees' work attitude and behavior. *Information & Management, 46*(8), 419–425. doi:10.1016/j.im.2009.06.006

Lin, L. (2021). Longitudinal associations of meaning in life and psychosocial adjustment to the COVID-19 outbreak in China. *British Journal of Health Psychology, 26*(2), 525–534. doi:10.1111/bjhp.12492 PMID:33217144

Li, Q., Miao, Y., Zeng, X., Tarimo, C. S., Wu, C., & Wu, J. (2020). Prevalence andfactors for anxiety during the coronavirus disease 2019 (COVID-19) epidemic among the teachers in China. *Journal of Affective Disorders*, *277*, 153–158. doi:10.1016/j.jad.2020.08.017 PMID:32828002

Liu, B., Song, M., Yang, G., Cheng, S., & Li, M. (2020). RETRACTED: Stimulus organism response model based analysis on consumers' online impulse buying behavior. *International Journal of Electrical Engineering Education*. Advance online publication. doi:10.1177/0020720920940585

Liu, C., & Long, F. (2014). The discussion of traditional teaching and multimedia teaching approach in college English teaching. *2014 International Conference on Management, Education and Social Science (ICMESS 2014)*. 10.2991/icmess-14.2014.9

Liu, X. S., Shi, Y., Xue, N. I., & Shen, H. (2022). The impact of time pressure on impulsive buying: The moderating role of consumption type. *Tourism Management*, *91*, 104505. doi:10.1016/j.tourman.2022.104505

Liu, X., & Ramsey, J. (2008). Teachers' job satisfaction: Analyses of the teacher follow up survey in the United States for 2000–2001. *Teaching and Teacher Education*, *24*(5), 1173–1184. doi:10.1016/j.tate.2006.11.010

Li, Y. (2015). Impact of impulsive buying behavior on postimpulsive buying satisfaction. *Social Behavior and Personality*, *43*(2), 339–351. doi:10.2224bp.2015.43.2.339

Lizana, P. A., & Vega-Fernadez, G. (2021a). Teacher teleworking during the covid-19 pandemic: Association between work hours, work–family balance and quality of life. *International Journal of Environmental Research and Public Health*, *18*(14), 7566. doi:10.3390/ijerph18147566 PMID:34300015

Lizana, P. A., Vega-Fernadez, G., Gomez-Bruton, A., Leyton, B., & Lera, L. (2021). Impact of the COVID-19 Pandemic on Teacher Quality of Life: A Longitudinal Study from before and during the health Crisis. *International Journal of Environmental Research and Public Health*, *18*(7), 3764. doi:10.3390/ijerph18073764 PMID:33916544

Liza, V. (2011). Stress management techniques: Evidence-based procedures that reduce stress and promote health. *Health Science Journal*, *5*(2), 74–89. https://www.itmedicalteam.pl/

Lloyd, K., & Pennington, W. (2020). Towards a theory of minimalism and well-being. *International Journal of Applied Positive Psychology*, 1-16. doi:10.1007/s41042-020-00030-y

Long Beach. (n.d.). *Data collection strategies II: Qualitative research*. California State University.

Lonska, J., Mietule, I., Litavniece, L., Arbidane, I., Vanadzins, I., Matisane, L., & Paegle, L. (2021b). Work–Life balance of the employed population during the emergency situation of COVID-19 in Latvia. *Frontiers in Psychology*, *12*, 1–15. doi:10.3389/fpsyg.2021.682459 PMID:34421734

Losda-Baltar, A., Jiménez-Gonzalo, L., Gallego-Alberto, L., Pedroso-Chaparro, M. D. S., Fernandes-Pires, J., & Márquez-González, M. (2020). "We're Staying at Home". Association of Self-Perceptions of Aging, Personal and Family Resources and Loneliness With Psychological Distress During the Lock-Down Period of COVID-19. *The Journals of Gerontology: Series B*, *76*(2), e10–e16. doi:10.1093/geronb/gbaa048

Lowe, H. (2018). Constructive Termination in Franchise Law. *Franchise Law Journal*, *38*(2), 267–284.

Luo, H., Chen, J., Li, S., Nie, Y., & Wang, G. (2021). Social exclusion and impulsive buying among Chinese college students: The mediating role of self-esteem and the moderating role of risk preference. *International Journal of Environmental Research and Public Health*, *18*(21), 11027. doi:10.3390/ijerph182111027 PMID:34769547

Luthans, B. C., Luthans, K. W., & Luthans, F. (2021). *Organizational Behavior: An Evidence-Based Approach* (14th ed.). Information Age Publishing, Incorporated.

Luthans, F., & Avolio, B. J. (2003). Authentic leadership development. *Positive Organizational Scholarship*, *241*(258), 1–26.

Lutz, C. E. (1978). The Oldest Library Motto: Ψγxhσ 'Iατρεῖον. *The Library Quarterly*, *48*(1). doi:10.1086/629993

MacBeth, A., & Gumley, A. (2012). Exploring compassion: A meta-analysis of the association between self-compassion and psychopathology. *Clinical Psychology Review*, *32*(6), 545–552. doi:10.1016/j.cpr.2012.06.003 PMID:22796446

Macdonald, A. (2020, September 30). *Obstacles Facing Cameroon's E-learning Drive. E-Learning in Cameroon.* iafrikan.com

Macey, W. H., & Schneider, B. (2008). The Meaning of Employee Engagement. *Industrial and Organizational Psychology: Perspectives on Science and Practice*, *1*(1), 3–30. doi:10.1111/j.1754-9434.2007.0002.x

Madden, W., Green, S., & Grant, A. M. (2020). A Pilot Study Evaluating Strengths-Based Coaching for Primary School Students. In *Coaching Researched* (pp. 297–312). John Wiley & Sons, Ltd. doi:10.1002/9781119656913.ch16

Mahapatra, B., & Bhorekar, K. K. (2021). Analyzing the Economic Depression Post-COVID-19 Using Big Data Analytics. In *Emerging Technologies for Battling Covid-19* (pp. 309–325). Springer. doi:10.1007/978-3-030-60039-6_16

Malik, N. A. A., Björkqvist, K., & Österman, K. (2017). Factors associated with occupational stress among university teachers in Pakistan and Finland. *Journal of Educational, Health and Community Psychology*, *6*(2), 1–14. doi:10.12928/jehcp.v6i2.7047

Malisch, J. L., Harris, B. N., Sherrer, S. M., Lewis, K. A., Shepherd, S. L., McCarthy, P. C., & Deitloff, J. (2020). Opinion: In the wake of COVID-19, academia needs new solutions to ensure gender equity. *Proceedings of the National Academy of Sciences of the United States of America*, *117*(27), 15378–15381. doi:10.1073/pnas.2010636117 PMID:32554503

Mansaray, H. E. (2019). The role of leadership style in organisational change management: A literature review. *Journal of Human Resource Management*, *7*(1), 18–31. doi:10.11648/j.jhrm.20190701.13

Marchiondo, K., Marchiondo, L., & Lasiter, S. (2010). Faculty incivility: Effects on program satisfaction of BSN students. *The Journal of Nursing Education*, *49*(11), 608–614. doi:10.3928/01484834-20100524-05 PMID:20509588

Margetić, B., Peraica, T., Stojanović, K., & Ivanec, D. (2021). Predictors of emotional distress during the COVID-19 pandemic; a Croatian study. *Personality and Individual Differences*, *175*, 110691. doi:10.1016/j.paid.2021.110691 PMID:33518867

Marinoff. (2021). *How to Have Self-Control and Be the Master of Your Life*. https://www.lifehack.org/844012/self-control

Marks, S. R. (1977). Multiple roles and role strain: Some notes on human energy, time and commitment. *American Sociological Review*, *42*(6), 921–936. doi:10.2307/2094577

Marks, S. R., & MacDermid, S. M. (1996). Multiple roles and the self: A theory of role balance. *Journal of Marriage and Family*, *58*(2), 417–432. doi:10.2307/353506

Markus, M. L. (1994). Electronic mail as the medium of managerial choice. *Organization Science*, *5*(4), 502–527. doi:10.1287/orsc.5.4.502

Martarelli, C. S., & Wolff, W. (2020). Too bored to bother? Boredom as a potential threat to the efficacy of pandemic containment measures. *Humanities and Social Sciences Communications*, *7*(1), 1–5. doi:10.105741599-020-0512-6

Martin, S., Seppala, E., Heineberg, Y., Rossomando, T., Doty, J., Zimbardo, P., Shiue, T.-T., Berger, R., & Zhou, Y. Y. (2015). Multiple Facets of Compassion: The Impact of Social Dominance Orientation and Economic Systems Justification. *Journal of Business Ethics*, *129*(1), 237–249. doi:10.100710551-014-2157-0

Maslach, C., & Leiter, M. P. (2022). *The burnout challenges*. Harvard Press.

Mas-Machuca, M., Berbegal-Mirabent, J., & Alegre, I. (2016). Work-life balance and its relationship with organizational pride and job satisfaction. *Journal of Managerial Psychology*, *31*(2), 586–602. doi:10.1108/JMP-09-2014-0272

Matos, M., McEwan, K., Kanovský, M., Halamová, J., Steindl, S. R., Ferreira, N., Linharelhos, M., Rijo, D., Asano, K., Márquez, M. G., Gregório, S., Vilas, S. P., Brito-Pons, G., Lucena-Santos, P., da Silva Oliveira, M., de Souza, E. L., Llobenes, L., Gumiy, N., Costa, M. I., ... Gilbert, P. (2022). Compassion Protects Mental Health and Social Safeness During the COVID-19 Pandemic Across 21 Countries. *Mindfulness*, *13*(4), 863–880. doi:10.100712671-021-01822-2 PMID:35003380

Mattke, S., Schnyer, C., & Van Busum, K. R. (2013). A review of the US workplace wellness market. *Rand Health Quarterly*, *2*(4), 7. PMID:28083279

Maunder, R. G., Lancee, W. J., Balderson, K. E., Bennett, J. P., Borgundvaag, B., Evans, S., Fernandes, C., Goldbloom, D., Gupta, M., Hunter, J., McGillis Hall, L., Nagle, L., Pain, C., Peczeniuk, S., Raymond, G., Read, N., Rourke, S., Steinberg, R., Stewart, T., ... Wasylenki, D. A. (2006). Long-term psychological and occupational effects of providing hospital healthcare during SARS outbreak. *Emerging Infectious Diseases*, *12*(12), 1924–1932. doi:10.3201/eid1212.060584 PMID:17326946

Maunder, R. G., Leszcz, M., Savage, D., Adam, M. A., Peladeau, N., Romano, D., Rose, M., & Schulman, R. B. (2008). Applying the lessons of SARS to pandemic influenza. *Canadian Journal of Public Health*, *99*(6), 486–488. doi:10.1007/BF03403782 PMID:19149392

Mayordomo-Rodríguez, T., Meléndez-Moral, J. C., Viguer-Segui, P., & Sales-Galán, A. (2015). Coping strategies as predictors of well-being in youth adult. *Social Indicators Research*, *122*(2), 479–489. doi:10.100711205-014-0689-4

Mazza, C., Ricci, E., Biondi, S., Colasanti, M., Ferracuti, S., Napoli, C., & Roma, P. (2020). A nationwide survey of psychological distress among Italian people during the COVID-19 pandemic: Immediate psychological responses and associated factors. *International Journal of Environmental Research and Public Health*, *17*(9), 3165. doi:10.3390/ijerph17093165 PMID:32370116

McCarthy, K. A. (2016). Is rudeness really that common? An exploratory study of incivility at work. *Journal of Organizational Computing and Electronic Commerce*, *26*(4), 364–374. doi:10.1080/10919392.2016.1228362

McCarty, R. (2016). The Fight-or-Flight Response: A Cornerstone of Stress Research. In G. Fink (Ed.), *Stress: Concepts, Cognition, Emotion, and Behavior* (pp. 33–37). Academic Press. doi:10.1016/B978-0-12-800951-2.00004-2

McEwen, B. S. (2004). Protection and damage from acute and chronic stress: Allostasis and allostatic overload and relevance to the pathophysiology of psychiatric disorders. *Annals of the New York Academy of Sciences*, *1032*(1), 1–7. doi:10.1196/annals.1314.001 PMID:15677391

McGouran, C., & Prothero, A. (2016). Enacted voluntary simplicity–Exploring the consequences of requesting consumers to intentionally consume less. *European Journal of Marketing*, *50*(1/2), 189–212. doi:10.1108/EJM-09-2013-0521

Mckenna, G. (2010). Patients' and Providers' Perspectives on Bibliotherapy in Primary Care. *Clinical Psychology & Psychotherapy*, *17*(6). doi:10.1002/cpp.679

Mehrabian, A., & Russell, J. A. (1974). *An approach to environmental psychology*. The MIT Press.

Mendes, J., Cabral, H., & Melo, F. (2021). Burnout em profissionais de Serviço Social durante a pandemia de COVID. *Revista Portuguesa De Investigação Comportamental E Social*, *7*(1), 25–40. doi:10.31211/rpics.2021.7.1.204

Merino-Soto, C., & Ruiz-del Castillo, C. G. (2018). Explorando el vínculo de la inteligencia emocional y la satisfacci_on con la vida en adultos peruanos. *Ansiedad y Estrés, 24*(2–3), 140–143. doi:10.1016/j.anyes.2018.03.004

Mesaglio, M. (2020, March). *4 actions to be a strong leader during COVID-19 disruption.* Retrieved from https://www.gartner.com/smarterwithgartner/4-actions-to-be-a-good-leader-during-covid-19-disruption/

Mesaglio. (2020). *4 Actions to Be a Strong Leader During COVID-19 Disruption.* https://www.gartner.com/smarterwithgartner/4-actions-to-be-a-good-leader-during-covid-19-disruption

Miao, L., & Mattila, A. S. (2013). Impulse buying in restaurant food consumption. *Journal of Foodservice Business Research, 16*(5), 448–467. doi:10.1080/15378020.2013.850379

Mihić, M., & Kursan, I. (2010). Assessing the situational factors and impulsive buying behavior: Market segmentation approach. *Management, 15*(2), 47–66. https://hrcak.srce.hr/62289

Milkie, M. A., Kendig, S. M., Nomaguchi, K. M., & Denny, K. E. (2010). Time with children, children's Wellbeing, and work–family balance among employed parents. *Journal of Marriage and Family, 72*(5), 1329–1343. doi:10.1111/j.1741-3737.2010.00768.x

Ming, J., Jianqiu, Z., Bilal, M., Akram, U., & Fan, M. (2021). How social presence influences impulse buying behavior in live streaming commerce? The role of SOR theory. *International Journal of Web Information Systems, 17*(4), 300–320. doi:10.1108/IJWIS-02-2021-0012

Ministry of Health Republic of Turkey (MoH-TR). (2022, January 22). *COVID-19 web page.* https://covid19.saglik.gov.tr/

Miranda, S. C. C. (2011). *Stress ocupacional, burnout e suporte social nos profissionais de saúde mental* [Master's Thesis, Universidade Católica Portuguesa]. http://hdl.handle.net/10400.14/8796

Mishna, F., Muskat, B., & Cook, C. (2012). Anticipating Challenges: School-Based social work intervention research. *Children & Schools, 34*(3), 135–144. doi:10.1093/cs/cds002

Mishra, L., Gupta, T., & Shree, A. (2020). Online teaching-learning in higher education during lockdown period of COVID-19 pandemic. *Int. J. Educ. Res. Open, 1*, 1–8. doi:10.1016/j.ijedro.2020.100012 PMID:35059663

MoH-TR. (2022). *Ministry of Health, Republic of Turkey.* Available at https://covid19.saglik.gov.tr/TR-66935/genel-koronavirus-tablosu.html

MoI. (2022). *Ministry of Interior (Turkey).* Available at https://www.icisleri.gov.tr/koronavirus-salgini-yeni-tedbirler

MoI. (2022). *Ministry of Interior (Turkey).* https://www.icisleri.gov.tr/81-il-valiligine-kademeli-normallesme-tedbirleri-genelgesi-gonderildi

Mongey, S., & Weinberg, A. (2020). *Characteristics of Workers in Low Work-From-Home and High Personal-Proximity Occupations.* White Paper.

Monk-Turner, E., & Fogerty, R. (2010). Chilly environments, stratification, and productivity differences. *The American Sociologist, 41*(1), 3–18. doi:10.100712108-009-9083-0

Monopolis, A. N. (2010). *Voluntary simplicity, authentic happiness, and ecological sustainability [PhD]. University of California.*

Monroe, S. M., & Slavich, G. M. (2016). Psychological Stressors: Overview. In G. Fink (Ed.), *Stress: Concepts, Cognition, Emotion, and Behavior* (pp. 109–115). Academic Press. doi:10.1016/B978-0-12-800951-2.00013-3

Monteiro, A. P., Cunha, P., Simões, M., & Relva, I. (2021). Conflitos Psicossociais e saúde mental em período de pandemia. In P. Cunha & A. P. Monteiro (Eds.), *Gestão de conflitos na saúde* (pp. 197–212). Pactor.

Morales-Vives, F., Dueñas, J. M., Vigil-Colet, A., & Camarero-Figuerola, M. (2020). Psychological variables related to adaptation to the COVID-19 lockdown in Spain. *Frontiers in Psychology, 11*, 2438. doi:10.3389/fpsyg.2020.565634 PMID:33041929

Morawski, C. M., & Gilbert, J. N. (2000). Developmental interactive bibliotherapy. *College Teaching, 48*(3).

Moreira-Almeida, A., Neto, F. L., & Koenig, H. G. (2006). Religiousness and mental health: A review. *RevistaBrasileira de Psiquiatria, 28*(3), 242–250. PMID:16924349

Moreta, R., Lopez, C., Gordon, P., Ortiz, W., & Gaibor, I. (2018). Satisfaction with life, psychological and social well-being as predictors of mental health in Ecuadorians. *Actualidades en Psicología, 32*(124), 111–125.

Morgan. (2021). *5 Components of Emotional Intelligence*. https://thefutureorganization.com/5-components-of-emotional-intelligence/

Morgul, E., Bener, A., Atak, M., Akyel, S., Aktaş, S., Bhugra, D., Ventriglio, A., & Jordan, T. R. (2021). COVID-19 pandemic and psychological fatigue in Turkey. *The International Journal of Social Psychiatry, 67*(2), 128–135. doi:10.1177/0020764020941889 PMID:32650681

Motowidlo, S., & Kell, H. (2012). Job Performance. In *Handbook of Psychology* (pp. 82–103). Wiley Online Library.

Mousavi, M., & Jafari, F. (2019). Virtual education in the era of corona virus, opportunities and challenges. *The First National Conference of Applied Research in Education Processes*.

Muis, M., Nai'em, M. F., Arsin, A. A., Darwis, A. M., Thamrin, Y., & Hans, N. A. P. (2021). The effect of multiple role conflicts and work stress on the work performance of female employees. *Gaceta Sanitaria, 35*, S90–S93. doi:10.1016/j.gaceta.2020.12.025 PMID:33832638

Mullins, L. J. (2007). *Management and organisational behaviour*. Pearson education.

Munir, S., Gondal, A. Z., &Takov, V. (2019). *Generalized Anxiety Disorder*. Academic Press.

Muralidhar, B., Prasad, K., & Rao Mangipudi, M. (2020). Association Among Remote Working Concerns and Challenges on Employee Work-Life Balance: An Empirical Study Using Multiple Regression Analysis With Reference To International Agricultural Research Institute, Hyderabad. *International Journal of Advanced Research in Engineering and Technology, 11*(6), 281–297. doi:10.34218/IJARET.11.6.2020.025

Muris & Petrocchi, N. (2017). Protection or Vulnerability? A Meta-Analysis of the Relations Between the Positive and Negative Components of Self-Compassion and Psychopathology: Self-compassion: Protection or vulnerability? *Clinical Psychology and Psychotherapy, 24*(2), 373–383. doi:10.1002/cpp.2005

Murphy, L. R. (1996). Stress management in work settings: A critical review of the health effects. *American Journal of Health Promotion, 11*(2), 112–135. doi:10.4278/0890-1171-11.2.112 PMID:10163598

Murray, L. K. (2020). *How to lead with emotional intelligence in the time of COVID-19*. Johns Hopkins Bloomberg School of Public Health.

Myers, J. E. (1998). Bibliotherapy and DCT: Co-constructing the therapeutic metaphor. *Journal of Counseling and Development, 76*(3).

Myers, J. E. (2003). Coping With Caregiving Stress: A Wellness-Oriented, Strengths-Based Approach for Family Counselors. *The Family Journal (Alexandria, Va.)*, *11*(2), 153–161. doi:10.1177/1066480702250162

Mysirlaki, S., & Paraskeva, F. (2020). Emotional intelligence and transformational leadership in virtual teams: Lessons from MMOGs. *Leadership and Organization Development Journal*, *41*(4), 551–566. doi:10.1108/LODJ-01-2019-0035

Naeem, M. (2020). Understanding the customer psychology of impulse buying during COVID-19 pandemic: Implications for retailers. *International Journal of Retail & Distribution Management*, *49*(3), 377–393. doi:10.1108/IJRDM-08-2020-0317

Nafukho, F. M., Muyia, M. H., Farnia, F., Kacirek, K., & Lynham, S. A. (2016). Developing emotional intelligence skills among practicing leaders: Reality or Myth? *Performance Improvement Quarterly*, *29*(1), 71–87. doi:10.1002/piq.21215

Namie, G. (2003). Workplace bullying: Escalated incivility. *Ivey Business Journal*, *68*(2), 1–6.

Nam, T. (2014). Technology use and work-life balance. *Applied Research in Quality of Life*, *9*(4), 1017–1040. doi:10.100711482-013-9283-1

Nastasa, M., Golu, F., Buruiana, D., & Oprea, B. (2020). Teachers' work – home interaction and satisfaction with life: the moderating role of core self- evaluations life: The moderating role of core self-evaluations. *Educ. Psychol*, 1–16.

National Commission for the Protection of Human Subjects of Biomedical and Behavioral Research. (1979). *The Belmont Report: Ethical Principles and Guidelines for the protection of Human Subjects of Research*. Author.

Naumann, E. (1993). Antecedents and consequences of satisfaction and commitment among expatriate managers. *Group & Organization Management*, *18*(2), 153–187. doi:10.1177/1059601193182003

Neal, M. B., & Hammer, L. B. (2017). *Working couples caring for children and aging parents: effects on work and Well-being*. Psychology Press. doi:10.4324/9781315083865

Neff, K. D. (2011). *Self-compassion: Stop beating yourself up and leave insecurity behind.* William Morrow.

Neff, K. D., & Germer, C. K. (2013). A Pilot Study and Randomized Controlled Trial of the Mindful Self-Compassion Program. *Journal of Clinical Psychology*, *69*(1), 28–44. doi:10.1002/jclp.21923 PMID:23070875

Nel, E. (2019). The impact of workplace bullying on flourishing: The moderating role of emotional intelligence. *SA Journal of Industrial Psychology*, *45*(0). Advance online publication. doi:10.4102ajip.v45i0.1603

Netolicky, D. M. (2020). School leadership during a pandemic: Navigating tensions. *Journal of Professional Capital and Community*, *5*(3/4), 391–395. doi:10.1108/JPCC-05-2020-0017

Nevins. (2020). *Why A Post-Covid World Demands Greater Emotional Intelligence*. https://www.forbes.com/sites/hillennevins/2020/09/29/why-a-post-covid-world-demands-greater-emotional-intelligence/?sh=3d259d0e6bbd

Newman, S. A., & Ford, R. C. (2021). Five steps to leading your team in the virtual COVID-19 workplace. *Organizational Dynamics*, *50*(1), 100802. doi:10.1016/j.orgdyn.2020.100802 PMID:36536689

Newman, S. A., Ford, R. C., & Marshall, G. W. (2020). Virtual team leader communication: Employee perception and organizational reality. *International Journal of Business Communication*, *57*(4), 452–473. doi:10.1177/2329488419829895

Ngulube, P. (2015). Qualitative data analysis and interpretation: systematic search for meaning. *Addressing research challenges: Making headway for developing researchers, 131*, 156.

Nguyen, B., Chang, K., Rowley, C., & Japutra, A. (2016). Organizational citizenship behavior, identification, psychological contract and leadership frames: The example of primary school teachers in Taiwan. *Asia-Pacific Journal of Business Administration*, *8*(3), 260–280. doi:10.1108/APJBA-01-2016-0010

Nguyen, J., & Brymer, E. (2018). Nature-Based Guided Imagery as an Intervention for State Anxiety. *Frontiers in Psychology*, *9*, 1–10. doi:10.3389/fpsyg.2018.01858 PMID:30333777

Nguyen, T. M., & Le, G. N. H. (2021). The influence of COVID-19 stress on psychological well-being among Vietnamese adults: The role of self-compassion and gratitude. *Traumatology*, *27*(1), 86–97. doi:10.1037/trm0000295

Niemiec, R. M. (2013). VIA Character Strengths: Research and Practice (The First 10 Years). In H. H. Knoop & A. Delle Fave (Eds.), *Well-Being and Cultures: Perspectives from Positive Psychology* (pp. 11–29). Springer Netherlands. doi:10.1007/978-94-007-4611-4_2

Nikoubakht, A., & Kiamanesh, A. (2019). The comparison of the effectiveness of computer-based education and traditional education on the numerical memory in students with mathematics disorder. *J. Psychol Sci*, *18*(73), 55–65.

Ni, Y. L., Kuo, C. C., Wu, C. H., Chang, W. H., & Chen, L. H. (2022). How Can We Cope with Self-Control Demands and Enhance Proactive Vitality Management? The Role of Leisure Crafting and Supervisor Recreational Sports Support. *Journal of Happiness Studies*, *23*(8), 3961–3980. doi:10.100710902-022-00572-9

Norelli, S. K., Long, A., & Krepps, J. M. (2022). Relaxation Techniques. In *StatPearls*. StatPearls Publishing. https://www.ncbi.nlm.nih.gov/books/NBK513238/

Nowell, L. S., Norris, J. M., White, D. E., & Moules, N. J. (2017). Thematic analysis: Striving to meet the trustworthiness criteria. *International Journal of Qualitative Methods*, *16*(1), 1–13. doi:10.1177/1609406917733847

Nunnally, J. C. (1978). *Psychomtietrictheory*. McGraw-Hill.

O'Driscoll, M., Brough, P., & Kalliath, T. (2004). Work-family conflict, psychological Well-being, satisfaction and social support: A longitudinal study in New Zealand. *Equal Opportunities International*, *23*(1/2), 36–56. doi:10.1108/02610150410787846

O'Driscoll, M., Brough, P., & Kalliath, T. (2006). Work-family conflict and facilitation. In F. Jones, R. J. Burke, & M. Westman (Eds.), *Work-life balance: A psychological perspective* (pp. 117–142). Psychology Press.

O'Sullivan, P. B., & Flanagin, A. J. (2003). Reconceptualizing flaming and other problematic messages. *New Media & Society*, *5*, 67–93.

Oates, K. (2021). *Leader Empathy, Emotional Intelligence Behaviors and Years of Federal Employment: Predictability of Employee Well-Being* [Doctoral dissertation]. Capella University.

Obuobisa-Darko, T., & Ameyaw Domfeh, K. (2016). Authentic Leadership and Employee Engagement the Mediating Role of Trust: A Framework for Future Research and Practice. *International Journal of Business and Management*, *4*(9), 312–320.

Obuobisa-Darko, T., & Domfeh, K. A. (2019). Leader behaviour to achieve employee engagement in Ghana: A qualitative study. *International Journal of Public Leadership*, *15*(1), 19–37. doi:10.1108/IJPL-04-2018-0018

Odriozola-González, P., Planchuelo-Gómez, Á., Irurtia, M. J., & de Luis-García, R. (2020). Psychological effects of the COVID-19 outbreak and lock-down among students and workers of a Spanish university. *Psychiatry Research*, *290*, 113108. doi:10.1016/j.psychres.2020.113108 PMID:32450409

Office of the Surgeon General. (2022). *The U.S. Surgeon General's Framework for Workplace Mental Health & Well-Being*. Department of Health and Human Services.

Ohemeng, F. L., Obuobisa Darko, T., & Amoako-Asiedu, E. (2020). Employee engagement and task performance in state-owned enterprises in developing countries: The case study of the power sector in Ghana. *Journal of Public Affairs, 20*(2), e2021. doi:10.1002/pa.2021

Oruh, E. S., Mordi, C., Dibia, C. H., & Ajonbadi, H. A. (2021). Exploring compassionate managerial leadership style in reducing employee stress level during COVID-19 crisis: The case of Nigeria. *Employee Relations: The International Journal, 43*(6), 1362–1381. doi:10.1108/ER-06-2020-0302

Osikominu, J., & Bocken, N. (2020). A voluntary simplicity lifestyle: Values, adoption, practices and effects. *Sustainability, 12*(5), 1903. doi:10.3390u12051903

Ott-Holland, C. J., Shepherd, W. J., & Ryan, A. M. (2019). Examining wellness programs over time: Predicting participation and workplace outcomes. *Journal of Occupational Health Psychology, 24*(1), 163–179. doi:10.1037/ocp0000096 PMID:28872333

Ozamiz-Etxebarria, N., Dosil Santamaría, M., Idoiaga Mondragon, N., & Berasategi Santxo, N. (2021a). Estado emocional del profesorado de colegios y universidades en el norte de España ante la COVID-19. *Revista Espanola de Salud Publica, 95*(1), e1–e8.

Özer, L., & Gultekin, B. (2015). Pre-and post-purchase stage in impulse buying: The role of mood and satisfaction. *Journal of Retailing and Consumer Services, 22*, 71–76. doi:10.1016/j.jretconser.2014.10.004

Özgül, E. (2011). Tüketicilerin sosyo-demografik özelliklerinin hedonik tüketim ve gönüllü sade yaşam tarzları açısından değerlendirilmesi. *Ege Akademik Bakış, 11*(1), 25–38. doi:10.21121/eab.2011119578

Pace, F., D'Urso, G., Zappulla, C., & Pace, U. (2021). The relation between workload and personal well-being among university professors. *Current Psychology (New Brunswick, N.J.), 40*(7), 3417–3424. doi:10.100712144-019-00294-x

Pak, A., Adegboye, O. A., Adekunle, A. I., Rahman, K. M., McBryde, E. S., & Eisen, D. P. (2020). Economic consequences of the COVID-19 outbreak: The need for epidemic preparedness. *Frontiers in Public Health, 8*, 241. doi:10.3389/fpubh.2020.00241 PMID:32574307

Palmer, B. C., Biller, D. L., Rancourt, R. E., & Teets, K. A. (1997). Interactive bibliotherapy: An effective method for healing and empowering emotionally-abused women. *Journal of Poetry Therapy, 11*(1).

Pande, N., & Naidu, R. K. (1992). Anāsakti and health: A study of non-attachment. *Psychology and Developing Societies, 4*(1), 89–104. doi:10.1177/097133369200400106

Pandey, S., & Sharma, V. (2016). Understanding Work-Related Stress, Job Conditions, Work Culture and Workaholism Phenomenon as Predictors of HR Crisis: An Empirical Study of the Indian IT Sector. *International Journal of Human Capital and Information Technology Professionals, 7*(2), 13. doi:10.4018/IJHCITP.2016040105

Panis, E. (2022). Implementation of School Learning Continuity Plan (SLCP) in Selected Public Secondary Schools of Aborlan North District in the Division of Palawan. *Journal of World Englishes and Educational Practices, 4*(3), 1-13.

Pardeck, J. T. (1993). Literature and adoptive children with disabilities. *Early Child Development and Care*, 91.

Pardeck, J. T. (1994). Using literature to help adolescents cope with problems. *Adolescence, 29*(114).

Park, C. L., Russell, B. S., Fendrich, M., Finkelstein-Fox, L., Hutchison, M., & Becker, J. (2020). Americans' COVID-19 stress, coping, and adherence to CDC guidelines. *Journal of General Internal Medicine*, *35*(8), 2296–2303. doi:10.100711606-020-05898-9 PMID:32472486

Park, J., & Lennon, S. J. (2006). Psychological and environmental antecedents of impulse buying tendency in the multichannel shopping context. *Journal of Consumer Marketing*, *23*(2), 56–66. doi:10.1108/07363760610654998

Parsad, C., Prashar, S., Vijay, T. S., & Sahay, V. (2019). Role of in-store atmospherics and impulse buying tendency on post-purchase regret. *Journal of Business and Management*, *25*(1).

Patton, M. Q. (2002). Two decades of developments in qualitative inquiry: A personal, experiential perspective. *Qualitative Social Work: Research and Practice*, *1*(3), 261–283. doi:10.1177/1473325002001003636

Paudel, P. (2021). Online education: Benefits, challenges and strategies during and after COVID-19 in higher education. *International Journal on Studies in Education*, *3*(2), 70–85. doi:10.46328/ijonse.32

Pavlov, I. P. (1927). *Conditioned reflexes: An investigation of the physiological activity of the cerebral cortex* (1st ed., G. V. Anrep, Trans.). Oxford University Press.

Pearson, C. M., & Porath, C. L. (2005). On the nature, consequences and remedies of workplace incivility: No time for "nice"? Think again. *The Academy of Management Executive*, *19*(1), 7–18. doi:10.5465/ame.2005.15841946

Pehrsson, D. E., & Bruneau E.K (2006, June). *Benefits of utilizing bibliotherapy with play therapy*. Academic Press.

Peiró, J. M., Montesa, D., Soriano, A., Kozusznik, M. W., Villajos, E., Magdaleno, J., . . . Ayala, Y. (2021). Revisiting the happy-productive worker thesis from a Eudaimonic perspective: A systematic review. *Sustainability*, *13*(6), 3174.

Penado Abilleira, M., Rodicio-García, M. L., Ríos-de Deus, M. P., & Mosquera-González, M. J. (2021). Technostress in Spanish university teachers during the COVID-19 pandemic. *Frontiers in Psychology*, *12*, 496. doi:10.3389/fpsyg.2021.617650 PMID:33732187

Peng, L., Xia, X., & Su, X. (2020, November). The Effect of Consumer's Loneliness on Impulse Buying in the Internet era: A Model Based on Para-social Interaction. In *2020 2nd International Conference on Economic Management and Model Engineering (ICEMME)* (pp. 843-848). IEEE. 10.1109/ICEMME51517.2020.00173

Peng, C., & Kim, Y. G. (2014). Application of the Stimuli Organism-Response (S-O-R) framework to online shopping behavior. *Journal of Internet Commerce*, *13*(3-4), 159–176. doi:10.1080/15332861.2014.944437

Pérez, V. M. O. (2003). Estrés y ansiedad en los docentes. *Pulso: revista de educación*, (26), 9-22.

Peterson, C., Park, N., & Sweeney, P. J. (2008). Group Well-Being: Morale from a Positive Psychology Perspective. *Applied Psychology*, *57*(s1), 19–36. doi:10.1111/j.1464-0597.2008.00352.x

Petriglieri. (2020). *The Psychology Behind Effective Crisis Leadership*. https://hbr.org/2020/04/the-psychology-behind-effective-crisis-leadership

Pfattheicher, S., Nockur, L., Böhm, R., Sassenrath, C., & Petersen, M. B. (2020). The Emotional Path to Action: Empathy Promotes Physical Distancing and Wearing of Face Masks During the COVID-19 Pandemic. *Psychological Science*, *31*(11), 1363–1373. doi:10.1177/0956797620964422 PMID:32993455

Picó-Pérez, M., Ferreira, S., Couto, B., Raposo-Lima, C., Machado-Sousa, M., & Morgado, P. (2021). Sociodemographic and lifestyle predictors of mental health adaptability during COVID-19 compulsory confinement: A longitudinal study in the Portuguese population. *Journal of Affective Disorders*, *295*, 797–803. doi:10.1016/j.jad.2021.08.150 PMID:34517254

Pieh, C., O' Rourke, T., Budimir, S., & Probst, T. (2020). Relationship quality and mental health during COVID-19 lockdown. *PLoS One*, *15*(9), e0238906. doi:10.1371/journal.pone.0238906 PMID:32915878

Pierce, M., Hope, H., Ford, T., Hatch, S., Hotopf, M., John, A., Kontopantelis, E., Webb, R., Wessely, S., McManus, S., & Abel, K. M. (2020). Mental health before and during the COVID-19 pandemic: A longitudinal probability sample survey of the UK population. *The Lancet. Psychiatry*, *7*(10), 883–892. doi:10.1016/S2215-0366(20)30308-4 PMID:32707037

Pignata, S., Boyd, C., Gillespie, N., Provis, C., & Winefield, A. (2014). Awareness of organizational stress-reduction interventions: The impact on employee wellbeing and attitudes. *Stress and Health*, *32*, 231–243. doi:10.1002mi.2597 PMID:25066108

Piron, F. (1993). *A comparison of emotional reactions experienced by planned, unplanned and impulse purchasers.* ACR North American Advances.

Pluskota, A. (2014). The application of positive psychology in the practice of education. *SpringerPlus*, *3*(1), 147. doi:10.1186/2193-1801-3-147 PMID:24790805

Polizzi, C., Lynn, S. J., & Perry, A. (2020). Stress and coping in the time of COVID-19: Pathways to resilience and recovery. *Clinical Neuropsychiatry*, *17*(2), 59. doi:10.36131/CN20200204 PMID:34908968

Pollock, E. D., Kazman, J. B., & Deuster, P. (2015). Family Functioning and Stress in African American Families: A Strength-Based Approach. *The Journal of Black Psychology*, *41*(2), 144–169. doi:10.1177/0095798413520451

Porath, C., & Pearson, C. (2012). Emotional and behavioral responses to workplace incivility and the impact of hierarchical status. *Journal of Applied Social Psychology*, *42*, 326–357. doi:10.1111/j.1559-1816.2012.01020.x

Porges, S. W. (2011). *The polyvagal theory: Neurophysiological foundations of emotions, attachment, communication, and self-regulation.* W W Norton & Co.

Pounder, C. (1998). Homeworking: No longer an easy option? *Computers & Security*, *17*(1), 27–30. doi:10.1016/S0167-4048(97)80246-5

Power, K. (2020). The COVID-19 pandemic has increased the care burden of women and families. *Sustainability: Science, Practice and Policy*, *16*(1), 67–73.

Prasada, K. D. V., Vaidyab, R. W., & Mangipudic, M. R. (2020). Effect of occupational stress and remote working on psychological well-being of employees: An empirical analysis during covid-19 pandemic concerning information technology industry in Hyderabad. *Indian Journal of Commerce & Management Studies*, *XI*(2), 1. doi:10.18843/ijcms/v11i2/01

Preacher, K., & Hayes, A. (2008). Asymptotic and resampling strategies for assessing and comparing indirect effects in multiple mediator models. *Behavior Research Methods*, *40*(3), 879–891. doi:10.3758/BRM.40.3.879 PMID:18697684

Prensky, M. (2001a). Digital Natives Digital Immigrants. *Horizon*, *9*(5), 1–6. doi:10.1108/10748120110424816

Prentice, C., Chen, J., & Stantic, B. (2020). Timed intervention in COVID-19 and panic buying. *Journal of Retailing and Consumer Services*, *57*, 102203. doi:10.1016/j.jretconser.2020.102203

Prieto, M., & Bermejo, L. (2006). Contextolaboral y malestardocente en unamuestra de profesores de Secundaria.*Rev. Psicol. TrabajolasOrganiz.*, *22*, 45–73.

Probst, T. M., Lee, H. J., & Bazzoli, A. (2020). Economic stressors and the enactment of CDC-recommended COVID-19 prevention behaviors: The impact of state-level context. *The Journal of Applied Psychology*, *105*(12), 1397–1407. doi:10.1037/apl0000797 PMID:33271028

Proctor, C., Tsukayama, E., Wood, A. M., Maltby, J., Eades, J. F., & Linley, P. A. (2011). Strengths Gym: The impact of a character strengths-based intervention on the life satisfaction and well-being of adolescents. *The Journal of Positive Psychology*, *6*(5), 377–388. doi:10.1080/17439760.2011.594079

Proto, E. (2016). Are happy workers more productive? *IZA World of Labor: Evidence-Based Policy Making*, *315*. Advance online publication. doi:10.15185/izawol.315

Puertas-Molero, P., Zurita-Ortega, F., Chacón-Cuberos, R., Martínez-Martínez, A., Castro-Sánchez, M., & González-Valero, G. (2018). An explanatory model of emotional intelligence and its association with stress, burnout syndrome, and non-verbal communication in the university teachers. *Journal of Clinical Medicine*, *7*(12), 524. doi:10.3390/jcm7120524 PMID:30544532

Purohit, M. (2013). a Comparative Study of Work Life Balance in Various Industrial Sectors in Pune Region. *International Journal of Marketing, Financial Services & Management Research*, *2*(3), 198–206.

Rachman, S. (2010). Betrayal: A psychological analysis. *Behaviour Research and Therapy*, *48*(4), 304–311. doi:10.1016/j.brat.2009.12.002 PMID:20035927

Raghavendra, H. K., & Raghunandan, M. V. (2018). Women engineers and work life balance a case study of women working in manufacturing industries in Mysuru city. *International Journal of Mechanical Engineering and Technology*, *9*(1), 752–755.

Rajeev, A., & Hebbani, S. (2020). Anasakti and resilience in older adults in south India: a correlation study. *International Journal of Indian Psychology, 8*(4), 1534-1544. Doi:10.25215/0804.166

Ralph, P., Baltes, S., Adisaputri, G., Torkar, R., Kovalenko, V., Kalinowski, M., Novielli, N., Yoo, S., Devroey, X., Tan, X., Zhou, M., Turhan, B., Hoda, R., Hata, H., Robles, G., Milani Fard, A., & Alkadhi, R. (2020). Pandemic programming: How COVID-19 affects software developers and how their organizations can help. *Empirical Software Engineering*, *25*(6), 4927–4961. doi:10.100710664-020-09875-y PMID:32952438

Ramos, M. A. S. (2005). *Crianças, tecnologias e aprendizagem: contributo para uma teoria substantiva* [Doctoral Thesis, Universidade do Minho]. https://hdl.handle.net/1822/6914

Rana, S., & Tirthani, J. (2012). Effect of education, income and gender on impulsive buying among Indian consumer an empirical study of readymade garment customers. *Management*, *1*(12).

Randall, K., Ford, T. G., Kwon, K.-A., Sisson, S. S., Bice, M. R., Dinkel, D., & Tsotsoros, J. (2021). Physical activity, physical well-being, and psychological well-being: Associations with life satiscfaction duing the COVID 19 pandemic among early childhood educators. *International Journal of Environmental Research and Public Health*, *18*(18), 9430. doi:10.3390/ijerph18189430 PMID:34574354

Rao, M. S. (2016). Innovative tools and techniques to manage your stress to ensure work-life balance. *Industrial and Commercial Training*, *48*(6), 320–324. doi:10.1108/ICT-05-2015-0035

Rao, M., Prasad, K. D. V., & Vaidya, R. (2019). Employee competencies as the predictors of the performance management system: An empirical study in IT enabled service companies around *Hyderabad. International Journal of Management*, *10*(6), 33–44. doi:10.34218/IJM.10.6.2019.004

Rapanta, C., Botturi, L., Goodyear, P., Guàrdia, L., & Koole, M. (2020). Online university teaching during and after the covid-19 crisis: Refocusing teacher presence and learning activity. *Postdigital Sci. Educ.*, *2*(3), 923–945. doi:10.100742438-020-00155-y

Rapp, T. L., Bachrach, D. G., Rapp, A. A., & Mullins, R. (2014). The role of team goal monitoring in the curvilinear relationship between team efficacy and team performance. *The Journal of Applied Psychology*, *99*(5), 976–987. doi:10.1037/a0036978 PMID:24865579

Rashid, T., & McGrath, R. (2020). Strengths-based actions to enhance wellbeing in the time of COVID-19. *International Journal of Wellbeing*, *10*(4), 4. doi:10.5502/ijw.v10i4.1441

Rebouças, R., & Soares, A. M. (2021). Voluntary simplicity: A literature review and research agenda. *International Journal of Consumer Studies*, *45*(3), 303–319. doi:10.1111/ijcs.12621

Redondo-Fl´orez, L., Fern´andez-Lucas, J., & Clemente-Suarez, V. (2020). *Cultural differences in stress-related psychological, nutrition, physical activity, and oral health factors of professors*. Academic Press.

Reigada, C. (Ed.). (2020). *Boas Práticas do Assistente Social COVID-19 (Perspetiva: grupo de Assistentes Sociais de Cuidados Paliativos)*. https://drive.google.com/file/d/1ZMw0_KaeaDf2fkVOgLhS4p5gsAOwWgc5/view

Reio, T. Jr, & Ghosh, R. J. (2009). Antecedents and outcomes of workplace incivility: Implications for human resource development research and practice. *Human Resource Development Quarterly*, *20*(3), 237–264. doi:10.1002/hrdq.20020

Restubog, S. L. D., Garcia, P. R. J. M., Toledano, L. S., Amarnani, R. K., Tolentino, L. R., & Tang, R. L. (2011). Yielding to (cyber)-temptation: Exploring the buffering role of self-control in the relationship between organizational justice and cyberloafing behavior in the workplace. *Journal of Research in Personality*, *45*(2), 247–251. doi:10.1016/j.jrp.2011.01.006

Rezvani, A., & Khosravi, P. (2019). Emotional intelligence: The key to mitigating stress and fostering trust among software developers working on information system projects. *International Journal of Information Management*, *48*, 139–150. doi:10.1016/j.ijinfomgt.2019.02.007

Ricard, M. (2013). *Altruism: The power of compassion to change yourself and the world*. Bay Back Books.

Rice, E. L., & Fredrickson, B. L. (2017). Do positive spontaneous thoughts function as incentive salience? *Emotion (Washington, D.C.)*, *17*(5), 840–855. doi:10.1037/emo0000284 PMID:28206793

Rich, S. A., Hanna, S., & Wright, B. J. (2017). Simply satisfied: The role of psychological need satisfaction in the life satisfaction of voluntary simplifiers. *Journal of Happiness Studies*, *18*(1), 89–105. doi:10.100710902-016-9718-0

Ridwan, M., Mulyani, S. R., & Ali, H. (2020). Improving employee performance through perceived organizational support, organizational commitment, and organizational citizenship behavior. *Systematic Reviews in Pharmacy, 11*(12).

Riley, K. E., & Park, C. L. (2015). How does yoga reduce stress? A systematic review of mechanisms of change and guide to future inquiry. *Health Psychology Review*, *9*(3), 379–396. doi:10.1080/17437199.2014.981778 PMID:25559560

Rivers, S. E., Handley-Miner, I. J., Mayer, J. D., & Caruso, D. R. (2020). Emotional Intelligence. In R. J. Sternberg (Ed.), *The Cambridge handbook of intelligence* (pp. 709–735). Cambridge University Press. doi:10.1017/9781108770422.030

Robbins, S. P., & Judge, T. A. (2009). *Organisational behaviour* (13th ed.). Pearson, Prentice Hall.

Robbins, S. P., & Judge, T. A. (2017). *Organizational Behavior* (Global Edition). Pearson.

Robbins, S. P., Judge, T. A., & Breward, K. E. (2018). *Essentials of Organizational Behavior Ottawa*. Pearson.

Robert J. H. & Emmanuel C. & Amanah A., (2016). *Scientific Reports Supplementary Info*. License. CC BY 4.0.

Robertson, S. L., Robinson, M. D., & Reid, A. (2017). Electronic Health Record Effects on Work-Life Balance and Burnout Within the I3 Population. *Collaborative Journal of Graduate Medical Education*, *9*(4), 479–484. doi:10.4300/JGME-D-16-00123.1 PMID:28824762

Roca, P., Diez, G., McNally, R. J., & Vazques, C. (2021). The impact of compassion meditation training on psychological variables: A network perspective. *Mindfulness*, *12*(4), 873–888. doi:10.100712671-020-01552-x

Roca, V., Vazquez, C., Diez, G., Brito-Pons, G., & McNally, R. J. (2021). Not all types of meditation are the same: Mediators of change in mindfulness and compassion meditation interventions. *Journal of Affective Disorders*, *283*, 354–362. doi:10.1016/j.jad.2021.01.070 PMID:33578349

Rodrigues, C. B., Ribeiro, J. L., & Gomes, D. (2022). Emotional Intelligence and the Impact of the Covid-19 Pandemic on Pharmaceutical Professionals—An Exploratory Study. In *Organizational Management in Post Pandemic Crisis* (pp. 65–87). Springer International Publishing. doi:10.1007/978-3-030-98052-8_4

Rodriquez, J. (2018). The US minimalist movement: Radical political practice? *The Review of Radical Political Economics*, *50*(2), 286–296. doi:10.1177/0486613416665832

Rook, D. W. (1987). The buying impulse. *The Journal of Consumer Research*, *14*(2), 189–199. doi:10.1086/209105

Rook, D. W., & Fisher, R. J. (1995). Normative influences on impulsive buying behavior. *The Journal of Consumer Research*, *22*(3), 305–313. doi:10.1086/209452

Rotundo, M., & Sackett, P. R. (2002). The relative importance of task, citizenship, and counterproductive performance to global ratings of job performance: A policy-capturing approach. *The Journal of Applied Psychology*, *87*(1), 66–80. doi:10.1037/0021-9010.87.1.66 PMID:11916217

Roy, M., & Mandal, A. (2021). A Comparative Study on The Influence Of Job Satisfaction On Deviant Workplace Behavior In Private And Government Educational Institutes. *Psychology and Education Journal*, *58*(5), 2850–2862.

Rubin, G. J., Amlôt, R., Page, L., & Wessely, S. (2009). Public perceptions, anxiety, and behaviour change in relation to the swine flu outbreak: Cross sectional telephone survey. *BMJ (Clinical Research Ed.)*, *339*(3), b2651. Advance online publication. doi:10.1136/bmj.b2651 PMID:19574308

Rubin, R. J. (1978). *Using Bibliotherapy: a Guide to Theory and Practice*. Oryx Press.

Ruiz-Palomino, P., Yáñez-Araque, B., Jiménez-Estévez, P., & Gutiérrez-Broncano, S. (2022). Can servant leadership prevent hotel employee depression during the COVID-19 pandemic? A mediating and multigroup analysis. *Technological Forecasting and Social Change*, *174*, 121192. doi:10.1016/j.techfore.2021.121192 PMID:34538969

Russell, D., Peplau, L. A., & Ferguson, M. L. (1978). Developing a measure of loneliness. *Journal of Personality Assessment*, *42*(3), 290–294. doi:10.120715327752jpa4203_11 PMID:660402

Russo, D., Hanel, P. P., Altnickel, S., & Van Berkel, N. (2021). The Daily Life of Software Engineers during the COVID-19 Pandemic. doi:10.1109/ICSE-SEIP52600.2021.00048

Russo, M., Shteigman, A., & Carmeli, A. (2016). Workplace and family support and work–life balance: Implications for individual psychological availability and energy at work. *The Journal of Positive Psychology*, *11*(2), 173–188. doi:10.1080/17439760.2015.1025424

Ryerson, N. C. (2020). Behavioral and psychological correlates of well-being during COVID-19. *Psychological Reports*, *125*(1), 200–217. doi:10.1177/0033294120978160 PMID:33302799

Ryff, C. D. (1989). Happiness is everything, or is it? Explorations on the meaning of psychological well-being. *Journal of Personality and Social Psychology*, *57*(6), 1069–1081. doi:10.1037/0022-3514.57.6.1069

Sageder, M., & Feldbauer-Durstmüller, B. (2019). Management control in multinational companies: A systematic literature review. *Review of Managerial Science*, *13*(5), 875–918. doi:10.100711846-018-0276-1

Saglam, Y. C., Çankaya, S. Y., Golgeci, I., Sezen, B., & Zaim, S. (2022). The role of communication quality, relational commitment, and reciprocity in building supply chain resilience: A social exchange theory perspective. *Transportation Research Part E, Logistics and Transportation Review*, *167*, 102936. doi:10.1016/j.tre.2022.102936

Sahito, Z., & Vaisanen, P. (2020). A literature review on teachers' job satisfaction in developing countries: Recommendations and solutions for the enhancement of the job. *Review of Education*, *8*(1), 3–34. doi:10.1002/rev3.3159

Sahoo, S. R. (2016). Management of Stress at Workplace. *Global Journal of Management and Business Research. Administrative Management*, *16*(6), 1–8.

Sahu, P. (2020). Closure of universities due to coronavirus disease 2019 (COVID-19): Impact on education and mental health of students and academic staff. *Cureus*, *12*, e7541. doi:10.7759/cureus.7541 PMID:32377489

Sakellarides, C. (2020). National Health Service: Responding to Current Challenges Through Necessary Transformations. *Acta Medica Portuguesa*, *33*(2), 133–142. doi:10.20344/amp.12626 PMID:32035499

Saleem, F., Malik, M. I., & Qureshi, S. S. (2021). Work stress hampering employee performance during COVID-19: Is safety culture needed? *Frontiers in Psychology*, *12*, 655839. doi:10.3389/fpsyg.2021.655839 PMID:34512434

Saleh, M. A. H. (2012). An investigation of the relationship between unplanned buying and post-purchase regret. *International Journal of Marketing Studies*, *4*(4), 106. doi:10.5539/ijms.v4n4p106

Salzberg, S. (2002). *Lovingkindness: The Revolutionary Art of Happiness*. Shambhala.

Sanchez-Ruiz, M. J., Tadros, N., Khalaf, T., Ego, V., Eisenbeck, N., Carreno, D. F., & Nassar, E. (2021). Trait emotional intelligence and wellbeing during the pandemic: The mediating role of meaning-centered coping. *Frontiers in Psychology*, *12*, 648401. doi:10.3389/fpsyg.2021.648401 PMID:34054650

Santini, F. D. O., Ladeira, W. J., Vieira, V. A., Araujo, C. F., & Sampaio, C. H. (2019). Antecedents and consequences of impulse buying: A meta-analytic study. *RAUSP Management Journal*, *54*(2), 178–204. doi:10.1108/RAUSP-07-2018-0037

Santomauro, D. F., Mantilla Herrera, A. M., Shadid, J., Zheng, P., Ashbaugh, C., Pigott, D. M., Abbafati, C., Adolph, C., Amlag, J. O., Aravkin, A. Y., Bang-Jensen, B. L., Bertolacci, G. J., Bloom, S. S., Castellano, R., Castro, E., Chakrabarti, S., Chattopadhyay, J., Cogen, R. M., Collins, J. K., ... Ferrari, A. J. (2021). Global prevalence and burden of depressive and anxiety disorders in 204 countries and territories in 2020 due to COVID-19 pandemic. *Lancet*, *398*(10312), 1700–1712. doi:10.1016/S0140-6736(21)02143-7 PMID:34634250

Santos, M. F. J. (2017). *A Prática Profissional Do Assistente Social Em Contexto De Cuidados De Saúde Primários Infantojuvenis* [Master's Thesis, Instituto Superior de Serviço Social do Porto]. http://hdl.handle.net/10400.26/22393

Santos-Ruiz, A., Robles-Ortega, H., Pérez-García, M., & Peralta-Ramírez, M. I. (2017). Effects of the Cognitive-Behavioral Therapy for Stress Management on Executive Function Components. *The Spanish Journal of Psychology*, *20*, 1–30. doi:10.1017jp.2017.10 PMID:28190412

Savard, Y. P. (2023). Work-family spillover of daily positive affect onto performance: The moderating role of domain identity salience. *European Review of Applied Psychology*, *73*(2), 100819. doi:10.1016/j.erap.2022.100819

Savitsky, B., Findling, Y., Ereli, A., & Hendel, T. (2020). Anxiety and coping strategies among nursing students during the covid-19 pandemic. *Nurse Education in Practice*, *46*, 102809. doi:10.1016/j.nepr.2020.102809 PMID:32679465

Sbarra, D. A., Smith, H. L., & Mehl, M. R. (2012). When leaving your ex, love yourself: Observational rating of self-compassion predict the course of emotional recovery following marital separation. *Psychological Science*, *23*(3), 261–269. doi:10.1177/0956797611429466 PMID:22282874

Schlegel, K., & Mortillaro, M. (2019). The Geneva Emotional Competence Test (GECo): An ability measure of workplace emotional intelligence. *The Journal of Applied Psychology*, *104*(4), 559–580. doi:10.1037/apl0000365 PMID:30346195

Schnell, T., & Krampe, H. (2020). Meaning in life and self-control buffer stress in times of COVID-19: Moderating and mediating effects with regard to mental distress. *Frontiers in Psychiatry*, *11*, 983. doi:10.3389/fpsyt.2020.582352 PMID:33173525

Schutt, R. K. (2013). Using Bibliotherapy to Enhance Probation and Reduce Recidivism. *Journal of Offender Rehabilitation*, *52*(3). doi:10.1080/10509674.2012.751952

Schwantes. (2020). *Steve Jobs: 'Technology is nothing'—here's what he said it really takes to achieve great success*. https://www.cnbc.com/2019/10/05/apple-ceo-steve-jobs-technology-is-nothing-heres-what-it-takes-to-achieve-great-success.
html

Schwarz, N., & Clore, G. L. (1988). How do I feel about it? Information functions of affective states. *Affect, Cognition and Social Behavior,* 44-62.

Schwarz, N. (1990). *Feelings as information: Informational and motivational functions of affective states*. The Guilford Press.

Schwarz, N., & Clore, G. L. (1983). Mood, misattribution, and judgments of well-being: Informative and directive functions of affective states. *Journal of Personality and Social Psychology*, *45*(3), 513–523. doi:10.1037/0022-3514.45.3.513

Seaward, B. L. (2019). *Essentials of Managing Stress* (2nd ed.). Jones & Bartlett Learning.

Selye, H. (1950). Stress and the General Adaptation Syndrome. *British Medical Journal*, *1*(4667), 1383–1392. doi:10.1136/bmj.1.4667.1383 PMID:15426759

Semenets-Orlova, I., Klochko, A., Shkoda, T., Marusina, O., & Tepliuk, M. (2021). Emotional intelligence as the basis for the development of organizational leadership during the covid period (educational institution case). *Studies of Applied Economics*, *39*(5). Advance online publication. doi:10.25115/eea.v39i5.5074

Sendjaya, S. (2015). *Servant leadership research. In Personal and Organizational Excellence through Servant Leadership*. Springer. doi:10.1007/978-3-319-16196-9

Serrão, C., Duarte, I., Castro, L., & Teixeira, A. (2021). Burnout and Depression in Portuguese Healthcare Workers during the COVID-19 Pandemic—The Mediating Role of Psychological Resilience. *International Journal of Environmental Research and Public Health*, *18*(2), 636. doi:10.3390/ijerph18020636 PMID:33451083

Shahjehan, A., Zeb, F., & Saifullah, K. (2012). The effect of personality on impulsive and compulsive buying behaviors. *African Journal of Business Management*, *6*(6), 2187–2194. doi:10.5897/AJBM11.2275

Shama, A. (1981). Coping with staglation: Voluntary simplicity. *Journal of Marketing*, *45*(3), 120–134. doi:10.1177/002224298104500310

Shama, A. (1985). The voluntary simplicity consumer. *Journal of Consumer Marketing*, *2*(4), 57–63. doi:10.1108/eb008146

Shandel Group. (2017). *Worry-is-a-false-sense-of-control*. Group Leadership Blog.

Shechtman, Z. (2009, June). *Treating child and adolescent aggression through bibliotherapy*. Academic Press.

Shell, E. M., Teodorescu, D., & Williams, L. D. (2021). Investigating Race-related Stress, Burnout, and Secondary Traumatic Stress for Black Mental Health Therapists. *The Journal of Black Psychology*, *47*(8), 669–694. doi:10.1177/00957984211033963

Sherman, G. D., Lee, J. J., Cuddy, A. J., Renshon, J., Oveis, C., Gross, J. J., & Lerner, J. S. (2012). Leadership is associated with lower levels of stress. *Proceedings of the National Academy of Sciences of the United States of America*, *109*(44), 17903–17907. doi:10.1073/pnas.1207042109 PMID:23012416

Sheth, J. (2020). Impact of Covid-19 on consumer behavior: Will the old habits return or die? *Journal of Business Research*, *117*, 280–283. doi:10.1016/j.jbusres.2020.05.059 PMID:32536735

Shevlin, M., Nolan, E., Owczarek, M., McBride, O., Murphy, J., Gibson Miller, J., Hartman, T. K., Levita, L., Mason, L., Martinez, A. P., McKay, R., Stocks, T. V. A., Bennett, K. M., Hyland, P., & Bentall, R. P. (2020). COVID-19-related anxiety predicts somatic symptoms in the UK population. *British Journal of Health Psychology*, *25*(4), 875–882. doi:10.1111/bjhp.12430 PMID:32458550

Shin, J. T., Jeong, M., Oh, H., & Tierney, E. (2017). Exploring determinants of meeting planners' commitment to the business relationships with destination management companies. *Journal of Convention & Event Tourism*, *18*(2), 135–158. doi:10.1080/15470148.2016.1237317

Sieber, S. D. (1974). Toward a theory of role accumulation. *American Sociological Review*, *39*(4), 567–578. doi:10.2307/2094422

Siegel, R. D., & Germer, C. K. (2012). Wisdom and compassion: Two wings of a bird. In C. K. Germer & R. D. Siegel (Eds.), *Wisdom and compassion in psychotherapy: Deepening mindfulness in clinical practice*. Guilford.

Sinding, K., & Waldstrom, C. (2014). *Organisational Behaviour*. McGraw-Hill Education.

Singh, R., & Bansal, R. (2020). Industry 4.0 in India: Challenges & opportunities. *New Paradigm in Business & Education, 160*.

Singhal, T. (2020). A Review of Coronavirus Disease-2019 (COVID-19). *Indian Journal of Pediatrics*, *87*(4), 281–286. doi:10.100712098-020-03263-6 PMID:32166607

Singh, K., & Raina, M. (2015). Development and validation of a test on Anasakti (non-attachment): An Indian model of well-being. *Mental Health, Religion & Culture*, *18*(9), 715–725. doi:10.1080/13674676.2015.1084612

Singh, R., & Bansal, R. (2020). Study of privatisation in Indian higher education: Pros & cons. *New Horizons in Commerce, IT & Social Sciences*, 91.

Sirajudeen, M. S., Alaidarous, M., Waly, M., & Alqahtani, M. (2018). Work-related musculoskeletal disorders among faculty members of college of Applied Medical Sciences, Majmaah University, Saudi Arabia: A cross-sectional study. *International Journal of Health Sciences*, *12*(4), 18. PMID:30022899

Sirgy, M. J., & Lee, D. J. (2018). Work-life balance: An integrative review. *Applied Research in Quality of Life*, *13*(1), 229–254. doi:10.100711482-017-9509-8

Skalski S. B. (2022). Resilience and Mental Well-Being During the COVID-19 Pandemic: Serial Mediation by Persistent Thinking and Anxiety About Coronavirus. *Front. Psychiatry, Sec. Public Mental Health, 12*. doi:10.3389/fpsyt.2021.810274

Slickdeals. (2022, January 22).) *Slickdeals Survey: Americans Are Spending More During the Coronavirus Pandemic.* https://slickdeals.net/article/news/pandemic-impulse-spending-survey-2020/

Sliter, M., Jex, S., Wolford, K., & McInnerney, J. (2010). How rude! Emotional labor as a mediator between customer incivility and employee outcomes. *Journal of Occupational Health Psychology*, *15*(4), 468–481. doi:10.1037/a0020723 PMID:21058859

Smidt, A.M., Adams-Clark, A.A., & Freyd, J.J. (2023) Institutional courage buffers against institutional betrayal, protects employee health, and fosters organizational commitment following workplace sexual harassment. *PLoS ONE, 18*(1). doi:.pone.027883 doi:10.1371/journal

Smite, D., Wohlin, C., Gorschek, T., & Feldt, R. (2010). Empirical evidence in global software engineering: A systematic review. *Empirical Software Engineering*, *15*(1), 91–118. doi:10.100710664-009-9123-y

Smith, M. & Boxall, R. (2020). *Managing Worry Group Handbook.* Academic Press.

Smith, C., & Freyd, J. (2014). Institutional Betrayal. *The American Psychologist*, *69*(6), 575–587. doi:10.1037/a0037564 PMID:25197837

Sneath, J. Z., Lacey, R., & Kennett-Hensel, P. A. (2009). Coping with a natural disaster: Losses, emotions, and impulsive and compulsive buying. *Marketing Letters*, *20*(1), 45–60. doi:10.100711002-008-9049-y

Solnet, D., Subramony, M., Golubovskaya, M., Snyder, H., Gray, W., Liberman, O., & Verma, R. (2020). Employee wellness on the frontline: An interactional psychology perspective. *Journal of Service Management*, *31*(5), 939–952.

Song, K., Xu, R., Stratton, T. D., Kavcic, V., Luo, D., & Hou, F. (2020). (Preprint). Sex differences and psychological stress: Responses to the COVID-19 epidemic in China. *MedRxiv*. Advance online publication. doi:10.1101/2020.04.29.20084061

Songsangyos, P., & Iamamporn, S. (2020). Remote Working with Work-life Balance. International. *Journal of Applied Computer Technology and Information Systems*, *9*(2), 85–88.

Sood, Schroeder, & Gorman. (2014). *Bibliotherapy to decrease stress and anxiety and increase resilience and mindfulness: A pilot trial.* doi:10.1016/j.explore.2014.04.002

Sousa, I. (2015). Serviço Social em debate: Que referenciais genéricos? *Intervenção Social*, *42/45*, 11–23.

Spadafora, N., Frijters, J. C., Molnar, D. S., & Volk, A. A. (2020). Do little annoyances relate to bullying? The links between personality, attitudes towards classroom incivility, and bullying. *The Educational and Developmental Psychologist*, *37*(1), 30–38. doi:10.1017/edp.2019.20

Spikins, P. (2017). Prehistoric origins: The compassion of far distant strangers. In P. Gilbert (Ed.), *Compassion: Concepts, research, and applications*. Routledge. doi:10.4324/9781315564296-2

Spreitzer, G. M. (1995). Psychological empowerment in the workplace: Dimensions, measurement, and validation. *Academy of Management Journal*, *38*(5), 1442–1465. doi:10.2307/256865

Sridhar, D., & Vaughn, S. (2000). Bibliotherapy for all. *Teaching Exceptional Children*, *33*(2).

Stachteas, P., & Stachteas, C. (2020). The psychological impact of the COVID-19 pandemic on secondary school teachers. *Psychiatriki*, *31*(4), 293–301. doi:10.22365/jpsych.2020.314.293 PMID:33361059

Steigleder, J., Buhr, L., Ehm, J. H., Gawrilow, C., & von Suchodoletz, A. (2023). Changes in subjective stress experiences and self-efficacy beliefs of preschool teachers in Germany: A longitudinal study during 12 months of the COVID-19 pandemic. *Teaching and Teacher Education*, *124*, 104015. doi:10.1016/j.tate.2023.104015 PMID:36628186

Steiner, A. M., & Gengoux, G. W. (2018). Strength-Based Approaches to Working with Families of Children with ASD. In M. Siller & L. Morgan (Eds.), *Handbook of Parent-Implemented Interventions for Very Young Children with Autism* (pp. 155–168). Springer International Publishing. doi:10.1007/978-3-319-90994-3_10

Stellar, J. E., Cohen, A., Oveis, C., & Keltner, D. (2015). Affective and physiological responses to the suffering of others: Compassion and vagal activity. *Journal of Personality and Social Psychology, 108*(4), 572–585. doi:10.1037/pspi0000010

Steven M. S. (2014). *Resilience definitions, theory, and challenges: interdisciplinary perspectives.* doi:10.3402/ejpt.v5.25338

Stock, R. M., Bauer, E. M., & Bieling, G. I. (2014). How do top executives handle their work and family life? A taxonomy of top executives' work–family balance. *International Journal of Human Resource Management, 25*(13), 1815–1840. doi:10.1080/09585192.2013.860383

Stress archives. (2021, June 8). *Evolve.* Retrieved December 28, 2022, from https://evolveinc.io/mental-health/stress/

Strosahl, K. D., Robinson, P. J., & Gustavsson, T. (2015). *Inside this moment: A clinician's guide to promoting radical change using acceptance and commitment therapy.* Context Press.

Sultana, U. S., Tarofder, A. K., Darun, M. R., Haque, A., & Sharief, S. R. (2020). Authentic Leadership effect on Pharmacists Job stress and satisfaction During COVID-19 Pandemic: Malaysian Perspective. *Talent Development & Excellence, 12,* 1824–1841.

Sun, X., Su, W., Guo, X., & Tian, Z. (2021). The impact of awe induced by COVID-19 pandemic on green consumption behavior in China. *International Journal of Environmental Research and Public Health, 18*(2), 543. doi:10.3390/ijerph18020543 PMID:33440719

Suppawittaya, P., Yiemphat, P., & Yasri, P. (2020). Effects of social distancing, self-quarantine and self-isolation during the COVID-19 pandemic on people's well-being and how to cope with it. *International Journal of Science and Healthcare Research, 5*(2), 12–20.

Suresh, Sharma, & Beulah. (2018). A Conceptual Analysis on Work Life Balance. *Journal of Management, 5*(4), 97–100.

Suryavanshi, N., Kadam, A., Dhumal, G., Nimkar, S., Mave, V., Gupta, A., Cox, S. R., & Gupte, N. (2020). Mental health and quality of life among healthcare professionals during the COVID-19 pandemic in India. *Brain and Behavior, 10*(11), e01837. doi:10.1002/brb3.1837 PMID:32918403

Sutton. (2021). *Assertiveness in Leadership: 19 Techniques for Managers.* https://positivepsychology.com/assertiveness-in-leadership/

Sutton, A., Williams, H. M., & Allinson, C. W. (2015). A longitudinal, mixed method evaluation of self-awareness training in the workplace. *European Journal of Training and Development, 39*(7), 610–627. doi:10.1108/EJTD-04-2015-0031

Swaim. (2022). *How to Improve Your Self-Control.* https://www.verywellmind.com/psychology-of-self-control-4177125

Tal, A. I. (2006). *Pregnant women's self-efficacy for integrating multiple roles* [Unpublished doctoral dissertation]. Fordham University.

Tallis, F., Davey, G. C. L., & Capuzzi, N. (1994). *The phenomenology of non-pathological worry: A preliminary investigation. In Worrying: Perspectives on theory, assessment, and treatment.* Wiley.

Tambe, P., Cappelli, P., & Yakubovich, V. (2019). Artificial intelligence in human resources management: Challenges and a path forward. *California Management Review, 61*(4), 15–42. doi:10.1177/0008125619867910

Tang, H. W. V., Yin, M. S., & Nelson, D. B. (2010). The relationship between emotional intelligence and leadership practices: A cross-cultural study of academic leaders in Taiwan and the USA. *Journal of Managerial Psychology*, *25*(8), 899–926. doi:10.1108/02683941011089143

Tan, S. Y., & Yip, A. (2018). Hans Selye (1907–1982): Founder of the stress theory. *Singapore Medical Journal*, *59*(4), 170–171. doi:10.11622medj.2018043 PMID:29748693

Tari, S., & Amonkar, G. (2021). Impact of covid on higher education in India. *Educational Resurgence Journal*, *2*(5), 22–27.

Tarkar, P. (2020). Impact of COVID-19 Pandemic on Education System. *International Journal of Advanced Science and Technology*, *29*(9), 3812–3814.

Tatzel, M. (2002). 'Money worlds' and well-being: An integration of money dispositions, materialism and price-related behavior. *Journal of Economic Psychology*, *23*(1), 103–126. doi:10.1016/S0167-4870(01)00069-1

Taute, H., & McQuitty, S. (2004). Feeling good! Doing good! An exploratory look at the impulsive purchase of the social good. *Journal of Marketing Theory and Practice*, *12*(2), 16–27. doi:10.1080/10696679.2004.11658516

Taylor, S., Landry, C. A., Paluszek, M. M., Fergus, T. A., McKay, D., & Asmundson, G. J. (2020a). COVID stress syndrome: Concept, structure, and correlates. *Depression and Anxiety*, *37*(8), 706–714. doi:10.1002/da.23071 PMID:32627255

Taylor, S., Landry, C. A., Paluszek, M. M., Fergus, T. A., McKay, D., & Asmundson, G. J. (2020b). Development and initial validation of the COVID Stress Scales. *Journal of Anxiety Disorders*, *72*, 102232. doi:10.1016/j.janxdis.2020.102232 PMID:32408047

Taylor, S., Paluszek, M. M., Landry, C. A., Rachor, G. S., & Asmundson, G. J. (2021). Predictors of distress and coping during pandemic-related self-isolation: The relative importance of personality traits and beliefs about personal threat. *Personality and Individual Differences*, *176*, 110779. doi:10.1016/j.paid.2021.110779 PMID:36540361

Temiz, Z. (2020). Nursing students' anxiety levels and coping strategies during the COVID-19 pandemic. *International Archives of Nursing and Health Care*, *6*(4), 150. doi:10.23937/2469-5823/1510150

Terjesen, M., Jacofsky, M., Froh, J., & Digiuseppe, R. (2004). Integrating positive psychology into schools: Implications for practice. *Psychology in the Schools*, *41*(1), 163–172. doi:10.1002/pits.10148

Terry, D. J., Nielsen, M., & Perchard, L. (1993). Effects of work stress on psychological well-being and job satisfaction: The stress-buffering role of social support. *Australian Journal of Psychology*, *45*(3), 168–175. doi:10.1080/00049539308259135

TGA. (2022, January 22). Türkiye tourism promotion and development agency. *Fight against COVID-19 in Turkey*. https://www.tga.gov.tr/fight-against-covid-19-in-turkey/

The Lancet. (2020). Research and higher education in the time of COVID-19. *Lancet*, *396*(10251), 583.

Thewellnesssociety. (2020). *Coronavirus anxiety workbook*. Author.

Thoits, P. A. (1986). Multiple identities: Examining gender and marital status differences in distress. *American Sociological Review*, *51*(2), 259–272. doi:10.2307/2095520

Thompson, A., & Gaudreau, P. (2008). From optimism and pessimism to coping: The mediating role of academic motivation. *International Journal of Stress Management*, *15*(3), 269–288. doi:10.1037/a0012941

Tirch, D., Schoendorff, B., & Silberstein, L. R. (2014). *The ACT practitioner's guide to the science of compassion*. New Harbinger.

Torres, R., & Fernández, M. J. (2020). La políticaeconómicaespañola y el COVID-19. *Funcas. Cuadernos de InformaciónEconómica, 275*, 1–7.

Tosun, P., & Sezgin, S. (2021). Voluntary simplicity: A content analysis of consumer comments. *Journal of Consumer Marketing, 38*(5), 484–494. doi:10.1108/JCM-04-2020-3749

Toussaint, L., Nguyen, Q. A., Roettger, C., Dixon, K., Offenbächer, M., Kohls, N., Hirsch, J., & Sirois, F. (2021). Effectiveness of Progressive Muscle Relaxation, Deep Breathing, and Guided Imagery in Promoting Psychological and Physiological States of Relaxation. *Evidence-Based Complementary and Alternative Medicine, 2021*, e5924040. doi:10.1155/2021/5924040 PMID:34306146

Tsai, J. C. A., & Kang, T. C. (2019). Reciprocal intention in knowledge seeking: Examining social exchange theory in an online professional community. *International Journal of Information Management, 48*, 161–174. doi:10.1016/j.ijinfomgt.2019.02.008

Tsui, P. L. (2021). Would organizational climate and job stress affect wellness? An empirical study on the hospitality industry in Taiwan during COVID-19. *International Journal of Environmental Research and Public Health, 18*(19), 10491. doi:10.3390/ijerph181910491 PMID:34639791

Türkoglu, D., Ozbey, S., & Büyüktanir, A. (2014). Analysis of the satisfaction with life of preschool prospective teachers according to some variables. *Procedia: Social and Behavioral Sciences, 116*, 4175–4181. doi:10.1016/j.sbspro.2014.01.912

Tutzer, F., Frajo-Apor, B., Pardeller, S., Plattner, B., Chernova, A., Haring, C., Holzner, B., Kemmler, G., Marksteiner, J., Miller, C., Schmidt, M., Sperner-Unterweger, B., & Hofer, A. (2021). Psychological distress, loneliness, and boredom among the general population of Tyrol, Austria during the COVID-19 pandemic. *Frontiers in Psychiatry, 12*, 921. doi:10.3389/fpsyt.2021.691896 PMID:34177672

Tyler, K. (2014). Listening Skills. *HRMagazine, 59*(2), 42–43.

Tynes, B. (2020, March). The Importance of Diversity and Inclusion for Today's Companies. *Forbes Magazine.*

Uggla, Y. (2019). Taking back control: Minimalism as a reaction to high speed and overload in contemporary society. *Sociologisk Forskning, 56*(3–4), 233–252. doi:10.37062f.56.18811

UNESCO COVID-19 Initiatives. (2020). *A film about teenagers surviving COVID in different countries*. UNESCO.

UNESCO COVID-19 Initiatives. (2020). *Creatives against COVID-19: The photography edition*. UNESCO.

UNESCO. (2020). *COVID-19 Educational disruptions and response, 2020*. UNESCO.

UNESCO. (2020). *Turning the threat of COVID-19 into an opportunity for greater support to document heritage*. UNESCO.

Ungar, M. (Ed.). (2012). The social ecology of resilience: A handbook of theory and practice. Springer Science + Business Media. doi:10.1007/978-1-4614-0586-3

UNO. (2020). *Education during COVID-19 and beyond.* UNESCO.

Uresha, K. I. (2020). Influence of telecommuting on work-life balance and employee happiness: An empirical study of Sri Lankan employees. *Int. J. Manag. Excell, 15*, 2234–2243.

Ustun, G. (2021). Determining depression and related factors in a society affected by COVID-19 pandemic. *The International Journal of Social Psychiatry, 67*(1), 54–63. doi:10.1177/0020764020938807 PMID:32605422

Utama, A., Sawıtrı, H. S. R., Haryanto, B., & Wahyudı, L. (2021). Impulse buying: The influence of impulse buying tendency, urge to buy and gender on impulse buying of the retail customers. *Journal of Distribution Science*, *19*(7), 101–111. doi:10.15722/jds.19.7.202107.101

Valcour, M. (2007). Work-based resources as moderators of the relationship between work hours and satisfaction with work–family balance. *The Journal of Applied Psychology*, *92*(6), 1512–1523. doi:10.1037/0021-9010.92.6.1512 PMID:18020793

Valence, G., d'Astous, A., & Fortier, L. (1988). Compulsive buying: Concept and measurement. *Journal of Consumer Policy*, *11*(4), 419–433. doi:10.1007/BF00411854

Van der Zwan, J. E., De Vente, W., Huizink, A. C., Bögels, S. M., & de Bruin, E. I. (2015). Physical Activity, Mindfulness Meditation, or Heart Rate Variability Biofeedback for Stress Reduction: A Randomized Controlled Trial. *Applied Psychophysiology and Biofeedback*, *40*(4), 257–268. doi:10.100710484-015-9293-x PMID:26111942

Van Dierendonck, D. (2011). Servant leadership: A review and synthesis. *Journal of Management*, *37*(4), 1228–1261. doi:10.1177/0149206310380462

Vargas Rubilar, N., & Oros, L. B. (2021). Stress and burnout in teachers during times of pandemic. *Frontiers in Psychology*, *12*, 756007. doi:10.3389/fpsyg.2021.756007 PMID:34899498

Varga, S., Mistry, T. G., Ali, F., & Cobanoglu, C. (2021). Employee perceptions of wellness programs in the hospitality industry. *International Journal of Contemporary Hospitality Management*, *33*(10), 3331–3354. doi:10.1108/IJCHM-12-2020-1417

Varma, P., Junge, M., Meaklim, H., & Jackson, M. L. (2021). Younger people are more vulnerable to stress, anxiety and depression during COVID-19 pandemic: A global cross-sectional survey. *Progress in Neuro-Psychopharmacology & Biological Psychiatry*, *109*, 110236. doi:10.1016/j.pnpbp.2020.110236 PMID:33373680

Veena, J. (2016). Short-term exposure to enriched environment rescues chronic stress-induced impaired hippocampal synaptic plasticity, anxiety, and memory deficits. *Journal of Neuroscience Research*, *95*(8), 1602–1610. PMID:27862185

VIA Character Strengths Survey & Character Reports. (n.d.). Retrieved December 21, 2022, from https://www.viacharacter.org/

Viswesvaran, C., & Ones, D. S. (2000). Perspectives on models of job performance. *International Journal of Selection and Assessment*, *8*(4), 216–226. doi:10.1111/1468-2389.00151

Voydanoff, P. (2002). Linkages between the work-family interface and work, family, and individual outcomes: An integrative model. *Journal of Family Issues*, *23*(1), 138–164. doi:10.1177/0192513X02023001007

Wafula, M., & Nyaboga, E. (2019). Stress management and employee performance: Use of psychotherapy as mitigation in selected schools (School of business and economics and Health sciences) in Kisii University, Kenya. *Merit Research Journal of Business and Management*, *7*(3), 19–27.

Walker, E., Wang, C., & Redmond, J. (2008). Women and work-life balance: Is home-based business ownership the solution? *Equal Opportunities International*, *27*(3), 258–275. doi:10.1108/02610150810860084

Walumba, F. O., Wang, P., Wang, H., Schaubroeck, J., & Avolio, B. J. (2010). Psychological processes linking authentic leadership to follower behaviours. *The Leadership Quarterly*, *21*(5), 901–914. doi:10.1016/j.leaqua.2010.07.015

Walumbwa, F., Avolio, B., Gardner, W., Wensıng, T., & Peterson, S. (2008). Authentic leadership: Development and validation of a theory-based measure. *Journal of Management*, *34*(1), 89–126. doi:10.1177/0149206307308913

Wang, C., Pan, R., Wan, X., Tan, Y., Xu, L., Ho, C. S., & Ho, R. C. (2020). Immediate psychological responses and associated factors during the initial stage of the 2019 coronavirus disease (COVID-19) epidemic among the general population in China. *International Journal of Environmental Research and Public Health, 17*(5), 1729. doi:10.3390/ijerph17051729 PMID:32155789

Wang, F., & Shi, W. (2020). The effect of work-leisure conflict on front-line employees' work engagement: A cross-level study from the emotional perspective. *Asia Pacific Journal of Management, 39*(1), 225–247. doi:10.100710490-020-09722-0

Wang, S. (2005). A conceptual framework for integrating research related to the physiology of compassion and the wisdom of Buddhist teachings. In P. Gilbert (Ed.), *Compassion: Conceptualisations, research and use in psychotherapy*. Routledge.

Wang, S., Liu, Y., Du, Y., & Wang, X. (2021). Effect of the COVID-19 pandemic on consumers' impulse buying: The moderating role of moderate thinking. *International Journal of Environmental Research and Public Health, 18*(21), 1–19. doi:10.3390/ijerph182111116 PMID:34769636

Warr, P., & Nielsen, K. (2018). *Wellbeing and work performance. In Handbook of well-being*. DEF Publishers.

Waters, L. (2015). The Relationship between Strength-Based Parenting with Children's Stress Levels and Strength-Based Coping Approaches. *Psychology, 6*(6), 6. doi:10.4236/psych.2015.66067

Waterschoot, J., Van der Kaap-Deeder, J., Morbée, S., Soenens, B., & Vansteenkiste, M. (2021). "How to unlock myself from boredom?" The role of mindfulness and a dual awareness-and action-oriented pathway during the COVID-19 lockdown. *Personality and Individual Differences, 175*, 110729. doi:10.1016/j.paid.2021.110729 PMID:36540053

Wayne, J., Musisca, N., & Fleeson, W. (2004). Considering the role of personality in the work-family experience: Relationship of the Big Five to work-family conflict and facilitation. *Journal of Vocational Behavior, 64*(1), 108–130. doi:10.1016/S0001-8791(03)00035-6

Wehrenberg, M. (2005). *10 Best-Ever Anxiety-Management Techniques*. Academic Press.

Weiss, H. M., & Cropanzano, R. (1996). Affective Events Theory: A theoretical discussion of the structure, causes and consequences of affective experiences at work. In B. M. Staw & L. L. Cummings (Eds.), *Research in organizational behavior: An annual series of analytical essays and critical reviews* (Vol. 18, pp. 1–74). Elsevier Science/ JAI Press.

Weissinger, E., Caldwell, L. L., & Bandalos, D. L. (1992). Relation between intrinsic motivation and boredom in leisure time. *Leisure Sciences, 14*(4), 317–325. doi:10.1080/01490409209513177

Wheeler, D. W. (2012). *Servant leadership for higher education: Principles and practices*. John Wiley & Sons.

WHO. (2020). *WHO Director-General's opening remarks at the media briefing on COVID-19*. WHO.

WHO. (2022, January 22). *WHO Coronavirus (COVID-19) Dashboard*. https://covid19.who.int/

Wilson, C. B. (1991). US businesses suffer from workplace trauma. *The Personnel Journal, 70*(7), 47–50.

Wolff, W., Martarelli, C. S., Schüler, J., & Bieleke, M. (2020). High boredom proneness and low trait self-control impair adherence to social distancing guidelines during the COVID-19 pandemic. *International Journal of Environmental Research and Public Health, 17*(15), 5420. doi:10.3390/ijerph17155420 PMID:32731369

Wood, M. (1998). Socio-economic status, delay of gratification, and impulse buying. *Journal of Economic Psychology, 19*(3), 295–320. doi:10.1016/S0167-4870(98)00009-9

Woodworth, R. (1929). *Psychology* (revised edition). Henry Holt.

World Health Organization. (2004). *Promoting mental health: Concepts, emerging evidence, practice: Summary report.* World Health Organization.

World Health Organization. (2014). *Constitution.* https://www.who.int/about/who-we-are/constitution

World Health Organization. (2019). *Burn-out an "occupational phenomenon": International Classification of Diseases.* https://www.who.int/news/item/28-05-2019-burn-out-an-occupational-phenomenon-international-classification-of-diseases

World Health Organization. (2021). *Stress.* Retrieved December 15, 2022, from https://www.who.int/news-room/questions-and-answers/item/stress

World Health Organization. (2022). *Mental health: Strengthening our response.* https://www.who.int/en/news-room/fact-sheets/detail/mental-health-strengthening-our-response

World Health Organizations Regional Office for the Western Pacific. (2001). *Health research methodology: A guide for training in research methods* (2nd ed). WHO regional Office of the Western Pacific.

Wren, S., Somers, T. J., Wright, M. A., Goetz, M. C., Leary, M. R., Fras, A. M., Huh, B. K., Rogers, L. L., & Keefe, F. J. (2012). Self-Compassion in Patients with Persistent Musculoskeletal Pain: Relationship of Self-Compassion to Adjustment to Persistent Pain. *Journal of Pain and Symptom Management*, *43*(4), 759–770. doi:10.1016/j.jpainsymman.2011.04.014 PMID:22071165

Wright, T. A., Cropanzano, R., & Bonett, D. G. (2007). The moderating role of employee positive well-being on the relation between job satisfaction and job performance. *Journal of Occupational Health, 12*(2), 93–104.

Wright, T. A., Cropanzano, R., Denney, P. J., & Moline, G. L. (2002). When a happy worker is a productive worker: a preliminary examination of three models. *Canadian Journal of Behavioural Science/Revue canadienne des sciences du comportement, 34*(3), 146-150.

Wright, M., & Hill, L. (2015). Academic incivility among health sciences faculty. *Adult Learning*, *26*(1), 14–20. doi:10.1177/1045159514558410

Wu, C. H., Chen, I. S., & Chen, J. C. (2017). A study into the impact of employee wellness and job satisfaction on job performance. *International Journal of Organizational Innovation*, *10*(2), 253–269.

Xiao, H., Zhang, Z., & Zhang, L. (2020). A diary study of impulsive buying during the COVID-19 pandemic. *Current Psychology (New Brunswick, N.J.)*, 1–13. doi:10.100712144-020-01220-2 PMID:33250615

Xu, J., & Thomas, H. C. (2011). How can leaders achieve high employee engagement? *Leadership and Organization Development Journal*, *32*(4), 399–416. doi:10.1108/01437731111134661

Yang, D. J., Huang, K. C., & Feng, X. (2011). A study of the factors that affect the impulsive cosmetics buying of female consumers in Kaohsiung. *International Journal of Business and Social Science*, *2*(24), 275–282.

Yang, S. Y., Chen, S. C., Lee, L., & Liu, Y. S. (2021). Employee Stress, Job Satisfaction, and Job Performance: A Comparison between High-technology and Traditional Industry in Taiwan. *The Journal of Asian Finance. Economics and Business*, *8*(3), 605–618.

Yan, L., Gan, Y., Ding, X., Wu, J., & Duan, H. (2021). The relationship between perceived stress and emotional distress during the COVID-19 outbreak: Effects of boredom proneness and coping style. *Journal of Anxiety Disorders*, *77*, 102328. doi:10.1016/j.janxdis.2020.102328 PMID:33160275

Yan, T., Chan, C. W. H., Chow, K. M., Zheng, W., & Sun, M. (2020). A systematic review of the effects of character strengths-based intervention on the psychological well-being of patients suffering from chronic illnesses. *Journal of Advanced Nursing*, *76*(7), 1567–1580. doi:10.1111/jan.14356 PMID:32187708

Yarnell, A. M., & Grunberg, N. E. (2017). Developing "allostatic leaders": a psychobiosocial perspective. In *Leader development deconstructed* (pp. 23–50). Springer. doi:10.1007/978-3-319-64740-1_2

Yasmin, H., Khalil, S., & Mazhar, R. (2020). COVID 19: Stress management among students and its impact on their effective learning. *International Technology and Education Journal, 4*(2), 65-74.

Yeow, J., & Martin, R. (2013). The role of self-regulation in developing leaders: A longitudinal field experiment. *The Leadership Quarterly*, *24*(5), 625–637. doi:10.1016/j.leaqua.2013.04.004

Yin, R. K. (2013). Validity and generalization in future case study evaluations. *Evaluation*, *19*(3), 321–332. doi:10.1177/1356389013497081

Yoav, B. (2006). The Association Between Psychological Distance and Construal Level: Evidence From an Implicit Association Test. *Journal of Experimental Psychology. General*, *135*(4), 609–622. doi:10.1037/0096-3445.135.4.609 PMID:17087576

Yu, B., Funk, M., Hu, J., Wang, Q., & Feijs, L. (2018). Biofeedback for Everyday Stress Management: A Systematic Review. *Frontiers in ICT (Lausanne, Switzerland)*, *5*, 1–22. doi:10.3389/fict.2018.00023

Yufek, B. (2021). *Holiday classes: MINESEC boss visits schools in Yaoundé*. Academic Press.

Yuh, J., & Choi, S. (2017). Sources of social support, job satisfaction, and quality of life among childcare teachers. *The Social Science Journal*, *54*(4), 1–8. doi:10.1016/j.soscij.2017.08.002

Yu, Y., She, R., Luo, S., Xin, M., Li, L., Wang, S., Ma, L., Tao, F., Zhang, J., Zhao, J., Li, L., Hu, D., Zhang, G., Gu, J., Lin, D., Wang, H., Cai, Y., Wang, Z., You, H., ... Lau, J. T. F. (2021). Factors influencing depression and mental distress related to COVID-19 among university students in China: Online cross-sectional mediation study. *JMIR Mental Health*, *8*(2), e22705. doi:10.2196/22705 PMID:33616541

Zammuto, R. F., & Krakower, J. Y. (1991). *Quantitative and qualitative studies of organizational culture*. JAI Press.

Zavestoski, S. (2002). The social–psychological bases of anticonsumption attitudes. *Psychology and Marketing*, *19*(2), 149–165. doi:10.1002/mar.10007

Zelenski, J. M., Murphy, S. A., & Jenkins, D. A. (2008). The happy-productive worker thesis revisited. *Journal of Happiness Studies, 9*(4), 521-537.

Zessin, U., Dickhäuser, O., & Garbade, S. (2015). The relationship between self-compassion and well-being: A meta-analysis. *Applied Psychology, 7,* 340–364. doi:10.1111/aphw.12051

Zhang, S. X., Wang, Y., Rauch, A., & Wei, F. (2020). Unprecedented disruption of lives and work: Health, distress and life satisfaction of working adults in China one month into the COVID-19 outbreak. *Psychiatry Research*, *288*, 112958. doi:10.1016/j.psychres.2020.112958 PMID:32283450

Zhang, S., Gates, D., Nealy, C., & Stark, J. (2009). *Managerial communication: Theory and application*. The Publishing House of South-China University of Technology.

Zhang, T. C., Kandampully, J., & Choi, H. Y. (2014). The role of employee wellness programme in the hospitality industry: A review of concepts, research, and practice. *Research in Hospitality Management*, *4*(1 & 2), 45–54. doi:10.1080/22243534.2014.11828313

Zheng, L. (2022). *DEI deconstructed: Your no-nonsense guide to doing the work and doing it right*. Berrett-Hoehler.

Zhou, X., & Yao, B. (2020). Social support and acute stress symptoms (ASSs) during the COVID-19 outbreak deciphering the roles of psychological needs and sense of control. *European Journal of Psychotraumatology*, *11*(1), 1779494. doi:10.1080/20008198.2020.1779494 PMID:33062202

Znazen, H., Slimani, M., Bragazzi, N. L., & Tod, D. (2021). The Relationship between Cognitive Function, Lifestyle Behaviours and Perception of Stress during the COVID-19 Induced Confinement: Insights from Correlational and Mediation Analyses. *International Journal of Environmental Research and Public Health*, *18*(6), 3194. doi:10.3390/ijerph18063194 PMID:33808777

About the Contributors

Rohit Bansal is working as Associate Professor in Department of Management Studies in Vaish College of Engineering, Rohtak. He is a perseverant, passionate academician cum seasoned professional. He obtained Ph.D. in Management from Maharshi Dayanand University, Rohtak. With a rich experience of 15 years, he has achieved growth through robust and proactive academic initiatives. He has authored & edited 19 books with renowned national & international publishers including IGI Global USA, Scrivener-Wiley Publishing, De Gruyter, Weser Books, Scholar's Press, Germany etc. In addition to, Dr. Rohit has published 120 research papers and chapters in journals of repute including Scopus indexed as well as edited books. He has also presented papers in 45 conferences and seminars. His area of interest includes marketing management, organizational behaviour, services marketing, customer engagement, digital marketing, human resource management and organizational development. He is on Editorial Advisory Board as a member in 125 national and international peer reviewed journals. He has acted as session chair in many international conferences.

* * *

Deepanshi Aggarwal is a Research Scholar in the Department of Commerce at Maharshi Dayanand University, Rohtak. She has completed her B. Com Honours and M. Com Honours from Maharshi Dayanand University and became the Gold Medalist of the respective programmes. Currently she is pursuing a Ph.D. from the department of Commerce in the Marketing field. She has qualified UGC NET- JRF in 2018. She has also published few research papers in reputed National and International journals (including UGC care listed Journal) and has presented many research papers in conferences and seminars. Furthermore, she has also attended many workshops. Apart from that, she is a determined and hardworking individual who has a keen research interest.

Elif Aralık is a PhD student at the Department of Business Administration in Gebze Technical University. Her main research interests include consumer behavior and sustainable consumption.

Helen Chwienui Ghogomu Gayelle currently teaches Literature in English and English Language at the British Isles International School in Yaoundé. She holds a BA in African Literature from the University of Yaoundé I and a M.Ed. from the University of the People at Pasadena in the USA.

İnci Dursun studied the MSc in Business Administration and Ph.D. in Business Administration specializing in marketing management at Gebze Technical University (GTU). Currently, she is working at GTU as an Associate Professor. Her research interests are in the areas of on consumer behavior and social marketing. Specifically, she focuses on sustainable consumption and change of nonfunctional consumer attitudes and behaviors. She lectures on marketing management, consumer behaviors, research methodology.

Denise Gates is an educator, author, and consultant from the United States, specializing in strategic management, organizational socialization, and employee engagement. Her research has been published and presented globally. She has authored and co-authored several books and a plethora of academic articles. However, she is most known for her organizational socialization model that was published in 2009 by The Publishing House of South-China University of Technology. Her model has been utilized in her work with talent optimization to help leaders position key people as a competitive advantage. Ultimately, Dr. Gates strives to help leaders draw the greatest value out of people.

Justin D. Henderson is co-director and assistant professor of Professional Mental Health Counseling – Addictions at Lewis & Clark College. He is also faculty in the Eating Disorders Certificate. He is a licensed psychologist and a National Certified Counselor. Dr. Henderson has clinical expertise in mindfulness, acceptance, and compassion-based therapeutic modalities (e.g., Acceptance and Commitment Therapy; Compassion Focused Therapy). Dr. Henderson is a Certified Compassion Cultivation Training (CCT)™ Teacher through the Compassion Institute and the Center for Compassion and Altruism Research and Education at Stanford University. He is a professional member of the Compassion Institute, Compassion Education Alliance, and Compassionate Mind Foundation. Dr. Henderson's scholarship focuses on compassion, wellbeing, burnout, and addiction.

Esmaeil Jafari is an assistant professor at the Faculty of Education and Psychology of Shahid Beheshti University. Jafari graduated with a PhD in curriculum planning. Virtual education, virtual curriculum, MOOCs and educational technologies are his favorite research fields. He is currently the manager of human resource and support at Shahid Beheshti University and has published more than 40 scientific research articles in national and international conferences and journals. He authored a chapter of the international book titled "E-Learning in the Middle East and North Africa (MENA) Region".

Abirami K. is a Research Scholar (Part Time) in Department of Business Management, Erode Arts and Science College (Autonomous), Erode. Working as an Assistant Professor with the experience of four years in Department of Business Management (SF), Erode Arts and Science College (Autonomous), Erode.

Chandra Kumari is working as Professor and Head in the department of Home Science for the past 24 years. She possesses teaching and research experience of 26 years. She has completed several sponsored projects and has expertise in the area of Human Development. Currently, she is working on a book based on Research Methods and Contemporary Issues in Human Development.

Rajnish Kumar Misra is currently Head of Academics at Jaypee Business School. He has more than 23 years' experience in academics. He is also Adjunct faculty by invitation to Indian Institute of Management Kozhikode (IIMK). He has conducted several training programs for both services and manufacturing companies like Reserve Bank of India, United Bank India, BHEL, IFFCO, Mahanadi

Coal Fields, JK Tyres, HAL; and delivered lectures in Patni Computers Ltd., Hindustan Aeronautics Ltd. (HAL – Sunabeda) and Areva T&D (ALSTOM) Limited on "Emerging Trends in Executive Career". His research interest area are Bullying, Employer Branding, Self & Leadership Development, Career Management.

Divya Nair is currently working at School of Education and Research, MIT Art Design and Technology University, Pune, Maharashtra as an Assistant Professor. Her academic qualifications include M.Sc. Microbiology, M.A. Psychology, M.Ed., NET with JRF and Post Graduate Diploma in Mass Media. She has an experience of 6 years and is currently pursuing her Ph.D. in the interdisciplinary area encompassing of positive psychology, cognitive psychology and education. Her PhD work is titled as, "Developing a strength based program and studying its effectiveness for enhancing critical and creative thinking among teacher trainees." Her work "Active Inquisitive Model [AIM] for Multicultural Education" is copyright registered under the number L-112269/2022. Her two book chapters namely, Techno Pedagogical Concepts with Digital Skills and National Education Policy 2020: A Landmark in India's History of Education have been published by CRC Press, Taylor and Francis. Another book chapter of hers titled, "Augmenting Cybersecurity: A Survey of Intrusion Detection Systems in Combating Zero Day Vulnerabilities" is in the final stages of publication under Scopus indexed publication Emerald, Taylor and Francis. Her chapter on chatbots has been accepted for publication by Wiley Publications. She has participated in various International, National and State Level Conferences and also published research papers in peer-reviewed journals. She has won many national and state level competitions including a gold medal for her research work. Educational Psychology, Clinical Psychology, ICT and Research are her domains of expertise. Her other areas of interest include classical dancing, singing, writing poems and short stories.

Theresa Obuobisa-Darko holds a PhD in Public Administration and Policy Management and an MBA in Human Resource Management both from University of Ghana and an MA in Organisational Development from University of Cape Coast. Theresa is a Professor in Human Resource Management in the Department of Human Resource Management in her University. She has experience in teaching and research. Her research interest includes Leadership in Organisation, Performance Management, Conflict Management, Employee Health and Safety, and Employee Engagement. Theresa has published in peer reviewed journals and presented papers at both international and national conferences.

Seema Rathee is currently working as an Assistant Professor at Department of Commerce, Maharshi Dayanand University, Rohtak. She has completed her Ph.D. from the Department of Commerce. Her areas of specialization are Accounting and Finance. She has qualified UGC Net in Commerce. She has approximately 11 years of experience in teaching and research. She has published several research papers in National and International journals. She has presented many research papers at conferences and seminars. She has also organized various academic activities in the form of workshops, seminars, extension lectures, and conferences at the National and International levels. She has attended many workshops and faculty development programs in her academic career.

Jayasudha S. M. is working as an Assistant Professor in Department of Business Management, Erode Arts and Science College (Autonomous), Erode with the experience of 30 Years of this noble service.

Organised many student development programs and published many articles related management titles. Completed a UGC sponsored Minor research project - IQAC coordinator of this institution.

Divya Sharma is currently working with Lloyd Business School as an Associate Professor. She has more than 10 years of industry and academic experience to teach/train a variety of courses. She has participated and presented papers in various national and international conferences held in India. Her research interests include Workplace bullying, incivility, abusive supervision, and negative behavior. She has authored case studies and research papers which got published in reputed journals like Inderscience, and The Case Centre (formerly ECCH, European Case Clearing House). She has been awarded with a Best-Case Award from The Case Centre UK for paper titled "Kwality Glass: Store tmospherics", 2017. She has worked on a Project of Competency Mapping of NSPCL (a joint venture of NTPC and SAIL) employees and has conducted an in-company training programme on "Leadership Development" for NTPC Employees assigned by BIMTECH, Greater Noida.

Evans Sokro holds a PhD in Human Resource Management from Federation University Australia. He was a recipient of Federation University Australia postgraduate research scholarship and a special overseas student scholarship award in 2014. Evans is currently a Senior lecturer and Head, Department of Human Resource Management at Central Business School, where he teaches courses in HRM at the MBA and undergraduate levels. He is also a member of Chartered Institute of Human Resource Management, Ghana. His research interests include expatriation in sub-Saharan Africa, organisational culture and values, high performance work systems and emotions at work. Evans has published in peer review journals and has presented papers at several conferences both locally and internationally.

Ebru Tumer Kabadayi, PhD, is a professor of marketing at Gebze Technical University. She obtained her Ph.D. in Marketing from Gebze Technical University in 2001. Her research interests focus on brand management, consumer behavior, and relationship marketing. Her research studies have been published in Journal of Business Research, Journal of Marketing Management, and in numerous Turkish language scholarly journals.

Hediye Yürüyen Kılıç is currently working as a research assistant at the Department of Business Administration in Gebze Technical University. Her main research interests include sustainability, green consumption, social marketing.

Index

E

F

G

H

I

J

L

M

N

O

P

Q

R

S

T

U

V

W

www.ingramcontent.com/pod-product-compliance
Lightning Source LLC
LaVergne TN
LVHW060407300926
849162LV00006B/1366